HERBAL MEDICINE IN TREATING GYNAECOLOGICAL CONDITIONS VOLUME II

HERBAL MEDICINE IN TREATING GYNAECOLOGICAL CONDITIONS VOLUME II

Specific Conditions and Management Through the Practical Usage of Herbs

Part 2 of *Herbal Medicine in Treating Gynaecological Conditions*

Hananja Brice-Ytsma
with
Nathalie Chidley

AEON

First published in 2024 by
Aeon Books

Copyright © 2024 by Hananja Brice-Ytsma

Photographs © 2024 Peter Jarrett

The right of Hananja Brice-Ytsma to be identified as the author of this work has been asserted in accordance with §§ 77 and 78 of the Copyright Design and Patents Act 1988.

All rights reserved. No part of this publication may be reproduced, stored in a retrieval system, or transmitted, in any form or by any means, electronic, mechanical, photocopying, recording, or otherwise, without the prior written permission of the publisher.

British Library Cataloguing in Publication Data

A C.I.P. for this book is available from the British Library

ISBN-13: 978-1-80152-005-8

Typeset by Medlar Publishing Solutions Pvt Ltd, India

www.aeonbooks.co.uk

CONTENTS

INTRODUCTION   ix

ACKNOWLEDGEMENT   xiii

SECTION ONE: SPECIFIC CONDITIONS

CHAPTER 1
Dysmenorrhoea   3
    1.1 Primary and secondary dysmenorrhoea   3
    1.2 Pathophysiology of primary dysmenorrhoea   10
    1.3 Herbal management of primary dysmenorrhoea   12
    1.4 Dietary and lifestyle recommendations   26

CHAPTER 2
Menorrhagia   28
    2.1 Menorrhagia definition and differential diagnosis   28
    2.2 Dysfunctional uterine bleeding (DUB)   33
    2.3 Herbal management of dysfunctional uterine bleeding   36
    2.4 Dietary and lifestyle recommendations   42

CHAPTER 3
Amenorrhoea and oligomenorrhoea — 46
   3.1 Presentation/symptoms, differential diagnosis and investigations — 46
   3.2 Functional hypothalamic amenorrhoea (FHA) — 52
   3.3 Herbal management of functional hypothalamic amenorrhoea — 55
   3.4 Dietary and lifestyle recommendations — 63

CHAPTER 4
Infertility — 66
   4.1 Presentation/symptoms, differential diagnosis and investigations — 66
   4.2 Herbal management of infertility — 78
   4.3 Dietary and lifestyle recommendations — 89

CHAPTER 5
Vaginal discharge — 94
   5.1 Presentation/symptoms, differential diagnosis and investigations — 94
   5.2 Vaginal and upper reproductive tract infections — 96
   5.3 Herbal treatment of vaginal infections — 104
   5.4 Dietary and lifestyle recommendations — 114

CHAPTER 6
Ovarian cysts — 118
   6.1 Presentation/symptoms, differential diagnosis and investigations — 118
   6.2 Pathophysiology of ovarian cysts — 121
   6.3 Herbal management of ovarian cysts — 123

CHAPTER 7
Polycystic ovarian syndrome (PCOS) — 125
   7.1 Presentation/symptoms, differential diagnosis and investigations — 125
   7.2 Pathophysiology of PCOS — 128
   7.3 Herbal management of PCOS — 130
   7.4 Dietary and lifestyle recommendations — 149

CHAPTER 8
Endometriosis   154
- 8.1 Presentation/symptoms, differential diagnosis and investigations   154
- 8.2 Pathophysiology of endometriosis   156
- 8.3 Herbal management of endometriosis   160
- 8.4 Dietary recommendations   176

CHAPTER 9
Uterine fibroids (uterine leiomyomas)   180
- 9.1 Presentation/symptoms, differential diagnosis and investigations   180
- 9.2 Pathophysiology of uterine fibroids   182
- 9.3 Herbal management of uterine fibroids   184
- 9.4 Dietary and lifestyle recommendations   194

CHAPTER 10
Cervical dysplasia   198
- 10.1 Presentation/symptoms, differential diagnosis and investigations   198
- 10.2 Herbal management of cervical dysplasia   203
- 10.3 Dietary and lifestyle recommendations   211

CHAPTER 11
Benign breast disorders   215
- 11.1 Presentation/symptoms, differential diagnosis and investigations   215
- 11.2 Pathophysiology of benign breast disorders   221
- 11.3 Herbal management of benign breast disorders   222
- 11.4 Dietary and lifestyle recommendations   226

CHAPTER 12
Lichen sclerosus   231
- 12.1 Presentation/symptoms, differential diagnosis and investigations   231
- 12.2 Herbal management of lichen sclerosus (LS)   233
- 12.3 Dietary and lifestyle recommendations   237

CHAPTER 13
Premenstrual syndrome (PMS) 239

CHAPTER 14
Menopause 243

SECTION TWO: MONOGRAPHS OF HERBS FREQUENTLY USED IN WOMEN'S HEALTH, WITHOUT A HORMONAL REPUTATION

Achillea millefolium	249
Alchemilla vulgaris	255
Anemone pulsatilla	260
Angelica sinensis	266
Capsella bursa-pastoris	271
Caulophyllum thalictriodes	276
Leonurus cardiaca	282
Mitchella repens	286
Rubus idaeus	289
Thuja occidentalis	294
Viburnum prunifolium	300

APPENDIX	303
Vitamins, minerals and other important nutrients	303
NOTES	313
INDEX	507
HERB INDEX	525

INTRODUCTION

This is the second book in the series of **Herbal Medicine in Treating Gynaecological Conditions**. The first book, subtitled 'Herbs, Hormones, Pre-Menstrual Syndrome and Menopause' (Aeon Books, 2020), covered the hormonal background and herbs, with an in-depth exploration of menopause and PMS. The herbs included were those mainly thought of as 'hormonal', such as *Actaea racemosa, Vitex agnus-castus* etc. We refer to this first book in the present text as 'book 1'.

In this new book, subtitled 'Specific Conditions and Herbal Management', we focus on gynaecological conditions, none of which are simply 'hormonal' as multifactorial causes are the rule. We find very often that herbal books contain oversimplifications in this area, where a gynaecological condition is seen as a hormonal condition and all it needs is a hormonal herb. We hope the complexity of hormones has been untangled in the first book. Now it is time to look, as far as we can, into mechanisms and discover how these can be influenced by herbs.

This book consists of two sections: the first focuses on conditions typically seen in clinical practice and the second on herbs traditionally used in women's health. Very little research can be found on these herbs, however, but the ways in which the herbs have been traditionally used can be revealing, and this is often confirmed by what research there is.

We have tried to lay out this book in a way that is user-friendly for those in practice to find the relevant information easily.

In each chapter we start by outlining the condition, the symptoms, any relevant aetiology and pathophysiology, where we feel this aids understanding, plus any other information we think is useful for herbalists. We also touch on investigations and conventional treatment options.

In the section on herbal management we first consider broad treatment aims and strategies. We then move on to 'Key herbs used in clinical practice'. This part reflects herbs that we have used successfully in clinical practice for that condition. We have collated clinical research that corresponds directly to the way each specific herb acts in or on a particular condition.

For each of the key herbs in each section we have included only the relevant studies, along with any relevant traditional use related to the chapter's condition, as opposed to whole monographs. We delve into detail where we feel it may be enlightening or interesting and, on occasion, go down side alleys to correct popular misunderstandings.

Sometimes these herbs have direct clinical research, sometimes actions are inferred from constituents and sometimes we rely on traditional and/or our empirical experience. At the end of the chapter we include evidence from clinical trials on herbs, constituents and combinations.

Where we give herb dosages, the daily dose usually corresponds to that found in the *British Herbal Pharmacopoeia (BHP) 1983,* by the British Herbal Medicine Association's Scientific Committee (Bournemouth: BHMA) or Kerry Bone's 2003 book, *A Clinical Guide to Blending Liquid Herbs: Herbal Formulations for the Individual Patient* (Edinburgh: Churchill Livingstone [1st edition]).

Weekly dosages can be taken as representative within a herbal mixture, unless otherwise stated, and reflect those used in clinical practice by most herbalists, but ultimately are guided by our own experience.

In the dietary and lifestyle sections we have collated research relevant directly to each condition, to enable a practitioner to make informed, evidence-based recommendations.

The second section of the book concentrates on monographs of 'nonhormonal herbs' traditionally used in female health. These are herbs with a long tradition of use in gynaecology that were not covered in the first book.

In the text we make reference to traditional medicine, going back to our herbal roots, Hippocrates, Gerard and Culpeper, as well as looking at texts from the Eclectics. Eclectic medicine was a branch of North American medicine that made use of predominantly Native American remedies in the late 19th and early 20th centuries. They were eclectic in the sense that they integrated whatever worked in terms of herbal medicine and homeopathy. The Eclectics included doctors Milton Scudder, John King, John Felter and Finley Ellingwood, who were practising throughout the US and published a number of texts from their experiences, many focusing on gynaecology.

Our aim is to present a thoroughly researched, in-depth textbook on a herbal medicine approach to gynaecology. We hope to give an understanding of the physiological processes and deepen the reader's understanding of the herbs in the context of female health. Our passion is to integrate traditional knowledge and clinical research to better inform our practice.

Hananja and Nathalie

ACKNOWLEDGEMENT

The writing of this book took over three years (and longer once you count the patients I have seen over the last 35 years).

I would like to acknowledge the support from my husband, The Revd Paul Brice, who patiently cooked meals and supported me in this endeavour, including during our travels. He – together with my daughter, Zamira Brice (MChem, MSc) – helped with straightening out the English as well as the tedious workings of an Index.

A very special thanks must go to Nathalie Chidley (MNIMH) for many stimulating discussions while editing individual chapters and for translating technical language as well as my peculiar thinking into understandable English.

Thank you to Matthew Seal, who patiently went through the copy-editing, the countless references and detail, and to Peter Jarrett who provided the brilliant photo on the front cover as well as the photos in the book itself.

I also want to give a big thank you to all those individuals I have had the opportunity to support in their herbal treatment and become part of their journeys. They motivated me to delve deeper into herbal medicine and women's health.

Finally, thank you to the publishers Aeon, Alice Rathbone and Oliver Rathbone, who patiently supported me, dealt with the many delays (years'…), and without whom there would not be a book.

Hananja Brice-Ytsma FNIMH

SECTION ONE

SPECIFIC CONDITIONS

CHAPTER 1

Dysmenorrhoea

1.1 Primary and secondary dysmenorrhoea

The question uppermost in one's mind at the first visit of a patient is normally whether this is simple dysmenorrhoea, that is, is the problem the discomfort itself, or is it secondary to another cause? In these cases, questions around the history of the menstrual cycle are very helpful.

Information to gain in consultation

Age at onset

Primary dysmenorrhoea: occurs commonly in the first year after menarche and once ovulation is more regular.

Secondary dysmenorrhoea[1]
- Endometriosis: 20–30.
- Adenomyosis: 40+.
- Fibroids: 30+ (can be asymptomatic).
- Pelvic venous congestion: begins in adulthood secondary to pelvic venous varices.
- Ectopic pregnancy: after becoming sexually active.

In multiparous women, consider secondary causes especially if not present before childbirth.

Timing

Primary dysmenorrhoea
- Peaks 24 hours after onset, subsides after 2–3 days.[2]

Secondary dysmenorrhoea
- Pain of increasing severity over several menses.
- Pain increasing in severity during menses.
- Most common causes: endometriosis and adenomyosis.
- Endometriosis: the pain usually begins 1–2 weeks before menses.

Nature and severity

Primary dysmenorrhoea: central, supra-pubic pain, continual, dull, or sense of heaviness, plus episodic, cramping pain. Premenstrually the aching can extend to the groin and thighs with a heavy, dull sense of dragging in the vagina, a sense of fullness in bowel and/or the sensation that everything will fall out. It can be severe in the 20s and 30s, and often reduces with increasing age and childbirth.[3,4]

Secondary dysmenorrhoea: pain can present in different ways depending on the cause. The most common causes of dysmenorrhoea are endometriosis and adenomyosis.[5]
- Endometriosis: severe pain increasing severity or duration, onset 1–2 weeks before menses; peak pain occurs 1–2 days before, and during, menstruation.
- Adenomyosis: pain radiating to back and upper thighs, cramping or sharp, knife-like pain throughout menstruation, worsens with age.
- PID: bilateral/diffuse lower abdominal and pelvic pain, abdominal, uterine, adnexal; the pain is of increasing severity or duration.
- IUD: colicky pain, especially in the first three months after insertion, severe pain.
- Fibroids: mechanical effect of pressure caused by the size and position of the fibroid. This can manifest itself in different ways, e.g. urinary frequency, urinary retention, ureteral obstruction and hydronephrosis, a sensation of pressure.
- Pelvic venous congestion: dragging sensation, dull aching, worse on standing.
- Ectopic pregnancy: unilateral pain, pelvic tenderness on palpation.

Dyspareunia

- Not usually associated with primary dysmenorrhoea, but consider endometriosis, PID, adenomyosis, pelvic congestion, fibroids.

Associated symptoms

- Primary dysmenorrhoea: PMS such as: headache, malaise, fatigue, dizziness, nausea (sometimes vomiting), constipation, diarrhoea, lower back pain, urinary frequency, mood changes (tearfulness, irritability and depression).
- Endometriosis: infertility, menorrhagia, bloating, back pain, pelvic heaviness, cervical motion tenderness, dyspareunia.
- PID: dyspareunia, cervical motion tenderness, fever, malaise, offensive-smelling vaginal discharge. Chlamydia can be symptom-free.
- IUD: bleeding out of cycle, could be dislodged or an infection.
- Fibroids: urinary frequency, dyspareunia, urinary retention, ureteral obstruction and hydronephrosis.

Relieving or worsening factors

- Primary dysmenorrhoea: relieved by analgesics, OCP, exercise, childbirth.
- Secondary dysmenorrhoea: if not relieved by OCP, consider endometriosis. If not relieved by analgesics, consider PID.

<u>Sexual history</u>: if sexually active, consider PID

<u>Menstruation</u>: quality and quantity.

Primary: clots or casts can be present.

Secondary:
- Endometriosis: dark, tarry blood loss at beginning of menses, heavy periods, abnormal bleeding patterns.
- Adenomyosis: prolonged, menorrhagia, passing blood clots.
- PID: prolonged, menorrhagia, passing blood clots.
- IUCD can cause heavier, painful periods and bleeding between periods.
- Fibroids: menorrhagia.
- Ectopic: missed or late period, brown or watery discharge.

Family history:

Endometriosis, fibroids, and primary dysmenorrhoea[6] have a familial link.

Presence of pelvic pain unrelated to menses:

This may indicate other conditions. Consider: appendicitis, renal colic, UTI.

Investigate if the pain is:

- new
- sudden onset
- unremitting
- changing in character
- unilateral
- radiating
- worsens after end of period
- aggravated by pressure, bowel motions and sexual activity
- usual control measures not effective

Also investigate if:

- new symptoms accompany the pain
- missed period when pregnancy possible
- fever
- discharge

Recommended investigations:[7]

- FBC for anaemia if periods heavy.
- WCC and ESR in PID.
- Discharge: cervical cultures and cervical swab for chlamydia, to establish pathogen (PID).
- Ultrasound: for anatomical abnormalities, such as ovarian cysts, fibroids, endometriomas, ectopic pregnancy, localised pelvic masses, advanced endometriosis.
- Laparoscopy: DDx of PID and endometriosis can help to make definite diagnosis especially if history suggestive of secondary dysmenorrhoea. In half of laparoscopies no organic pathology is found.
- Pregnancy testing: intrauterine and ectopic pregnancy.

Table 1.1: Primary vs secondary dysmenorrhoea

Dysmenorrhoea	Onset	Aggravating/relieving factors	Accompanying symptoms	Nature of pain
Primary (no organic cause) On menstruation, or just before, peak 24 hours after onset, subsides after 2–3 days	First year after menarche, peaks aged 20s–30s, reduces with increasing age, childbirth	Relieved by analgesics, OCP, exercise, childbirth Worse with longer duration of periods[8]	PMS symptoms: headache, nausea, constipation, diarrhoea, lower back pain, urinary frequency, malaise, fatigue, vomiting, dizziness, mood changes IBS aggravates period pain, as well being aggravated by	Central, supra-pubic, continual, dull, sense of heaviness, plus episodic cramping pain, intensifies as flow heavier, or when clots are passed Premenstrually the aching can extend to groin, thighs; heavy dull sense of dragging in the vagina, sense of fullness in bowel, sensation that everything will fall out
Secondary (pathology) increasing in severity and duration over period	Usually 25 and over[9]	Not relieved by OCP; certain conditions do not respond to analgesics	As secondary conditions	As secondary conditions

Table 1.2: Secondary dysmenorrhoea differential diagnosis

Conditions	Timing and nature of pain	Accompanying symptoms	Flow	Other
Endometriosis 20–30 yo	Increasing severity or duration: can start 1–2 weeks before the onset of menses, can worsen upon menstrual flow; sacral and lower backaches during menses also can be present OCP/painkillers: no effect	Dyspareunia, infertility, bloating, back pain, pelvic heaviness	Dark, tarry blood at beginning of menses, menorrhagia	Dx: visualisation of implants
Adenomyosis over 40 yo	Radiating to back and upper thighs cramping or sharp, knife-like during and throughout menstruation, worsens with age	Dyspareunia	Prolonged, menorrhagia, passing blood clots	Enlarged uterus on examination
Pelvic inflammatory disease sexually active	Bilateral/diffuse lower abdominal or pelvic, increasing severity or duration Painkillers: no effect	Dyspareunia, cervical motion tenderness, fever, malaise, pelvic pain, smelly vaginal discharge	Abnormal bleeding and menorrhagia	WBC high, ESR high

DYSMENORRHOEA

Condition			
IUD (forgotten?)	Colicky, esp. first three months after insertion, severe bleeding		Menorrhagia, bleeding between periods	Mirena (progesterone releasing IUD) prescribed for heavy periods, effects may take up to 6 months to become apparent[10]
Fibroids over 30 yo	Occasional	Dyspareunia, mechanical effect of pressure, e.g. urinary frequency, urinary retention, ureteral obstruction and hydronephrosis	Menorrhagia	More common in African-Americans
Pelvic venous congestion	Dragging, dull, aching, worse on standing		Menorrhagia	Multiparous
Ectopic pregnancy sexually active	Unilateral, pelvic tenderness on palpation		Missed or late period Brown, watery discharge	

Less common conditions to consider: retroverted uterus, cervicitis, ovarian endometriomas, endometrial polyps.

Rare conditions: cervical stenosis, psychogenic onset after traumatic event. Pain around menarche may indicate a congenital outflow problem such as uterine, cervical or vaginal outflow obstructions.[11]

Ovarian cysts or tumours: are usually symptom-free till quite large. These more typically present with pressure-related symptoms such as alteration in bowel and/or bladder habits.

1.2 Pathophysiology of primary dysmenorrhoea

Several factors have been put forward as contributing to primary dysmenorrhoea, such as abnormal and increased prostanoid and eicosanoid secretion, elevated leukotrienes, reduced prostacyclin and elevated vasopressin. These are all partially under the influence of hormones.

Abnormal and increased prostanoid and eicosanoid secretion in the endometrium

Progesterone levels decline during the late luteal phase (post ovulatory) and precursors for the COX (cycloxygenous) and lipoxygenase pathways are generated. Prostaglandins and prostanoids are synthesised from arachidonic acid through the COX pathway. In primary dysmenorrhoea there is excessive endometrial secretion of the menstrual prostaglandins PGF2-alpha and PGE2, causing myometrial contractions leading to myometrial ischaemia, both giving rise to pain.[12]

The peak release of prostaglandins occurs in the first 48 hours of menstruation when symptoms are at their worst. The adverse influence of prostaglandins may contribute to other symptoms such as nausea, vomiting and diarrhoea. NSAIDs are used to inhibit COX enzymes therefore reducing prostaglandins PGF2-alpha and PGE2, and this will relieve primary dysmenorrhoea.

Elevated leukotriene levels

Leukotrienes are synthesised in the endometrium and myometrium, which increases the sensitivity of pain fibres in the myometrium and contribute to uterine hypercontractility.

Leukotrienes are produced by the 5-lipoxygenase enzyme pathway rather than the COX pathway, and this may account for some forms of primary dysmenorrhea that are not responsive to NSAIDs.[13]

Reduced prostacyclin

Prostacyclin is a potent vasodilator and uterine relaxant; this appears to be low in primary dysmenorrhea.

Elevated vasopressin

This is seen in women with primary dysmenorrhoea. Vasopressin is synthesised in the hypothalamus and stored in the posterior pituitary, and may play a role in increasing dysrhythmic uterine contractility, causing vasoconstriction and ischaemic pain. *Zingiber officinalis* powder reduced plasma vasopressin in healthy volunteers.[14] For further interest note that the alkaloids chelerythrine and sanguinarine, found in *Eschscholzia californica*, demonstrated an affinity for vasopressin V1 receptors in vivo and are competitive inhibitors of [3H]-vasopressin binding.[15]

Risk factors for primary dysmenorrhoea

- Alcohol and drug abuse
- Depression and anxiety
- Early menarche, before age 12
- Family history
- Lack of exercise
- Low body mass index, as well as obesity
- Menorrhagia
- Nulliparity
- PMS
- Prolonged menstruation
- Sexual abuse
- Smoking

Conventional treatment

NSAIDS: ibuprofen, naproxen, ketoprofen, mefenamic acid and nimesulide. NSAIDs are used to inhibit COX enzymes, therefore reducing prostaglandins PGF2-alpha and PGE2, and this relieves primary dysmenorrhoea.

The oestrogen-progestin oral contraceptive pills (OCPs) inhibit endometrial development and decrease menstrual prostanoids, reduce menstrual fluid volume and prostaglandins to within, or even below, normal range. Oral contraceptive pills may also lower elevated plasma vasopressin levels. Some 1% of women with dysmenorrhea do not respond to NSAIDs or OCPs.[16]

Calcium antagonists: nifedipine inhibits myometrial contractility by blocking calcium entry into smooth muscle cell, reducing intracellular free calcium and as a result contractions are reduced and vasodilatation promoted. As a point of interest Ca^{++} channel antagonist effects have been seen in *Achillea millefolium*,[17] *Anethum graveolens*,[18] *Matricaria chamomilla*,[19] *M. piperita* essential oil and *Valeriana officinalis*,[20] and all have been used in dysmenorrhoea.

Placebo is powerfully effective in up to 35–40% of women with dysmenorrhoea.[21]

1.3 Herbal management of primary dysmenorrhoea

Understanding the pathophysiology of primary dysmennorrhoea can explain the mechanism of action of herbs traditionally used for treatment. We have seen that several inflammatory pathways are involved and that our anti-inflammatory herbs can play a key role in reducing symptoms. Dysfunctional or dysrhythmic uterine contractions lead to an ischaemic endometrium, hence the use of spasmolytics and uterine tonics/emmenagogues to support circulation in the womb; many herbs traditionally used for dysmenorrhoea were also used for amenorrhoea for this reason. Endocrine herbs might also play a role, as the drop in progesterone is a trigger for some of the mechanisms of menstruation. If the progesterone/oestrogen ratio is out of sync this can also contribute to and complicate the picture. Some herbs tick many of the herbal action boxes at once, for example ginger is a circulatory and anti-inflammatory as well as reducing vasopressin levels.

In cases of secondary dysmenorrhoea we need to address the underlying cause (see appropriate chapters). However symptomatic relief can and should be given using uterine antispasmodics, analgesics and anti-inflammatories. This strategy will be most effective if given two or three days *before* the onset of menstruation.

Aims

Reduce pain: anti-inflammatories, antispasmodics, analgesics
Improve uterine function: uterine tonics/emmenagogues
Normalise hormonal levels: hormonal modulators

Anti-inflammatories:

Many of our herbs have anti-inflammatory activity: some inhibit prostaglandin biosynthesis, via inhibition of the cyclooxygenase and/or 5-lipoxygenase enzyme. For example, salicin (found in *Actaea racemosa*, *Salix alba*, *Viburnum prunifolium*, *Zingiber officinale*) inhibited the spasmodic and inflammatory action of prostaglandin F2alpha in a preclinical study.[22]

Anti-inflammatory herbs: *Actaea racemosa, Achillea millefolium, Anemone pulsatilla, Angelica sinensis, Chamomilla recutica, Cinnamomum zeylanicum, Dioscorea villosa, Foeniculum vulgare, Rosa damascena fructus, Salix alba, Salvia rosmarinus (Rosmarinus officinalis), Thymus vulgaris, Vaccinium myrtillus, Viburnum prunifolium, Zingiber officinale.*

Antispasmodics:

Antispasmodics achieve their outcomes in various ways:

- Increasing prostacyclin, a vasodilator and uterine relaxant, which inhibits COX activity. Prostacyclin tends to be reduced in those with primary dysmenorrhoea. Some herbs are found in preclinical studies to promote prostacyclin synthesis such as *Ginkgo biloba*.[23] Phenolic phyto-oestrogens such as those found in soya stimulated prostacyclin release in human endothelial cells.[24]
- Vasopressin reduction. Elevated vasopressin levels are found in women with primary dysmenorrhoea and is involved in uterine contraction and ischaemic pain. *Zingiber officinale* reduced plasma vasopressin in healthy adults.[25]
- Ca^{++} channel blocking activity. Inhibition of myometrial contractility by blocking Ca^{++} entry into smooth muscle cells, reducing intracellular free Ca^{++}, results in contractions being reduced and vasodilatation being promoted.

Herbs shown to have Ca^{++} channel blocking activity: *Achillea millefolium*,[26,27] *Anethum graveolens, Matricaria recutita*,[28] *Mentha piperita* essential oil,[29-31] *Valeriana officinalis*.

Other antispasmodic herbs: *Actaea racemosa, Atropa belladonna, Cinnamomum zeylanicum, Dioscorea villosa, Foeniculum vulgare, Melissa offinicalis, Paeonia lactiflora & Glycyrrhiza glabra in combination, Salvia rosmarinus (Rosmarinus officinalis), Thymus vulgaris, Viburnum prunifolium or opulus, Zingiber officinale.*[32]

Uterine tonics/emmenagogues: improve pelvic circulation and prevent uterine ischaemia. *Achillea millefolium, Actaea racemosa, Anemone pulsatilla, Angelica sinensis.*

Hormonal herbs: compensating for progesterone drop
- Dopaminergic herbs such as *Actaea racemosa, Paeonia lactiflora & Glycyrrhiza glabra* and *Vitex agnus-castus* will encourage the healthy functioning of the corpus luteum (producing both progesterone and oestrogen).
- Phenolic phytoestrogenic herbs such as *Foeniculum vulgare* and *Trigonella foenum-graecum* occupy oestrogen receptor sites, reducing endogenous oestrogen in oestrogen-rich environments and acting as oestrogen in deficient states.
- Steroidal saponin-rich herbs such as *Dioscorea villosa* encourage the endogenous production of oestrogen.

Analgesics for symptomatic relief: *Actaea racemosa, Anemone pulsatilla, Atropa belladonna, Rosa damascena fructus, Salix alba.*

Key herbs used in clinical practice

Anemone pulsatilla

Traditional use: the Eclectics used anemone for amenorrhoea due to cold or from emotional causes, and for dysmenorrhoea if symptoms included a sense of fullness, or weakness in the back and hips during bleeding, and also used it as an emmenagogue.[33]

Prof. Chandler wrote in 1919: *As a rule, for dysmenorrhoea of the virgin or the unmarried, I give the choice to pulsatilla; while to the married, before pregnancy or after its occurrence, I have preferred cimicifuga.*[34] It has spasmolytic, analgesic and sedative effects.

Dosage
Typical weekly dosage 15–20ml of 1:3 (dried).
 In acute attacks of dysmenorrhoea: 0.75ml–2ml given half hourly.
 The Eclectics suggest only the fresh herbs should be employed.[35]
 Fresh plant tincture (1:10): 1–5 drops t.i.d. or PRN for acute pain.

Valeriana officinalis

Traditional use: Dioscorides saw it as a 'warming' metabolic stimulant and employed it as a menstrual stimulant. In the 16th century it was seen as sedative and spasmolytic, and continued to be used as a stimulant. It is also used for insomnia, as an anxiolytic and to relieve digestive and other spasms of smooth muscle.

Preclinical studies: valerinic acid shows an antispasmodic activity on smooth muscles. A possible mechanism is that is able to inhibit contractions resulting from cellular depolarisation via calcium channel blocking and the opening of potassium channels.[36]

Clinical studies: *V. officinalis* has similar effect to that of mefenamic acid.[37] It has been shown to reduce the severity of dysmenorrhea and reduced the need of pain relievers.[38] *There was also a* reduction in fainting compared to placebo.[39,40]

Dosage
Typical dosage per day 4–12ml of 1:1.
    Typical dosage per week 20–40ml of 1:1.

Viburnum prunifolium (alternative Viburnum opulus)

Traditional use: dysmenorrhoea, false labour pains and threatened miscarriage. Apparently it was common practice for plantation owners to make their slaves drink an infusion of *Viburnum prunifolium* daily while pregnant to prevent abortion from taking Cottonroot.[41] The *British Pharmaceutical Codex* (1911) reports good results for dysmenorrhoea and spasmodic affections of plain muscle.[42]

Pharmacological studies: spasmolytic effects shown in vivo and ex vivo on uterine tissue.[43,44] Salicin and salicylic acid plus flavonoids may contribute to the anti-inflammatory effects. Scopoletin is thought to be important in relation to smooth muscle antispasmodic activity.[45]

Dosage: higher ethanol percentages do not always confer higher activity. French researchers found that *Viburnum prunifolium* bark extracted at 30% ethanol was five times more spasmolytic than a 60% extract.[46]
    Daily dosage 1–3ml 1:3.
    Typical weekly dosage 20–45ml of 1:3.
    For dysmenorrhoea in acute treatment: daily dose 2–7ml of 1:3.

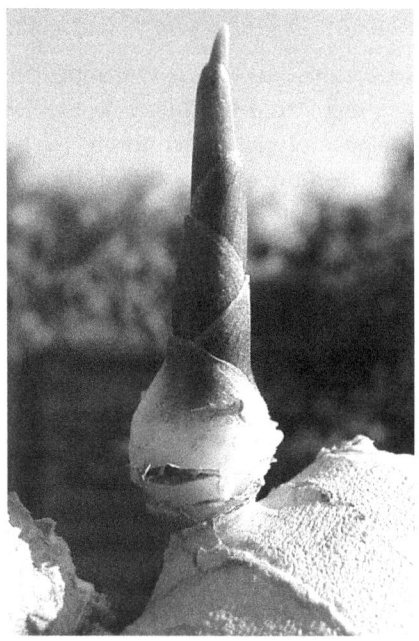

Zingiber officinale

Traditional use: digestive issues and general digestion, amenorrhoea and dysmenorrhoea. Used as carminative, anti-emetic, peripheral circulatory stimulant, spasmolytic and anti-inflammatory.

Preclinical studies: anti-inflammatory action by inhibition of prostaglandin synthesis,[47] inhibits both cyclooxygenase (COX) and lipooxygenase,[48] resulting in an inhibition of leukotriene[49] and prostaglandin[50] synthesis. On healthy volunteers it was shown to reduce vasopressin levels.

Clinical studies: effective for primary dysmenorrhoea. Systematic reviews and meta-analyses show ginger to be as effective as NSAIDs, mefenamic acid, ibuprofen and zinc sulphate in reducing pain severity as well as reducing accompanying nausea and diarrhoea.[51–67]

Dosage
Typical daily dosage 2.5–6ml of 1:3.
    Typical weekly dosage 5–10ml of 1:3.[68]
    Dosing 2 days before menstruation was significantly better at decreasing the duration of pain.[69]

Schedule 20 herb, for severe pain not controlled by any of the above:

Atropa belladonna fol contains tropane alkaloids such as atropine and antimuscarinics.

Traditional use: Gerard (1597) calls the plant the Sleeping Nightshade; the leaves moistened in wine vinegar and laid on the head induce sleep. The root was not used in medicine in England until 1860, when Peter Squire recommended it as the basis of an anodyne liniment.

The Eclectics also used belladonna for pain and spasm, including anal, biliary, uterine, intestinal and urethral.[70]

Weiss highly regards this plant, saying it is 'unsurpassed' as an antispasmodic drug for the GIT, can also be used for dysmenorrhoea.[71] It acts rapidly, with a lasting effect and suppresses secretions, e.g. hyperacidity.

Dosage: given for folia:
10 drops initially raised by 1–2 drops per dose every 2–3 hours thereafter until either symptoms are alleviated or the patient starts to develop a dry mouth and dry eyes.

Recommended initial weekly dose 2ml of 1:10, not to exceed 10ml per week.

Contraindications: tachycardia, paralytic ileus (may cause obstructions), glaucoma (may increase intra-ocular pressure, its action possibly accentuated by antidepressant drugs).[72]

Empirically proven acute mixture

While working at a training clinic for herbal degree students, we regularly provided acute medicine for dysmenorrhoea; students were often pleasantly surprised by how effective these herbs were! Our favourite combination is reproduced below.

Rx
Anemone pulsatilla 1:3   20ml
Valeriana officinalis 1:3   35ml
Viburnum prunifolium 1:3   35ml
Zingiber officinale 1:2   10ml
Sig. 5–10ml PRN

Other herbs commonly used

Achillea millefolium

Traditional use: the Physiomedicalist tradition classed yarrow as a diffusive vasostimulant affecting peripheral circulation, especially pelvic organs. The Eclectics traditionally used yarrow for atonic amenorrhoea, and *King's American Dispensatory* lists it for the relief of menorrhagia.[73]

Pharmacological studies, preclinical studies
Anti-inflammatory: COX-2 inhibitor.[74,75]
   Analgesic: contains salicylic acid derivatives, eugenol, menthol.
   Antispasmodic:[76] attributed to flavonoids, which would be found in tea. The mechanism is attributed in part to a Ca^{++} channel blocking activity and in part to mediator-antagonistic effects.[77]

Clinical studies: tea used for 3 days was effective in minimising pain severity in primary dysmenorrhoea.[78] In a study where *Achillea millefolium* was compared with *Matricaria chamomilla* taken every 8 hours during the first three days of menstruation, both were found effective, although *Achillea* was more effective at reducing the severity of dysmenorrhoea.[79]

Dosages: daily dose 3–12ml of 1:3.
   Typical weekly dose 20–30ml of 1:3.

Contraindications: people with known sensitivity to other members of the Compositae family (e.g. ragweed, daisies, chrysanthemums).

Actaea racemosa

Traditional use: dysmenorrhoea, ovarian pain, menorrhagia as well as rheumatic conditions. The Eclectics proposed a special affinity with the female reproductive organs, specifically for tensive, dragging pain.

Preclinical studies: dopaminergic activity/serotoninergic,[80] similar to *Vitex agnus-castus*. Also has an effect on the endogenous opioid system.[81] It is most likely that *Actaea* acts via multiple mechanisms: dopaminergic, serotonergic, antioxidative and anti-inflammatory.

The herb seems mainly to be researched for its action on menopausal symptoms, but in traditional use it has a much broader action for issues related to the whole female reproductive system.[82]

Dosage: as a powerfully acting herb low dosages are often all that is needed. Clinical trials used 80mg per day, which translates to 0.25ml of 1:3 per day.

Typical weekly dose: 5–10ml of 1:3.

The average weekly dose used in clinical trials is 1.8ml of a 1:3 per week. Most UK herbalists would use 10ml of a 1:3 per week.[83] Note: 60% alcohol is needed to extract the triterpene glycosides.

Dioscorea villosa

Traditional use: Native Americans have used *D. villosa* for pains associated with rheumatism and arthritis, colic and intestinal cramps, to relieve labour pains, for nausea and spasms during pregnancy, as well as for the treatment of bilious colic. It was one of the Eclectics' favourite herbs for spasmolytic activity and specific in bilious colic, but has also been used for dysmenorrhoea, quickly relieving muscular spasm.

Preclinical studies: *Dioscorea villosa* and diosgenin show anti-inflammatory and antinociceptive effect.[84]

Dosages according to Ellingwood (1919): *Five drops every hour or two can be given with good results in constantly recurring mild colicky pains without apparent cause. When given for the after pains of childbirth, it is usually best to give the tincture in ten drop doses in cold water every half hour or hour, as the hot infusion may cause too great relaxation of the uterine muscular structure, and permit severe haemorrhage.*[85]

Dosage: daily dose 4.5–9ml of 1:3.

Typical weekly dose 20–40ml of 1:3.

Matricaria chamomilla

Traditional use: popular in domestic medicine for the nervous system as well as GIT for its carminative and spasmolytic actions, it was also seen as of value in amenorrhoea and dysmenorrhoea with labour-like pains, and for the prevention of clot formation.

Pharmacological studies, preclinical studies
Anti-inflammatory effects shown by individual constituents chamazulene, alpha-bisabolol, apigenin, as well as the whole extract.[86–88] Multiple mechanisms are involved in having an influence on 5-lipoxygenase

activity, interleukin-6, tumour necrosis factor-alpha, lipid peroxidation, COX-2, iNOS, PGE$_2$ production and leukotrienes.[89–95]

Antispasmodic: inhibited cAMP-phosphodiesterases.[96] Antispasmodic as well as antidiarrhoeal, antisecretory activities are mediated through K$^+$ channels plus weak Ca^{++} channel antagonist-like pathways.[97]

Sedative and anti-anxiety effects: a papaverine-like activity is shown.[98] Individual flavonoids are shown to affect γ-amino butyric acid (GABA),[99] noradrenalin,[100] dopamine, and serotonin neurotransmission, modulating hypothalamic-pituitary-adrenocortical axis function.[101] The whole extract inhibited glutamic acid decarboxylase activity,[102] thereby influencing brain GABA levels and neurotransmission, and binds to benzodiazepine receptors in the brain,[103] exhibiting benzodiazepine-like hypnotic activity.[104]

Clinical studies: shown to be more effective than placebo for dysmenorrhoea if used before the pain begins, and more effective than mefenamic acid in reducing pain severity and haemorrhage.[105–107]

Chamomile tea taken as 2 cups a day, 1 week prior to menstruation and for the first five days of the menstruation cycle reduced dysmenorrhoea and anxiety.[108,109]

When compared with *Foeniculum vulgare*, *Matricaria* was more effective on pelvic and abdominal pain, depression and anger while *Foeniculum* was more effective in reducing fatigue and lethargy.[110]

Dosages: 5g infused for 10 minutes, making sure to keep covered so as not to lose the volatile oils via the steam.[111]

Daily dose 15ml of 1:3.

Typical weekly dose 25–50ml of 1:3.

Contraindications: Very rare cases of allergy.

Paeonia lactiflora and *Glycyrrhiza glabra*

Traditional use: while both have a long tradition of use in Traditional Chinese Medicine and other traditions for a variety of conditions, the combination of the two is what we focus on here.

Pharmacological studies, preclinical studies

Spasmolytic: paeony extracts interfere with acetylcholine release into the neuromuscular junctions and licorice extracts interfere with acetylcholine's activity in the neuromuscular junctions, providing a spasmolytic action.[112] While concentrations of paeoniflorin and glycyrrhizin were individually too low to inhibit muscle contraction, they were very active when applied simultaneously.[113] In vitro this combination may exert its action on dysmenorrhoea through preventing prostaglandin production.[114]

Dopaminergic: the combination also affects the modulation of the dopaminergic system, reducing prolactin levels and normalising progesterone level similar to the way *Vitex agnus-castus* has been shown to work.[115]

Anti-inflammatory: Paeonia with Glycyrrhiza were shown to suppress prostaglandin production in the myometrium (ex vivo) by inhibiting cytoplasmic phospholipase A2 activity.[116]

Clinical studies: reduced dysmenorrhea in women with uterine fibroids,[117] and inhibited contraction of uterine smooth muscles in pregnant women.[118]

Dosage: Japanese clinical trials used a Paeonia and licorice combination (extract equivalent to 4–6g/day of dried Paeonia root and 4–6g of *Glycyrrhiza glabra*); however, a hydro-ethanolic mix is a more effective solvent than water for many of the constituents.

Typical weekly dose 20–30ml of 1:1 of each herb.

Vitex agnus-castus

Traditional use: some argue that as *Vitex* indirectly stimulates progesterone, it could possibly aggravate dysmenorrhoea, but as its main effect is on the corpus luteum this also increases oestrogen secretion, not solely progesterone.

Pharmacological studies:
Dopaminergic: decreases of prolactin secretion by dopamine receptor agonism,[119] normalises corpus luteal function via its dopaminergic activity.

Affinity to certain opiate receptors: *mu* and *delta* opioid receptors.[120,121] This property may support the plant's efficacy in PMS.[122]

Anti-inflammatory: casticin and other constituents shown to have anti-inflammatory properties in vitro, and several mechanisms have been identified, including lipoxygenase inhibition.[123,124]

Increases melatonin levels: melatonin has been shown to have analgesic, antioxidant and anti-inflammatory effects.[125]

Clinical studies: *Vitex* reduced pain intensity in dysmenorrhoea[126] similar to that of ethinyl oestradiol/drospirenone in patients with severe primary dysmenorrhoea.[127]

In a trial on patients with endometriosis, *Vitex* improved sleep quality and reduced the need for analgesics.[128]

Dosage: daily dose can vary depending on underlying conditions, starting from around 0.54ml or 10 drops of 1:3 per day.
Typical weekly dose 4–5ml of 1:3.
For endometriosis up to 7.5ml per day of 1:3.
Typical weekly dose up to 50ml.[129]

Table 1.3: Other herbs shown to be effective in clinical trials

Herb	Studies (preclinical and clinical)
Anethum graveolens Traditional use as galactogogue, pain-relieving, anticonvulsant, anti-emetic.	**Preclinical studies:** spasmolytic, relaxant effect due to closing the voltage-dependent Ca^{++} channels.[130,131] **Clinical studies:** as effective as mefenamic acid in reducing the pain severity in primary dysmenorrhea.[131]
Angelica sinensis	**Clinical studies:** in Europe late 1800s,[132–134] relieved premenstrual pain and increased menstrual flow,[135] helpful for amenorrhoea.[136]
Cinnamomum zeylanicum Used for colic and cramp of the stomach, perhaps suggesting why it is also useful for dysmenorrhoea.	**Pharmacological studies, preclinical studies:** Cinnamaldehyde, eugenol show antispasmodic effects, eugenol inhibiting the biosynthesis of prostaglandins, thereby reducing inflammation.[137] **Clinical studies:** Reduced severity, intensity and duration of dysmenorrhoea, nausea and vomiting due to primary dysmenorrhea.[138–140]

(*Continued*)

Table 1.3: (Continued)

Herb	Studies (preclinical and clinical)
Foeniculum vulgare Most studies relate to the essential oil (EO). Iranian traditional medicine: anti-inflammatory, analgesic and antispasmodic effects on smooth muscle.[141]	**Preclinical studies:** Fennel EO inhibited the response of uterine tissue to oxytocin and prostaglandin E2, reducing frequency and intensity of contraction.[142] Anethole has a similar structure to dopamine, suggesting that it binds to dopamine receptors to decrease pain. A water extract of fennel showed antinociceptive effect, possibly mediated by the histamine H_1, H_2 receptors; in vivo the results were comparable to indomethacin on visceral pain.[143] **Clinical studies:** essential oil, compared to mefenamic acid,[144] placebo,[145,146] other herbs,[147] or vitamin E.[148,149] EO is effective for primary dysmenorrhea.[150] Compared to mefenamic acid: some more effective, some less potent.[151–155] Also reduced excessive bleeding,[156,157] decreased nausea, weakness, shortened the menstrual period, improved quality of life[158] and reduced lethargy.[159]
Mentha piperita: traditionally used as carminative	**Preclinical studies:** M. piperita oil inhibits contractions induced by cell depolarisation, blocks Ca^{++} channels and has antispasmodic properties on smooth muscle.[160] **Clinical studies:** extract reduced dysmenorrhoea.[161]

(Continued)

Table 1.3: (Continued)

Herb	Studies (preclinical and clinical)
Rosa damascena fructus Traditional use for abdominal and chest pain, strengthening the heart and for treatment of menstrual bleeding and digestive problems. Dried and fresh hips of R. damascena are used in Iran,[162] and decoctions of the flowers are used for painful menstrual bleeding.[163]	**Preclinical studies:** relaxant effect on tracheal chains,[164] analgesic and anti-inflammatory properties.[165] **Clinical studies:** tea reduced dysmenorrhoea, anxiety and improved psycho-physiologic well-being over 6 months.[166,167] R. damascena fruit 200mg and mefenamic acid had similar effects on the pain intensity of primary dysmenorrhea.[167,168]
Salvia rosmarinus (Rosmarinus officinalis) The Eclectics described it as an diffusively stimulating and relaxing, nervine, antispasmodic in 'mild hysteria', dysmenorrhoea.[169]	**Preclinical studies:** extract reduced the production of prostaglandins by reducing the IL β, TNF-α (tumour necrosis factor α) and cyclooxygenase-2.[170,171] **Clinical studies:** reduced menstrual bleeding and primary dysmenorrhea.[171]
Salix alba	**Preclinical studies:** anti-inflammatory activity associated with down regulation of tumour necrosis factor-α and nuclear factor-kappa B. **Clinical studies:** decreased dysmenorrhea.[172] Other: effective for chronic lower back, joint pain and osteoarthritis.[173]

(Continued)

Table 1.3: (Continued)

Herb	Studies (preclinical and clinical)
Thymus vulgaris Eclectic physicians considered thyme to be an emmenagogue and a tonic and prescribed the tea for 'hysteria' and dysmenorrhoea.	**Preclinical studies:** thymol and carvacrol components, effects are due to a reduction of prostaglandin synthesis.[174,175] **Clinical studies:** similar effects compared to Ibuprofen or placebo.[174,175] EO reduced the pain severity in primary dysmenorrhea.[176,177]
Trigonella foenum-graecum: used in ancient Egypt to facilitate childbirth and a galactogogue.	**Clinical studies:** effective in dysmenorrhea and mastalgia.[178] Decreasing the duration of pain, reduced systemic symptoms such as fatigue, headache, nausea, vomiting, lack of energy, syncope.[179]

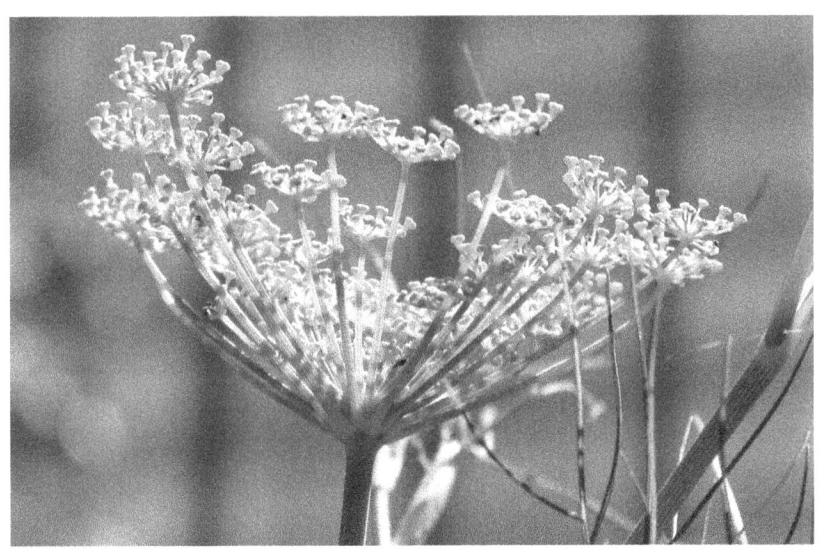

Foeniculum vulgare

1.4 Dietary and lifestyle recommendations

Supplementation by vitamins K, D, B1 and E and minerals calcium, magnesium, zinc sulfate and boron contribute effectively to dysmenorrhea pain management.

Vitamin E increases the production of vasodilator prostacyclin and prostaglandin E2 (PGE2), as well as a dose-dependent upregulation of phospholipase A2 and arachidonic acid release, but inhibits COX activity. Magnesium is a cofactor in delta-6 desaturase involved in anti-inflammatory prostaglandins (PGE1) and exerts a relaxing effect on the skeletal and smooth muscle cramping.

As usual, it is best to have a varied diet rich in nuts, seeds, good oils, vegetables (especially dark leafy greens and legumes), fruits, fish and whole grains. If in any doubt about nutritional intake supplements can be given, the closer to naturally occurring states the better. People are often deficient in vitamin D.

It may also be beneficial to include foods rich in anthocyanins. These are found in berries such as black elderberries, blueberries, blackberries, raspberries, strawberries and cherries, and fruit such as black plums, blood oranges, black or red grapes and pomegranates. A clinical study with 25% anthocyanin extract (310mg daily in 2 doses, used 3 days before and during menstruation) reduced the symptoms of dysmenorrhoea such as pelvic and lumbosacral pain, mammary tension, headache, nausea and heaviness of lower limbs.[181]

Table 1.4: Clinical trials on specific nutrients

Nutrient	Dose used in trials
Boron[182]	10mg daily
Calcium[183]	1200mg
Magnesium[184]	Dose and regime were widely variable
Omega 3[185,186]	2.5g per day
Vitamin B1[187]	100mg daily
Vitamin B6[188]	200mg daily
Vitamin D[189]	50,000 iu oral supplementation over 8 weeks. The benefits of vitamin D become apparent two months after intake begins.[190]
Vitamin E[191]	150mg per day

See Appendix for food sources.

Other recommendations

Exercise was associated with a reduction in dysmenorrhea symptoms,[192] and vigorous exercisers (more than 3 times per week) reported fewer physical symptoms during menstruation in comparison with a sedentary lifestyle.[193,194]

Hot water bottle: low-level topical heat therapy was as effective as ibuprofen, with a faster improvement in pain relief when heat was applied concurrent with ibuprofen.[195]

Aromatherapy: lavender oil.[196]

Lavender oil massage: decreased the severity of primary dysmenorrhea.[196]

CHAPTER 2

Menorrhagia

2.1 Menorrhagia definition and differential diagnosis

- Excessive duration (longer than 7–8 days), and/or abnormally heavy period (over 80ml or 16 soaked sanitary towels per menses).
- Saturating a super tampon or heavy pad more than every hour for 6–8 hours or more.
  - Flooding—an uncontrollable gush of blood.
  - Presence of clots, larger than about 2.5cm.
  - Polymenorrhagia: heavy bleeding that occurs at shorter intervals, with the cycle length being reduced.

Bleeding is controlled via a range of mechanisms—during the menstrual cycle there are a range of complex interactions between endocrine, paracrine, immunological and haemostatic factors on the endometrium.[1] Menorrhagia at every menses has a prevalence of about one in five women.[2] With the complexity of menstruation, the causes of menorrhagia can be many and multifactorial.

Control of normal menstrual bleeding

Endometrial function is under the control of oestrogen and progesterone via receptors; there is also involvement of ovarian androgens and glucocorticoids from the adrenal glands.

During the follicular phase, oestrogen, via oestrogen receptors (ER), increases endometrial responsiveness to ovarian hormones by upregulating oestrogen, progesterone and androgen receptors (ER, PR and AR respectively), causing cell proliferation, rebuilding and increasing the thickness of the endometrium.

During the luteal, or secretory phase, after ovulation, the production of progesterone by the corpus luteum is the trigger for change. This reduces endometrial ER, PR and AR expression and counteracts the oestrogen-driven mitotic activity of endometrial cells. The spiral arterioles within the stratum functionalis grow and acquire muscle.

During menstruation, the drop of progesterone levels, alongside declining oestrogen levels, cause stromal shrinkage and spiral arteriolar vasoconstriction. This leads to hypoxia in the functionalis layer, followed by acute inflammatory changes such as the influx of leucocytes and immune cells.[3] As a consequence, there is an increased synthesis of proinflammatory prostaglandins, cytokines, chemokines and proteases—destructive enzymes of the extracellular matrix, e.g. matrix metalloproteinases (MMP).[4] This causes tissue breakdown and bleeding.

The shedding of the 'old' stratum functionalis takes 1–2 days, and menstrual bleeding continues for several days during the proliferation and repair of the surface epithelium and tissue regeneration.[5]

Myometrial contractility is induced by increased endometrial production of prostaglandins such as $PGF_{2\alpha}$ and PGE_2,[6] to aid the clearing of the uterus and to control the bleeding. Cessation of menstrual bleeding involves platelet aggregation, fibrin deposition and thrombus formation.[7]

Most of the loss of blood occurs over the first three days. Normal menstrual loss is considered to be 20–80ml, while heavy is considered to be >80ml.

We must be mindful of an element of unreliable self-reporting. Many women may consider what is defined as a heavy bleed (>80ml) to be normal, and among women who present with menorrhagia, fewer than 50% have been objectively shown to have >80ml of menstrual loss.[8]

Menorrhagia is a relatively uncommon occurrence in younger women and has a prevalence of one in three women in the perimenopausal period.[9]

Many women may complain only of physical symptoms associated with anaemia (fatigue, lethargy and exertional dyspnoea) that interfere with normal daily life and may not consider that the underlying source may be menorrhagia.

Emergency

- Saturating pads every half hour.
- Symptoms of orthostatic hypotension: lightheadedness, dizziness, fainting.

Consider

- If the woman is young, has painless heavy periods and is generally well with a normal examination, consider dysfunctional uterine bleeding (DUB, see next section of this chapter).
- A single heavy period can be caused by factors such as excessive exercise or be stress-related, and so simply needs to be monitored over several cycles.
- Anovulatory cycle: heavy, often prolonged bleeding occurs 35 or more days apart.[10]

Information to gain in consultation

- Age
- Cycle: length, pattern i.e. regular or irregular
- Changes in menstrual patterns
- Contraception methods, including forgotten coil
- Flow: number of tampons and pads used and how often, saturation of tampons or pads, occurrence of flooding
- Frequency of occurrence
- Length of menstrual period
- PMH
- Pregnancy
- Presence of large blood clots (blood clots suggest significant heavy bleeding)
- Sexual history
- Signs of pelvic infection

MENORRHAGIA 31

Table 2.1: Differential diagnosis of menorrhagia

Condition	Dysmenorrhoea	On examination	Age	Cycle
Hormonal causes				
Dysfunctional uterine bleeding (DUB)	No	No tenderness	Commonly during puberty and perimenopause PCOS, obesity (endometrial hyperplasia)	Possibly long anovulatory cycles (35 days or more), heavy, often prolonged bleeding
Structural causes				
Cervical and endometrial polyp	Possible	No tenderness	20–40	Normal
Endometriosis Adenomyosis	Severe, plus dyspareunia, infertility	Tender, possibly enlarged uterus	Endometriosis, 20–30 years old, but anyone ovulating Adenomyosis, over 40 years	Normal
Fibroids	Pressure symptoms, dysmenorrhoea can be present.	No tenderness, enlarged uterus	Over 30	Normal
PID	Dysmenorrhoea, dyspareunia	Tenderness, vaginal discharge, possible raised temperature	Sexually active	Erratic bleeding

Red flags

- Chaotic, inter-menstrual and/or post-coital bleeding.
- Menorrhagia with secondary dysmenorrhoea, dyspareunia, pelvic tenderness on examination suggests endometriosis or chronic PID.
- Post-menopausal years: if not on hormone therapy, post-menopausal bleeding is abnormal, investigate for neoplastic lesions.

Other causes

- Cystic glandular hyperplasia: causes intermenstrual bleeding due to erratic and irregular shedding of the endometrium.
- Hypothyroidism and hyperthyroidism: these conditions can interfere with the feedback mechanism that regulates the secretion of gonadotrophin-releasing hormone from the hypothalamus and gonadotrophins from the pituitary and hormones from the ovary.
- IUCD: periods can become heavier and longer—it is thought that they elevate circulating levels of plasminogen activator, due to increased fibrinolytic activity. Conversely, progesterone releasing IUCDs are used to reduce blood loss.
- Iatrogenic (OCP, HRT).

Rare

- Adrenal disorders.
- Liver disease can interfere with the metabolism of oestrogen and cause a reduction of hepatically derived coagulation factors.
- Coagulation defects: adolescents with acute menorrhagia have a 20% to 30% incidence of a coagulation disorders (such as von Willebrand's disease, idiopathic thrombocytopenic purpurea, leukaemia).
- Endometrial carcinoma.

Investigations

- Pregnancy test.
- FBC: anaemia and thrombocytopenia.
- Serum ferritin: may be the first indication of decreased iron levels. Menstrual blood loss above 60ml is associated with negative iron balance in most cases. Chronic iron deficiency can lead to heavier bleeding.

- Thyroid function test: 2/3 of women with hypothyroidism develop abnormal menstruation.
- Liver function test.
- Clotting studies: history of abnormal bleeding, bruising.
- FSH, LH: menopause and/or premature menopause.
- Transvaginal ultrasound: fibroids, polyps, endometrial thickness.
- Vaginal swab: chronic PID with discharge.
- Other endocrine: hyperprolactinaemia and adrenal disorders.
- Occasionally D&C is diagnostic, but sometimes bleeding patterns return to normal after a procedure, endometrial sampling, hysteroscopy.

Conventional treatment

The combined oral contraceptive pill, levonorgestrel-releasing intra-uterine system, non-steroidal anti-inflammatory drugs, and anti-fibrinolytics have all been shown to have some degree of efficacy.[11]

2.2 Dysfunctional uterine bleeding (DUB)

Definition

Excessive, prolonged, unpatterned endometrial bleeding in the absence of organic disease.

Some 20% of cases occur in adolescent girls where normal hypothalamic function is not yet well established. It is also highly prevalent among perimenopausal women (one in three),[12] due to the reduction of oestrogen to levels not high enough to trigger the LH surge needed for ovulation and corpus luteum formation. There is a higher prevalence in obesity, due to increased conversion of androgens to oestrogens in fat cells. Hormones are influenced by high dietary fat intake, stress and exercise; the latter is associated with lighter menstrual loss. Some 5% to 10% of women will experience some form of DUB in their lifetime.

A summary of the possible causes of dysfunctional uterine bleeding:

- As the corpus luteum regresses progesterone levels fall, causing a local inflammatory response.
- There is reduced vasoconstriction of the spiral arterioles, causing more bleeding and transient hypoxia.
- The production of factors needed for endometrial repair is reduced.

- Haemostatic principles are reduced and are not able to control bleeding.

DUB with anovulatory cycles often presents with heavy, prolonged bleeding occurring 35 or more days apart.[13] It is common at the beginning and end of the reproductive years when oestrogen secretions may be less than normal and not opposed by progesterone. In anovulatory cycles, the corpus luteum does not get formed, and hence no progesterone is secreted. In the presence of unopposed oestrogen, the endometrium continues in its proliferative phase,[14] leading to endometrial hyperplasia.[15] As the follicle degenerates, oestrogen levels drop, and oestrogen withdrawal bleeding occurs.

Herbal approach: stimulating ovulation with herbs rich in steroidal saponins, as well as *Vitex agnus-castus*.

Anovulation can also be related to the hypothalamic-pituitary axis, and stress has a major impact on the hypothalamic/pituitary/ovarian axis, which leads to luteal phase defects, or prolactin excess. Consequently, the use of nervines and adaptogens can be of help in DUB.

DUB with ovulatory cycle is more common in women aged 35–44 and is thought to be due to inadequate production of progesterone by the corpus luteum. The period tends to be regular, heavy and painful, with bleeding occurring between days 21 and 32. It is commonly seen in PCOS and occasionally in endometriosis due to unknown mechanisms. PCOS can lead to hypersecretion of LH, and suppression of FSH, which can also cause chronic anovulation.

Herbal approach: treat relative oestrogen excess with foods rich in isoflavonoids and lignans such as soy and flaxseeds, and herbs that indirectly stimulate the corpus luteum and improve oestrogen/progestone ratio, e.g. *Actaea racemosa, Paeonia lactiflora* and *Glycyrrhiza glabra, Vitex agnus-castus*.

Other conditions associated with DUB include diabetes, androgen excess disorders, hypo and hyperthyroidism. Iron deficiency anaemia is a common cause of excessive menstrual flow as well as a consequence.

Contributing factors

Oestrogen dominance, corpus luteum deficiency: both ovulatory and anovulatory DUB are associated with oestrogen dominance, as oestrogen supports the ongoing proliferative activity in the endometrium even at the time of shedding. This can cause prolonged, heavy bleeding as well as incomplete cessation of bleeding.

Herbal approach: reduce excess oestrogen (work on elimination pathways and avoid xenoestrogens), reduce weight if appropriate.[16]

Fragility of the endometrium is a factor along with the lack of development of spiral arterioles; the endometrial tissue eventually becomes fragile and breaks down erratically.[17,18]

Fragility of the blood vessel walls due to abnormal or incomplete angiogenesis, resulting in abnormal blood vessels with fragile vessel walls,[19,20] which leads to reduced vascular smooth muscle cells.[21]

Herbal approach: these factors may explain the efficacy of herbs and foods rich in flavonoids that improve vascular fragility, e.g. *Achillea millefolium, Alchemilla vulgaris, Cinnamomum zeylanicum, Crataegus* spp., *Myrtus communis* berries.

Poor endometrial circulation: paradoxically, an association seems to exist between the flow impedance of uterine arteries and the amount of menstrual blood loss. Studies on menorrhagia without known cause suggested that women with lower uterine blood flow bleed more.[22]

Herbal approach: this would explain the use of uterine tonics and emmenagogues to increase blood flow[23] such as *Achillea millefolium, Alchemilla vulgaris* and *Angelica sinensis*.

Prostaglandin imbalance: women with high menstrual blood loss have relatively high levels of available arachidonic acid in their endometrium.[24,25] The increased arachidonic acid released during menstruation results in the increased production of series 2 prostaglandins, which may be a factor in menorrhagia as well as dysmenorrhoea.

The bleeding is also aggravated by the lack of certain prostaglandins and thromboxane, as the presence of these is relative to the secretion of progesterone.

Herbal approach: these factors may explain the use of anti-inflammatories such as *Achillea millefolium, Actaea racemosa, Alchemilla vulgaris, Capsella bursa-pastoris, Zingiber officinale* and flavonoid-rich herbs and foods. There is also a need to avoid inflammatory foods rich in arachidonic acid (animal products) and to increase anti-inflammatory foods such as fish, omega 3-rich foods and flavonoid-rich foods.

The quality of the microbiome within the endometrial cavity and endocervix in women with menorrhagia or dysmenorrhea might play a role.[26]

Other processes involved: Vascular endothelial growth factor (VEGF) produced by neutrophils plays a role in the development of the blood vessels.[27] Hypoxia, caused by contractions, causes induction of hypoxia-inducible factor (HIF-1α), which regulates VEGF, release of cytokines (TGF-α and IL-1β), which all play a role induction and sustaining levels of VEGF during menstruation.[28]

Conventional treatment

- Progestogen-releasing IUCD (levonorgestrel-releasing). This thins the endometrium and after 3 months' use leads to lighter periods (does not work so well in women with fibroids or polyps).
- Combined oral contraceptive pill, progesterone only pill.
- Mefenamic acid (prostaglandin inhibitor).
- Tranexamic acid (anti-fibrinolytic effect).
- Zoladex (gonadotrophin-releasing hormone agonist), leading to temporary medically induced menopause.
- Hysterectomy, hysteroscopic resection and ablations, cauterisation via hysteroscopy, or thermal balloon which destroys the endometrium.
- Iron supplementation.

2.3 Herbal management of dysfunctional uterine bleeding

DUB herbal management approaches can be divided into two categories:

Treatment of acute, non-life-threatening bleeding episodes: haemostatic/anti-haemorrhagic herbs (traditional and empiric evidence) alongside anti-inflammatories. Acute treatment can be effective for mild to moderate bleeding within a couple of hours. In cases of severe menorrhagia, the herbs need to be taken daily throughout the cycle, with an increase in dosage two or three days before the period.

Treatment and/or prevention of chronic dysfunctional uterine bleeding: normalising hormonal levels, uterine tonics/pelvic circulatories, iron tonics and improving vascular integrity.

Aims

Address the underlying factors, as well as endocrine dysregulation
Control bleeding, correct anaemia, address vascular instability and uterine tissue healing, improve pelvic circulation and uterine tone, reduce inflammation
Reduce the negative impact of stress

Address endocrine dysregulation

Hyperprolactinaemia, luteal deficiency, progesterone deficiency: dopaminergic herbs such as *Actaea racemosa, Paeonia lactiflora & Glycyrrhiza glabra, Vitex agnus-castus*.

Oestrogen excess/relative progesterone deficiency: there are multifactorial causes (see previous book for more detail).

- Nutritional deficiency: B vitamins, magnesium.
- Reduced liver metabolism: *Taraxacum radix*.
- Sluggish digestion leading to increase of oestrogen recycling: *Taraxacum radix*. Compromised microbiome affecting oestrogen recycling and inhibiting the effects of phytoestrogens in the diet: prebiotics such as inulin-rich herbs, probiotics, anti-microbial herbs.
- Environmental endocrine disruptor exposure: eat organic, avoid plastics in cooking and food wrapping.
- Weight control as excess weight can lead to increased androgen conversion to oestrogen; obesity has also been found to increase endometrial thickness independently.

Actaea racemosa, Paeonia & Glycyrrhiza, Vitex agnus-castus.

Phenolic phytoestrogens in the diet (soy, flaxseed, legumes, seeds and nuts).

Thyroid-stimulating herbs: there may be a subclinical insufficiency of thyroid hormone; patients with menorrhagia have been shown to have a positive response to thyroxine. Hypothyroidism leads to reduced levels of SHBG, which causes an increase in oestrogen availability. *Withania somnifera* and *Nigella sativa*, adaptogens in general.

Control the bleeding using anti-haemorrhagics

Achillea millefolium, Alchemilla vulgaris, Capsella bursa-pastoris, Cinnamomum zeylanicum. These herbs are often rich in polyphenols, including tannins, but it is likely the flavonoids that are of benefit here rather than tannins.

Correct anaemia using mineral-rich herbs and tonics: *Urtica* spp. *folia, Withania somnifera,* iron-rich foods.

Improve pelvic circulation and uterine tone with uterine tonics, emmenagogues: an atonic uterus can lead to excess bleeding. Improving weak smooth muscle activity will regulate contractions, aiding vasoconstriction. This strategy needs to be employed over some time to get results. *Achillea millefolium, Angelica sinensis* (although care needs to be taken with the timing of dosage, as angelica can increase bleeding when taken during menstruation), *Caulophyllum thalictroides, Chamaelirium luteum, Cinnamomum zeylanicum, Mitchella repens, Rubus idaeus.*

Address vascular instability using flavonoids-rich herbs: anthocyanin-rich foods and plants improve capillary fragility in blood vessels with fragile walls. Flavonoids also have an anti-inflammatory action and are often found in astringent plants. *Achillea millefolium, Alchemilla vulgaris, Crataegus* spp., citrus fruits, esp. the pulp, *Myrtus communis* berries, *Vaccinium myrtillus.*

Reduce inflammation with anti-inflammatories: correct increased synthesis of pro-inflammatory prostaglandins, cytokines and chemokines, which play a role in menorrhagia; omega 3, flavonoid-rich foods, and herbs, avoid animal products (high in arachidonic acids), *Achillea millefolium, Alchemilla vulgaris, Zingiber officinale.*

Reduce the negative impacts of stress with nervines, sedatives, adaptogens: stress has a negative impact on hormones as well as clotting mechanisms. Exercise also reduces the effects of stress. *Leonurus cardiaca, Matricaria chamomilla, Melissa officinalis, Withania somnifera.*

Key herbs used in clinical practice

Achillea millefolium

Traditional use world-wide, including historically for menorrhagia. Pliny the elder (AD23/24–79) reports its use for excessive menstruation, given as a sitz bath.[29] Dioscorides (c. AD40–90) recommends a decoction used as a douche for menstrual bleeding.[30]

According to the Eclectics it is one of the best agents for the relief of menorrhagia.[31] Best as a strong infusion and its use must be persisted with.[32] A diffusive vasostimulant, it exerts its influence mainly on the uterus and its circulation, clearing pelvic congestion, reducing uterine flooding and pain due to engorged pelvic veins, useful in uterine atony.

Preclinical studies
Anti-inflammatory: a COX-2 inhibitor,[33] inhibition of HNE and MMP-2 and -9,[34,35] antioxidant.[36]

Haemostyptic: accelerates the coagulation of blood and shortens recalcification time.[37]

Antispasmodic effect:[38] calcium-channel blocking activity and mediator-antagonistic effect.[39]

Vasoprotective: effects on vascular inflammation.[40]

Clinical study: one study looking at primary dysmenorrhea found it to be effective for this and reducing blood flow.[41]

Dosages
Daily dose 3–9ml of 1:3.
Typical weekly dosage 20–40ml of 1:3.

Cautions/contraindications: contact dermatitis as adverse effect, may be connected to sesquiterpenes.

Alchemilla vulgaris

Traditional use: menorrhagia, leucorrhoea, emmenogogue, promotes contraction during labour, used as an astringent, anti-haemorrhagic, anti-inflammatory. According to Andrés Laguna de Segovia (1499–1559) astringes parts for those who want to appear virginal.[42]

Preclinical studies: antibacterial, astringent, antioxidant, anti-inflammatory and wound-healing properties.[43–46]

Clinical study: clinical trial (open study) related to menorrhagia in teenage girls; using FE 50–60gtt 3–5 times per day, used 10–5 days before the period, the volume of flow reduced, cycle shortened, premenstrual administration prevented menorrhagia from recurring.[47]

Dosages
Daily dose 6–12ml of 1:3.
Typical weekly dose 15–30ml of 1:3.

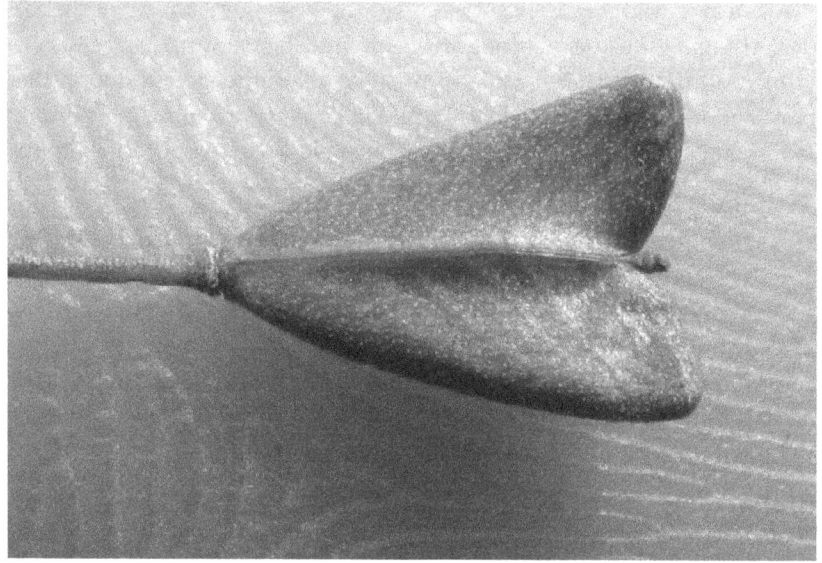

Capsella bursa-pastoris

Used world-wide as an emmenagogue, stimulates uterine contraction at birth,[48] and for menorrhagia.[49] According to Ellingwood (1898): "... uncomplicated chronic menorrhagia it has accomplished permanent cures".[50] Bombelon (1897): "prompt use to arrest bleedings and flooding". Mrs Grieve mentions its use during WWI as a substitute for ergot in uterine bleeding.[51,52]

Preclinical studies: a smooth muscle stimulant, acting similarly to oxytocin, it causes strong contractions of uterus,[53-55] reducing coagulation time,[56,57] anti-inflammatory,[58] reducing capillary permeability,[59] uterotonic effect,[60] moderating acetyl cholinesterase inhibitors.[61]

It may be that the effect on menorrhagia is mediated through an increased contraction of smooth muscles.

Clinical studies: studies using *Capsella* alongside orthodox treatment for menorrhagia, mefenamic acid,[62] and in postpartum haemorrhage alongside oxytocin,[63] found the combinations more effective than orthodox treatments by themselves.

Dosages: Dr Weiss states the maximum activity is reached 3 months after the manufacture date, as active principles form through the

conversion of other principles and are lost again on extended storage.[64] The Eclectics suggested that 'fresh is best'.
Daily dose 9–36ml of 1:3.
Typical weekly dosage 20–30ml of 1:3.

Cautions/contraindications: glucosinolates excrete into breastmilk. Use with caution in people with a history of kidney stones.

Cinnamomum zeylanicum

Preclinical studies: contains polyphenols, tannins (anti-inflammatory), essential oils: cinnamaldehyde (antispasmodic), eugenol (prevents the biosynthesis of prostaglandins and reduces inflammation).[65]

Clinical study: young college students with dysmenorrhoea given during the first three days of the menstrual cycle; reduced pain, the amount of menstrual bleed, nausea and vomiting.[66]

Dosages
Daily dose 4.5–9ml of 1:3.
Typical weekly dosage 15–30ml of 1:3.

Vitex agnus-castus

Has a long history of use: Hippocrates, c. 400BC: "If blood flows from the womb, let the woman drink dark wine in which the leaves of the chaste tree have been steeped."

Preclinical studies: intensively researched (see book 1). Luteal defects, for conditions resulting from unopposed oestrogen (perimenopause), during menarche, or latent hyperprolactinemia.[67]

Clinical studies: cystic hyperplasia,[68] menorrhagia, polymenorrhea; improvements noted within 2 to 3 months of treatment.[69]

In polymenorrhea the duration between periods lengthened; in patients with menorrhagia a significant shortening of menses was shown.[70]

Intrauterine device induced bleeding compared to mefenamic acid, both decreased bleeding;[71] *Vitex* in comparison with mefenamic acid had much fewer complications.[72]

In a range of abnormal bleeding patterns: polymenorrhea, oligomenorrhea, amenorrhea, dysmenorrhea, intermenstrual bleeding, hypermenorrhea, menometrorrhagia, ovulation bleeding, premenstrual or postmenstrual bleeding; found effective by physicians as well as patients.[73]

Dosages

Slow acting—there may not be an effect for 3–4 months. Low dosages are effective in hyper-prolactinaemia.

For menorrhagia doses up to 7.5ml of 1:3 can be given in 2–3 divided doses during and just before the period to symptomatically reduce bleeding.

Typical weekly dosage for menorrhagia: 10–20ml of 1:3.

Zingiber officinale

Preclinical studies: anti-inflammatory; inhibition of prostaglandin synthesis, also inhibits cyclooxygenase (COX) and lipooxygenase resulting in an inhibition of leukotriene and prostaglandin synthesis.[74]

Clinical study: high school girls with heavy menstrual bleeding; menstrual blood loss dramatically declined during all three intervention cycles in ginger-receiving group.[75]

Dosages

Daily dosage 1–3ml of 1:3.

Typical weekly dosage 5–10ml of 1:3.

2.4 Dietary and lifestyle recommendations

Broadly a diet rich in fruit and vegetables, nuts, whole grains, fish and healthy oils (Mediterranean diet), which includes all the nutrients below, is known to be of benefit.

Specific diet suggestions

- Reduce inflammatory foods: low in animal fat, red meat, processed meats, fried foods, refined carbohydrates, sugar, margarine (transfats).
- Include anti-inflammatory foods: rich in flavonoids, e.g. quercitin (red onions), vitamins, ginger, turmeric (golden milk), and other aromatic spices, colourful vegetables, green leafy vegetables, nuts, fatty fish, red and blue berries, coffee and tea, esp. green tea contain

polyphenols, high in fish oils and linolenic and linoleic acids from vegetable oil sources (olive oil).
- Foods shown to be of benefit in clinical trials: lemon juice, ginger, pomegranate, myrtle syrup, soya.

Punica granatum, Pomegranate

Avicenna (AD980–1037) uses *Punica granatum* (part not specified) for the treatment of abnormal uterine bleeding.[76]

Preclinical studies: all parts of the pomegranate are rich in flavonoids and have an inhibitory activity on biosynthesis of prostaglandins.

Clinical studies: *Punica granatum* flower capsules were as effective as tranexamic acid capsules in reducing menstrual bleeding in women with menorrhagia.[77] Pomegranate flower syrup was found to be the equal of tranexamic acid in menorrhagia due to fibroids and led to the reduction of uterine fibroid size and bleeding, plus an improvement in quality of life.[78]

Might be sufficient reason to include pomegranate in the diet.

Table 2.2: Specific nutrients: clinical evidence

Nutrient	Clinical evidence
Flavonoids improve capillary fragility. The effect might be due to suppression of endometrial prostaglandins E2, F2-alpha, thromboxane A2, and prostacyclin release.	A study showed a reduction in menorrhagia and dysmenorrhoea, with an improvement of haemoglobin. Another trial indicated a reduction in blood flow and duration and increased capillary strength.[79-81] Trial, with lemon juice showed that the concentration of PGF2α (vasoconstrictor) increased 60%, a decrease in menstrual bleeding.[82] Myrtle syrup: reductions of bleeding duration, decline of the intensity of bleeding, and improved quality of life.[83] Micronised flavonoids suppressed endometrial prostaglandins and improved abnormal uterine bleeding.[84]

(Continued)

Table 2.2: (Continued)

Nutrient	Clinical evidence
Isoflavones inhibit the effect of oestrogens on the endometrium due to competitive inhibition with endogenous oestrogen (see book 1).	Soy protein (60g containing 45mg isoflavones): a small study of the effect on premenopausal women showed increased follicular phase length and/or delayed menstruation with lighter and shorter periods.[85]
Iron: pay attention to ferritin levels as haemoglobin levels can be normal. Include vitamin C-rich foods alongside iron-rich foods.	Low iron level itself leads to menorrhagia. Loss of more than 60ml per period can make difficult to maintain healthy iron levels.
Vitamin A deficiency leads to impaired activity of enzyme 3 beta-dehydrogenase, needed for production of oestradiol.	Deficiency may be a contributing factor in the menorrhagia, serum levels lower than in those with menorrhagia; menorrhagia was alleviated in more than 92% of patients.[86]
Vitamin B complex A correlation shown between a deficiency of vitamin B and menorrhagia. With Vitamin B complex deficiencies, the liver loses its ability to inactivate oestrogen.	Two gynaecologists described the effect of B-12 and B-complex to treat anaemia in prolonged bleeding (bleeding more than 10 days); they noted with surprise that irregular bleeding stopped and in the following two cycles the bleeding pattern was normal.[87]
Vitamin C with flavonoids helps reduce heavy bleeding, improving the vasculature, preventing capillary fragility, increasing iron absorbency. Vitamin C: enhances iron absorption.[88,89] It captures non-heme iron and stores it in a form that is more easily absorbed.[90]	Small study: 16 out of 18 patients who had heavy menstrual bleeding showed bleeding improved with vitamin C and bioflavonoids use.[91]

(Continued)

Table 2.2: (Continued)

Nutrient	Clinical evidence
Vitamin E	In menorrhagia caused by IUDs a dose of 100mg/day on alternate days for 14 days showed a return to normal limits.[92]
Vitamin K is needed for normal blood clotting, although bleeding time and prothrombin levels in women with menorrhagia tend to be normal.	Case report of vitamin K deficiency associated with high intake of high-energy drinks and inadequate diet, presenting with severe menorrhagia without obvious causes.[93]

See Appendix for food sources.

CHAPTER 3

Amenorrhoea and oligomenorrhoea

3.1 Presentation/symptoms, differential diagnosis and investigations

Primary amenorrhoea definition:
- No menstruation by age 15 with normal growth and secondary sexual characteristics: consider causes as in secondary amenorrhoea as breast development only occurs in the presence of ovarian oestrogens.
- No menstruation by age 13 plus no development of secondary sexual characteristics: need to refer.

Usually there is no major physical problem as the onset of puberty has simply been delayed. However, this diagnosis needs to be confirmed and is a diagnosis of exclusion. Pelvic ultrasound, blood tests such as FSH, LH and prolactin are usual; these will be normal in delayed puberty.[1]

Secondary amenorrhoea and oligomenorrhoea definition: the absence or irregularity of menses for ≥6 months after the establishment of regular menstrual cycle.[2,3]

Amenorrhoea and oligomenorrhoea are often associated with low oestrogen levels, which in turn, will increase the risk of osteoporosis.

A prolonged time without menstruation, when oestrogen levels are 'normal' (e.g. as can be the case with PCOS), can lead to an increased risk of endometrial hyperplasia and uterine cancer, so both warrant treatment and preventative care for long-term problems. It is normal to occasionally miss a period as disruptions to routines, such as travel, working night shifts and stress, can cause women to miss a period, and often monitoring is all that is needed.

Control of menstrual cycle

The hypothalamus releases pulses of gonadotropin-releasing hormone (GnRH), which stimulates the pituitary to produce gonadotropins (follicle-stimulating hormone and luteinising hormone). These are released into the bloodstream, which causes ovulation and stimulates the ovaries to produce oestrogen (mainly oestradiol), androgens (mainly testosterone) and progesterone.

A malfunction on any level could cause anovulatory amenorrhoea.

- **Follicle-stimulating hormone (FSH)** activates aromatase in the granulosa cells around the developing oocytes to convert androgens to oestradiol.
- **Oestrogen** stimulates the endometrium leading to proliferation.
- **Luteinising hormone (LH)** surge promotes maturation of the dominant oocyte, the release of the oocyte and the formation of the corpus luteum, which produces progesterone as well as oestrogen.
- **Progesterone** changes the endometrium into a secretory structure and prepares it for egg implantation.

If there is no fertilisation, oestrogen and progesterone production decreases and the endometrium breaks down. It is then sloughed during menses, which normally takes place 14 days after ovulation.

Ovulatory amenorrhoea causes: physical obstruction

- *Asherman's syndrome:* intra-uterine adhesions usually following a curette or from a uterine infection.[4]
- *Cervical stenosis:* extreme narrowing or closure of the cervical canal, this can be caused by chronic infection, cone biopsy, cauterisation, cryosurgery, laser surgery or irradiation of the cervix.

Anovulatory amenorrhoea causes

Hypothalamic dysfunction: common (see next chapter).

Pituitary dysfunction
- *Pituitary lesions:* prolactinomas, which leads to hyperprolactinaemia.
- *Pituitary insufficiency* (rare): damage by lack of oxygen, blood clots or severe haemorrhage; FSH, LH and oestrogen levels are all low.
- *Empty sella syndrome:* rare.

Ovarian dysfunction
- *Premature ovarian failure.*
- *Polycystic ovarian syndrome.*
- *Breastfeeding:* high prolactin levels cause ovulation and menstruation to cease.
- *Thyroid conditions:* lower levels of SHBG increases availability of oestrogen along with a greater conversion of androgens to oestrogens.
- *Cushing's syndrome:* excess corticosteroids causing wide range of symptoms including obesity, thinning of the skin, abnormal fat distribution around the neck and upper back, high blood pressure, diabetes, hirsutism and amenorrhoea. Can be caused by adrenal or pituitary tumours or high-dose cortisone medication.
- *Other rare conditions:* congenital adrenal hyperplasia, androgen-secreting adrenal or ovarian tumours.
- *Destruction of ovarian tissue:* ovarian tissue can be damaged by impaired blood flow.

Information to gain

- Pregnancy.
- Regular periods in the past? If ongoing problem, consider PCOS, weight issues. If new consider functional hypothalamic anovulation, premature ovarian failure, perimenopause, menopause.
- Last normal menstrual period, to get idea of timescale.
- How long and how heavy was the menstruation as anovulatory cycles tend to be irregular, heavy, prolonged, etc. typically seen in adolescence and perimenopause.
- Dysmenorrhoea: if present suggests an ovulatory cycle.
- Presence of any cyclic breast tenderness and mood changes suggests ovulatory cycle; symptoms tend to be worse perimenopausal.[5]

- Temperature intolerance, vaginal dryness suggests low oestrogen, possibly peri/menopausal.
- Past procedures including obstetric history: this could hint at obstruction, due to scarring—Asherman's syndrome, see above.
- OCP use in the past: up to 80% of women start menstruation 3 months after stopping pill.[6]
- Family history: e.g. PCOS.
- Height and weight, body mass index (BMI): if underweight, consider hypothalamic dysfunction, hyperthyroid; overweight, consider PCOS, metabolic syndrome leading to amenorrhoea, oligomenorrhoea, hypothalamic dysfunction, hypothyroidism.
- Presence of galactorrhoea: breast feeding, pituitary adenoma, pregnancy, hyperprolactinaemia, certain drugs.
- Presence of cervical mucus with spinnbarkeit (a stringy, stretchy quality) indicates adequate oestrogen and ovulation.
- Symptoms of androgen excess: hirsutism, temporal balding, acne, voice deepening, increased muscle mass, are suggestive of PCOS, and also consider androgen-secreting tumour, Cushings, medication.
- Symptoms of other diseases: chronic illness can be an underlying cause.

Red flags

- Delayed puberty (primary amenorrhoea?).
- Impaired sense of smell: rare conditions such as Kallmann syndrome with delayed or absent puberty.
- Significant weight increase (hypothyroid) or decrease (hyperthyroid, malignancy, eating disorder), extreme dieting, exercise.
- Spontaneous galactorrhoea (pituitary adenoma).
- Virilisation: androgen excess, androgen-secreting tumour, Cushings, medication.
- Visual fields defects alongside galactorrhoea (pituitary adenoma).

Investigations

<u>Gonadotrophin and oestrogen</u>: low levels suggestive of functional hypothalamic anovulation (FHA).

LH and FSH

- high FSH level suggests ovarian dysfunction, perimenopause, premature ovarian failure.
- low FSH level suggests hypothalamic or pituitary dysfunction.
- Increased LH levels, might indicate PCOS.
- Occasionally: progestin challenge to check if uterine function is normal (only of use if oestrogen levels ok). The consequence of low circulating oestrogen will be lack of bleed following progestin administration and withdrawal.

Oestrogen levels: low in perimenopause, premature ovarian failure, functional hypothalamic amenorrhoea and low weight.

Prolactin: 50–100ng/mL (mildly elevated) consider medication, stress; if over >100ng/mL consider tumour.

Testosterone or DHEA: can be mildly elevated in women with hypothalamic or pituitary dysfunction and are sometimes normal in hirsute women with PCOS.

TSH: high in hypothyroidism, low in hyperthyroidism.

Hormone levels should be remeasured to confirm results, as there will be normal variations during the menstrual cycle.

Pelvic ultrasound to image obstructions, cysts, ovarian cyst, PCO, etc.

Table 3.1: Summary: common causes of amenorrhea

Condition	Tests	Symptoms
Functional hypothalamic anovulation (causes: excessive exercise, weight loss, eating disorder, stress, chronic illness)	Low levels gonadotrophin, low FSH and oestrogen Possibly mildly elevated levels of testosterone, DHEA or prolactin	Low BMI, signs of oestrogen deficiency, e.g. hot flushes, night sweats, vaginal dryness or atrophy. Hypothermia, hypotension, palpitations, bradycardia with electrolyte abnormalities, e.g. with eating disorders, anorexia, depression

(*Continued*)

Table 3.1: (Continued)

Condition	Tests	Symptoms
Hyperprolactinaemia (drugs, stress, hypothyroid)	Prolactin high, possibly high TSH	Can be asymptomatic, infertility, low libido, hot flushes, galactorrhea
Hyperthyroid	Greater conversion of androgen to oestrogens leading to ovarian failure. TSH low, high T4	Palpitations, anxiety tremor, heat intolerance, warm moist skin, tachycardia, underweight
Hypothyroid	Lower SHBG, increases oestrogen production leading to ovarian failure, TSH high, normal or low T4	Fatigue, low mood, weight gain, cold intolerance, coarse, thick skin, loss of eyebrow hair, bradycardia, delayed deep tendon reflexes, constipation
Menopause/ premature ovarian failure	FSH high, LH high and low oestrogen levels	Hot flushes, night sweats, vaginal dryness, sleep disturbance, low libido, fragility fractures, mood changes
PCOS	LH levels are often increased, increasing ratio of LH to FSH. Mildly elevated levels of testosterone or DHEAS, but not always. Ultrasound: 'pearl necklace' image of the ovaries	Amenorrhoea following weight gain, acne, hirsutism, deepening voice, high BMI, Acanthosis nigricans, insulin resistance
Pregnancy	Pregnancy test, US	Fatigue, urinary frequency, breast tenderness

(Continued)

Table 3.1: (Continued)

Condition	Tests	Symptoms
Post contraceptive pill		Long-term amenorrhoea could have been masking condition—up to 80% start menstruation 3 months after stopping the pill—changes in mood PMS, weight changes, acne, hirsutism, changes in libido
Prolactinoma, pituitary lesions	Prolactin over 100ng/mLCT scan Mildly elevated levels of testosterone or DHEA Low FSH	Headaches and decreased peripheral vision, visual defects, reduced libido, infertility, galactorrhea

3.2 Functional hypothalamic amenorrhoea (FHA)

The most common cause of both primary and secondary amenorrhoea is functional hypothalamic amenorrhoea (FHA). It is thought to be related to weight issues including dieting, low micro- and macronutrient intake, stress, sleep disorders and/or excessive exercise.[7-9]

Symptoms

Irregular menstruation, elongated cycles with spotting, eventually resulting in amenorrhoea, with or without PMT. If oestrogen is low, symptoms related to this can be seen such as vaginal dryness and hot flushes.

FHA typically presents as the absence or irregularity of menses for 6 months or missed menstruation over 3 cycles after the establishment of regular menstrual cycles.

FHA is a diagnosis of exclusion: see previous chapter.

Blood tests: low levels of gonadotrophin and oestrogen are highly suggestive.

Pathophysiology

The hypothalamus-pituitary gland-ovary/adrenal/thyroid axis are all involved, GnRH pulsatile activity is affected,[10] and decreased gonadotropin secretion from the pituitary gland leads to reduced oestradiol production in the ovary. If there is no ovulation there will be no progesterone. Long term this can lead to osteopenia, osteoporosis, cardiovascular problems, hypercholesteremia, depression, anxiety.[11] This range of long term consequences illustrates how important oestrogen is for normal function of the body.

The range of endocrine abnormalities associated with FHA are:

- Low levels of gonadotrophin and oestrogen.
- Low thyroid function; TSH levels are affected (lower end of normal) as well as T3, as conversion of T4 to T3 can be impaired.[12]
- Hyperprolactinaemia.
- Mild elevation of cortisol levels.

The deeper one delves the more one can get lost in a maze of neuropeptides, neurotransmitters and neurosteroids that affect GnRH pulsatile secretion.[13] Just to give a flavour of a few: kisspeptin,[14,15] neuropeptide Y (NPY), ghrelin, leptin, corticotropin-releasing hormone (CRH), b-endorphin and allopregnanolone.

As an example of the interactions: stress increases corticotropin-releasing hormone (CRH) secretion, which results in mild hypercortisolaemia and inhibits the release of GnRH and gonadotropins.[16,17] Mildly elevated levels of cortisol are found in those with FHA, and thyroid levels are also affected.[18] Chronically elevated cortisol levels cause a reduction in leptin, which leads to reduced glucose, insulin, insulin-like growth factor (IGF-1) and kisspeptin along with an elevation in ghrelin, growth hormone (GH), neuropeptide Y, peptide YY and beta-endorphin.

Further research may show that some of our herbs influence these neurochemicals either directly or indirectly. Preclinical studies suggest a range of possible effects:

- Neuropeptide Y is reduced in amenorrheic women:[19] *Eleutherococcus senticosus, Rhodiola rosea, Schisandra chinensis* stimulated the expression of NPY in vitro.[20] *Rhodiola rosea* used on patients with amenorrhea had successful outcomes.[21]

- Genistein found in soy affected GnRH secretion by modulating kisspeptin receptors.[22]
- *Schisandra chinensis* and *Rhodiola rosea* in vivo decreased the stress-induced elevation of corticotropin-releasing hormone CRH and cortisone levels, and showed an anti-stress effect in vivo by balancing the HPA axis.[23]

Factors affecting secretion of GnRH

Body weight: body fat affects oestrogen levels; for example, when body fat content is below 25% the low oestrogen levels cause amenorrhoea. However, FHA can be present in people with a wide range of body weight and body fat, suggesting that more is at play.[24,25]

Hyperprolactinaemia: stress and hypothyroidism (see above) cause an elevated prolactin level, which interferes with the pulsatile secretion of GnRH, decreasing levels of FSH and LH slightly, shortening luteal phase with lowered progesterone levels.[26]

Insomnia: the quality of sleep can influence the whole endocrine system, including cortisol and leptin levels. Obviously, a simple lack of sleep will affect mood and reduces one's ability to cope with stress.[27]

Post-pill amenorrhoea: about 80% of women start to menstruate within 3 months of stopping the OCP, but a few may experience long-term amenorrhoea. It might well be that OCP use has masked other conditions such as PCOS.

Night shift work, rotating shift work: can have a cumulative effect, causing irregular menstrual cycle and infertility.[28] Circadian rhythms, sleep disturbances,[29] altered melatonin production[30] might all interfere with homeostasis and coordination of the menstrual cycle.[31,32]

Rigorous and prolonged exercise: partly affects body fat, but there is more to it. Excessive exercise alongside lack of adequate food intake to compensate for energy loss causes a decrease in the pulsatile release of GnRH. High-intensity activity affects the functioning of the reproductive system even if the body weight is normal.[33] It is possible that physical stress triggers some of the same physiological responses as emotional stress.

Rigorous and or extreme dieting: leptin and ghrelin are regulators of energy homeostasis and influence the reproductive system. When on extreme or restricted diets leptin levels drop, and low levels cause amenorrhoea. In disordered eating patterns, even at normal weight, high ghrelin levels are seen. Type of food/energy intake will also make a difference. There is a possible evolutionary protective mechanism; in moments of famine, this would protect against pregnancy.[34] For this reason the distribution of both fat and carbohydrates throughout the day is important for normal hormone pulsation.

Severe prolonged illnesses such as chronic renal or liver failure can interfere with menstruation because of the effect on the hypothalamus. Autoimmune conditions may form part of the pathophysiology such as hyperprolactinaemia.[35]

Stress: both stress and hypothyroidism can cause hyperprolactinaemia. Elevated prolactin level stimulates an increase in dopamine secretion by the hypothalamus, which interferes with the pulsatile secretion of GnRH, so shortening luteal phase, with lowered progesterone levels.[36] It has been suggested that adolescents with FHA show dysfunctional attitudes, low self-esteem, depressive mood, anxiety and inability to cope with daily stress, and there may also be a genetic link.[37]

Subclinical hypothyroid can be part of the cascade that leads to hyperprolactinaemia.

Conventional treatment

Multidisciplinary treatment includes lifestyle changes, medical, dietary and mental health support, OCP.

3.3 Herbal management of functional hypothalamic amenorrhoea

Many old herbals mention herbs to bring on menses, known as emmenagogues. This may partly have referred to avoiding pregnancy but might also be because menstruation was seen as a crucial part of elimination, and thus the lack of menstruation was thought to contribute to ill health.

Very little clinical research is found related to herbs and functional amenorrhoea but, as usual, it is always important to treat underlying cause, and this needs to be multifaceted as stress, nutritional status, exercise and lifestyle all play a significant role.

Aims

Reduce impact of stress, support sleep
Ensure healthy body weight, support assimilation
Hormone modulation: address HPO axis, subclinical hyperprolactinaemia and subclinical hypothyroidism
Ensure healthy pelvic circulation

Support the ability to deal with stress by adaptogens and nervines

Nervines: *Leonurus cardiaca*, when anxiety and palpitations are present.
Adaptogens: *Angelica sinensis, Rhodiola rosea, Withania somnifera*.

Aid good-quality sleep: nervines that have multiple uses in this situation are *Actaea racemosa, Leonurus cardiaca, Vitex agnus-castus, Withania somnifera*.

Ensure healthy body weight: if underweight, support with anabolic herbs alongside bitters to increase appetite and ensure maximum use of food intake: *Serenoa serrulata, Withania somnifera*. For general debility and/or anaemia consider herbs such as *Angelica sinensis* and *Withania somnifera*, both specifically indicated where amenorrhoea and anaemia are present.

Support assimilation and stimulate appetite, if appropriate, with the aid of bitters to ensure proper uptake of nutrients: *Artemisia vulgaris, Leonurus cardiaca* and bitters in general. Stress may negatively affect digestive enzymes and gut microbiota, which may interfere with nutrient uptake.

Ensure healthy pelvic circulation, using uterine tonics/emenagogues to support normal function: *Actaea racemosa, Artemisia* spp. (wormwoods), *Caulophyllum thalictroides, Mitchella repens, Ruta graveolens* have all traditionally been used for amenorrhoea.

Normalise hypothalamic-pituitary-ovarian axis:

- <u>Dopaminergic agents to reduce prolactin levels</u>: *Actaea racemosa, Paeonia lactiflora & Glycyrrhiza glabra, Vitex agnus-castus*.
- <u>Steroidal saponin-rich herbs to stimulate ovarian ovulation</u>: *Asparagus racemosa, Chamaelirium luteum, Dioscorea villosa, Tribulus terrestris*. Some herbalists suggest dosing these from days 5 to 14 of the menstrual cycle for 2 to 3 months, or to use in the preovulatory phase

in combination with a conventional ovulation stimulant. This probably comes from research related to *Tribulus*.[38]
- Phenolic phytoestrogens (isoflavones and lignans) can combat low oestrogen levels. Interestingly the effects are broader; genistein found in soy affected GnRH secretion by modulating kisspeptin receptors.[39] A larger range of effects can be found in book 1.

Address subclinical hyperprolactinaemia: herbs with dopaminergic activity, *Paeonia lactiflora & Glycyrrhiza glabra, Vitex agnus-castus*.

Address subclinical hypothyroid: *Nigella sativa, Withania somnifera* and some adaptogens.

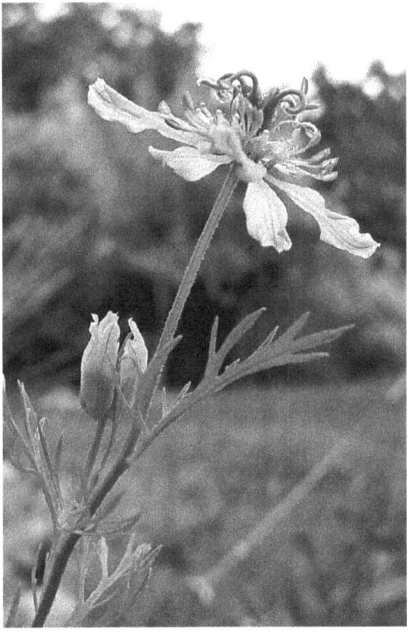

Nigella sativa

Key herbs used in clinical practice

Actaea racemosa (see book 1)

Traditionally used as a uterine tonic, emmenagogue, antispasmodic, and for amenorhoea. Ellingwood found it very efficacious in maladies of the female reproductive organs, including amenorrhoea.[40,41] The Eclectics regarded this as a primary remedy for menstrual irregularities, including sterility.

Preclinical studies: anti-inflammatory, antioxidant, antiproliferative; does not bind to the known oestrogen α or β receptors, but does show oestrogen-like effect, a neurotransmitter-mimetic shown to have dopaminergic, noradrenergic, serotoninergic and GABAergic effects.

Clinical studies: trials have indicated effects on improving FSH/LH ratio, decreasing LH, however in most trials on post-menopausal women there was no effect on LH. It lowered LH for women with PCOS receiving *Actaea racemosa* compared to clomiphene alone and gave favourable changes in FSH/LH ratio.

Dosage: daily dose in clinical trials 80mg per day; this translates to 0.25ml of 1:3 per day.
Typical weekly dose: 5–10ml of 1:3.
The average weekly dose used in clinical trials is 1.8ml of a 1:3 per week. Most UK herbalists would use 10ml of a 1:3 per week. Higher doses have not been found to be more effective for menopausal symptoms. Note: 60% alcohol is needed to extract the triterpene glycosides.

Alchemilla vulgaris

Parkinson and Culpeper both recommend taking it internally for 20 days to help conception, to retain the birth, as well as a sit in bath with a decoction of the herb.

Traditional and folk medicine: menorrhagia, leucorrhoea, emmenagogue, to promote contractions during labour, used as an astringent, antihaemorrhagic, anti-inflammatory.

Preclinical studies: antibacterial, astringent, antioxidant, anti-inflammatory and wound-healing properties.

Clinical study: no clinical trials on amenorrhoea; one clinical trial relates its effectiveness on menorrhagia in teenage girls.

Dosage: daily dose 6–12ml of 1:3.
Typical weekly dose 15–30ml of 1:3.

Angelica sinensis

In traditional use *Angelica sinensis* appears to normalise uterine activity, easing pelvic blood flow, which relieves pelvic congestion and pain.

Clinical studies: studies in the treatment of amenorrhoea and dysmenorrhoea in Europe published in 1899 and 1910[42–45] report the successful treatment of amenorrhoea. In a case report of a woman with atypical polypoid adenomyoma and infertility, oral use for 4 months corrected the endometrium to a normal secretory endometrium and pregnancy followed. It was suggested that *Angelica sinensis* may have acted as an ovulation inducer.[46]

Dosage: daily dose 6–12ml of 1:3.
Typical weekly dose 15–30ml of 1:3.

Artemisia vulgaris

Artemisia has a long tradition of use for amenorrhoea going back to Dioscorides and Pliny, and continued with Galen.

Dosage: daily dose 4.5–18ml of 1:3 per day.
Typical weekly dose 10–20ml.

Leonurus cardiaca

Has a reputation for use in amenorrhoea associated with anxiety and palpitation, as a nervine and mild uterine stimulant. Many famous herbalists in our history considered it a helpful herb for amenorrhoea. John Gerard (1598) says: "The powder in wine provoketh the monthly courses, also is good for them that it is hard travail with child." Nicholas Culpeper (1652): "Besides, it makes women joyful mothers of children, and settles their wombs as they should be, therefore we call it Motherwort." Native Americans used motherwort to treat gynaecological disorders. Felter similarly described *Leonurus* in *King's American Dispensatory* and *The Eclectic Materia Medica* as "emmenagogue, nervine, antispasmodic, and laxative", and recommended a warm infusion for amenorrhoea.

Preclinical studies: a stimulating effect on the uterus, leonurine is an uterotonic in vitro, on human myometrial strips, and ex vivo.

Stachydrine has oxytocic activity, anti-fibrotic properties (on various types of fibrosis), decreasing inflammatory and oxidative stress.

Clinical studies: no clinical studies in amenorrhoea.

Dosage: daily dose 6–12ml of 1:3.
Typical weekly dose 15–25ml of 1:3.

Rhodiola rosea

It seems that *Rhodiola rosea* may benefit those working night shifts, which can interfere with menstrual regularity; *Rhodiola rosea* 680mg per day reduced fatigue among those on night duty among young, healthy physicians.[47] This was contradicted by another, larger trial, although most participants were taking about half the recommended dose, 364mg/day.[48]

Preclinical studies: decreased the stress-induced elevation of corticotropin-releasing hormone CRH and peripheral cortisone level.[49]

Clinical studies: in a small study on amenorrhea using 100mg twice daily for two weeks, normal menses were restored in 25 women, 11 of whom became pregnant.[50] Lower basal serum neuropeptide Y is found in amenorrheic women;[51] studies with *Rhodiola rosea* stimulated the expression of NPY in vitro.[52]

Dosage: daily dose 200–680mg per day; 0.6ml–2ml of 1:3.
Typical weekly dose 5–15ml of 1:3.

Schisandra chinensis

In the Unani herbal tradition of Indian Ayurvedic medicine used for 'functional amenorrhoea' and irregular periods, but also as sedative, and well known as a liver herb.

Preclinical studies: *Schisandra chinensis* decreased the stress-induced elevation of corticotropin-releasing hormone CRH and peripheral cortisone level.[53] Lower basal serum neuropeptide Y (NPY) is found in amenorrhoeic women,[54] and interestingly in vitro *Schisandra* stimulated the expression of NPY.[55]

Dosage: daily dose 5.25–12.75ml per day of 1:3.
Typical weekly dose 20–50ml of 1:3.

AMENORRHOEA AND OLIGOMENORRHOEA

Vitex agnus-castus (see book 1)

Has a long history of use going back to Hippocrates; clinical studies have shown it has a dopaminergic effect, lowers prolactin levels, improves hormonal profiles, improves concentration of progesterone in luteal phase, normalises or shortens the luteal phase,[56] improves fertility.[57–59]

Clinical studies: suggested it to be effective in amenorrhea, found effective by physicians as well as patients. Slow acting, effects may not show until 3–4 months later. Low dosages will be effective in hyperprolactinaenemia.

Dosage: Low dose is used for irregular cycle, PMS, corpus luteal insufficiency, latent hyperprolactinaemia and associated infertility.
Daily dose 0.6–1.5ml of 1:3.
Typical weekly dose 5–10ml of 1:3.

Table 3.2: Eclectics' recommendations for treatment of amenorrhoea

Atropa belladonna	Ellingwood: stimulating normal ovulation, reported successful outcome in infertility. He suggests that it stimulates the capillary circulation of the ovary. He says: "If there are hysterical manifestations at the menstrual epoch, with deficient menstruation, *pulsatilla* may be used in conjunction with it."[60]
Caulophyllum thalictroides	The Eclectics regularly used this for amenorrhea, suggesting it gave "excellent and quick results", especially if due to pelvic congestion.
Serenoa serrulata	Ellingwood: "In simple cases where there is no organic lesion, this agent has an excellent reputation for restoring the ovarian action properly." He reported one physician saying that in five definite cases, pregnancy followed the use of this remedy where sterility was pronounced previously and thought to be incurable.[61]
Viburnum prunifolium	Ellingwood: use to restore normal functional ovarian activity, for menstrual irregularities, infertility; he reported when used pregnancy promptly occurred.[62]
Zingiber officinale	The Eclectics mention it for use in amenorrhoea to increase pelvic circulation, induce warmth and relaxation.

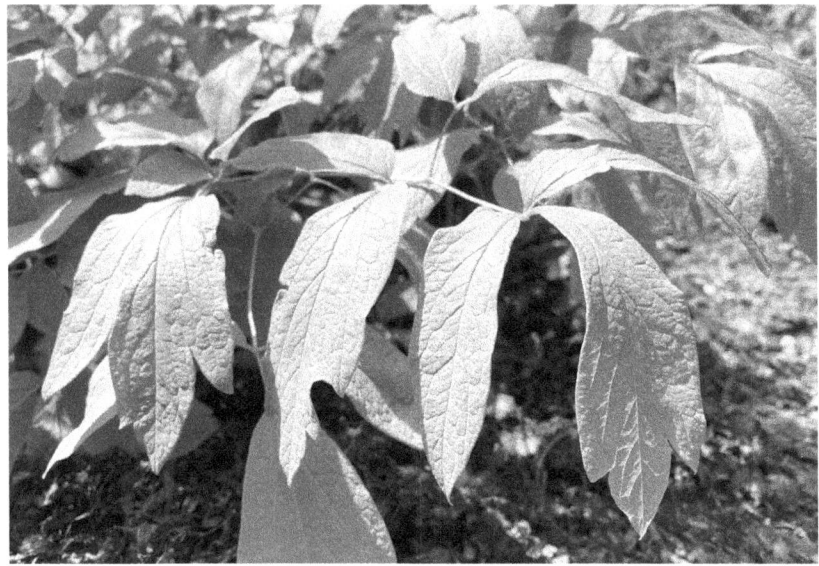

Caulophyllum thalictroides

Table 3.3: Herbs with research related to amenorrhoea

Herb	Clinical evidence
Cinnamomum cassia/ zeylanicum	Clinical trials with PCOS patients with an average intake 1.5g/day: normalised the menstrual cycles,[63,64] reduced anti-Müllerian hormone (AMH),[65] with a positive effect on hormonal status.[66,67] AMH promotes pre-antral follicle survival, and negatively impacts later stages of antral follicle maturation.[68]
Foeniculum vulgare	Resolved depot medroxyprogesterone acetate DMPA-induced amenorrhea.[69]
Linum sativum	Lengthens the luteal phase of the cycle and increases the frequency of ovulatory menstrual cycles.[70]
Mentha longifolia (horse mint) syrup Traditionally used in Iran as emmenagogue	The syrup induced bleeding and re-established regular bleeding in women with secondary amenorrhea and oligomenorrhea.[71] Tea: another trial in premature ovarian failure; decreased FSH and induced menstruation among patients with premature ovarian failure.[72]

(*Continued*)

Table 3.3: (Continued)

Herb	Clinical evidence
Paeonia lactiflora and *Cinnamomum cassia*	Clinical studies in luteal phase defects: decreased plasma luteinising hormone, increased 17 beta-oestradiol in the follicular phase, increased progesterone in the mid luteal phase. Increased development of the dominant follicle and endometrium. Prolongation and correction of the luteal phase, increased incidence of pregnancy.[73]
Paeonia lactiflora and *Glycyrrhiza glabra*	Increased oestrogen levels by increasing aromatase activity and prolactin lowering.[74] From clinical trials: hyperprolactinaemia induced by antipsychotic medication with oligomenorrhea or amenorrhea,[75] anovulatory,[76] aided menstrual resumption,[77,78] progesterone and oestrodiol increased.

3.4 Dietary and lifestyle recommendations

As is clear from the pathophysiology of dysfunctional hypothalamic amenorrhoea, nutritional intake and exercise can have a major impact on the cycle and need to be addressed where appropriate.

Broadly, ensure there are good sources of energy, optimising insulin/glucose metabolism and ensuring the caloric intake is adequate especially in those that exercise intensely. The diet should include fat, carbohydrates and protein, and the distribution of food throughout the day should be paid attention to as this encourages normal hormone pulsation.[79] It is possible that intermittent or other systems of fasting are not appropriate and would cause significant drops in glucose.[80] Recommendations would typically include a diet rich in colourful vegetables, fruit, legumes, seeds, nuts, healthy oils and fish.

Where nutritional restrictions and/or dieting are part of the history, a good multivitamin and mineral supplement alongside an omega 3 supplement might be warranted.

Increase intake of lignans and isoflavones

- Genistein, found in soy, affected GnRH secretion by modulating kisspeptin receptors.[81]

- *Sesamum indicum*, used by Avicenna, was effective in inducing bleeding in women with oligomenorrhoea (60g per day).[82]

Vitamins and minerals

Studies hint at shortages of the minerals Mg, Zn, Fe⁺ and vitamins A, B, C, D, E, K may be a factor in those with amenorrhoea.[83] It should also be noted that stress can deplete mineral and vitamin status.[84]

Table 3.4: Nutrients and their effects

Nutrient	Effect
B2, B6, and B12 and zinc	Affects methylation of DNA, a lower sensitivity of oocytes to FSH, reduced oocytes and reduced oestradiol production.[85]
Fe+	Levels can be lower in those with increased physical activity.[86]
Mg	Helpful for hormonal issues such as PMS.[87]
Omega 3 fatty acids	May improve fertility.[88]
Vitamin D3	Lower levels are associated with a longer follicular phase and overall longer menstrual cycles.[89]
Zn	Necessary for the normal synthesis of dopamine, vitamin B6 acts as a co-factor in the synthesis of dopamine.

See Appendix for food sources.

Other specific foods

Dark chocolate may boost endorphins and other feel-good chemicals, such as dopamine,[90] and is rich in polyphenolic compounds like flavonoids that trigger the brain to release endorphins. High-percentage (70%+) cocoa is recommended, and to stick to a few small squares per serving.

Avoid beer as this can stimulate prolactin secretion, both alcoholic as well as non-alcoholic, as the effects are due to polysaccharides from barley.[91]

Lifestyle, relaxation techniques and exercise

The importance of looking at more than just the physical is illustrated in that Cognitive Behavioral Therapy (CBT) has shown to be helpful in the return of menstrual function with ovulation, increased leptin and T3 concentrations, and decreased ghrelin and cortisol levels, all achieved without changes in body weight.[92]

The impact of excessive exercise might need to be discussed in cases where there is reason to believe this may be a factor.

Be sure to share a wide range of appropriate tips and resources to deal with stress, so that the patient can find something that 'clicks' for them.

CHAPTER 4

Infertility

4.1 Presentation/symptoms, differential diagnosis and investigations

Definition: no conception after one year of trying to conceive.

Conception usually occurs within 3 months for 50% of women, within 6 months for 75%, and within 12 months for 90%. Most pregnancies occur within three years.

Optimal fertility is before the age of 30–31 for women and decreases with increasing age, more quickly after the age of 35; into their 40s half of women have lost the ability to conceive, while adverse pregnancy outcomes increase on a similar time scale.[1]

Women will have around 300,000 follicles at menarche, around 360–400 of which will mature, the remainder being lost or undergoing degeneration. Ageing and smoking will speed up the degeneration process, reducing the quantity and quality of follicles in the ovaries, thereby reducing the ability to conceive.

Male fertility also declines with age, with the optimal age between 16 and 40.

It is important to evaluate both partners in cases of infertility.

Evaluation sooner than 12 months:

- The woman is >35
- There is a decreased ovarian reserve (e.g. because there is only one ovary)
- Infrequent menses
- The presence of structural abnormality of the uterus, fallopian tubes or ovaries
- The man is known to be sub-fertile or is at risk of sub-fertility; men >45 are less fertile than younger men

Information to gain:

- Age of both
- How long trying to conceive
- Previous pregnancies, outcome
- Menstrual cycle
- Past use of contraception, duration without contraception
- Intercourse timing, coinciding with the time most fertile (the fertile window is a six-day period ending on the day of ovulation)
- Surgeries, hospitalisations, illnesses, PID, STIs, Pap smear history
- System enquiry, e.g. thyroid problems, nipple discharge, signs of excess androgens (facial hair, acne and hair loss)
- Medications, allergies
- Family medical history
- Lifestyle: smoking history, alcohol use, recreational drug use, exercise
- Height and weight

Infertility occurrence among women is about 9%.[2,3] The most common cause is PCOS, followed by tubal issues caused by infection and or inflammation, uterine fibroids, thyroid disorders.

Unexplained infertility is quoted at around 30%,[4] and the proportion is increasing.[5]

Male causes: sperm disorders in 30–45% of couples, men >45 are less fertile; underlying causes include production of viable sperm, motility, morphology, count and DNA integrity. Investigations: semen analysis, sperm motility, sperm count (low counts can be related to age, addiction, smoking, alcohol).[6]

Table 4.1: Infertility causes in women

Cause	Symptoms	Underlying cause	Investigations
Ovarian causes			
Ovulatory dysfunction: see amenorrhoea	Absent, irregular menses (less than 9 menses/yr) Heavy bleeding, no dysmenorrhoea Rarely PMS	PCOS (common), hyperprolactinaemia, thyroid disease (hypo and hyper) Obesity: just a little weight loss can restore ovulation and give better outcomes in IVF. Obesity is linked to increased risk of miscarriage, birth defects, complications of premature delivery, stillbirth Underweight: will take time to normalise menstrual cycle once healthy weight Luteal phase defect (short luteal phase) Use of anti-oestrogens (Depo-Provera, danazol)	Menstrual history Check for ovulation signs: basal body temperature, mucous testing, cervix os Home testing kits (increase in urinary luteinising hormone (LH) 24 to 36 hours before ovulation, daily testing around mid-cycle, beginning day 9) Serum progesterone 1 week before onset of the next menstrual period indicates ovulation occurred Serial pelvic ultrasonography to monitor ovarian follicle diameter and rupture

Decreased ovarian reserve	Menopausal symptoms	Ovarian reserve decreases at age 30, more rapidly after 40, premature ovarian failure	Low anti-Müllerian hormone (early predictor of declining ovarian function) Antral follicle count (total number of follicles of 2 to 10mm during the early follicular phase) FSH levels >10mIU/mL, and oestradiol levels <80pg/mL (day 3 of menstrual cycle), suggests decreased ovarian reserve Clomiphene citrate challenge test
Hypothyroidism	Increased risk for miscarriage, premature delivery, and stillbirth Symptoms of hypothyroid	Miscarriage is increased in the presence of the thyroid antibodies as well as affecting ovulation	TSH, T4, T3

(Continued)

INFERTILITY 69

Table 4.1: (Continued)

Cause	Symptoms	Underlying cause	Investigations
Hyperthyroidism	Menstrual irregularities, and symptoms of hyperthyroid	Miscarriage is increased in the presence of any of the thyroid antibodies, correlating with immune modulation requirements of gestation (i.e. implantation and throughout the first trimester at individual increments)	TSH, T4, T3
Immune system involvement	Recurrent implantation failure with IVF or recurrent pregnancy losses	Intolerance to semen leading to local and/or systemic immune response. Implantation process of embryo is partly foreign and development relies on tolerance of the immune system	The relationship between the immune system and infertility is poorly understood, apart from antiphospholipid syndrome (cause of recurrent pregnancy loss, treatment with aspirin and heparins) Theory: ABO blood type incompatibility results in 'cervical hostility' between the man's blood type antigens, present in his sperm, and the woman's opposing antibodies, present in the mucus[7]

Tubal and pelvic causes

Abnormal cervical mucus (5%): inhibiting penetration or increased destruction of sperm	Cervical mucus changes from thick and impenetrable to thin and stretchable by an increase in oestradiol levels during the follicular phase	Abnormal mucus, e.g. due to vaginal bacteria (e.g. bacterial vaginosis), chronic cervicitis or smoking Mucus contains sperm antibodies (rarely) Cervicitis: cervical exudate (purulent or mucopurulent) or cervical friability	Normal changes in cervical fluid: inserting finger into vagina, the fluid should be like egg white. Fertile-quality cervical fluid is produced 3 to 5 days before ovulation (increasing estrogen levels before the luteinising hormone (LH) surge). Sperm survives for 5 to 6 days in the presence of fertile-quality cervical fluid
Cervical stenosis due to prior treatment for cervical intraepithelial neoplasia		Complete cervical stenosis is diagnosed if a 1- to 2-mm diameter probe cannot be passed into the uterine cavity	Signs of fertility: softening, opening of the cervical os, increased wetness from cervical fluid and a lengthening of the vaginal canal as the cervix shortens away from the vaginal opening Signs of infertility include a closed os, hardening, shortening and dryness

(*Continued*)

Table 4.1: (Continued)

Cause	Symptoms	Underlying cause	Investigations
Endometriosis associated with infertility and miscarriage, severity of lesions does not correlate with infertility	See specific condition	Cause not known, suggested theories: 1. Dysbiosis affecting tubal transport of fertilised egg 2. Tubal scarring, adhesions and unruptured follicles are common 3. Excessive amounts of free radicals 4. Alterations of eutopic endometrium 5. Autoantibodies, including those to sperm 6. Inflammatory environment of the pelvis causing poor ovulation and affect tubal transport and implantation of the fertilised egg	Hysterosalpingography: see below Laparoscopy: see below

Tubal and pelvic lesions (second most common cause)	PMH	Inflammation; endometriosis
		Infection: hence crucial to diagnose PID early, sexually transmitted diseases, pelvic TB
		Pelvic adhesions due to the above and surgical history (e.g. fibroids), ectopic pregnancy, ruptured appendix
		Structural; fibroids, malformations
		Hysterosalpingography (fluoroscopic imaging of the uterus and fallopian tubes) 2 to 5 days after menstruation: fertility in women appears to be enhanced after procedure if test result is normal
		Sonohysterography (isotonic fluid through the cervix into the uterus during ultrasonography)
		Laparoscopy: during the procedure pelvic adhesions can be lysed, or pelvic endometriosis can be fulgurated or ablated by laser. Pregnancy rates after laparoscopic treatment of pelvic abnormalities are low (25%)
		Hysteroscopy during which adhesions can be lysed, and submucous fibroids and intrauterine polyps removed, treatment of intrauterine abnormalities is often successful

Recurrent miscarriage: although a high percentage of pregnancies end up in miscarriage very few women have recurrent miscarriages. Most often this occurs straight after implantation and may seem to be a late or heavy period.

Causes include chromosomal abnormalities, age of mother (incidence increases over age 40), luteal deficiencies (often seen in PCOS, hyperprolactinaemia), metabolic abnormalities (diabetes, PCOS), structural abnormalities of uterus, deficiencies in nutrients and general health, antiphospholipid syndrome, immune intolerance, thrombophilias, male factors. In the majority of cases there is no known cause.

Factors that affect fertility

Alcohol: associated with an increased risk of miscarriage, alcohol intake during the week of conception increases the risk of early pregnancy loss and is associated with reduced fertility. The association is dose dependent.

Excessive alcohol consumption is known to have adverse effects on oocyte retrieval and thus a lower chance of successful IVF treatment.

Alcohol intake increases oestrogen and prolactin, and causes a reduction in FSH secretion, suppressing folliculogenesis so causing anovulation and infertility; it may also exacerbate age-related infertility.

Caffeine: overall the research is not conclusive, but it may impair oestrogen production or the metabolism of oestrogens. Substances other than caffeine in coffee, tea and other beverages may also be responsible for reduced fertility, e.g. tannins. In animal experiments, tannins have reduced fertility in mice and hens.[8]

Endocrine: all women who experience conception difficulties should have a basic screen for hypothyroidism.

Environmental pollution: chemical exposure; herbicides and organophosphate pesticides.[9] Air pollutants exposure is associated with slightly higher rates of infertility and increased rates of miscarriage.[10]

Gluten: avoidance has been shown to improve fertility rates in sensitive patients. Asymptomatic coeliac disease can be the cause of unexplained infertility or repeated miscarriage. There might be signs of anaemia and/or general nutritional deficiencies.

Sleep patterns: shift work affects the menstrual cycle.

Smoking: more than 10 cigarettes per day is associated with reduced fertility in women, higher rates of ectopic pregnancies and increased risk of miscarriage, greater rates of stillbirths and infant mortality. Mothers who quit smoking in the first trimester showed the same rates of stillbirth and infant mortality as non-smoking women. When Ireland banned smoking in the workplace, the rates of preterm births dropped by 25%. Smoking is also associated with earlier menopause.

Stress hormones: have inhibitory effects on the reproductive system, suppressive effects on the fertility of both the male and female, and are likely to have effect on gonadotropin release (FSH, LH). Prolonged stress is associated with higher levels of premenstrual tension and lower pregnancy rates.

Vigorous exercise: defined as more than four hours per week, may interfere with the success of in vitro fertilisation (IVF). Moderate regular exercise is probably indicated for most individuals. The intensity of the exercise is not the issue, but the lack of adequate nutrition, specifically total calories and protein.

Overweight: issues with ovulation and miscarriages; normal body weight increases the success of assisted reproductive therapies.

No difference found if diet was high-carbohydrate or high-protein: both groups who stuck to low calorie diets and lost weight had improved menstrual cycles and fertility.

Increase in abdominal fat → decreases insulin sensitivity, which is related to ovulation dysfunction. A weight loss of 5% can be significant in helping to normalise menses and ovulation, especially in cases of PCOS.

Underweight: worse if alongside an eating disorder or excessive exercise → infrequent or no ovulation.

Table 4.2: Investigations

Assessment	Time of cycle to be tested	Role	Result
Follicle-stimulating hormone (FSH)	Day 2–3	Stimulates follicle development	High: menopause, declining fertility, ovarian failure Reduced oocyte numbers: serum FSH >11 U/L PCOS: suspected when LH:FSH (U/L) >2:1. Correlate any findings with a day 7 ultrasound PCOS: requires additional treatment, increased miscarriage risk Low oocyte numbers: risk of early menopause; IVF may be indicated if also infertile
Luteinising hormone (LH)	Day 2–3 or pre-ovulation (day 13)	Surge causes ovulation	High: PCOS
Progesterone	Day 21 (7 days post-ovulation)	Level of progesterone	If present, ovulation takes place. If low, luteal-phase defect
Prolactin	Any day	Inhibits ovarian production of oestrogen, progesterone	Note: stress increases prolactin, so when blood is taken the patient needs to be relaxed to get a conclusive result

(*Continued*)

Table 4.2: (Continued)

Assessment	Time of cycle to be tested	Role	Result
Oestradiol	Day 2–3	Stimulates egg maturation and endometrial maturation for implantation	Responsible for quality cervical fluid
Testosterone (TT), free androgen index (FAI), androstenedione	Any day		High: PCOS or testosterone dominance
Specific hormone-binding globulin (SHBG)	Any day		Affects free testosterone and free oestrogen
Anti-Müllerian hormone (AMH)	Any day	Ovarian follicle/ cyst status, ovarian reserve	Combine with US with antral follicle count AMH levels correlate with the number of ovarian follicles and cysts, related to the severity of hyperandrogenism and oligo-anovulation in PCOS Reduced: failing ovarian reserve Increased: might be PCOS, although controversial

Conventional treatment

Clomiphene (anti-oestrogen), Letrozole (aromatase inhibitor) and gonadotropins can lead to ovarian hyperstimulation syndrome: in 10 to 20% of patients the ovaries become massively enlarged and intravascular fluid volume shifts into the peritoneal space, causing potentially life-threatening ascites and hypovolaemia.

4.2 Herbal management of infertility

For conception to occur one needs to ensure viable sperm, a healthy genital tract of both male and female and that ovulation occurs with a healthy egg as well as a receptive uterus.

Aims

Treat any underlying cause, including male health
Hormone level modulation, regulate ovarian function, support the corpus luteum, stress management
Promote uterine and endometrial health, promote the health of the cervical mucus and microbiome

Check ovulation is occurring: ovulation occurs about 14 days before the menstrual period, and fertility charting is helpful to check if ovulation is taking place and to assess the lengths of the follicular and luteal phases. This can also be used as pregnancy prevention, and many apps exist for this purpose.

- **Morning basal body temperature:** taken immediately on waking, temperature decreases when about to ovulate; an increase of ≥0.5°C indicates ovulation has just occurred.
- **Cervical fluid changes:** the vaginal fluid/discharge should stretch between the fingers like egg white; many online resources exist to identify and track cervical mucous changes. Fertile-quality cervical fluid is produced 3 to 5 days before ovulation, as a consequence of the increased levels of oestrogen seen just before ovulation.
- Sperm can survive up to 6 days in healthy fertile-quality cervical fluid, which protects the sperm from the acidic pH of the vagina and is a medium for travel as well as nourishment. The fertile window is a six-day period ending on the day of ovulation,[11] however the most reliable indicator is cervical mucus quality regardless of timing relative to ovulation.[12]
- **Cervical position:** (can also be affected by bowel movements)
  <u>Signs of fertility</u>: softening, opening of the cervical os, increased wetness from cervical fluid, and a lengthening of the vaginal canal.
  <u>Signs of infertility</u>: closed os, hardening, shortening and dryness.

- **Urine LH prediction test kits:** LH surge occurs 24 to 36 hours before ovulation. False positives can occur, and the tests are not thought to be helpful in PCOS as LH is already increased and the short surge can be missed. Can also be misleading in those with hyperprolactinaemia and other conditions that affect FSH/LH secretion.

Establish if there is a specific cause of infertility and treat accordingly: refer to chapters on PCOS, endometriosis, PID, bacterial vaginosis.

Herbal support for IVF: any treatment should begin a minimum of 4 months before an in vitro fertilisation (IVF) cycle, or intended pregnancy. Primary follicle development from primordial follicle needs 4 months, so a similar length in pre-conception care for both partners will be helpful; it is a chance to focus on a healthy diet, and possibly to use supplements high in antioxidants and crucial nutrients.

- Identify any causative or contributing factors and treat, consider other health issues.
- Ovulation detection (see above).

Herbal management

Hormone level modulation: phenolic phytoestrogenic-rich herbs, steroidal saponin-rich herbs, dopaminergic herbs affecting the thyroid. Soya, flaxseed, *Actaea racemosa, Asparagus racemosus, Dioscorea villosa, Paeonia lactiflora, Tribulus terrestris, Vitex agnus-castus*. Thyroid-supporting herbs: *Nigella sativa, Withania somnifera*.

Support the corpus luteum to maintain pregnancy: *Vitex agnus-castus*, apart from regulating regular cycle can also reduce the risk of miscarriage as it supports the corpus luteum in the crucial first three months of pregnancy.

Regulate ovarian function: steroidal saponins such as diosgenin bind to oestrogen receptors in the hypothalamus, competing with endogenous oestrogens. As the steroidal saponin effects are weak compared to endogenous oestrogens, the body responds as though the oestrogen levels are lower than they really are by increasing FSH and oestrogen. It has therefore been suggested that herbs rich in steroidal saponins may regulate ovulation and enhance fertility.

There is a strong traditional application of steroidal saponin herbs in the regulation of ovarian function, and they are particularly indicated to assist in the regulation of menstrual issues experienced in the first half of the cycle. Some herbalists suggest giving these herbs from days 5 to 14 of the menstrual cycle for 2 to 3 months or to use in the pre-ovulatory phase in combination with a conventional ovulation stimulant. This probably comes from the research related to *Tribulus*.[13] In addition they may use *Paeonia* & *Glycyrrhiza* or *Vitex* during the corpus luteum phase. In our clinical experience to use *Vitex* and *Paeonia* & *Glycyrrhiza* in this manner is ill-informed and does not seem to have any greater effect than using them continuously. The herbs are more than just directly hormonal and work more holistically; they have many other additional beneficial properties. Having said that, pulsing the steroidal saponin herbs, if there is no clear cycle present, seems reasonable.

Asparagus racemosus, Chamaelirium luteum, Dioscorea villosa, Tribulus terrestris.

Promote uterine and endometrial health using uterine tonics and emmenagogues[14] and improve pelvic circulation. There is a need to ensure a healthy endometrium for the implantation and establishment of early pregnancy as the risk of miscarriage is highest immediately after implantation. The normal endometrium is >5mm thick, a thick endometrium is found in hyperplasia or polyps, a thin endometrium can be seen in endometritis. *Achillea millefolium, Alchemilla vulgaris, Angelica sinensis, Artemisia vulgaris, Leonurus cardiaca.*

Treatment suggestions for a thin endometrium: *Actaea racemosa* is shown to enhance success rates alongside clomiphene, having a thicker endometrium compared to when not used. It also has a beneficial role on the vaginal pH, which might encourage a healthy microbiome. Phytoestrogens may also reverse the anti-oestrogen effects of clomiphene citrate.[15,16] Consider also pelvic circulation.

Treatment suggestions for a thick endometrium: this can be related to relative oestrogen excess, therefore consider *Vitex, Glycyrrhiza glabra & Paeonia lactiflora* and isoflavone-rich herbs such as soy, flaxseed, *Trifolium pratense*. Consider also pelvic circulation.

Promote the health of the cervical mucus as well as the microbiome: as this can be affected by hormonal issues, consider an alkaline diet (low protein, high in fruit and vegetables); see also the chapter on infectious vaginitis for more details on promoting a healthy vaginal microbiome.

Alkalinising herbs: *Apium graveolens, Urtica dioica.*

Oestrogen-promoting herbs: *Asparagus racemosus, Dioscorea villosa* and *Tribulus terrestris*, which will help to stabilise vaginal flora.

Reduce the negative impacts of stress: stress can be a major contributory factor and needs to be addressed. Stress can affect hormonal levels via the hypothalamic-pituitary-ovarian/adrenal axis and increase prolactin levels with a negative effect on fertility. Nervines and adaptogens are appropriate along with other lifestyle suggestions. *Leonorus cardiaca, Verbena officinalis* (which, interestingly, is in the same family as *Vitex*).

Thyroid-supporting herbs: hypothyroidism affects the menstrual cycle and fertility, and needs to be checked. If it may be subclinical consider *Nigella sativa, Rhodiola rosea, Panax ginseng, Withania somnifera*.

Key herbs used in clinical practice

Actaea racemosa

The Eclectics spoke highly of *Actaea* in relation to fertility. Ellingwood writes: "Alone, I have found this resin very efficacious in maladies of the female reproductive organs, in chronic ovaritis, endometritis, menstrual derangements, menorrhea, dysmenorrhea and menorrhagia, frigidity, sterility, threatened abortion, uterine sub-involution and to relieve severe after pains."[17,18] Felter and Lloyd write: "When there is a disordered action or lack of functional power in the uterus, giving rise to *sterility*, cimicifuga often corrects the impaired condition and cures."[19]

Clinical studies: clinical trials have reported improved pregnancy rates using *Actaea* plus clomiphene.[20] One trial comparing *Actaea* and clomiphene had favourable results.

Clomiphene has an anti-oestrogenic effect on the cervical mucous and endometrium, a reason for possible low pregnancy rates in clomiphene induction cycles.

Patients with unexplained infertility and recurrent clomiphene citrate induction failure: adding *Actaea* improved endometrial thickness, serum progesterone, clinical pregnancy rates higher. Also improved the pregnancy rate and cycle outcomes.[21]

Follicular phase ethinyl oestradiol plus clomiphene compared to *Actaea* plus clomiphene: *Actaea* improved cycle characteristics more so than oestradiol, with fewer days for follicular maturation and a thicker endometrium. Similar pregnancy rates were seen across both groups.[22]

PCOS with infertility, *Actaea racemosa* plus clomiphene: adding *Actaea* to clomiphene-induction cycles with timed intercourse improved cycle outcomes and pregnancy rates. Improvements were seen in serum levels of mid-luteal and mid-cycle oestradiol and LH as well as mid-luteal progesterone, plus higher clinical pregnancies per cycle.[23]

PCOS, comparing clomiphene (100mg daily for 5 days) to *Actaea* 20mg daily for 10 days: favourable changes were seen in LH levels and FSH/LH ratios, and progesterone levels were higher from the first treatment cycle, indicating better ovulation, and greater endometrial thickness. The pregnancy rate was higher in the *Actaea* group (not statistically significant).[24]

Dosage: the average weekly dose used in clinical trials is 1.8ml of a 1:3 per week. Most UK herbalists would use 10ml of a 1:3 per week. Higher doses have not been found to be more effective for menopausal symptoms. Note: 60% alcohol is needed to extract the triterpene glycosides.

Daily dose clinical trials used 80mg per day; this translates to 0.25ml of 1:3.

Typical weekly dose 5–10ml of 1:3.

Alchemilla vulgaris

In medieval times *Alchemilla* was regarded as a panacea for almost any illness. Several writers in the past suggest that it will firm up the breasts, possibly repeating Gerard from 1597. Both Parkinson and Culpeper recommended to take it internally for 20 days to help conception, retain the birth, as well as sit in a bath with a decoction of the herb. Parkinson adds: "as women that are barren, and cannot conceive, or retain the birth after conception, through too much humidity of the matrice, and fluxe of moist humours there unto, causing the seeds not to abide but to passe away without fruit, will reduce their bodies to so good and comfortable an estate, that they shall thereby be made more fit and able to retain the conception and bear out their children, if they do also sit sometimes as in a bath, in the decoction made of the herb."[25]

Dosage
Daily dose 6–12ml of 1:3.
Typical weekly dose 15–30ml of 1:3.

Angelica sinensis

Clinical studies: studies on the treatment of amenorrhoea and dysmenorrhoea stretch back to Europe in the late 1800s,[26] where 5ml of a fluid extract of the roots three times daily before meals for 1 week before menstruation for amenorrhoea and dysmenorrhoea is recommended.[27] No abortifacient activity was observed in two pregnant women treated.[28]

Case report: a woman with atypical polypoid adenomyoma and infertility. Oral use for 4 months corrected the endometrium to a normal secretory endometrium. Pregnancy followed. Her doctors suggested that Dong Quai may have acted as an ovulation inducer.[29]

Dosage
Daily dose 6–12ml of 1:3.[30]
 Typical weekly dose 15–30ml of 1:3.

Asparagus racemosus

Shatavari is the main Ayurvedic rejuvenative tonic for women, and in the ancient classical Ayurvedic literature is recommended in cases of threatened miscarriage; many other steroidal saponin-rich herbs have similar historic use.

Traditionally used for promoting conception, sexual debility and infertility in both sexes.

Dosage
Up to 20–30g of powder per day. Lower doses are used by infusion or decoction.
 Weekly dose 30–60ml of 1:2.

Dioscorea villosa

Wild yam has some oestrogenic effects on the body, probably mediated by the HPA axis due to feedback effects. The amount of diosgenin absorbed in the body is probably fairly small but the effects on the hypothalamus can be relatively significant nonetheless.

Dosage: daily dose 4.5–9ml of 1:3.
Typical weekly dose 20–40ml of 1:3.

Linum sativum

Clinical studies: shown to lengthen the luteal phase of the cycle and increase the frequency of ovulatory menstrual cycles.[31]

In a clinical study in PCOS, 15g of flaxseed powder daily reduced the ovarian volume, reduced the number of follicles in the ovaries and improved the frequency of menstrual cycles.[32]

Vitex agnus-castus

Studies related to latent hyperprolactinaemia and irregular cycle: lowered prolactin in those with hyperprolactinaemia, improved the hormonal profile, improved concentrations of progesterone in the luteal phase, shortened the cycle, normalised a shortened luteal phase, improved menstrual cyclicity in menstrual irregularity, such as polymenorrhoea, oligomenorrhoea, secondary amenorrhoea, and improved fertility.[33–35] Regularity of cycle was achieved better in those with oligomenorrhea as opposed to amenorrhoea, the pregnancy rate increased.[36]

Clinical trials:
A comparison with low dose oral contraceptive in those with PCOS. Both led to normalisation of menstrual cycle duration, free testosterone levels, DHEA-S and prolactin serum levels.[37]

Oligomenorrhoea in those with PCOS: 3.2–4.8mg of dried extract of *Vitex agnus-castus* and metformin for 3 months were found to be equally effective.[38]

Dosage
Daily dose 0.6–1.5ml of 1:3.
Typical weekly dose 5–10ml of 1:3.

Table 4.3: Clinical studies: herbs and actions

Action	Herb
AMH, lowering	*Cinnamomum cassia*[39]
Endometrial thickness, increase	*Actaea racemosa*[40]
	Anethum graveolens & Asparagus racemosus[41]
LH:FSH ratio lowering	PCOS trial
	Actaea racemosa[42]
	Apium graveolens & Pimpinella anisum[43]
	Foeniculum vulgare EO[44]
	Paeonia lactiflora & Glycyrrhiza glabra[45]
	Paeonia lactiflora & Cinnamomum cassia[46]
	Soya flour[47]
	Trigonella foenum-graecum (increases both LH and FSH)[48]

(Continued)

Table 4.3: (Continued)

Action	Herb
LH, reduce	*Actaea racemosa*[49] *Paeonia lactiflora & Cinnamomum cassia*[50] Combination of *Cinnamomum verum, Glycyrrhiza glabra, Hypericum perforatum, Paeonia lactiflora, Tribulus terrestris*[51]
Luteal deficiency	*Vitex agnus-castus, Paeonia lactiflora & Glycyrrhiza glabra* Flaxseed: lengthened the luteal phase of the cycle[52]
Prolactin levels, lowering	*Paeonia lactiflora & Glycyrrhiza glabra*[53] *Vitex agnus-castus*[54–57]
Menstrual cycle regulation, increasing ovulation, improving fertility	Clinical studies in PCOS *Actaea racemosa*[58] *Anethum graveolens & Asparagus racemosus*[59] *Apium graveolens and Pimpinella anisum*[60] *Cinnamomum cassia*[61–64] *Foeniculum vulgare* tea[65] and EO[66] *Grifola frondosa*[67] *Nigella sativa*[68] *Paeonia lactiflora and Cinnamomum cassia*[69,70] *Paeonia lactiflora & Glycyrrhiza glabra*[71,72] *Tribulus terrestris* (infertility oligo anovular)[73] (possibly other steroidal saponin-rich herbs might help similarly: *Asparagus racemosus, Chamaelirium luteum, Dioscorea villosa*) *Trigonella foenum-graecum*[74] *Vitex agnus-castus*[75–80] Combination of *Cinnamomum verum, Glycyrrhiza glabra, Hypericum perforatum, Paeonia lactiflora, Tribulus terrestris*[81] **Preclinical studies** *Linum usitatissimum*[82] *Paeonia lactiflora & Glycyrrhiza glabra*[83,84] *Trifolium pratense*[85] *Aloe vera*[86] *Glycyrrhiza uralensis*[87] Isolated constituents: Gymnemic acid (with myo-inositol, and l-methylfolate)[88]

Eclectic texts

Atropa belladonna: Ellingwood writes: "A few years ago a number of writers were quite enthusiastic concerning the action of belladonna in stimulating normal ovulation and thus overcoming sterility. In a number of cases where one-eighth of a grain of the extract was given before meals or four or five times a day, cases which had previously been sterile, found that the condition was entirely removed. Its influence in stimulating the capillary circulation of the ovaries in stasis renders it of value in the treatment of sterility from inactivity of those organs. If there are hysterical manifestations at the menstrual epoch, with deficient menstruation, *pulsatilla* may be used in conjunction with it."[89]

Serenoa repens: was also suggested for female sterility. Ellingwood again: "In simple cases where there is no organic lesion on the part of the patient, this agent has an excellent reputation for restoring the ovarian action properly and assisting in putting the patient into an excellent condition. One conscientious reliable lady physician assures me that in five definite cases, pregnancy has followed the use of this remedy where sterility was pronounced previously, and thought to be incurable."[90]

Viburnum prunifolium: Ellingwood writes, in *King's Dispensatory*, for use in menstrual irregularities in sterile females. He reported that pregnancy promptly occurred and suggested it restores normal functional ovarian activity. In the past it had been suggested that spasm of tubes might affect fertility, possibly a reason why antispasmodics like *Viburnum prunifolium* were thought to be of help.[91]

Table 4.4: Other clinical trials: herbs, herb combinations and isolated compounds

Herb	Clinical trial
Apium graveolens & Pimpinella anisum	4.5g/day of both seed powders taken for 15 days from beginning of follicular phase/or in amenorrhoea for 15 days, compared to metformin on oligomenorrhea in PCOS. Regulated menstrual cycles and reduced total serum testosterone and LH/FSH ratio, the result suggesting the combination was superior to metformin.[92]

(Continued)

Table 4.4: (Continued)

Herb	Clinical trial
Anethum graveolens and *Asparagus racemosus*	A combination trial used orally, rectally as an enema (not a common way to give herbs in the UK), or both given to PCOS patients. All showed reduced ovarian volumes compared with pre-treated stages. Endometrial thickness improved, and those taking it rectally as well as orally had the most improvement.[93]
Berberine (isolated)	Improved the menstrual pattern and ovulation rate.[94]
Foeniculum vulgare	Clinical trials PCOS patients with oligomenorrhoea using tea plus cupping vs metformin, reduced the days between the cycle and pain.[95] In amenorrhoea: efficacy of daily 60mg fennel EO.[96] The trial was only 21 days.
Cinnamomum cassia/ zeylanicum	Clinical trials with PCOS patients average intake 1.5g/day normalised the menstrual cycles,[97,98] reduced anti-Müllerian hormone (AMH),[99] and had a positive effect on hormonal status.[100,101] AMH promotes preantral follicle survival, and negatively impacts the later stages of antral follicle maturation.[102]
Paeonia lactiflora & Cinnamomum cassia	In those with luteal phase defects: decreased plasma luteinising hormone and increased 17 beta-oestradiol in the follicular phase, increased progesterone in the midluteal phase. Increased development of the dominant follicle and endometrium. Prolongation and correction of the luteal phase, leading to increased incidence of pregnancy.[103] Studies on women with PCOS: anovulatory women with high plasma LH levels; decreased plasma LH in polycystic ovary syndrome and non-polycystic ovary syndrome. Plasma oestradiol levels increased. Significant development of the dominant follicle observed in patients, improved menstrual cyclicity, increased ovulation.[104]

(Continued)

Table 4.4: (Continued)

Herb	Clinical trial
Glycyrrhiza glabra & *Paeonia lactiflora*	Prolactin lowering effects. Clinical trials in those with hyperprolactinaemia induced by antipsychotic medication with oligomenorrhea or amenorrhea,[105] anovulatory,[106] aided menstrual resumption,[107,108] progesterone and oestrodiol levels increased.[109] Clinical studies in women with PCOS: lowered serum testosterone levels and induced regular ovulation and pregnancy in oligomenorrheic and hyperandrogenic patients.[110,111] LH to FSH ratio was lower, and the pregnancy rate increased.[112]
Grifola frondosa **Maitake mushroom**	Clinical trials with Maitake extract to induce ovulation in patients with PCOS increased ovulation when used alone as well as in combination with clomiphene.[113]
Panax ginseng	In vivo *Panax ginseng* improved hypothyroid-induced deterioration in trophic and gonadal hormones.[114] In vivo: KRG saponins positive effects on oocyte quality, decreasing the proportion of abnormal oocytes, improved the hormonal profiles during the ovulatory cycle. Plus stimulates antioxidant enzymes in embryos.[115]
Rhodiola rosea	In vivo: enhanced fertility, enhanced thyroid function, enhanced egg maturation.[116] Trial in women with amenorrhea and infertility, rhodiola (100mg) given twice daily for two weeks. Normal menses were restored in the majority, and 25% became pregnant.[117]
Silymarin (isolated)	IVF: 4 out of the 20 women ovulated; the effects were greater in women treated with silymarin and metformin combined.[118]

(*Continued*)

Table 4.4: (Continued)

Herb	Clinical trial
Tribulus terrestris	Oligo/anovular infertility: *Tribulus terrestris* (Tribestan®) compared with several medications to induce ovulation over 3 months. Ovulation rates were highest with epimestrol (74%), followed by *Tribulus terrestris* (60%), clomiphene (47%) and cyclofenil (24%), little information given on baseline characteristics. The authors suggested the results were better if used on certain days during the cycle. *Tribulus* and ovulation stimulant on days 5 to 14 was better than treatment with either single agent.[119] In healthy women: increased serum FSH concentration, return to pre-treatment levels on cessation of treatment.[120] *Tribulus terrestris* alongside other herbs: *Cinnamomum verum, Glycyrrhiza glabra, Hypericum perforatum, Paeonia lactiflora,* on overweight PCOS patients using herbs alongside lifestyle changes, or lifestyle changes only. *Tribulus* taken from menstrual cycle day 5 for 10 days, or within 1 week of trial for women with amenorrhoea. In combination with lifestyle changes this resulted in a reduction of the number of days of the menstrual cycle, oestradiol and LH, and improved fasting insulin levels, blood pressure, conception rates and quality of life. The live birth rate was similar.[121]
Trigonella foenum-graecum **seed**	Clinical studies, patients Dx with PCOS. *Trigonella foenum-graecum* seed extract, 2 capsules of 500mg each/day); reduction in ovary volume. Regulated menstrual cycle, pregnancy rate increased as well as increases in LH and FSH.[122] Alongside metformin in oligo-anovulatory: decrease in polycystic appearing ovaries and improved menstrual cyclicity.[123]

4.3 Dietary and lifestyle recommendations

Good preconception care and health status increase the likelihood of a successful pregnancy and a healthy baby. Broadly this would include stopping smoking, reducing alcohol intake, working towards a healthy weight, addressing stress and anxiety, and focusing on the diet to ensure optimum intake of micronutrients. It is essential to start treatment two to three months before conception as a minimum because health before conception is strongly linked to the outcome of pregnancy. The months before conception are critical while gametes mature. These are sensitive to exposure from environmental factors, while primary follicle development from the primordial follicle takes 4 months. For the prevention of neural tube defects, a minimum of 4–6 weeks of folic acid supplementation is required to reach adequate levels before neurulation, three weeks after conception, to reduce the risk of neural tube defects.[124]

Cohort studies have suggested that diet can have a major influence up to three years before pregnancy and is associated with a reduced risk of gestational diabetes, hypertensive disorders of pregnancy and preterm birth.[125] A high intake of fruit, vegetables, legumes, nuts and fish, and low intake of red and processed meat are associated with positive outcomes. Oxidative balance is thought to be important in relation to unexplained infertility,[126] so a healthy, colourful diet rich in flavonoids, vitamins and minerals would also be a sensible strategy to follow. A good-quality multivitamin and mineral supplements might be indicated for the same reasons.

Weight: maternal obesity is associated with an inability to conceive and poor maternal and perinatal outcomes.[127] Paternal obesity has been linked to impaired fertility affecting sperm quality and quantity,[128] and increased chronic disease risk in offspring.[129] In assisted reproductive therapy there is an increased success rate in those with optimal body weight.

Importance of exercise: higher levels of preconception physical activity were associated with a lower risk of gestational diabetes and pre-eclampsia; walking at a brisk pace for four hours or more per week before pregnancy was also associated with lower risk of gestational diabetes.[130]

Healthy diets, some of the evidence

Mediterranean diet is associated with better fertility, higher birth rate and helpful in preconception care, and linked with increased successful outcome in IVF treatment. Higher intake of omega 3 fatty acids and diets rich in fish, seafood, poultry, whole grains, fruits and vegetables are related to better fertility in women and better semen quality in men.[131] Better fertility has also been linked to a diet rich in MUFAs, olive oil, legumes, low intake of snacks, higher intakes of protein from vegetable sources,[132] full fat dairy, iron and the use of multivitamins and minerals.[133-135]

High-fat (or unadulterated foods) dairy foods: low-fat dairy foods have a negative effect on fertility, increasing the risk of anovulatory infertility. It was suggested that the fat-soluble substances in full-fat dairy foods might be important to aid fertility.[136]

Multivitamin use: there appears to be an inverse association between the frequency of multivitamin use and ovulatory infertility. Folic acid appeared to explain part of the association.[137] Several formulations of multivitamins and minerals with different combinations have been studied. Results suggest increased ovulation and pregnancy rates[138] as well as a reduction of pre-eclampsia incidence.[139,140]

Soy food: has a beneficial effect among women undergoing infertility treatment.[141,142]

Environmental pollutants: affect reproductive health.[143] Exposure in the pre-conceptional period affects conception as well as neonatal health.[144]

Caffeine: has been suggested to have negative effect on fertility, but despite it being intensively studied it has not been confirmed, and caffeine use is not associated with diminished fertility.[145] There are concerns of increased risk of pregnancy loss with caffeine intake.[146]

Other: cigarette smoking, alcohol consumption and/or drug abuse have negative impacts, particularly on female fertility.[147] Epidemiological studies suggest exposure to tobacco, alcohol and stress are factors influencing foetal development, including miscarriages.[148]

Avoiding gluten: patients with coeliac disease are at higher risk of spontaneous abortion, low new-born birth weights, reduced duration of lactation,[149] a higher incidence of PCOS and endometriosis.[150] Undiagnosed coeliac disease is a risk factor for infertility.[151]

Diet low in glycaemic load: associated with a lower risk of ovulatory disorder infertility, and lower risk of infertility due to other causes.[152]

Table 4.5: Vitamin and minerals, studies on individual nutrients

Arginine: a precursor of nitric oxide synthesis, it is required for angiogenesis, embryogenesis, hormone secretion and fertility in general.	Arginine supplementation improved ovarian response, endometrial receptivity and pregnancy rates.[153]
Calcium	Low levels are related to reduced male fertility. Ca^+ supplementation before and early in pregnancy seemed to reduce the risk of pre-eclampsia or pregnancy loss.[154]
Coenzyme Q10: synthesised in most human tissues using pantothenic acid (B5) and pyridoxine (B6); around 25% of plasma CoQ10 is derived from food sources.[155]	Pretreatment with CoQ10 improved ovarian response to stimulation in young women with poor ovarian reserve in IVF-ICSI cycles, increasing the number of retrieved oocytes, higher fertilisation rate and more high-quality embryos.[156]
Folic acid and vitamin B12	Higher levels increase fertility and live birth rates in IVF; high folate status increases the likelihood of twin births after IVF.[157] Adequate folic acid also reduces the risk of pre-eclampsia, miscarriage, low birth weight and stillbirth.[158]
Iron (Fe)	Intake is associated with an increased chance of conception among women who had heavy menses or short menstrual cycles.[159]
L-carnitine	Given in conjunction with clomiphene citrate, significantly improved both the ovulation and pregnancy rates of women with clomiphene-resistant PCOS. Women with functional hypothalamic amenorrhea given l-carnitine showed increased LH plasma levels.[160]

(Continued)

Table 4.5: (Continued)

Magnesium (Mg)	Mg supplement during pregnancy reduced occurrence of many complications.[161]
Melatonin found in the follicular fluid; reduced levels are found in those with unexplained infertility.	Melatonin supplementation is shown to rebalance intrafollicular oxidative status, improve oocyte quality and slightly enhance IVF success rates in those with unexplained infertility.[162]
Probiotics	Taken orally as well as vaginally (cf. vaginal infections chapter). Any infection in the female reproductive system could affect fertility and implantation rates in assisted reproductive technology. Higher pregnancy rates after IVF cycles were seen in patients with vaginal microbiomes consisting of *Lactobacillus* spp.[163] Colonising the embryo catheter tip with *Lactobacillus* spp. at the time of embryo transfer may lead to higher implantation rate and live birth rates, by lowering the intrauterine infection rate.[164]
Selenium (Se)	Selenium deficiencies may lead to gestational complications, miscarriages, pre-eclampsia, pre-term labour, gestational diabetes and obstetric cholestasis and low birth weights.[165] A deficiency can also affect the quality of semen and sperm motility.[166]
Vitamin A, alongside carotenoids	Low levels are associated with anovulation, and levels are decreased in women with habitual miscarriage. Vitamin A supports both male and female reproduction as well as embryonic development, and is needed for the maintenance of the male genital tract as well as spermatogenesis.[167]

CHAPTER 5

Vaginal discharge

5.1 Presentation/symptoms, differential diagnosis and investigations

The healthy vaginal microbiome

Healthy vaginal flora consists of a wide variety of anaerobic and aerobic bacteria, the dominant organisms in health being *Lactobacillus* genus (most commonly *L. crispatus, L. iners, L. gasseri, L. jensenii*); other bacteria present in varying population amounts are *Staphylococcus* species, *Gardnerella vaginalis, Streptococcus* species, *Bacteroides* species, *Mobiluncus* and *Candida* species. Factors that contribute to the maintenance of a healthy vaginal environment are glycogen, oestrogen, local pH and the metabolic by-products of both 'normal' flora and pathogens.

Glycogen is produced by vaginal mucosal cells, which are in turn affected by hormone levels tending to peak after ovulation. These glycogens are fed on by *Lactobacillus* spp., which produce bacteriocins, lactic acid and hydrogen peroxide. These are in part responsible for regulating the acidic (anti-pathogenic) vaginal environment[1]—maintaining the vaginal pH at ≤4.5 inhibits overgrowth of pathogens,[2] especially anaerobic bacteria.[3,4] *Lactobacillus crispatus* has a positive effect on the urinary system; high levels are associated with a significant reduction in recurrent UTI.[5]

Secreted by vaginal and cervical cells, vaginal discharge provides lubrication and a protective layer; amounts, colour and odour will vary from person to person, with diet and within the menstrual cycle. This may also change in response to hormone levels in pregnancy and with oral contraceptive use. Broadly a 'healthy' discharge will be clear to white, slippery to slightly sticky depending on the phase of the cycle and amount to around a teaspoon per day.

Causes of changes in discharge

Infection/overgrowth: the most common are bacterial vaginosis, candidiasis and trichomoniasis. About 30% of women of childbearing age have bacterial vaginosis and 3% have trichomoniasis. Nearly 75% of all adult women have had at least one yeast infection in their lifetime.[6-8]

Bacterial vaginosis (BV) caused by an overgrowth of *Gardnerella vaginalis*: thin, frothy, grey, unpleasantly 'fishy' discharge.

Vulvo vaginal candidiasis (VVC), aka thrush, caused by opportunistic overgrowth of *Candida albicans*: cottage cheese-like discharge, yeasty smell. DDx metabolic or immune compromised as underlying cause when recurrent.

Trichomoniasis caused by the *Trichomonas vaginalis* parasite: fishy smell, yellow–green, frothy or bubbly discharge, with pruritis, dysparunia, dysuria and occasionally abdominal pain.

Chlamydia, a bacterial infection: can be asymptomatic, pain on urination, pain on intercourse, strong-smelling yellow discharge, abdominal pain.

Gonorrhoea, a bacterial infection: can be asymptomatic, pain on urination, yellow or bloody discharge, bleeding between periods.

Others: *mycoplasma, campylobacter* and even parasites like pinworms and *giardia*.

Hormonal vaginitis: atrophic vaginitis, usually in postmenopausal or postpartum women, but occasionally before puberty. Symptoms arising from lack of moisture: dryness, dysuria, dysparunia.

Irritant vaginitis: allergies to latex in condoms, spermicides, deodorants, soaps. Symptoms are of inflammation: sore, swollen, red, pruritis, dysuria.

Non-infectious causes of vaginal discharge: foreign body such as forgotten tampons or diaphragms, malignancy.

Risk factors

Any factors that affect the pH balance of the vagina are likely to be contributory factors associated with high vaginal pH (alkaline), age, frequency of douching and menopausal status.

Endogenous
- Health of mucous membranes, e.g. atrophic tissue in post-menopausal.
- Hormonal influences (cyclic changes), high or low oestrogen states such as pregnancy, menopause, hormonal dysregulation.
- Underlying conditions: obesity, diabetes, immunosuppression, endocrine disorders.

Lifestyle factors
- Diet
- Poor sleep
- Stress

External factors
- Sexual intercourse: causing friction leading to damage of the local tissue and inflammation.
- Lubricants and semen, which can alkalise the vaginal environment.
- Feminine hygiene products: douches, chemicals in soaps, panty liners, sanitary pads, tampons.

Medication
- Contraceptive devices, OCP, HRT
- Antibiotic use
- Systemic steroids

5.2 Vaginal and upper reproductive tract infections

Bacterial vaginosis

This is the most common of the conditions affecting the vagina and also the most resistant to treatment. Bacterial vaginosis (BV) is found to be present in about 25% of pregnant women;[9] 50% of infections are asymptomatic.

Pathophysiology

As mentioned earlier, vaginal *Lactobacilli* maintain the healthy vaginal environment at an acid pH, which inhibits the overgrowth of other microorganisms, especially anaerobic bacteria[10,11] such as *Gardnerella vaginalis, Mycoplasma hominis* and *Prevotella* species, which are naturally present within the vaginal biome.[12,13] Bacterial vaginosis is not an infection caused by a single microorganism. It should instead be understood as an imbalance either due to reduction in pH, favouring anaerobic organisms that prefer a more alkaline environment, and/or due to the reduction of *Lactobacillus*, with the same result.[14] As the anaerobic organisms become more dominant they further influence pH, making the environment even less favourable to *Lactobacillus* species. This imbalance can become persistent but can also resolve spontaneously, perhaps in response to endogenous or exogenous changes.

Gardnerella vaginalis is often the dominant pathogen and produces a poly-microbial biofilm.[15] Levels of sialidase, an enzyme that removes protective gel layer of the vaginal and cervical epithelium, are increased in women with BV.[16] This lack of protection exposes the epithelium to other organisms and causes 'clue cells' that line the vagina and have clusters of bacteria adhered to their surface. These can be seen under the microscope and are unique to BV and thus diagnostic.

Other local effects: upregulation of inflammatory cytokines, the absence or rare presence of white blood cells in the vaginal discharge, a decrease in naturally protective molecules like secretory leukocyte protease inhibitor.

Diagnosis relies on three positive criteria out of four:

1. Discharge: thin, frothy, grey/milky smelly, especially after intercourse or during menstruation.[17]
2. A fishy odour, especially after intercourse. The odour is due to increased vaginal fluid concentrations of diamines, polyamines and organic acids. This is often tested by adding potassium hydroxide to the discharge.
3. Vaginal pH over 4.5.
4. Presence of 'clue cells'.
5. Persistent or recurrent.

Complications associated with untreated/undertreated BV:

- Increased risk of miscarriage, premature labour and increased incidence of perinatal death.[18]

- Increased incidence of abnormal Pap smear, PID, infertility and endometriosis.
- Increased incidence of complications such as post-surgical gynaecological infections.[19]

Risk factors

In addition to those mentioned earlier affecting the vaginal biome, also consider IUD, numerous sexual partners, smoking. Hormonal contraceptive use is associated with a decreased risk of BV,[20] and this may underline the need to correct hormonal imbalances.

Conventional treatment

With metronidazole, however, reoccurrence seems to be common. As the underlying cause is not one particular organism but the lack of healthy vaginal microbiome, reoccurrence is very likely if this is not corrected alongside conventional drug treatment.[21]

Antibiotic treatment can eradicate BV in pregnancy, although a review suggested there is little evidence that screening and treating all pregnant women with asymptomatic BV will prevent pre-term birth.[22]

Candida vaginitis

The second most common cause of vaginitis is *Candida albicans*. However, this is often misdiagnosed by patients (by self-diagnosis) as well as by practitioners.

Typical organisms involved are *Candida albicans, C. glabrata, C. tropicallis* and *C. krusei*. As with many other infections, there is development of resistance to over-the-counter treatment medications.

If there are four or more confirmed candida symptomatic infections within one year, this must be investigated as there are likely to be systemic causes.

Symptoms

- Discharge: white, yellow–white cottage cheese-like in character (watery to thick), yeasty smell.
- Normal vaginal pH ≤4.5.

- Microscopic findings are not helpful as *candida* is part of the normal flora.
- Pruritis can be present without discharge, especially premenstrually.
- Vaginal inflammation: soreness, irritation, vulvar burning, dysparunia and urinary discomfort.
- Worse before onset of menses, relieved after.

Risk factors

- Allergy.
- High-oestrogen medication (hormones), contraceptive devices.
- Immuno-compromised individuals, leukaemia, diabetes, endocrine conditions (Cushing's, Addison's, hypo- or hyperthyroidism).
- Impaired glucose tolerance.
- Medications (cytotoxic drugs, immunosuppressive drugs, radiotherapy, or chemotherapy), frequent antibiotic use.
- Pregnancy, commonly in late pregnancy.
- Type and fit of clothing (tight fitting, non-breathable).

The incidence of candida infections rises in late pregnancy. In Germany treatment is recommended in the third trimester of pregnancy, as the rate of oral thrush and diaper dermatitis in healthy newborns is increased as babies become infected during vaginal delivery. Vaginal clotrimazole treatment in the first trimester of pregnancy has shown to reduce the rate of pre-term births in two studies.[23]

DDx: vulvar hyperplasia, vestibulitis (inflammation of the tissue surrounding the opening to the vagina), genital ulcerations, lichen sclerosis, other dermatitis conditions.

Conventional treatment

OTC anti-fungal oral and/or topical, should clear within 7–14 days.

Trichomonas vaginalis

A motile flagellate protozoan, passed via direct sexual contact. *T. vaginalis* in men causes non-gonococcal urethritis and can have negative impact on fertility.[24] In women *T. vaginalis* usually affects the vagina and urethra but can also infect the Bartholin glands and bladder.

Symptoms

- Can be asymptomatic.[25]
- Discharge: frothy, bubbly, white to green, yellow–green discharge, or colourless present in 50 to 75%, malodorous.
- pH greater than 4.5.
- Dyspareunia, bleeding on intercourse, dysuria.
- Vulvovaginal pruritus, burning, irritation, vulvar redness and swelling.
- Occasional: lower abdominal pain.
- Can be present alongside other sexually transmitted disease such as gonorrhoea.
- Diagnostic: 'strawberry cervix' (cervix with small haemorrhages), however only present in 2%.

Dx: microscopic (wet prep) evaluation detects 60 to 80% of cases; culture is more sensitive for diagnosis. Pap smears are not sensitive in testing trichomoniasis.

Complications

- Cervical dysplasia.[26]
- Female infertility.[27]
- Pelvic inflammatory disease (PID), and increased risk of postoperative infection.
- Postpartum infection.[28]
- Pre-term delivery and low-birth weight infants.[29]

It is important that this infection is treated, symptomatic or not. Sexually transmitted infections such as gonorrhoea, chlamydia and trichomoniasis can lead to complications including pelvic inflammatory disease (PID), chronic pelvic pain and infertility, and can increase the possibility of transmission of other infections such as human immunodeficiency virus (HIV) and genital herpes.

Conventional treatment

Metronidazole, tinidazole

Treatment with metronidazole, tinidazole does clear most cases though there are strains that are drug resistant.[30] If these drugs are prescribed, ensure the patient also takes probiotics and adds either live yogurt or *L. acidophilus* vaginally as well as internally, to make the treatment more effective. As with many of these infections, it is important to treat both partners.

The decision to treat during pregnancy is not very clear. A Cochrane analysis found there was no benefit from antimicrobial treatment during pregnancy, and indeed there was possible harm; the largest trial was stopped due to an increased risk of pre-term labour with the use of metronidazole.[31] Treatment of pregnant women with asymptomatic trichomoniasis does not prevent pre-term delivery, and researchers concluded that routine screening and treatment of asymptomatic pregnant women for this condition cannot be recommended.[32]

Pelvic inflammatory disease (PID)

PID is an inflammation of the upper reproductive tract due to an infection. PID can be acute, chronic or subclinical and is often underdiagnosed. Typically caused by sexually transmitted infections, the most commonly involved pathogens are *N. gonorrhoea* and *C. trachomatis*, although other cervical, enteric, bacterial vaginosis-associated and respiratory pathogens may be involved. Vaginal inflammation and bacterial vaginosis assist in the upward spread of vaginal microorganisms.[33]

Infections can affect the cervix, uterus, fallopian tubes and, if severe, can also affect the ovaries and spread to the peritoneum (peritonitis). Pus may collect and an abscess can form (tubo-ovarian abscess).

The infection also causes inflammatory damage, scarring, adhesions and obstruction of the fallopian tubes. This inflammation and subsequent tissue damage can result in the loss of the ciliated epithelial cells in the fallopian tube, affecting fertility, as well as increasing the risk of ectopic pregnancy. Adhesions can lead to chronic pelvic pain.[34]

Many with PID have very few or no symptoms. Diagnosis is made primarily on clinical suspicion, hence a clear and thorough history is crucial along with a physical examination. PID should be suspected in those presenting with lower abdominal or pelvic pain and reproductive tract tenderness, who are sexually active. Referral will be necessary as urgent treatment is required to reduce complications. Long-term complications can lead to chronic pelvic pain, impaired fertility and ectopic pregnancy.

Symptoms

Infection with *N. gonorrhoea* presents acutely and causes more severe symptoms. PID due to chlamydia is less likely to cause symptoms and is more likely to result in subclinical PID with consequent long-term complications.

- Abnormal uterine bleeding: heavier and/or delayed menses, spotting, and bleeding after sex.
- Cervical motion tenderness.
- Dyspareunia.
- Dysuria.
- Fever, anorexia, nausea, vomiting.
- Lower abdominal pain, unilateral or bilateral adnexal.
- Mucopurulent cervical discharge.

If the cervix is involved, i.e. cervicitis, the cervix is red and bleeds easily. The mucopurulent discharge is yellow–green.

If the infection travels further, such as in salpingitis, there is lower abdominal pain (although this can also be upper abdominal) bilaterally but may also be unilateral. Nausea and vomiting (with severe pain). Irregular bleeding caused by endometrial inflammation. Fever is present in 1/3 of patients. In the early stages, signs are mild or absent. Later symptoms of cervical motion tenderness, guarding and rebound tenderness may appear.

Complications

<u>Tubo-ovarian or pelvic abscess</u>: may be palpable, although extreme tenderness may limit examination. This is a red flag that should be referred for appropriate treatment.

Increased likelihood of an abscess is related to incomplete or late treatment and can also occur with chronic PID. Other symptoms are pain, fever and peritoneal signs. The abscess may rupture, causing severe symptoms and can lead to septic shock.[35]

Hydrosalpinx: damage and blockage at the end part of the fallopian tube causes tubal distention with non-purulent fluid. Presents asymptomatically but can cause pelvic pressure, chronic pelvic pain, dyspareunia and/or infertility.

Chronic pelvic pain: present in 1/3 of women with PID, it is caused by tubal scarring and adhesions, with infertility and an increased risk of ectopic pregnancy.

Infertility: infections can cause damage to the fallopian tubes, loss of the ciliary epithelial cells of the fallopian tube and occlusion. Increased incidence is related to chlamydia as infectious cause, a delay in treatment, recurrent episodes, as well as the severity of PID.

Ectopic pregnancy: related to damage of the fallopian tubes.

Fitz-Hugh-Curtis syndrome (perihepatitis, upper right quadrant pain): infections may become chronic, characterised by intermittent exacerbations and remissions. Symptoms may mimic acute cholecystitis.

Risk factors

- Douching.
- Multiple or new sex partners or a partner who does not use a condom.
- Previous PID.
- Presence of bacterial vaginosis and/or any sexually transmitted infection.
- Younger age (occurs most frequently in women aged 15 to 25 years).

Differential diagnosis

It is important to bear PID in mind where there are similar presentations.
Other conditions that mimic PID:

- Appendicitis
- Cystitis
- Diverticulitis
- Ectopic pregnancy
- Endometriosis
- Ovarian cyst rupture
- Ovarian torsion
- Pyelonephritis
- Traumatic injury

Investigations

- Pregnancy test to rule out ectopic pregnancy.
- Laboratory tests may help to confirm diagnosis, but will take time, and negative results do not exclude the diagnosis, nor will an ultrasound (thickened, fluid-filled tubes, or tubo-ovarian mass) or CT. Treatment is started regardless of findings to avoid delay.
- In uncertain diagnoses a laparoscopy is usually performed. Purulent peritoneal material noted during laparoscopy is the diagnostic gold standard.

Conventional treatment

Early diagnosis and treatment can potentially prevent complications and should be started, based on clinical suspicion and a referral with urgency.[36] Antibiotics. Sexual partners should also be treated to prevent immediate reinfection.

Herbal treatment alongside conventional treatment can be helpful to support the health of the vaginal microbiome and give immune support. See the chapter on treatment for vaginal discharge and trichomoniasis.

5.3 Herbal treatment of vaginal infections

Common general principles related to treatment of any infectious vaginitis

Aims

Restore a healthy vaginal environment: microbiome, mucous, pH and pelvic circulation
Treat infection: antimicrobial, support immune system
Soothing and calm infected areas: anti-inflammatories

Prevention as well as treatment

Re-establish the lactobacillus-dominant vaginal flora: use probiotics internally, which can also be used vaginally, e.g. yogurt. As mentioned earlier *Lactobacillus* species produces lactic and acetic acid as well as hydrogen peroxide (H_2O_2), which helps to maintain a healthy pH in the vagina. A diet rich in vegetables, fruit, fermented foods and garlic, and avoiding sugar/refined carbohydrates and known allergenic foods, will help maintain a healthy gut microbiome, which will, in turn, influence the vaginal microbiome.

Restore pH to less than 4.5 to prevent reoccurrence of infection, wash external area with cider vinegar, 2 tablespoons to a pint of water. Re-establish vaginal flora, as above. *Actaea racemosa* increases the amount of superficial cells (in vaginal smear tests), which leads to lower pH in the vagina. Lower pH levels prevent ascending infection.

Promote a healthy mucous membrane in the vagina: *Althea officinalis, Asparagus racemosus* as demulcents, *Hydrastis canadensis* as a mucous membrane restorative. Consider use of simple cocoa butter pessary to nourish local tissues.

Adequate oestrogen levels to maintain an acidic as well as a moist vaginal environment as recurrent infections tend to flare up in second half of cycle when both progesterone and oestrogen are produced by the corpus luteum. Oral contraceptives reduce the risk of BV. *Actaea racemosa, Paeonia lactiflora & Glycyrrhiza glabra, Vitex agnus-castus*, steroidal saponin-rich herbs such as *Asparagus racemosus*.

Support healthy pelvic circulation, which will ensure healthy hydration of pelvic area, with uterine tonics/emmenagogues. *Achillea millefolium, Actaea racemosa, Alchemilla vulgaris, Artemisia* spp., *Calendula officinalis*, etc.

For treatment of infection

As above plus any of the following, as needed.

Anti-inflammatories to reduce discomfort as anaerobic bacteria produce inflammatory proteins: *Calendula officinalis* pessaries, *Curcuma longa*, etc.

Antimicrobials internally and vaginally.

Internal antimicrobials: *Allium sativum, Arctostaphylos uva ursi, Myrtus communis, Thymus vulgaris*, berberine-rich herbs such as *Berberis vulgaris, Hydrastis canadensis*.

Pessaries vaginally: *Calendula officinalis, Foeniculum vulgare* EO, *Lavandula angustifolia* EO, *Melaleuca alternifolia* EO, *Thymus* CT linalool EO.

Immune and lymphatic system support to fight infections: *Andrographis paniculata, Baptisia tinctoria, Calendula officinalis, Echinacea* spp., *Phytolacca decandra, Thuja occidentalis*.

Prevention is always easier than cure: condom use (semen raises pH), treat partner to reduce reinfection, use gentle feminine hygiene products (if at all) and gentle soaps as well as gentle washing powder, wear loose clothing of natural fibres, ensure toilet hygiene (wiping front to back), maintain vaginal biome.

Repeat treatment as often as needed to ensure a healthy vaginal flora has been established to maintain a healthy vaginal environment.

Douching is not recommended as douching disrupts the vaginal flora. There was a significant 21% increase in risk of bacterial vaginosis for participants who used vaginal douches.[37,38]

Key herbs used in clinical practice

For internal prescriptions we recommend using 4–6 x a day, for pessaries one every night, for 2 weeks. This should be enough to clear any symptoms. If not, continue till symptom-free, and repeat after 2-week break.

This treatment combination is effective on a range of causes of vaginitis. In our clinic a patient was referred to us by the nearby Sexual Health Clinic, Dx with a chlamydia infection that was not responding to antibiotics. Legally we herbalists are required to refer onwards anyone with a sexually transmitted disease, however as they were maintained under the care of the Sexual Health Clinic, we were able to proceed with the above protocol and within 6 weeks they were clear of symptoms.

Allium sativum

Preclinical studies:
In vitro, antibacterial, antiprotozoal[39,40] including *Trichomonas vaginalis*.[41,42]

Clinical studies:
In BV a vaginal cream as effective as metronidazole.[43]

Vulvovaginal candidiasis (VVC): a vaginal douche effective in relieving and clearing symptoms.[44]

Garlic and thyme cream had a similar effect to clotrimazole cream for VVC.[45]

Vaginal application: the safest mode of application would be to use a non-broken clove, to avoid the risk of contact burns.

Typical oral doses: 2–4g per day, 1–3 cloves a day.

Arctostaphylos uva ursi

Actions: antimicrobial, astringent and anti-inflammatory effects in the genitourinary tract.

Historical use: used by Native Americans in the form of a tea to treat venereal disease, inflammation of the genitourinary tracts and as a urinary antiseptic.[46] The Eclectics also used it for menorrhagia, leucorrheoa, chronic gonorrhoea and suggested it had specific influence upon the urinogenital structures.[47,48] One writer suggested it cured several cases of lingering gonorrhoea in females and stated that it tones the uterus. It was used in the treatment of leucorrhea, especially when connected with a flaccid condition of the womb and vagina, and with prolapse.[49,50]

In the past it had been suggested that alkaline urine was needed to deconjugate hydroquinone from arbutin, which has antibacterial effects. However, later research suggests that pH is not important. Instead, it appears that the process is catalysed by enzymes present in bacterial cytoplasm.[51]

Preclinical studies: hydroquinone is a phenolic antiseptic and antibacterial. Arbutin is antimicrobial, including against *Candida albicans* and bacteria associated with non-gonococcal urethritis.

Extract of the whole plant is antimicrobial, including against *Candida albicans*,[52] and an hydroethanolic extract effective against *Neisseria gonorrhoeae*.

Dosages: 4.5–12g per day, a cold-water extract of leaves gives the best levels of arbutin and lower levels of tannins compared to hot water extraction.

Daily dose: 13.5–36ml of 1:3.
Typical weekly dose: 15–30ml of 1:3.

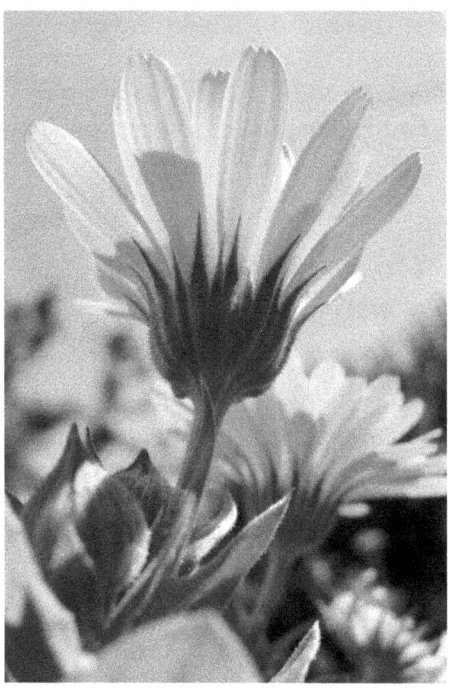

Calendula officinalis

Preclinical: in vitro ethanol extracts have antifungal and antimicrobial activity.[53] Aqueous extracts show antibacterial effect against both Gram-positive and Gram-negative strains.[54]

Clinical studies:
BV: local application of extract of *C. officinalis* was as effective as metronidazole.[55]

VVC: Calendula vaginal cream was effective, with a delayed but greater long-term effect compared to clotrimazole.[56]

Dosages: used in pessaries, cream or as a local wash.

Echinacea angustifolia/purpurea, Baptisia tinctora and Thuja occidentalis

Clinical studies (not related to infectious vaginitis):
The combination is more effective than the individual herbs, and all have slightly different actions so the sum total is more than the

individual. It is found to be effective for acute and chronic infections of the upper respiratory infections and common cold,[57,58] and as an adjuvant to antibiotics in severe bacterial infections such as bronchitis, pharyngitis, otitis media and sinusitis.[59] Although no studies are related specifically to vaginal infections, the support of non-specific immunity seems commonsense.

Dosages
Echinacea angustifolia/purpurea radix mix: daily dose 4.5–9ml of 1:3 60%.
Typical weekly dose 20–50ml of 1:3.
Baptisia tinctora: daily dose 3–9ml of 1:3 60%.
Typical weekly dose 15–25ml of 1:3.
Thuja occidentalis: daily dose 1.5–3ml of 1:5 60%.
Typical weekly dose 10–15ml of 1:3.

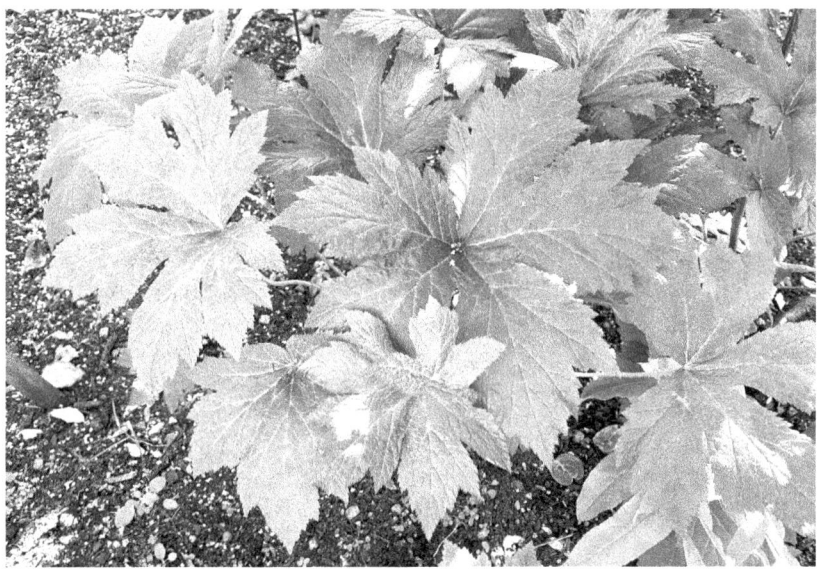

Hydrastis canadensis: endangered so only use cultivated sources.

Goldenseal belongs to the buttercup family *Ranunculaceae*, which also includes *Anemone pulsatilla* and *Actaea racemosus*, herbs regularly utilised in gynaecological treatment.

Actions: anti-haemorrhagic, anti-catarrhal, mucous membrane trophorestorative, antimicrobial, antibacterial, bitter tonic, anti-inflammatory, possibly oxytocic.

Historical use: early settlers of America learnt of the virtues of Goldenseal from the Native Americans. It was a very popular herb mentioned in the *Eclectic Dispensatory of the United States* (now *American Dispensatory*) in 1852; traditionally the rhizome and rootlets are the parts used, and extensive harvesting alongside destruction of their woodland habitat led to Goldenseal becoming endangered by the 1900s.

The Eclectics suggest that it decreased congestion of the genitourinary tract by action upon the mucous and glandular structures, indicated in disorders of a sub-acute character and in atonic states with increased flow of mucus. Thought to have beneficial action in 'fungoid endometritis, lacerated cervix, and pelvic cellulitis', used both locally (externally) and internally. Effective in '*leucorrhoea*, as well as for *gonorrhoea*. For this purpose it may frequently be combined with aqueous thuja.'[60]

Preclinical studies: *H. canadensis* extracts in vitro against MRSA, the leaves demonstrated a more potent antimicrobial activity than the alkaloid berberine alone; *H. canadensis* leaf extracts possess a mixture of constituents that act against MRSA via several different mechanisms.[61]

Berberine: in vitro inhibits growth of *Candida albicans*,[62] *Trichomoniasis vaginalis*,[63] and BV. In vivo increased the effectiveness of amphotericin in the treatment of systemic candidiasis.[64]

Clinical studies: none with *H. canadensis*, but a study using *Berberis vulgaris* vaginally in BV showed a better response when combined with metronidazole gel, with no relapse, compared to the metronidazole alone.[65]

Dosages: mainly used internally in practice for vaginal infection, rather than externally.
Daily dose 3–6ml of 1:5 60%.
Typical weekly dose 10–25ml of 1:5.

Melaleuca alternifolia EO

Preclinical: a fungicidal activity was shown against all strains of *Candida* and only a slightly negative effect on the beneficial vaginal microbiota.[66]

A broad antimicrobial activity against bacteria, fungi and viruses as well as microorganisms that are resistant to conventional drugs.[67]

A small study using a combination of tea tree EO for vaginal *Candida*, alongside vaginal probiotics, showed positive results.[68]

Dosage

5% dilution pessary per vagina to clear infections, not to be used long term.

Caution: may cause skin irritation at higher concentrations and allergic reactions in predisposed individuals.

Thymus vulgaris

Actions: antibacterial, antifungal, antimicrobial.

Historical use: typically used as a lung herb, the Eclectics also used *Thymus* as a mild emmenagogue[69] and for dysmenorrhoea.[70]

Preclinical studies (in vitro):
Thymus vulgaris EO showed a broad spectrum of antibacterial and antifungal activity on bacteria involved in upper respiratory tract infection.[71,72]

Aqueous and ethanolic extracts had an inhibitory effect on *H. pylori*[73] as well as against methicillin resistant staphylococcus aureus.[74]

BV: 90% of subjects with BV show the growth of bacteria in the form of biofilms;[75] thymol demonstrated an inhibition of mature biofilm. Multiple mechanisms of thymol may be acting on different steps in the evolution of biofilm.[76]

Thyme essential oil and thymol alone or in combination with antifungal drugs effective against drug-resistant strains of *Candida* species.[77]

Clinical research: confined to vaginal application and on a range of thymus species.

VVC
Zataira multiflora vaginal cream was as effective as clotrimazole cream.[78]

Vaginal cream containing garlic and thyme as effective as clotrimazole.[79]

VVC and BV
A vaginal gel containing *Thymus vulgaris* and *Eugenia caryophyllus* with *Lactobacillus fermentum* and *L. plantarum* effective for BV as well as VVC.[80]

Other clinical studies of interest: after a single oral dose of thyme dry extract, thymol sulfate could be detected in the human plasma for up to 38 hours, and renal elimination was completed within 24 hours,[81,82] suggesting effective absorption and the ability for systemic action.

Dosages: vaginal pessaries using *Thymus CT (chemotype) linalool EO* 1%; this is a cultivar with low phenolic constituents.
Daily dose 3.6–10ml of 1:3 45%.
Typical weekly dose 10–30ml of 1:3.

Cautions/Contraindications: vaginal applications should avoid *Thymus vulgaris CT thymol*, which contains high levels of highly irritating phenolic constituents.

Probiotics

Preclinical studies
BV
In vivo: probiotics *S. cerevisiae, Clostridium butyricum* reduced the capacity of *G. vaginalis* to bind to vaginal epithelial cells and improved the *lactobacilli* growth to normalise the vaginal microecological balance.[83,84]

VVC
In vitro: *lactobacilli* inhibit the growth of *Candida albicans* and/or its adherence on the vaginal epithelium.[85]

Clinical studies
BV
Women in the first trimester of pregnancy using intravaginal application of live yogurt, led to correction of vaginal pH and *lactobacillus* flora.[86]

Intravaginal application of 5ml of commercial yogurt showed decreases of vaginal discharge, redness and lowered vaginal pH three days after application; all 14 strains of Gram-negative bacteria disappeared.[87]

Oral use of probiotics (*L. rhamnosus* and *L. reuteri*) restored the health of vaginal microbiota,[88] and meta-analysis suggest probiotic regimes in a mixture of oral and vaginal use are helpful for BV treatment.[89]

VVC
Oral and or intravaginally: *lactobacilli*, especially *L. acidophilus, L. rhamnosus* and *L. fermentum* prevented the colonisation and infection of the vagina by *C. albicans*, although not all studies confirm this.[90]

Table 5.1: Clinical studies: other herbal vaginal applications

Herb	Clinical evidence	Condition
Achillea millefolium	Vaginal cream of aqueous extract as effective as clotrimazole.[91]	VVC
Anethum graveolens	Suppositories effective in reducing clinical and microbiological symptoms of VVC.[92]	VVC
Commiphora molmol	Small trial: pts with metronidazole and tinidazole resistant Trichomoniasis were given *C. molmol* 2 × 300mg/capsule for 6 to 8 days showing promising results.[93] 10–11.5ml of 1:5 90%, short-term use would be fine.	Trichomoniasis
Curcumin	Curcumin-based vaginal 10% cream effective for vaginal discharge, itching, vulvovaginal irritation, and abnormal smear results.[94] [Preclinical, in vivo: antifungal.[95–97]]	VVC
Myrtus communis	Combination of metronidazole vaginal gel with *Myrtus* extract for bacterial vaginosis, better than metronidazole vaginal gel alone and showed a reduction in recurrence of infection.[98] More effective than clotrimazole vaginal creams for vaginal candida, improvement in vaginal itching and reduction in vaginal discharge.[99,100] Combined with *Quercus infectoria* (oak gall) for treatment of vaginitis; improved vaginal discharge (BV, trichomoniasis) and pH, reverse whiff test.[101] [Preclinical, in vitro: antibacterial.[102–104] In vivo: analgesic and anti-inflammatory effects.[105]]	BV, VVC, trichomoniasis

(Continued)

Table 5.1: (Continued)

Herb	Clinical evidence	Condition
Nigella sativa	Use of oral black cumin capsule with clotrimazole vaginal cream, compared to cream by itself. The combination had a greater effect on the reduction of discharge as well as on the symptoms and signs of vaginitis.[106,107]	VVC
Propolis	Vaginal cream using 10% propolis was similar to clotrimazole in terms of dropped colony count.[108]	VVC
Tribulus terrestris, Myrtus communis, Foeniculum vulgare, Tamarindus indica	Pessary: showed improvement of pH, vaginal discharge, whiff test, presence of clue cells and Gram staining; pelvic pain and cervical inflammation were decreased.[109]	BV
Salvia officinalis	A vaginal tablet: effective against VVC.[110]	VVC
Zingiber officinalis	Cream combined with clotrimazole, more effective than clotrimazole alone.[111] [Preclinical, in vitro: induces apoptosis in T. vaginalis[112]]	VVC In vitro: T. vaginalis

Other preclinical studies of interest

<u>Herbal treatment for trichomoniasis</u> in vitro methanol extracts of P. granatum fructus, black tea, green tea, grape seed and resveratrol extracts found to have anti-parasitic activity.[113]

<u>Verbascum thapsus</u> induction of apoptosis in T. vaginalis.[114]

5.4 Dietary and lifestyle recommendations

Promoting a healthy gut microbiome: Lactobacilli colonising the rectum may be a reservoir for vaginal lactobacilli and may contribute to the maintenance of vaginal microflora.[115]

- Avoid sugar and refined carbohydrates.
- Diet rich in fibre, vegetables and fruits.
- Fermented foods (yogurt, kefir, sauerkraut).
- High-fat diets are thought to have a negative effect, possibly because this alters the composition of the gut microbiome, affecting the pH.[116]
- Prebiotics to stimulate the growth of the body's indigenous lactobacilli, which affects the composition of the intestinal microflora and its metabolic activity (garlic, chicory, artichokes, asparagus, onions, bananas, etc.)

Table 5.2: Clinical studies: bacterial vaginosis and specific foods

Diet and nutrient	Studies with BV
Increase fibre, fruit and vegetables	Low fibre intake was associated with increased incidence of BV.[117]
Reduce dietary fat intake	The risk of severe BV was higher in women with higher total fat intake.[118] High fat may increase vaginal pH, thereby increasing the risk of BV, and/or may alter the vaginal microflora, which may increase the vaginal pH and increase the risk of BV.
Increase intake of folate, vitamin A, C, E, beta carotene, calcium	Increased intake of folate, vitamin A and calcium may decrease the risk of severe BV.[119] Low serum folate is associated with impaired T cell and neutrophil function, and deficiency of folate is associated with an increased risk of BV in pregnancy.[120] Lower concentrations of vitamins A, C, E and beta-carotene were associated with an increased risk of BV in women with HIV.[121,122]
Ensure healthy iron levels in the diet	Subclinical iron deficiency (measured based on soluble transferrin receptor) can be a significant predictor of BV.[123]
Serum vitamin D	Conflicting results, some studies associated low vitamin D with increased risk of BV. A lower mean plasma concentration of 25-OH-D and folate among women diagnosed with BV during pregnancy.[124]

(Continued)

Table 5.2: (Continued)

Diet and nutrient	Studies with BV
Diet low in glycaemic load	Diet high in glycaemic load is associated with greater BV prevalence and an increase in BV persistence and acquisition.[125]
Diet rich in betaine: bran and wheatgerm, goji berries, spinach or beets, seafood (especially marine invertebrates), quinoa	Higher intake of betaine reduces the risk of BV and BV-related symptoms;[126] like folate and vitamin B12 it is a 'methyl donor'.[127] Betaine protects cells, proteins and enzymes from environmental stress and, as a methyl donor, plays an important role in hepatic, cardiovascular and renal health.

See Appendix for food sources.

Table 5.3: Clinical studies: vulvovaginalis candidiasis

Diet and nutrient	Studies with VVC
Live yogurt and probiotics	Vaginal inflammation in a group that consumed yogurt was decreased threefold.[128]
Avoid sweets and sweet drinks	Avoidance showed a protective effect. This may contribute to the fact that increased glucose concentrations in vaginal secretions could promote the adherence of *Candida* to epithelial cells and further stimulate its development.[129]

Other factors

Stress factors: stress and any sleep disorders can have an impact on the immune system and the pH of the vagina as well as the microflora, regardless which organism is causing the vaginitis. Morning rise salivary cortisol level is blunted in women with recurrent vaginal candidiasis.[130]

Clothing: wearing tights is risk factor for VVC.[131] Other risk factors for VVC involved synthetic underclothing, frequently wearing tight underpants.[132] As VVC often coexists with other infections, including BV, it is good general advice to avoid this in any form of vaginitis.

Contraceptive use: condom use was a protective factor helping to prevent against VVC as well as other infections, partly due to sperm altering the vaginal pH, but also because it reduces exposure to infectious organisms.

There is a possible link between IUD use and VVC;[133] all parts of the IUD allow the adherence of yeasts. This might be helpful to keep in mind with other infections.

Exercise: sedentary life increases the susceptibility to VVC almost eightfold; one could speculate that increasing exercise relieves stress, as well as a positively influencing pelvic circulation and the immune system.[134]

CHAPTER 6

Ovarian cysts

6.1 Presentation/symptoms, differential diagnosis and investigations

Ovarian cysts are sacs usually filled with fluid, in an ovary or on its surface. Ovarian cysts can be benign or malignant. If they become large, the increased weight may cause the ovary to rotate on itself (ovarian torsion), cutting off the blood supply, and may result in rupture and/or haemorrhage. This presents with extreme abdominal pain and is an emergency, as it can cause destruction of ovarian tissue, infection such as peritonitis, and infertility.

Most of us are familiar with PCOS, but these are not the only kind of ovarian cysts!

Their prevalence is unknown as they are usually asymptomatic and undiagnosed, discovered incidentally on imaging. It is postulated that about 20% of women develop at least one ovarian cyst in their lifetime.[1]

An ultrasound will not be able to distinguish between benign and malignant cysts; a biopsy is needed for a definitive Dx. Cysts in post-menopausal women have a higher risk of malignancy and should always be investigated further.[2]

Symptoms

Most cysts do not cause symptoms, but larger ovarian cysts can cause:

- Adnexal or cervical motion tenderness.
- Irregular cycle and/or abnormal vaginal bleeding in hormone-producing cysts.
- Other symptoms arising from complications, see below.
- Unilateral pelvic pain: a dull or sharp ache in the lower abdomen, intermittent or constant.
- Symptoms related to pressure: tenesmus or urinary frequency.
- Underlying malignancy: weight loss/cachexia, lymphadenopathy, abdominal discomfort, fullness, heaviness, bloating, indigestion, heartburn, or quickly feeling full after eating.

Complications

<u>Torsion, rupture and haemorrhage</u>: complete or partial twisting of the ovarian vessels resulting in obstruction of blood flow to the ovary, which can be associated with trauma, exercise or coitus. Symptoms: sudden, sharp, unilateral pelvic pain, which can lead to peritoneal signs, abdominal distension and bleeding, hyperpyrexia, tachycardia and hypotension.

<u>Some cysts can become malignant</u>: this may cause symptoms of weight loss/cachexia, lymphadenopathy, abdominal discomfort, fullness, heaviness, bloating, indigestion, heartburn or feeling full after eating.

Risk factors for ovarian cysts[3]

- Endometriosis
- Hypothyroidism
- Infertility treatment (Clomid): ovarian hyperstimulation syndrome.
- Pelvic infection, if spread to the ovaries can cause cysts.
- Pregnancy as ovarian cysts may form in the second trimester when hCG levels peak.[4]
- Previous ovarian cyst
- Smoking
- Tamoxifen

- Tubal ligation sterilisation has been associated with functional cysts.[5]

Investigations

- Cancer antigen 125 (CA125) protein is found on the cell membrane of healthy ovarian tissue as well as on ovarian carcinomas. It tends to be elevated in advanced epithelial ovarian cancers. However, early on, this is often within normal range. It can also be mildly elevated in endometriosis, fibroids, pelvic inflammatory disease, pregnancy, peritonitis, cholecystitis and pancreatitis.
- Endocervical swabs to rule out infection, such as PID.
- Laparotomy and laparoscopy, also enabling a biopsy, which will enable a definitive diagnosis of all ovarian cysts.
- Physical examination: palpation on abdominal examination may find a mass/tenderness (ascites may interfere with palpation).
- Transvaginal ultrasonography.
- Urinalysis to rule out UTI, kidney stones.

It is helpful to have a full medical history, including gynaecological history and family history.

Differential diagnosis of acute symptoms related to torsion rupture:
- Appendicitis
- Diverticulitis
- Ectopic pregnancy
- Nephrolithiasis
- Psoas abscess
- UTI

Conventional treatment

Monitor, unless the woman is postmenopausal: in these cases intervention is warranted.

OCP is often given for recurrent functional cysts, as they prevent ovulation. The positive side to OCP use is that long-term use is associated with a lower risk of developing ovarian cancer.

If cyst does not resolve, and begins or continues to grow, surgery might be recommended.

6.2 Pathophysiology of ovarian cysts

There are many kinds of cysts, often found incidentally on ultrasound (US). The increasing incidence may be due to more widespread use of US. Depending on the size, the usual method would be to observe over several cycles—a 'wait and see' approach is usually appropriate to smaller cysts.

Functional or physiologic cysts: these occur during the reproductive years and not after the menopause. In a normal cycle numerous follicles are formed with one dominant follicle maturing and undergoing ovulation.

- **Follicular cysts:** larger than 2.5cm in diameter are common. This can be a consequence of either the most mature follicle failing to release its ovum and continuing to grow, forming a cyst, or one/some of the other developing follicles failing to disintegrate and forming a cyst. A possible cause of an ovum not being released may be excessive FSH stimulation or absence of the normal LH surge at mid-cycle so that growth continues. As a consequence excess oestradiol production may cause decreased frequency of menstruation. A follicular cyst will usually be reabsorbed without causing any problems. They do occasionally rupture, however, as they are small and tend not to contain blood; a rupture may not cause significant pain.
- **Corpus luteal cysts:** can grow to 3cm. In this case, fluid accumulates inside the follicle, causing the corpus luteum to grow into a cyst. A luteal cyst can cause dull pain on one side. If large enough, they may occasionally rupture, causing mild pain, but no treatment is needed. Luteal cysts may interfere with progesterone production and can cause irregularities in the cycle, delaying the onset of menstruation, or cause an alteration in blood loss during the period. Luteal cysts usually disappear after one cycle.
- **Haemorrhagic cysts:** both follicular cysts and luteal cysts can turn into haemorrhagic cysts. Usually they are asymptomatic and will spontaneously resolve without treatment.[6] Large blood-filled cysts can be associated with pain and may be confused with ruptured ectopic pregnancy or other causes of abdominal pain.

Polycystic ovary syndrome (PCOS): this is defined as a clinical syndrome and not by the presence of ovarian cysts. Ovaries may be enlarged, with many 2 to 6mm follicular cysts, seen on imaging as a characteristic 'string of pearls'.

Endometriomas: this is endometriosis on the ovaries, commonly referred to as 'chocolate cysts' as they contain dark, thick, gelatinous aged blood products. They tend to grow with each period and are prone to rupture, even when quite small, causing severe pain.

Theca lutein cysts: luteinised follicle cysts, caused by overstimulation in elevated hCG levels in pregnancy, gestational trophoblastic disease, multiple gestation and ovarian hyperstimulation.

Neoplastic cysts: overgrowth of cells within the ovary, malignant or benign.

Dermoid cysts (teratomas): cells that produce ovum develop abnormally and contain elements from all three germ layers—mainly from ectodermal, but also mesodermal and endodermal—and can produce structures including hair, teeth, bones and skin fragments. These will not resolve spontaneously. Mostly benign but can become malignant in 1–2% of cases.[7]

Hormone-producing cysts (functioning cysts): cells that normally produce hormones develop abnormally, interfering with the cycle and fertility.

Cystadenomas: developing on the surface of an ovary, these are filled with a watery or mucous material and can become large, sometimes attached to the ovary by a stem or pedicle. Torsion will lead to extreme pain, vomiting and rupture. Incomplete or intermittent torsion usually causes episodic pain. There is a risk of ovarian damage due to ischaemia; these rarely reabsorb.

Cystadenocarcinoma: malignant.

Fibromas: slow-growing connective tissue tumours, these are usually <7cm in diameter, occasionally can produce oestrogen.

Brenner tumours: rare ovarian tumours developing from the surface ovarian epithelium and sometimes associated with abnormal periods. These are small and benign, but can become malignant and are more common in post-menopausal women.

Ovarian cancer: rare and symptom-free until it is relatively advanced. Ovarian cysts in post-menopausal women should always be regarded as suspicious.

6.3 Herbal management of ovarian cysts

Herbal treatment is not always appropriate; always refer post-menopausal women.

Functional cysts under 5cm: 'wait and see', as these will usually resolve within two cycles. If the cyst does not resolve after several menstrual cycles, it is unlikely to be a functional cyst and further investigation is needed.[8]

For larger persistent ovarian cysts surgical removal may need to be considered to prevent infertility as a consequence of torsion and rupture.

Pregnancy-associated cysts usually resolve by 14 to 16 weeks of gestation.[9]

Aims

Treat the relevant underlying condition
Prevent recurrence by encouraging clearance by supporting immune and lymphatic systems
Ensure and encourage ovulation using hormone modulators and improving pelvic circulation

Herbal management

Improve pelvic circulation using uterine tonics and/or emmenagogues, as the development of recurrent cysts suggests stagnation, especially of the pelvic area.

Achillea millefolium, Alchemilla vulgaris, Angelica sinensis, Artemisia absinthum, Artemisia vulgaris, Cinnamomum zeylanicum, Zingiber officinalis.

Promote elimination and support the immune system using anti-inflammatories, lymphatics and immune modulators.

Anti-inflammatories: *Achillea millefolium, Actaea racemosa, Alchemilla vulgaris, Curcuma longa.*

Immune modulators: *Astragalus membranaceus, Echinacea angustifolia/purpurea, Thuja occidentalis.*

Lymphatics: *Calendula officinalis, Phytolacca decandra, Thuja occidentalis.*

Address any hormonal influences: reduce FSH, LH and possibly oestrogen, ensure clearance of excess hormones.

Hormonal modulators: *Actaea racemosus, Vitex agnus-castus.*

Hormone clearance: Promote a healthy gut flora with fibre, flax seed, *Artemisia absinthum, Berberis vulgaris, Carduus marianus* and *Tarax* radix.

Ensure proper ovulation

Steroidal saponin-rich herbs: *Chamaelirium lutea, Dioscorea villosa,* etc.

There is one clinical study of interest using Ziziphus jujuba: comparing high-dose contraceptive pill with jujube on functional ovary cyst regression. It was found to be as effective as the oral contraceptive, but as functional cysts commonly will disappear on their own, one would need to check and compare reoccurrence.[10]

CHAPTER 7

Polycystic ovarian syndrome (PCOS)

7.1 Presentation/symptoms, differential diagnosis and investigations

This is a complex condition: first, it should be understood that polycystic ovary syndrome (PCOS) is a metabolic/endocrine disorder, related to elevated androgens, fasting insulin and an abnormal relative ratio of LH and FSH. This leads to disordered ovarian folliculogenesis, chronic anovulation, clinical signs of hyperandrogenism and metabolic syndrome.[1]

It has been suggested that the condition has beneficial effects during times of famine, as those with PCOS may maintain fertility better when calorie intake is reduced.[2]

Some 5 to 10% of women of reproductive age are thought to have PCOS; it is a common cause of anovulatory infertility.

Symptoms

- Amenorrhoea, oligomenorrhoea or an unpredictable menstrual cycle: eight or fewer menstrual cycles per year. There can be excessive bleeding due to anovulatory cycles.

- Hyperandrogenism: hirsutism and/or thinning of the head hair or male pattern balding, acne vulgaris, deeper voice and change in body structure.
- Hyperinsulinaemia: overweight, difficulty losing weight, especially around trunk, an apple body shape. Acanthosis nigricans, a pigmented velvety lesion, which is a marker of insulin resistance.
- Infertility, recurrent miscarriages.
- Multiple ovarian follicles on ultrasound: high levels of androgens inhibit FSH, affecting development and maturation of the follicles,[3] thereby increasing the number of immature follicles causing the typical US 'string of pearls' morphology.[4]

Family history

- Baldness on the male side of the family
- Diabetes
- Menstrual irregularities

Long-term issues

- Increased risk of endometrial cancer as a result of long-standing unopposed oestrogen stimulation.
- Increased risk of CVD, abnormalities in lipid profiles.

Diagnosis

The diagnostic criteria for PCOS requires two of the following:

1. Oligo-ovulation or anovulation, infertility.
2. Clinical and/or biochemical hyperandrogenism.
3. Polycystic ovary morphology on ultrasound: >10 follicles per ovary, usually occurring on the periphery and resembling a string of pearls.

Differential diagnosis

At puberty it is normal to have some anovulatory cycles and relative excess androgen and LH as a result of spurts in growth hormone. However, it is possible that early weight gain can be a factor in the development of PCOS.[5]

Exclude:
- Adrenal virilism
- Cushing's syndrome
- Other causes of amenorrhoea (see relevant chapter)

Investigations

Blood tests

- Decreased SHBG.
- Increased fasting insulin or fasting glucose: fasting insulin levels of 10–14 IU/L are indicative, >20 IU/L are diagnostic.
- Increased LH and serum LH:FSH ratio >2.
- Increased oestrone levels; oestradiol can be increased but typically is low or normal.
- Increased prolactin in some cases.
- Increased serum androgen.

Ultrasound, polycystic ovary morphology.

Conventional treatment

Clomiphene (this is an oestrogen agonist or antagonist, depending on the target tissue): inhibits oestrogen negative feedback at the hypothalamus, enhancing the pituitary's production of FSH to improve ovulation and fertility for those wishing to conceive.

Metformin (hypoglycaemic): reduces fasting insulin levels, blood pressure and low-density lipoprotein cholesterol, ameliorates hyperandrogenism. Also decreases serum LH concentration and increases sex hormone-binding globulin (SHBG) concentration.[6] Side effects include: nausea, vomiting, diarrhoea, bloating and abdominal pain, loss of appetite, metallic taste in the mouth, lactic acidosis and deficiency of vitamin B12.

OCP: used for acne, hirsutism and irregular menses. It increases levels of SHBG, as well as decreasing androgen secretion. The combined pill can negatively affect insulin resistance.

Progesterone: to trigger withdrawal bleeding.

Spironolactone (diuretic, aldosterone antagonist): for acne and hirsutism. It inhibits binding of dihydrotestosterone (DHT) to receptors at the hair follicle sites.

7.2 Pathophysiology of PCOS

Metabolic/Endocrine syndrome

This is a complex condition. First of all, it should be understood that PCOS is a metabolic/endocrine disorder related to elevated androgens and fasting insulin, and an abnormal relative ratio of LH and FSH. This leads to disordered ovarian folliculogenesis, chronic anovulation, clinical signs of hyperandrogenism and metabolic syndrome.[7]

Excess weight: not all of those with PCOS are obese but many will have an element of insulin resistance, affecting serum LH and androgen levels.[8] An increase in fatty tissue leads to the conversion of androgens to oestrone via aromatisation, increasing the levels of acyclic oestrogens.

Insulin resistance, leading to hyperinsulinaemia: insulin actions are mediated by insulin receptors found in the ovary and the adrenal cortex. Insulin resistance causes higher pulsatile output of LH[9] and elevated LH to FSH ratio (2:1).[10] Excessive LH decreases hepatic SHBG synthesis.[11] LH alongside elevated insulin levels stimulates mainly ovarian androgen secretion and some adrenal androgen secretion.[12]

Leptin: leptin is a 'satiety hormone' made by adipose cells to regulate energy balance by inhibiting hunger. Higher leptin levels correlate with insulin resistance, metabolic disorder, infertility and increased cardiovascular disease risk.[13] Women with PCOS tend to have increased serum levels of leptin.[14] Involved in regulating energy homeostasis, leptin concentrations fluctuate during the menstrual cycle,[15] which has been shown to affect follicular maturation[16] and the development of obesity.[17] It is possible that insulin stimulates leptin secretion.[18]

Hormone dysregulation

Hyperprolactinemia: some PCOS patients have elevated prolactin levels resulting from abnormal feedback via the pituitary gland. Prolactin has an inhibitory effect on the production of FSH and elevates the production of LH, reducing aromatase activity, increasing androgens and worsening the scenario for women with PCOS. Elevated prolactin can also contribute to lower progesterone,[19] and prolactin can increase with stress.

Hyperandrogenism: mainly ovarian in origin, although both the ovaries and adrenal glands produce androgens. This inhibits FSH, so affecting development and maturation of the follicles,[20] thereby increasing the number of immature follicles causing the typical US 'string of pearls' morphology seen in PCOS.[21]

DHEA (an adrenal androgen) is elevated in some with PCOS due to stimulation by ACTH, produced by the pituitary in response to stress; stress can contribute to elevated androgen levels.[22] Aromatisation increases the conversion of androgen to oestrogens (a process stimulated by FSH), especially in the fat cells. Peripheral aromatisation increases with body weight, causing chronic hyper-oestrogen production (oestrogen dominance).

Oestrogen dominance: as a consequence of aromatisation detailed above. Oestrogen levels can be normal but tend not to be fluctuating, that is, not cyclic, compared to a normal menstrual cycle.

HPO axis: the negative feedback mechanism is affected, and it is suggested that those with PCOS require higher progesterone and oestradiol concentrations.[23]

Subclinical hypothyroidism: hypothyroidism has overlapping features with PCOS; polycystic-appearing ovaries are a clinical feature of hypothyroidism.[24]

Anti-Müllerian hormone (AMH): concentrations are often higher in women with PCOS, especially in those who are obese.[25] AMH reflects ovarian reserve and correlates to the number of growing follicles.[26] AMH is essential for normal cyclic ovulation; promoting preantral follicle survival, it negatively impacts later stages of antral follicle maturation.[27]

Endogenous opioids

These are involved in the regulation of pancreatic function, hepatic insulin clearance and glucose metabolism. There is an interaction between the sex steroids and the opioid system in both GnRH secretion and glucose metabolism. A dysregulation of the opioid system might play a part in PCOS. The opioid system effects on glucose metabolism also appear to be modulated by obesity.[28]

It is interesting to note that herbs that have been classified as influencing hormones have also been shown to have an effect on the opiate receptors.

Vitex agnus-castus: acted as an agonist at the mu-opiate receptor, supporting its beneficial action in PMS.[29,30]

Actaea racemosa: contains active principle(s) that activates mu-opiate receptor, supporting its beneficial role in alleviating menopausal symptoms.[31]

Decreased microbiome diversity

Women with PCOS often show a lack of gut microbiome diversity, which has been linked with hyperandrogenism.[32] There is a connection between intestinal bacteria and sex hormones, insulin resistance, hyperandrogenism and chronic low-grade inflammation. Raised inflammatory factors are part of the clinical picture of obesity and PCOS (increased TNF-α, IL-6).[33] Pro and pre-biotics are associated with improved effects on metabolic, hormonal and inflammatory issues.

7.3 Herbal management of PCOS

As a complex condition it is important to address multiple targets using a range of herbs. There will be an overlap in the areas of treatment identified below. Addressing insulin resistance will also have an element of hormone modulation, as will the regulation of menstruation. There will be some inevitable overlap also in the action of the herbs; all will have slightly different mechanisms of action and multiple target areas.

Aims

Treat any underlying insulin resistance/metabolic syndrome, regulate menstruation/ovulation, modulate hormones
Improve pelvic circulation, ensure effective elimination
Protect against the negative effects of stress

Herbal management

Treat insulin resistance/metabolic syndrome and address weight issues

Losing even a small amount of weight can make a difference in regularity of cycle as well as symptoms related to androgen excess. Metformin, commonly given to PCOS patients, improves insulin resistance, weight, regulates ovulation and has been shown to reduce serum levels of oestradiol, LH, insulin and androgens. This illustrates the interconnectedness of hormones and insulin. Similarly, many herbs are known to work on glucose metabolism and insulin resistance, using multiple pathways, and have been shown to have a positive effect on the ovaries and ovulation.

Hypoglycaemic herbs: *Cinnamomum zeylanicum, Galega officinalis, Gymnema sylvestris, Panax ginseng, Trigonella foenum-graceum.*

Herbs with potential effects on leptin:

Preclinical studies: *Actaea racemosa* reduced serum leptin concentration in vivo.[34] *Vitex* leaf[35] and *Vitex* fructus reduced leptin in vivo.[36]

Clinical study: *Linum sativum* in a controlled trial on 14 women with PCOS showed a range of positive effects including reduced leptin.[37]

Hormone modulation

Treat relative oestrogen excess: Polyphenolic phytoestrogenic herbs (*Linum sativum*, soya, *Trifolium repens*) can be used to displace endogenous oestrogen and reduce relative excess. Treat the liver to encourage oestrogen metabolism, maintain healthy gut microbiome to aid increased absorption of phytoestrogens and improve digestive function to inhibit endogenous oestrogens reentering the circulation (see book 1).

Increase SHBG, which binds to both oestrogen and androgen; an increase of SHBG will reduce free circulating levels of both. Include support of the thyroid, as low function reduces synthesis of SHBG.

Linum sativum, Urtica radix.

Herbs to modulate thyroid function: *Fucus vesiculosus* (if there is an iodine deficiency), *Nigella sativa, Turnera diffusa, Withania sominfera,* and adaptogens such as *Panax ginseng, Rhodiola rosea.*

Stimulate ovulation with steroidal saponin-rich herbs: *Asparagus racemosa, Chamaelirium luteum, Tribulus terrestris.*

Dopaminergic herbs to lower prolactin levels, and regulate the cycle. It is interesting to note that some of the herbs typically used as hypoglycaemics, such as *Galega officinalis, Trigonella* would also be used as galactagogues, suggestive of an effect on prolactin levels. *Vitex*, beside being a dopaminergic herb, is also a galactogogue.

Actaea racemosa, Paeonia lactiflora & Glycyrrhiza glabra, Vitex agnus-castus.

Stress increases prolactin levels, so the use of nervines, adaptogens, lifestyle adaptations, alongside dopaminergic herbs can be of benefit. Hyperprolactinamia will inhibit aromatisation activity, reducing the androgen to oestrogen conversion.

Anti-androgenic herbs to treat the symptoms related to androgen excess, such as acne and hirsutism.

It is frequently stated that *Paeonia lactiflora & Glycyrrhiza glabra* reduce androgen levels by stimulating aromatase activity, reinforced by reducing prolactin levels. The overall effect increases the potential for ovulation and therefore indirectly increases progesterone levels.

Herbs with anti-androgenic effect: *Mentha spicata, Paeonia lactiflora & Glycyrrhiza glabra, Serenoa serrulata, Urtica dioica* radix.

Reduce AMH concentrations

Preclinical study: flaxseed and *Foeniculum vulgare* in vivo.[38]

Clinical study in women with PCOS: the combination of *Lagerstroemia spesiosa & Cinnamomum burmannii*[39] reduced AMH levels.

Regulate menstruation (see chapters on amenorrhoea and infertility)

Ensure healthy pelvic circulation

Uterine tonics/emmenagogues to support normal function: *Actaea racemosa, Artemisia spp., Caulophyllum thalictroides, Mitchella repens, Ruta graveolens.*

Ensure effective elimination and healthy digestive function

Increase microbiome diversity, support liver and other digestive organs.

Clinical study: a PCOS meta-analysis showed that SHBG and nitric oxide concentration increased significantly in pro and pre-biotic groups.[40]

- Berberine-rich herbs plus *Artemisia absinthum*
- Inulin-rich herbs and food such as *Arctium lappa, Asparagus racemosus, Cynara scolymus, Taraxacum* radix
- Fermented foods
- Pro and pre-biotics

Support the ability to deal with stress

Adaptogens: *Angelica sinensis, Rhodiola rosea, Withania somnifera.*
Nervines: *Leonurus cardiaca* when anxiety and palpitations are present, *Verbena officinalis.*

Table 7.1: Clinical studies: herbs

Effects	Clinical studies	Preclinical
Decrease fasting blood sugar levels, improve insulin resistance	*Aloe vera*[41–43] *Camellia sinensis*[44,45] *Cinnamomum zeylanicum*[46] Flaxseed[47] *Glycyrrhiza* spp.[48,49] *Grifola frondosa*[50] *Matricaria chamomilla*[51–53] *Nigella sativa*[54] *Panax ginseng*[55–57] *Origanum majorana*[58] Soya isoflavones[59] *Tribulus terrestris*[60] *Trigonella foenum-graecum*[61] *Zingiber offinalis*[62,63]	*Actaea racemosa* (diabetic and menopausal models)[64–66] *Galega officinalis*[67] *Gymnema sylvestre*[68–70]
Improve lipid levels	*Aloe vera*[71] *Cinnamomum zeylanicum* Flaxseed[72] *Glycine max*[73] *Glycyrrhiza* spp.[74] *Gymnema silvestre*[75] *Matricaria chamomilla*[76–78] *Nigella sativa* oil[79] *Panax ginseng*[80,81] *Trigonella foenum-graecum*	*Actaea racemosa* (diabetic and menopausal models)[82–84] *Tribulus terrestris*[85] *Glycyrrhiza glabra*[86]
Weight loss	*Aloe vera* (diabetic patients)[87,88] *Cinnamomum zeylanicum*[89] *Camellia sinensis*[90,91] Flaxseed[92] *Glycyrrhiza* spp.[93,94] *Gymnema sylvestre*[95] Soya	*Actaea racemosa* (diabetic and menopausal models)[96]

(Continued)

Table 7.1: (Continued)

Effects	Clinical studies	Preclinical
Reduce androgen levels	*Apium graveolens* & *Pimpinella anisum*[97] *Camellia sinensis*[98,99] Flaxseed (case studies)[100–102] *Glycyrrhiza* spp.[103] *Matricaria chamomilla* *Mentha spicata*[104,105] *Origanum majorana* (reduced the levels of adrenal androgens)[106] *Paeonia lactiflora* & *Glycyrrhiza glabra*[107–111] Soya isoflavones[112]	*Actaea racemosa* with vitamin C,[113] *Vitex agnus-castus*[114] Clinical study showing *Vitex* helpful in acne vulgaris,[115] *Serenoa repens*[116]
Regulate menstrual cycle, increase ovulation, improve fertility	*Actaea racemosa*[117] *Anethum graveolens* & *Asparagus racemosus*[118] *Apium graveolens* & *Pimpinella anisum*[119] *Cinnamomum cassia*[120–123] *Grifola frondosa*[124] *Nigella sativa*[125] *Paeonia lactiflora* & *Cinnamomum cassia*[126,127] *Paeonia lactiflora* & *Glycyrrhiza glabra*[128,129] *Trigonella foenum-graecum*[130] *Vitex agnus castus*[131–136]	Flaxseed,[137] *Glycyrrhiza uralensis*,[138] *Paeonia lactiflora* & *Glycyrrhiza glabra*,[139,140] *Trifolium pratense*,[141] *Tribulus terrestris*[142]
Improve progesterone levels	*Actaea racemosa*[143,144] *Paeonia lactiflora* & *Glycyrrhiza glabra*[145] *Vitex agnus castus*	Flaxseed,[146] *Foeniculum vulgare*[147] Intraperitoneal use of *Zingiber officinale*[148]
Lower prolactin levels	*Paeonia lactiflora* & *Glycyrrhiza glabra*[149] *Vitex agnus castus*[150–153]	*Serenoa serrulata*[154,155]

(Continued)

Table 7.1: (Continued)

Effects	Clinical studies	Preclinical
Effect on leptin		*Actaea racemosa*,[156] flaxseed,[157] *Vitex agnus-castus*[158]
Reduce LH	*Actaea racemosa*[159] *Paeonia lactiflora & Cinnamomum cassia*[160]	*Vitex agnus-castus*[161]
LH:FSH ratio lowered	*Actaea racemosa*[162] *Apium graveolens & Pimpinella anisum*[163] *Foeniculum vulgare*[164] *Matricaria chamomilla*[165] *Paeonia lactiflora & Glycyrrhiza glabra*[166]	
Lower AMH	*Lagerstroemia spesiosa* (Pride of India, Rose of India, Queen's Crape Myrtle) & *Cinnamomum burmannii*[167]	
Decrease ovarian volume, reduce cyst number	*Anethum graveolens & Asparagus racemosus*[168,169] *Linum usitatissimum*[170] *Stachys lavandulifolia*[171] *Trigonella foenum-graecum*[172,173]	*Glycyrrhiza uralensis*,[174] *Linum usitatissimum*,[175] *Mentha spicata & Trifolium pratense*,[176] *Tribulus terrestris*[177]
Reduce hirsutism	*Anethum graveolens & Asparagus racemosus*[178] *Mentha spicata*[179,180] Flaxseed case report[181–183] *Foeniculum vulgare* cream[184–186] *Glycyrrhiza* spp. topical use[187]	

Key herbs used in clinical practice

Actaea racemosa (see book 1)

The Eclectic physicians used it for amenorrhoea, dysmenorrhoea, ovarian pain and menorrhagia.

Preclinical

PCOS model: the combination of *Actaea racemosa* with vitamin C was found to be more effective than *Actaea* by itself, reversing the dysregulated levels of testosterone and LH. It regulated both ovarian and hepatic malondialdehyde and glutathione (GSH) levels, with histological improvement observed in the liver and ovaries.[188]

Menopausal and diabetic models: lowered LH,[189,190] reduced leptin, cholesterol and glucose levels,[191,192] reduced and prevented body weight gain, reduced intra-abdominal fat accumulation, improved glucose metabolism and insulin sensitivity.[193,194]

Clinical trials

PCOS with infertility:
Adding *Actaea* to clomiphene with timed intercourse improved cycle outcomes and pregnancy rates. Improvements seen in serum levels of mid-luteal and mid-cycle oestradiol and LH as well as mid-luteal progesterone, plus higher clinical pregnancies per cycle.[195]

Comparing clomiphene (100mg daily for 5 days) to *Actaea* (20mg daily for 10 days): favourable changes seen in LH level and FSH/LH ratio; progesterone level was higher from the first treatment cycle, indicating better ovulation and greater endometrial thickness. The pregnancy rate was higher in the *Actaea* group (though not statistically significant).[196]

Dosage: The average dose used in clinical trials is 1.8ml of a 1:3 per week. Most UK herbalists would use 10ml of a 1:3 per week. Higher doses have not been found to be more effective for menopausal symptoms. Note: 60% alcohol is needed to extract the triterpene glycosides.

Daily dose clinical trials used 80mg per day; this translates to 0.25ml of 1:3.

Typical weekly dose 5–10ml of 1:3.

Cinnamomum zeylanicum

Clinical studies related to diabetes type 1 and 2 have shown that cinnamon has a beneficial effect on glycaemic control (both HbA1c and FPG).[197] It reduced insulin resistance and levels of fasting plasma glucose, as well as total cholesterol, LDL-cholesterol and triglycerides, and modestly increased levels of HDL-cholesterol.[198]

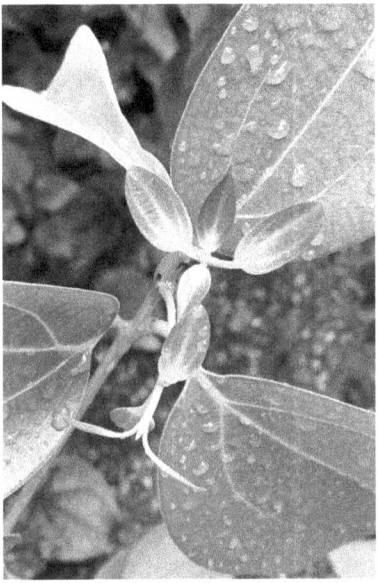

Cinnamomum verum

Preclinical studies in PCOS models
Cinnamomum was compared to metformin; both improved insulin resistance, lowered testosterone and LH.[199]

Clinical studies with PCOS patients normalised menstrual cycles, enabled PCOS patients to manage their metabolic parameters, and had a positive effect on hormonal status. Improvement was seen in glucose metabolism and lipid profile, with a reduction in insulin resistance.[200–205] A clinical study, where *Cinnamomum* was used alongside *Lagerstroemia spesiosa* (Pride of India, Rose of India, Queen's Crape Myrtle) showed reduced anti-Müllerian hormone.[206]

Dosage: 500mg to 6g per day used in trials.[207]
Daily dose 4.5–9ml of 1:3.
Typical weekly dose 10–25ml of 1:3.

Glycyrrhiza spp.

Ancient Hindus believed that licorice increased sexual vigour, which could be contradictory as it has been shown to reduce testosterone levels. Studies indicated that *Glycyrrhiza* has anti-androgenic effects and blocks

17-hydroxysteroid dehydrogenase, which catalyses the conversion of androstenedione to testosterone and also blocks 17,20-lyase in the ovaries and the adrenals.[208] *Glycyrrhiza* has been shown to decrease the secretion of testosterone in healthy women.[209] Glycyrrhizin and glycyrrhetinic acid are also known to suppress 5 beta-reductase and thus delay the clearance of corticosteroids and prolong the biological half-life of cortisol.[210]

Preclinical studies

Diabetic model: improved glucose tolerance by enhancing insulinotropic action.[211]

PCOS model: reduced free and total testosterone, increased oestradiol. It was suggested that this occurred primarily in the ovary via enhanced aromatisation of testosterone to 17-beta oestradiol and increased ovulation rates.[212,213]

Clinical studies

Clincial study in healthy women: licorice reduced body fat mass without any change in body mass index,[214] improved lipid profile and reduced systolic blood pressure by 10%.[215] In healthy young women (22–26yrs), it showed anti-androgen activity, decreasing plasma testosterone during the luteal phase of the menstrual cycle.[216,217]

Clinical study PCOS: licorice alongside spironolactone, combination indicated a synergistic effect on androgen excess.[218]

Topical use in idiopathic hirsutism: adding topical licorice is more effective than laser treatment alone.[219]

Dosage

Daily dosage 3–12ml of 1:1.

Typical weekly dosage 15–30ml of 1:1.

Gymnema sylvestre

This contains gymnemic acids and gurmanin (peptide), which bind to receptors on the taste buds, preventing receptor activation by sugar molecules and removing the ability to taste sugar.[220,221]

Preclinical studies in diabetic models: reduced intestinal absorption of glucose,[222] inhibited active glucose transport in the small intestine,[223,224] increased glucose uptake and use in the cells, and increased insulin levels.[225] It also increased the number of islets of Langerhans and number of pancreatic beta cells,[226] reducing body weight and food intake.[227]

It reduced blood sugar levels in diabetic models but did not affect blood sugar levels in normal models.[228,229]

Clinical studies on diabetes: in healthy adults it reduced sweetness perception by 50%, reduced caloric consumption for 1.5 hours after the sweetness-numbing effect stopped.[230] In obese adults it reduced body weight[231] and lowered VLDL values.[232]

In T2 diabetics: reduced raised insulin, fasting blood sugar levels, HbA1c, glycosylated plasma protein levels.[233]

When used alongside orthodox hypoglycaemic medication (glibenclamide or tolbutamide) some participants were able to reduce medication and maintain blood glucose homeostasis with *Gymnema* alone.[234]

Clinical studies with overweight PCOS patients: a combination of gymnemic acid, myo-inositol, l-methylfolate improved menstrual cycle regularity, along with a reduction in BMI, a decrease of total testosterone as well as an increase of SHBG serum levels, total cholesterol and homocysteine levels.[235]

Dosage: To reduce sweet cravings the tincture can be dropped onto the tongue, repeating every 2–3 hours.

Daily dose 3–6ml/day of 1:3.

Typical weekly dosage 10–20ml of 1:3; the best results come after 6 to 12 months of continuous use.

Mentha spicata

Preclinical studies
In vivo (male): *Mentha piperita* and *M. spicata* oral intake increased FSH and LH levels, whereas total testosterone levels decreased.[236]

Clinical studies
PCOS: spearmint tea, twice a day for 30 days, led to a reduction of free and total testosterone levels, alongside increased LH and FSH levels.[237] According to the patients, hirsutism had reduced, although no difference was observed in the Ferriman-Galwey ratings of hirsutism. Realistically the trial was too short to make a difference as the cycle of hair growth is at least three months.

In a trial in women with hirsutism, half were Dx with PCOS: using an infusion of *M. spicata* for 5 days twice a day decreased free testosterone, increased LH, FSH and oestradiol.[238]

Dosage: lovely as an infusion.
Daily dose 15ml of 1:3.
Typical weekly dosages 15–25ml 1:3.

Paeonia lactiflora & *Glycyrrhiza glabra* (see book 1)

This combination is effective for treatment of hyperprolactinaemia induced by antipsychotic medication with oligomenorrhea or amenorrhea.[239,240] The combination aided menstrual resumption,[241,242] increasing progesterone and oestradiol.[243] There were beneficial effects for those with acne vulgaris (a typical symptom in those with PCOS), where it was noted that it decreased serum-free testosterone and the number of comedomes.[244]

Preclinical research on PCOS: reduced free and total testosterone, increased oestradiol. Hormonal effects occurred primarily in the ovary via enhanced aromatisation of testosterone to 17-beta oestradiol. In oophorectomised models no changes in serum testosterone were seen, thus the action is due to the effect on the ovary via increased aromatase activity.[245]

Clinical research with oligomenorrheic and hyperandrogenic PCOS patients: decreased serum-free T levels and achieved pregnancy in patients with PCOS.[246,247] The efficacy may vary according to the type of polycystic ovary syndrome treated, general cystic or peripheral cystic; higher efficacy was found in the peripheral cystic pattern.[248]

Dosage: Japanese clinical trials with the paeony and licorice combination used an extract equivalent to 4–6g/day of each, but aqueous ethanol is a more effective solvent than water for many of the constituents.
Typical weekly dose: 20–30ml of 1:1 of each herb.

Serenoa repens/serrulata

Most of the research relates to benign prostatic hyperplasia (BHP):[249–253] *Serenoa* was found to have antiandrogenic properties by inhibiting testosterone and DHT binding.[254] Inhibits 5-alpha-reductase, which converts testosterone into the more potent 5-alpha-dihydrotestosterone,[255–257] antioestrogenic,[258] reduced hyperprolactinemia.[259,260]

Alopecia in men: improvement in 60% for those that took it orally,[261] and was also found to be beneficial topically.[262,263]

Due to the above studies many herbalists started using *Serenoa* for the treatment of androgenic symptoms of PCOS. There are no studies related to PCOS and only one study looked at topical use of *Serenoa* in women with idiopathic facial hirsutism, which led to improvement as well as reduced need for hair removal.[264]

Dosage
Daily dose 4.5–9ml of 1:3.
Typical weekly dose 20–30ml of 1:3.

Vitex agnus-castus (see book 1)

Its use goes back a long way as Dioscorides says that it 'makes the menses come on earlier'. It is regularly used by UK herbalists for acne, which is a common symptom of PCOS. *Vitex* has been shown in clinical trials to improve menstrual cyclicity in those with polymenorrhoea, oligomenorrhoea, amenorrhoea,[265] and increases fertility.[266,267] In hyperprolactinaemia it improved concentrations of progesterone in the luteal phase, shortening the cycle, and normalised a shortened luteal phase and menstrual regularity.[268]

Preclinical study in diabetic model: *Vitex* led to higher levels of serum LH, FSH, oestrogen and progesterone,[269] and reduced serum leptin.[270]

Preclinical studies with a PCOS model: *Vitex* increased serum levels of progesterone and decreased serum testosterone levels.[271]

Clinical trials on PCOS: In a comparison of low-dose oral contraceptive with *Vitex agnus-castus*, both led to normalisation of the menstrual cycle, as well as normalising testosterone levels, DHEA-S, and prolactin serum levels.[272] In a comparison with metformin, *Vitex agnus-castus* was equally effective, although more side effects were found in the metformin group.[273]

Dosage
In cases of moderate prolactin or androgen excess: daily dose 0.6–3ml of 1:3 per day.
Typical weekly dose 5ml of 1:3.
In cases of higher prolactin or androgen levels: daily dose 3–7.5ml of 1:3.
Typical weekly dose 10–20ml of 1:3.

Table 7.2: Clinical studies: other herbs, combinations of herbs, individual constituents

Herb	Clinical and preclinical studies
Apium graveolens & *Pimpinella anisum*	**Clinical trial in oligomenorrhea in PCOS:** increased bleeding episodes, reduced testosterone and LH/FSH ratio; celery and anise combination regulated menstrual cycles and improved oligomenorrhea in polycystic ovary syndrome patients superiorly to metformin.[274] 750mg each for 15 days from the beginning of the follicular phase, if no bleeding given for 15 days.
Asparagus racemosus with *Anethum graveolens*	**Clinical trial with PCOS:** given orally or rectally as an enema, or both. All groups resulted in reduced ovarian volumes, improved endometrial thickness, reduced hirsutism and regulated menstrual cycle. The most improvement was observed when taken both rectally and orally.[275]
Berberine[276] *Berberis vulgaris* contains 6% berberine, *Hydrastis canadensis* 2% to 4.5%, *Coptis chinensis* 7% to 9%.[277] Bioavailability of berberine is low, absorption in intestinal tract is poor.[278]	**Preclinical:** insulin sensitising and insulinotropic agent,[279] glucose-lowering.[280] **Clinical studies in PCOS:** Berberine (900–1500mg) with metformin; induced ovulation, regularised menstruation,[281] enhanced pregnancy rate, live birth.[282] Reduces visceral adipose tissue including for those without weight loss,[283,284] Reduced glycosylated haemoglobin, insulin resistance, total cholesterol, triglycerides and low-density lipoprotein cholesterol.[285] Berberine or metformin before the IVF cycle increased pregnancy rate, reduced incidence of severe ovarian hyperstimulation syndrome.[286,287] The combination of metformin and berberine had a higher ovulation rate compared to metformin by itself.[288]
Camellia sinensis	**Clinical studies with obese women with PCOS:** weight loss, a decrease in fasting insulin and a decrease in the level of free testosterone were seen.[289] Not all trials show consistent results. Some studies suggest possible beneficial effects on obesity[290] and type 2 diabetes.[291]

(Continued)

Table 7.2: (Continued)

Herb	Clinical and preclinical studies
Curcumin only	**Clinical trials in PCOS:** (1500mg curcumin TDS), increased activity of the glutathione peroxidase, hence an efficient reducer of oxidative stress,[292] decreased fasting plasma glucose and dehydroepiandrosterone levels, non-significant increase in oestradiol levels.[293] Trial, with 500mg/day curcumin; beneficial effects on body weight, glycemic control, serum lipid.[294] **Clinical studies patients with type 2 diabetes, obesity, and metabolic syndrome:** curcumin (300–1500mg per day) improved fasting blood glucose and triglyceride,[295] reduced glycosylated hemoglobin (HbA_{1c}), C-reactive protein (CRP), and inflammatory markers (TNF-α, IL-6).[296–298]
Foeniculum vulgare	**Preclinical studies with PCOS:** reduced serum estrogen level, increased serum progesterone level and endometrial thickness.[299] **Clinical trials with PCOS:** fennel plus cupping, vs metformin reduced days between the cycle, and pain.[300] Effective in amenorrhoea.[301] Changes in FSH levels.[302] Topically for Idiopathic Hirsutism; cream containing 2%[303] reduced thickness of facial hair.[304]
Matricaria chamomilla	**Preclinical research PCOS models:** decreased number of cysts in ovarian tissue, increased number of dominant follicles,[305] improved endometrial tissue.[306] **Clinical studies with PCOS patients** decrease in total testosterone levels.[307] **Clinical studies related to diabetes:** positive effects on glycemic control, reduced total cholesterol, serum LDL cholesterol, triglycerides,[308] lowered glycosylated hemoglobin, serum insulin levels.[309]

(*Continued*)

Table 7.2: (Continued)

Herb	Clinical and preclinical studies
Nigella sativa	**Preclinical in PCOS models:** effects on ovarian ovulation.[310] **Preclinical and clinical studies related to diabetes:** insulinotropic properties,[311] beneficial effect on fasting blood sugar levels and ameliorative effect on regeneration of pancreatic islets.[312] **Clinical studies with PCOS:** menstrual cycle intervals decreased. Serum cholesterol, triglycerides, FBS, insulin, AST, LH and HOMA-IR index improved.[313]
Origanum majorana	**Preclinical diabetes:** glycation inhibitory activity.[314] **Clinical studies with PCOS patients:** improved insulin sensitivity, reduced the levels of adrenal androgens.[315]
Paeonia lactiflora & Cinnamomum cassia	**Clinical trial with PCOS:** infertile women, including those with PCOS and/or oligo/amenorrhoea, resulted in increased oestradiol, reduced LH. Ovulation was confirmed in 30 out of 42 oligo/amenorrheic women with PCOS.[316]
Silymarin (single compound found in Silybum marianum)	**Clinical study in PCOS:** comparing silymarin (750mg per day) with metformin, or together. Combination treatment while also receiving IVF reduced proportion of early apoptosis and total apoptosis of granulosa cells,[317] improved blood glucose, insulin, progesterone and insulin resistance in women; 4 of the 20 women ovulated; the effects were greater in combination treatment.[318] Clinical studies showed reduction in fasting blood glucose levels and HbA1c levels.[319]
Trigonella foenum-graecum	**Preclinical diabetes:** reduced intestinal absorption of glucose, postprandial blood glucose,[320] enhanced utilisation of glucose.[321]

(Continued)

Table 7.2: (Continued)

Herb	Clinical and preclinical studies
	Clinical studies with PCOS patients: an extract enriched with furostanolic saponins reduced ovary volume/cyst size. Increased LH and FSH levels, slight decrease in the LH/FSH ratio. Regulated menstrual cycle, 12% of study population got pregnant.[322] **Combined with metformin:** ultrasound scans showed decrease in polycystic appearing ovaries and improved menstrual cyclicity.[323] **Clinical studies on diabetes:** indicated a positive effect in diabetes type 1 and 2, prediabetic states, reduced fasting blood sugar levels and symptoms of diabetes, improved glucose tolerance,[324,325] increased insulin sensitivity,[326] insulinotropic.[327] In diabetes (type 1 and 2) the effects are slow but sustained.[328] Hypocholesterolaemic.[329] Combination with Rx sulfonylureas improved glycaemic control, reduced blood glucose levels and ameliorated clinical symptoms in type 2 diabetes.[330]
Tribulus terrestris	**Preclinical study, diabetic model:** decreased blood glucose level, improved lipid profile.[331] **PCOS model:** the number of corpora lutea, primary and secondary follicles increased, and the number of ovarian cysts decreased. In the PCOS model it was found best used on days 5 to 14 of the menstrual cycle to restore menstrual regularity.[332] **Clinical studies, diabetic women:** lowered blood glucose.[333] **Oligo/anovular infertility:** Tribestan® was compared with several medications to induce ovulation; ovulation rates were highest with epimestrol (74%), followed by Tribestan® (60%), clomiphene (47%) and cyclofenil (24%).[334]

(Continued)

Table 7.2: (Continued)

Herb	Clinical and preclinical studies
Tribulus terrestris from menstrual cycle day 5 for 10 days, plus regular use of *Cinnamomum verum*, *Glycyrrhiza glabra*, *Hypericum perforatum*, and *Paeonia lactiflora*	**A clinical trial on overweight PCOS patients:** combining herbs alongside lifestyle changes was more effective in reducing length of menstrual cycle, oestradiol and LH, and improved fasting insulin levels, blood pressure, conception rates and quality of life. The live birth rate was similar.[335] Some herbalists suggest dosing all steroidal saponin-rich herbs from days 5 to 14 of the menstrual cycle for 2 to 3 months or to use in the preovulatory phase in combination with conventional ovulation stimulants. This probably comes from the research related to *Tribulus*.

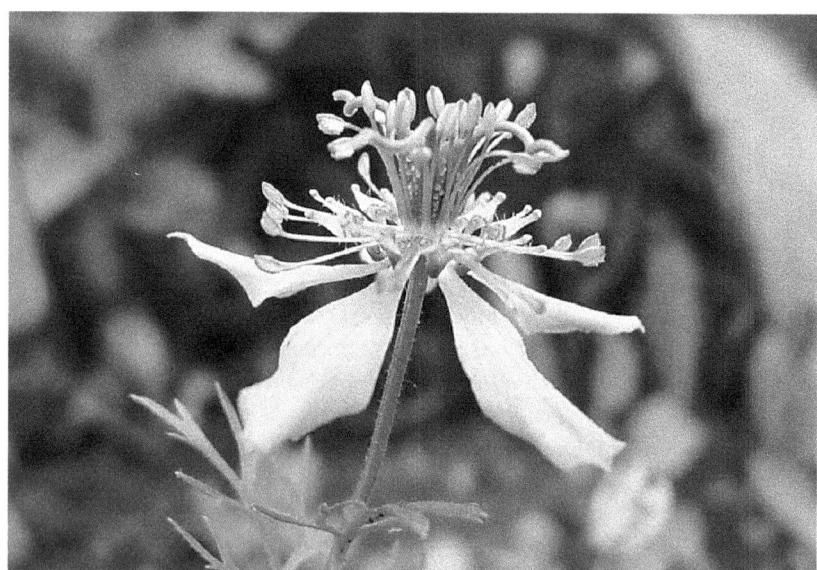

Nigella sativa

Preclinical studies in PCOS models

Aloe vera gel	**Preclinical study in PCOS model:** restored oestrus cyclicity, glucose sensitivity and steroidogenic activity,[336] reduced plasma triglyceride, LDL cholesterol levels, increased HDL cholesterol.[337] **Clinical study in diabetics:** reduced fasting blood glucose, HbA1c, triglycerides and LDL-C, and increased HDL-C, showed positive effect on glycaemic control, reduced body weight, body fat mass.[338-342]
Galega officinalis	**Preclinical research PCOS models (in vivo):** the hydroalcoholic extract increased serum levels of aromatase and oestradiol, decreased the levels of LH, FSH, testosterone, fasting blood sugar and insulin. It also decreased the number of cystic follicles and increased the number of normal follicles.[343] Guanidine potentiates the effects of insulin by promoting cell uptake of glucose, inhibits glucose absorption in the intestines, inhibits gluconeogenesis and lowers blood glucose. By the late 1990s, dimethylbiguanide was rediscovered and used for management of hyperglycaemia in type 2 diabetes under the name Metformin.[344]
Mentha spicata and flaxseed	**Preclinical study in vivo PCOS model:** increase in progesterone, decrease in testosterone and oestradiol, no change of DHEA, increase in primary, pre-antral and antral follicles, number of cystic follicles decreased. A combination of flaxseed and spearmint extract improved the endocrine profile and the histomorphometric features of the ovary; combination was better than either of them used on their own.[345]

(*Continued*)

(Continued)

Panax ginseng	**Preclinical studies:** it normalised ovarian morphology, lowered the high numbers of antral follicles and increased the number of corpora lutea in the polycystic ovaries. As a preventative it has the potential to inhibit the elevation of body and ovary weights. It inhibited the increase in number and size of ovarian cysts, and prevented the elevation of serum testosterone and oestradiol levels.[346-349] **Clinical studies in diabetic and prediabetic patients:** ginseng and ginsenosides lowered blood glucose, increased insulin sensitivity and regulated lipid metabolism,[350] improved fasting blood glucose, with a modest effect on lowering blood pressure.[351,352]
Trifolium pratense	**Preclinical studies with PCOS:** decreased testosterone levels, increased oestradiol, increased HDL and decreased LDL, reduced ovarian weight, volumes of ovarian, medulla, cortex and number of cysts and increased number of oocytes.[353]
Urtica dioica rad	Relevant studies showed *Urtica rad* inhibits both 5-alpha-reductase and aromatase, reduces the binding activity of SHBG and exerts anti-proliferative effects, found to be of help in BHP.[354] **Preclinical study PCOS:** improved antioxidant capacity, oocyte and embryo quality.[355]
Zingiber officinalis	**Preclinical study in PCOS model:** applied intraperitoneally and compared to clomiphene, *Zingiber* lowered the levels of LH and oestrogen, and increased the levels of FSH and progesterone.[356] **Clinical trials in patients with type 2 diabetes:** improved insulin sensitivity and reduced total cholesterol and triglycerides, reduced C-reactive protein and prostaglandin E2, and beneficial effect on serum glucose.[357]

7.4 Dietary and lifestyle recommendations

Several studies related to a range of different diets in PCOS agree that the key component that makes them effective is weight loss, although the importance of exercise should not be ignored.[358] Weight loss improves the presentation of PCOS regardless of which specific diet is followed.[359,360]

A small to moderate weight loss (5–10%) improves insulin resistance, restores ovulation, improves menstrual regularity and conception rates, and reduces hyperandrogenism, hirsutism and dyslipidemia.[361]

From clinical research

Strategies for weight loss could include increased meal frequency,[362] regular meal timing, and consuming the majority of carbohydrates at lunch time,[363] avoiding a high-carbohydrate breakfast.[364] The best outcomes are seen using these methods in the management and treatment of PCOS.[365,366]

All diets used in clinical trials for PCOS agree on the need for the diet to be rich in vegetables and to avoid foods high in sugar and refined carbohydrates.[367]

Chronic inflammation alters hormone secretion, and inflammatory markers are increased in obesity.[368] Hyperglycemia by itself will worsen inflammation. Glucose ingestion induces an inflammatory response that is independent of obesity.[369] Anti-inflammatory foods include berries, fatty fish, leafy greens and extra virgin olive oil

DASH diet (Dietary Approaches to Stop Hypertension): this consists of a low-GI, low-energy-density, high in complex carbohydrates, high-fibre diet. Comprising 52% carbohydrates, 18% proteins and 30% total fats, it is rich in fish, poultry, fruits, vegetables, whole grain and low-fat dairy produce, and low in saturated fats, cholesterol, refined grains and sweets.

Trials with PCOS patients showed beneficial effects on AMH and lipid profiles, a reduction in serum insulin,[370] c-reactive protein,[371] and serum androstenedione, and increased antioxidant status and SHBG,[372] along with beneficial effects on BMI.[373]

The DASH diet is also associated with better fertility in women and better semen quality in men.[374-376]

Mediterranean diet: this anti-inflammatory diet, rich in complex carbohydrates, fibre and high in monounsaturated fats, has beneficial effects for women with PCOS.[377]

DASH and Mediterranean-style diets are both rich in dietary fibre, antioxidants and anti-inflammatory nutrients and lead to greater satiety, having anti-hyperlipidemic, antihypertensive and antidiabetic effects.[378]

Ketogenic diet (KD): KD is a high-fat, adequate-protein and very low-carbohydrate content diet. With fasting or carbohydrate restriction (as in KD), blood insulin concentration decreases and glucagon increases to maintain the normal blood glucose level. The physiological ketosis caused by KD reduces the levels of circulating insulin and IGF-1, suppresses the stimulus for the production of ovarian and adrenal androgens. It also reduces circulating lipids, low-grade inflammation and oxidative stress.[379]

Low-carbohydrate and/or low-glycaemic index diet: a low-carbohydrate and/or low glycaemic index (GI) diet avoids insulin spikes. Foods to include are whole grains, legumes, nuts, seeds, fruits and vegetables (unprocessed, low-carbohydrate foods). A moderate reduction in dietary carbohydrates reduced fasting and post-challenge insulin concentrations among women with PCOS,[380] with improved menstrual regularity, reduced free androgen index, improved lipid profiles and improved quality of life.[381,382]

High-protein diets: these seem to improve glycaemic control, although it is not clear if the effects are due to the higher protein or lower carbohydrate intake.[383]

Trials with PCOS suggested that protein intake suppressed ghrelin significantly longer than glucose, which suggests prolonged satiety.[384]

Table 7.3: Supplements in trials for PCOS

Nutrient	Clinical studies: PCOS
Omega 3: eicosapentaenoic acid [EPA] and docosahexaenoic acid [DHA]) 2 and 4g per day	Reduced serum total testosterone levels[385–387] (antiandrogenic effect[388]) and blood lipids. Reduced production of inflammatory cytokines (TNF-α, IL-6) and increased secretion of the anti-inflammatory hormone adiponectin.[389] Decreased interval between periods.[390]

(Continued)

Table 7.3: (Continued)

Nutrient	Clinical studies: PCOS
Vitamin D	Supplementation decreased total testosterone without any effects on serum SHBG and free testosterone.[391] There appears to be an inverse association between vitamin D status and insulin resistance in women with PCOS.[392]
Selenium	Beneficial effects on sugar metabolism as well as effect on lipid profile.[393]
Zinc	Beneficial effects on sugar metabolism, as well as lipid profile.[394]
Folate	Beneficial effects on inflammatory factors and reduction of oxidative stress.[395]
Chromium Inconsistent findings in reviews of chromium and glycemic control	Unclear if beneficial in PCOS as results inconclusive,[396] though one study indicated it improved glucose tolerance in PCOS patients.[397] It is proposed that chromium binds to an oligopeptide, a chromium-binding substance that binds to and activates the insulin receptor to promote insulin action.
N-acetylcysteine (NAC) or cysteine or the acetylated form of cysteine, the rate-limiting nutrient in glutathione synthesis	Intake by women with PCOS, including clomiphene citrate (CC)-resistant PCOS, increased pregnancy rates as well as live-birth rates.[398] NAC as adjuvant to letrozole and clomiphene citrate increased ovulation and pregnancy rates in PCOS patients,[399] also with some beneficial impacts on endometrial thickness.[400,401]

See Appendix for food sources.

More helpful diet advice

High-fibre foods (flaxseed, legumes including soy, lentils, etc.) have a beneficial effect in reducing CVD risk factors in general,[402] as well as improving the health of the gut microbiome; the gut microbiota have critical role in metabolic diseases.[403–404] Soluble fibre can help with blood sugar control and weight loss by delaying the absorption of glucose by delaying gastric emptying.

Glycine max

Clinical trials in diabetics: soy protein and isoflavone moderates hyperglycemia, lowered hyperlipidemia and hyperinsulinemia, and reduced body weight.[407–409]

Clinical studies in PCOS
Soy isoflavones (50mg/d): improved markers of insulin resistance, reduced free androgen and serum triglycerides, reduced biomarkers of oxidative stress (increase glutathione, decrease in malondialdehyde levels).[410]

Soy bread consumption (70g/d soy flour, a loaf of soy bread): caused changes in the levels of FSH, oestradiol, and testosterone.[411]

As a rule it is always better to use the whole soy bean as a food, rather than isolated isoflavone supplements on their own.

Linum usitatissimum

Relevant preclinical studies to PCOS: elevated leptin levels in vivo (a hormone that suppresses appetite).[412]

Preclinical studies in PCOS
It decreased the level of testosterone, increased progesterone, and improved the histomorphometric features of the ovary.[413]

Clinical studies
PCOS: 15g flax seed powder daily reduced the ovarian volume and the number of follicles in the ovaries, and improved the frequency of menstrual cycles, although no change in hirsutism, blood sugar level and body weight was seen.[414]

Post-menopausal women: increased SHBG, reduced testosterone,[415,416] inhibited aromatase enzyme activity,[417,418] reduced serum levels of 17-β-oestradiol and oestrone sulphate.[419] Also inhibited 5-α-reductase, the enzyme responsible for converting testosterone into dihydrotestosterone, the more biologically active and potent form.[420]

Type 2 diabetics: reduced fasting blood glucose, haemoglobin A1C (HbA1C) and markers of inflammation,[421,422] improved lipid profile,[423] reduced calorie intake.[424]

Camellia sinensis

Clinical studies

Obese women with PCOS: weight loss, a decrease in fasting insulin and a decrease in the level of free testosterone were seen.[425] Not all trials had consistent results.

Some studies suggest possible beneficial effects on obesity and type 2 diabetes.[426,427]

Tomato juice

In people with metabolic syndrome tomato juice led to an improvement in endothelial function and improved fasting insulin resistance. Serum LDL-cholesterol levels were significantly decreased from baseline after 2 months' consumption.[428]

CHAPTER 8

Endometriosis

8.1 Presentation/symptoms, differential diagnosis and investigations

Endometriosis is a condition caused by misplaced endometrial cells. All endometrial tissues are under the influence of hormones,[1] specifically oestrogen, which causes proliferation of endometrial tissue.

In the luteal phase under the influence of progesterone, endometrial tissue develops microscopic glandular structures; before menstruation this causes an increase in the volume of endometriotic tissue. It is this that can give rise to premenstrual symptoms of bloating, discomfort and pelvic pain, depending on the site of the tissue. At the onset of menstrual shedding the endometrial tissue breaks down and can shed into the pelvic cavity and/or between the muscle fibres of the uterus, in a related condition called adenomyosis.

A large number of patients with dysmenorrhea may suffer from undiagnosed endometriosis.[2,3] The prevalence of the disease increases up to 30% in patients presenting with infertility, and up to 45% in patients presenting with chronic pelvic pain.[4]

There is also a genetic element, so a family history may be present. The typical age of onset is between the ages of 12 and 30.

Symptoms

Typically, there is a triad of dysmenorrhoea, dysparunia and infertility, which can be accompanied by menorrhagia. There is no relationship between the extent of the lesions and the severity of symptoms; some remain asymptomatic.

Severe debilitating dysmenorrhoea, after several years of relatively pain-free menses. The pain is cyclic, specifically preceding or during menses, and can be progressive. The severity of the pain can cause diarrhoea, nausea, vomiting.

Symptoms often lessen or resolve during pregnancy, and tend to become inactive after menopause.

Table 8.1: Symptoms vary, depending on location

Location	Symptom
Bladder	Dysuria Haematuria Suprapubic or pelvic pain Urge incontinence Urinary frequency
Large intestine	Abdominal bloating Pain during defecation Diarrhoea Constipation Rectal bleeding during menses
Ovaries	Endometriomas increase in size every month, leading to symptoms related to pressure. Tendency to rupture, even when small. Rupture of the cysts occurs typically just after menses, causing: acute abdominal or unilateral iliac fossa pain with shock. Occasionally they do shrink spontaneously due to deprivation of blood supply. Atrophied cysts can cause ovarian scarring.
Adnexal structures	Adhesions result in a pelvic mass and/or pain.
Extrapelvic structures	Sometimes vague abdominal pain

Differential

- GIT issues including appendicitis
- Ovarian cysts leading to torsion
- Pelvic inflammatory disease
- Sexually transmitted diseases (Chlamydia, gonorrhoea)
- Urinary tract infections

Investigations

Women can walk around with the condition for years before being diagnosed. The only reliable diagnosis is by laparoscopy with biopsy for histological confirmation of lesions, as well as simultaneous treatment. Consider the possibility of endometriosis if no relief with nonsteroidal anti-inflammatory drugs (NSAIDs) or oral contraceptive therapy.

Conventional treatment

- Aromatase inhibitors: letrozole and anastrozole, to inhibit the endometrial and endometriotic aromatase enzyme, to reduce local production of oestrogen.
- Combined oral contraceptive pills (COCPs): reduces menstrual flow and decidualisation of the ectopic endometrium, with decreased cell proliferation and increased apoptosis.[5]
- Cyclooxygenase (COX)-2 inhibitors and other NSAIDs.
- Gonadotropin Releasing Hormone agonists (GnRH-a).
- MMP-inhibitors, recombinant human TNF-α binding proteins, anti-VEGF therapy and interferon (IFN)-alpha-2b.
- Progestogens, especially non-androgenic progestogens.[6]

Surgical management

- Laparoscopic pelvic ablation: in 50% of these patients symptoms have recurred by the time of their one-year follow-up.
- Hysterectomy

8.2 Pathophysiology of endometriosis

Multiple mechanisms are involved in the condition and the aetiology is not completely understood.

Proposed aetiologies

Coelomic metaplasia: hormonal or immunological factors are thought to stimulate the transformation of normal peritoneal tissue/cells into endometrium-like tissue.[7]

Endometrial stem cell implantation: tissue derived from stem cells, the dissemination of these cells by different mechanisms such as retrograde menstruation, lymphatic and vascular dissemination, direct migration or a combination of all.

Lymphatic and vascular metastasis: endometrial cells and tissue fragments are transported from the uterine cavity through blood or lymph vessels to colonise distant ectopic sites.

Müllerian embryonic remnant abnormalities: Müller's duct cells undergo a process of disordered differentiation and proliferation, then spread to localised sites outside the expected area of Müller's duct development.

Retrograde menstruation: the most accepted theory, which seems to explain most types of endometriosis.

Pathophysiology

In the early stages of endometriosis high levels of inflammatory cytokines, lymphocytes and macrophages are found in the peritoneal fluid, implicating inflammation and the immune system. Later on, in established endometriosis, macrophage activity is reduced, which is associated with the reduced ability to suppress growth.

Once the endometrial tissue is established,[8] we enter a cycle of hormonally stimulated endometriosis caused by the upregulation of aromatase in endometrial tissue, which increases oestrogen, alongside an increase in the inflammatory prostaglandin E2. This leads to an increase in muscle spasm, inflammation, dilating blood vessels and increasing blood loss (for more details, see chapter on dysmenorrhoea[9]).

Retrograde menstruation

Retrograde menstruation through the fallopian tubes into the peritoneal cavity is common in all menstruating women (it occurs in 76–90%).[10] However, this process is not considered pathological, as not all women develop endometriosis. More factors must therefore be involved.

Early menarche, menstrual length, menorragia, shortened menstrual cycle: a higher incidence of endometriosis is associated with early menarche, menstrual length of more than 7 days, menorrhagia and a short cycle. Cell-mediated immunity is involved to clear retrograde menstrual debris, but too great a 'menstrual flow' might initiate the problem, alongside reduced immune surveillance.[11]

Dysmenorrhoea: in severe dysmenorrhoea the extreme contractions increase retrograde flow alongside prostaglandin imbalance generating inflammatory markers (IL-I, IL-6 and TNF alpha); these promote proliferation, adhesions and angiogenesis.

IUCD use increases the risk, possibly due to retrograde flow and an alteration of prostaglandin levels. This is not the case with the Mirena coil (progesterone medicated coil).

Strenuous exercise during menstruation has been suggested to contribute to retrograde menstruation, although those that do exercise have a lower risk due to lower oestrogen levels.

Immune system involvement, inflammatory response

Impaired cell-mediated immunity affects the clearance of retrograde menstruation and contributes to the progression of disease. Oestradiol reduces the activity of natural killer cells, interfering with their ability to detect and clear retrograde endometrial cells.[12,13]

Oxidative stress is involved in the initiation and progression of endometriosis by causing inflammatory responses in the peritoneal cavity.[14,15] On a cellular level inflammation results in adhesions, invasion, angiogenesis, reduced apoptosis[16] and proliferation.[17] Certain markers of inflammation cause the upregulation of metalloproteinases (MMPs), prostaglandins, cytokines and chemokines. The persistent inflammation results in the survival and growth of ectopic endometrial cells.

The range of individual components involved with endometriosis is endless and becomes a maze to become lost in, for example, integrins, membrane MMPs involved with endometrial adhesion and angiogenesis.[18-20] Angiogenesis is stimulated by inflammation, hypoxia,[21] NF-κB pathway—the main activator of VEGF.[22,23]

Reduced apoptosis: in a healthy menstrual cycle, apoptosis increases during the menstrual cycle to make sure the old cells are removed from the functional layer of the endometrium.[24] The rate of apoptosis is decreased in endometrial cells.[25] Macrophages have a reduced ability to clear away apoptotic cells in those with endometriosis.

Immune dysregulation: there is a higher incidence of autoimmune conditions and atopy among women with endometriosis.[26]

Hormonal involvement

Oestrogen

Oestrogen in relative excess causes increased endometrial thickness and heavy bleeding. Oestrogens influences, directly or indirectly, numerous factors and processes that cause or contribute towards cell survival, invasion, differentiation and adhesion, and tissue remodelling: macrophages,[27] pro-inflammatory cytokines (TNF-alpha, and IL-1, IL-6, IL-8,…), prostaglandins (PGE2, COX), transcription factors (NF-lB, AP-1), angiogenesis (VEGF, nitric oxide), MMPs,[28,29] and cell adhesion molecules (VCAM1, CD-44, ICAM-1, integrin and cadherins).[30–33]

Increased aromatase activity: endometrial cysts and ectopic endometriotic lesions express high levels of aromatase and therefore increased conversion of testosterone to oestrogen. As mentioned, early endometriosis is transformed into late hormonally stimulated endometriosis by the upregulation of aromatase. As aromatase activity is stimulated by insulin, normalisation of insulin and glucose metabolism is critical.

Lower levels of 17beta hydroxysteroid dehydrogenase type 2, which converts oestradiol into the weakly active oestrone.[34]

Progesterone receptors

Progesterone resistance: progestin treatment is often prescribed but is sometimes unhelpful in endometriosis. It has been suggested that this is due to progesterone resistance, from suppressed expression of the intracellular progesterone receptor in the ectopic endometrium.[35,36]

Environmental oestrogens

Pesticides and plastics, e.g. dioxin and polychlorinated biphenyls (PCBs). These mimic oestrogen and may contribute to endometriosis. However, no epidemiological evidence exists so far.

Tampons: dioxin is a by-product of the chlorine bleaching process. Although studies are conflicting, it is sensible to avoid chlorine-bleached tampons, where possible.[37–40]

OCP: possibly higher incidence in former OCP users, compared to those who have never taken OCP.

Family history/genetic causes

There is a genetic component.[41–43]

Fertility

In those with minimal/mild endometriosis, 50% conceive without treatment. In those with moderate disease, 25% will conceive without treatment. Only a few spontaneous conceptions occur in cases of severe endometriosis.

Infertility may be due to the to any of the following:

- Anti-endometrial antibodies, immune system deficiencies affect implantation and may increase incidence of miscarriage. Excessive amounts of free radicals and/or changes in cytokine profiles negatively affect the oocyte, spermatozoa and embryo.
- Dysfunctional uterotubal motility, inflammation causing scarring and adhesions.
- Disturbed folliculogenesis, luteinised unruptured follicle, luteal defect, progesterone resistance.[44]

8.3 Herbal management of endometriosis

There are very few clinical trials investigating the herbal treatment of endometriosis. Most research is in the form of preclinical studies.[45–47] While these studies might not necessarily give answers, they do suggest mechanisms as to why particular herbs, classically used in the treatment of endometriosis, might be helpful, reflecting clinical experience.

As with herbal treatments for any condition, the herbal approach to endometriosis needs to be aimed at several targets, often simultaneously, as outlined below.

Aims

Improve pelvic circulation, reduce pain, bleeding, inflammation and scarring
Support the immune system
Modulate hormones and aid fertility, if required

Herbal management

Reduce pain using anti-inflammatories, analgesics, antispasmodics: *Anemone pulsatilla, Viburnum prunifolium, Zingiber officinale*; see also chapter on dysmenorrhoea.

Reduce bleeding using anti-haemorrhagics, anti-inflammatories: *Achillea millefolium, Alchemilla vulgaris, Vitex agnus-castus, Zingiber officinale*, see chapter on menorrhagia.

Reduce inflammation using anti-inflammatories: *Actaea racemosa, Alchemilla vulgaris, Anemone pulsatilla, Viburnum prunifolium, Zingiber officinale*.

Reduce scarring using anti-fibrotics, anti-inflammatories and circulatories: *Calendula officinalis, Hydrocotyle asiatica*.

Support immune system and lymphatic clearance: *Calendula officinalis, Echinacea* spp., *Phytolacca decandra, Thuja occidentalis*.

Improve pelvic circulation using pelvic and general circulatories: *Actaea racemosa, Achillea millefolium, Alchemilla vulgaris, Calendula officinalis, Zingiber officinale*.

Aid fertility if required: *Actaea racemosa, Alchemilla vulgaris, Vitex agnus-castus*.

Modulate hormones and improve metabolism (see also oestrogen excess; elimination, hepatics, digestion): *Acteae racemosa, Vitex agnus-castus*.

Reduce the effects of stress using nervines and adaptogens: stress interferes with many pathways involved in the immune system and liver function, the disruption hypothalamic and pituitary gland function, and increased oestrogen levels. *Astragalus membranaceus, Matricaria chamomilla, Schisandra chinensis, Valeriana officinalis* (works well with *Viburnum prunifolium*), *Withania somnifera*.

Table 8.2: Specific mechanisms involved in endometriosis, with possible herbal activity

Agent and function	Herbs: mostly from preclinical research
Angiogenesis: process by which new blood vessels form, required for growth and development as well as the healing of wounds.	Inhibited by *Actaea racemosa, Andrographis paniculata, Camellia sinensis, Curcuma longa,* EGCG, *Glycyrrhiza glabra, Hydrocotyle asiatica,* isoflavones in soya, naringenin in citrus fruits, *Panax ginseng,* resveratrol, *Vitex agnus-castus, Zingiber officinale*
Anti-inflammatory	*Actaea racemosa, Andrographis paniculata, Anemone pulsatilla, Angelica sinensis, Calendula officinalis, Camellia sinensis, Capsella bursa-pastoris, Curcuma longa, Echinacea angustifolia/purpurea, Hydrocotyle asiatica, Paeonia lactiflora, Paeonia lactiflora & Glycyrrhiza glabra, Panax ginseng,* resveratrol, *Scutellaria baicalensis, Tanacetum parthenium, Uncaria tomentosa, Vitex agnus-castus, Zingiber officinale*
Antioxidant	*Actaea racemosa, Alchemilla vulgaris, Anemone pulsatilla, Andrographis paniculata, Angelica sinensis, Calendula officinalis, Camellia sinensis, Capsella bursa-pastoris, Centella asiatica, Curcuma longa, Echinacea angustifolia/purpurea, Glycyrrhiza glabra, Paeonia lactiflora, Paeonia lactiflora & Glycyrrhiza glabra,* resveratrol, *Uncaria tomentosa, Vitex agnus-castus, Zingiber officinale*
Apoptosis: the death of cells, which occurs as a normal and controlled part of an organism's growth or development.	Induced by *Actaea racemosa, Anemone pulsatilla, Camellia sinensis, Centella asiatica, Curcuma longa, Echinaceae angustifolia/purpurea, Glycyrrhiza glabra,* naringenin in citrus fruit, *Paeonia lactiflora,* resveratrol, *Uncaria tomentosa, Zingiber officinale*

(Continued)

Table 8.2: (Continued)

Agent and function	Herbs: mostly from preclinical research
Aromatase: enzyme responsible for conversion of androgens to oestrogens.	Inhibited by resveratrol, stimulated by *Paeonia lactiflora* & *Glycyrrhiza glabra*
Cell adhesion: the ability of a single cell to stick to another cell or an extracellular matrix (ECM), determines the polarity and the physiological function of cells within tissues. On every cell, adhesion molecules facilitate interactions within the cell microenvironment that consist of other cells and the extracellular matrix.	Inhibited by *Camellia sinensis*, *Curcuma longa*, *Viburnum opulus* and *prunifolium*, *Zingiber officinale*
Cell proliferation: in healthy tissue development is regulated, but can have unsystemic proliferation into mere cell masses.	Inhibited by *Actaea racemosa*, *Andrographis paniculata*, *Anemone pulsatilla*, *Alchemilla vulgaris*, *Angelica sinensis*, *Capsella bursa-pastoris*, *Camellia sinensis*, *Curcuma longa*, *Glycyrrhiza glabra*, *Hydrocotyle asiatica*, *Panax ginseng*, resveratrol, *Salvia miltriorrhiza*, *Tanacetum parthenium*, *Uncaria tomentosa*, *Zingiber officinale*
Cyclooxygenase-2 (COX-2): an enzyme is involved in the production of prostaglandins that mediate pain and support the inflammatory process.	Inhibited by *Actaea racemosa*, *Andrographis paniculata*, *Calendula officinalis*, *Curcuma longa*, *Glycyrrhiza glabra*, resveratrol, *Vitex agnus-castus*, *Zingiber officinale*
IL-1 Interleukin-1 (IL-1): cytokine key signalling molecules in both the innate and adaptive immune systems, mediating inflammation in response to a wide range of stimuli.	Reduced by *Echinaceae* spp., *Hydrocotyle asiatica*, *Tanacetum parthenium*, *Uncaria tomentosa*, *Zingiber officinale*

(Continued)

Table 8.2: (Continued)

Agent and function	Herbs: mostly from preclinical research
Interleukin 6 (IL-6): a cytokine that is produced in response to infections and tissue injuries, contributes to host defence through the stimulation of acute phase responses, hematopoiesis and immune reactions.	Reduced by *Actaea racemosa, Calendula officinalis, Hydrocotyle asiatica, Curcuma longa, Echinacea* spp., *Hippophae rhamnoides* & *Hypericum perforatum, Panax ginseng,* resveratrol, *Uncaria tomentosa, Viburnum opulus* & *prunifolium*
Interleukin-8 (IL-8): a cytokine that attracts and activates neutrophils in inflammatory regions.	Reduced by *Curcuma longa,* resveratrol, *Uncaria tomentosa, Zingiber officinale*
Interleukins, other	*Angelica sinensis* (IL-2), *Paeonia lactiflora* & *Glycyrrhiza glabra* (IL-2), *Paeonia lactiflora* (IL-2), *Tanacetum parthenium* (IL-2, and IL-4), *Uncaria tomenosa* (IL-2)
Matrix metalloproteinases (MMPs): play an important role in tissue remodelling such as morphogenesis, angiogenesis, tissue repair and metastasis. In the endometriotic peritoneum of women there is overproduction of MMPs, which have a role in implant progression and angiogenesis. Normally, MMP endometrial expression is low in the follicular stage, declines in the early luteal phase, increases in the late luteal phase. Progesterone is one of the major inhibitors of MMP expression; MMPs are controlled by different hormones, cytokines and growth factors.	Inhibited by curcumin, *Glycyrrhiza glabra, Panax ginseng,* pycnogenol, melatonin (so potentially also *Vitex agnus-castus*), resveratrol, *Salvia miltiorrhiza*

(Continued)

Table 8.2: (Continued)

Agent and function	Herbs: mostly from preclinical research
Nuclear factor-kappa B (NF-κB) is a transcription factor that is involved in inflammatory, immune responses. The NF-κB pathway regulates the proliferation, apoptosis and inflammation processes. In normal endometrium, the NF-κB pathway is downregulated whereas its expression is increased under the various endometriosis stages.[48] Activated NF-κB pathway leads to activation of IL-6 and IL-8 in endometriosis.[49,50] Also, a main activator of VEGF, to stimulate cell proliferation and angiogenesis in endometriosis.	Reduced by *Actaea racemosa, Andrographis paniculata, Curcuma longa*, EGCG, *Glycyrrhiza glabra, Hydrocotyle asiatica*, resveratrol, *Scutellaria baicalensis, Tanacetum parthenium, Zingiber officinale*
Prostaglandin E2; inflammatory mediator that is generated by cyclooxygenase 2 (COX_2) conversion of arachidonic acid, promoting angiogenesis, stimulating tumour-cell proliferation, and protecting tumour cells from apoptosis.	Inhibited by *Actaea racemosa, Angelica sinensis, Calendula officinalis,* curcumin, *Paeonia lactiflora* & *Glycyrrhiza glabra, Tanacetum parthenium, Uncaria tomentosa, Zingiber officinale*
Tumour necrosis factor alpha (TNF-α): a mediator of inflammatory and immune functions, regulates growth and differentiation of a wide variety of cell types. TNF-α is selectively cytotoxic for many transformed cells. Inappropriate or excessive activation of TNF-α signalling is associated with chronic inflammation.	Reduced by *Actaea racemosa, Calendula officinalis, Curcuma longa, Echinacea* spp., *Glycyrrhiza glabra, Hippophae rhamnoides* & *Hypericum perforatum, Hydrocotyle asiatica, Panax ginseng,* resveratrol, *Salvia miltiorrhiza, Tanacetum parthenium, Uncaria tomentosa, Viburnum opulus* and *prunifolium, Zingiber officinale*

(Continued)

Table 8.2: (Continued)

Agent and function	Herbs: mostly from preclinical research
Vascular endothelial growth factor (VEGF): considered the regulator of angiogenesis during growth and development, upregulated in many tumours.	Down regulation by *Actaea racemosa, Andrographis paniculata, Angelica sinensis, Camellia sinensis, Curcuma longa,* EGCG, naringenin in citrus fruits, *Panax ginseng,* resveratrol, soy (isoflavones), *Viburnum opulus* and *prunifolium, Vitex agnus-castus, Zingiber officinale*

Key herbs used in clinical practice

Actaea racemosa (see also book 1)

Preclinical: anti-inflammatory, inhibits IL-6, TNF-alpha, COX pathways, prostaglandin production,[51] modulates transcription factor NF-κB activities, dopaminergic, serotonergic,[52] analgesic. No direct binding effects on oestrogen receptors (ERα, ERβ), hence will not aggravate endometriosis. Induced apoptosis and suppressed E2-induced cell proliferation in endometrial adenocarcinoma cells.[53-55]

Dopaminergic effect: see under *Vitex agnus-castus* for detail on the relevance to endometriosis.

Clinical studies not related to endometriosis but found to improve FSH/LH ratio, decreasing LH in menopausal women,[56] and improved pregnancy rates in women with unexplained infertility.[57,58]

Dosage: the average weekly dose used in clinical trials is 1.8ml of 1:3 per week. Most UK herbalists would use 10ml of a 1:3 per week. Higher doses have not been found to be more effective for menopausal symptoms. Note: 60% alcohol is needed to extract the triterpene glycosides.

Daily dose in clinical trials of 80mg, which equates to 0.25ml of 1:3.
Typical weekly dose 5–10ml of 1:3.

Alchemilla vulgaris

Traditionally used as an antihaemorrhagic, anti-inflammatory

Preclinical: *Alchemilla mollis,* the garden variety of Alchemilla, has been investigated and found to reduce endometriosis formation in vivo.[59]

Dosage
Daily dose 6–12ml of 1:3.
Typical weekly dose 15–30ml of 1:3.

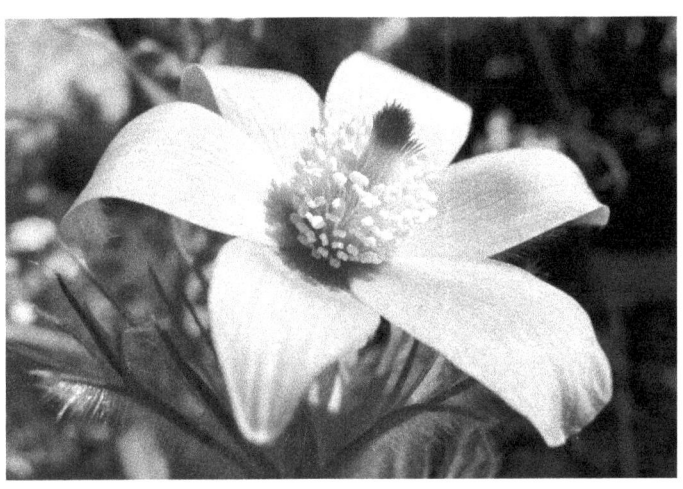

Anemone pulsatilla

Preclinical: there are no specific investigations into endometriosis, as yet, but it does induce apoptosis, and is anti-inflammatory, immunomodulating, antioxidant.[60]

Individual constituent detail:

Triterpenoid saponins: anticancer activity cell cycle arrest and apoptosis induction, anti-inflammatory, slight haemolytic effect, immunomodulatory enhanced specific antibody and cellular response,[61] antioxidant.[62]

Anemonin: anticancer activity,[63,64] anti-inflammatory, antioxidant, reducing endothelin-1, and soluble intercellular adhesion molecule,[65,66] inhibits apoptosis pathway,[67] sedative and central nervous system depressant (tyrosinase inhibitor).[68,69]

Dosage
Dried plant tincture, daily dose 0.9–3ml of 1:10.
Typical weekly dose 6.3–21ml of 1:10.
In acute dysmenorhoea doses of 0.75–2ml given half-hourly.

Contraindications and cautions: in pregnancy and when breastfeeding. Use with caution!!!

Calendula officinalis

Preclinical: anti-inflammatory, reduces levels of proinflammatory cytokines IL-1beta, IL-6, TNF-alpha and IFN-gamma, acute phase protein, C-reactive protein (CRP) and inhibits cyclooxygenase-2 (Cox-2) and subsequent prostaglandin synthesis.[70,71] Triterpenes such as faradiol and taraxasterol are inhibitors of tumour growth.[72]

Endometriosis model: *Calendula* not effective.[73]

Dosage: low percentage alcohol (25–45%).
Daily dose 4.5–9ml of 1:3.
Typical weekly dose 15–30ml of 1:3.

Echinacea angustifolia/purpurea

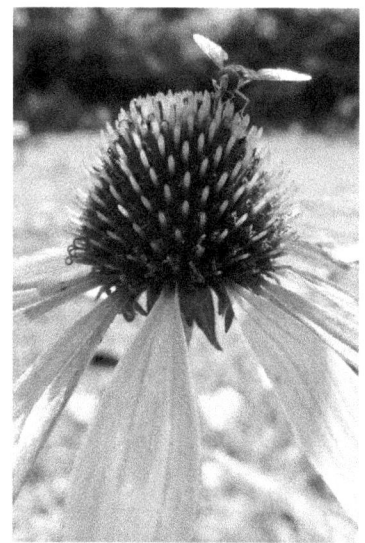

Studies, relevant but not specific to endometriosis:

Increases the number and activity of natural killer (NK) cytotoxicity, inhibits the products secreted by macrophages, including TNF-α and IL-1,[74,75] so reducing cytokines (TNF- and IL-1), decreasing inflammation and weakening the response of macrophages to immune stimulus.[76]

Lozenges of *E. purpurea* decreased TNF-α and IL-6 in six healthy volunteers.[77]

Echinacea affects the phagocytic immune system, not the acquired immune system.[78]

Alkamides bind with CB1 and CB2, possible mechanisms of their immunomodulatory action.[79-82]

Echinacea increases NF-κB, which regulates the expression of certain genes in innate immune responses like macrophages, neutrophils,[83] and is linked with apoptosis regulation.[84]

In the absence of immune issues (e.g. injury, stress, LPS, viral and microbial pathogens, cytokines or growth factors), the extract of the root has no effect on NF-κB expression.[85]

In vitro: virus-induced stimulation of pro-inflammatory cytokines was reversed or alleviated.[86]

Dosage: *Echinacea angustifolia/purpurea radix* mix
Daily dose 4.5–9ml of 1:3 60%.
Typical weekly dose 20–50ml of 1:3.

Glycyrrhiza glabra

Individual constituent detail

Triterpenes and flavonoids decreased TNF, MMPs, PGE2 and free radicals.[87]

Glycyrrhetinic acid decreases cell proliferation, inhibits the expression of angiogenic and inflammatory proteins and induces cell cycle arrest or apoptosis.[88,89]

Licoricidin: inhibition of phospholipase A2 activity, resulting in inhibition of cyclooxygenase activity and prostaglandin formation.[90-93]

Preclinical tests in experimental endometriosis: an extract of licorice decreased the growth and histopathologic grades of auto-transplanted endometrial implants in vivo.[94]

Glycyrrhizin suppressed TNF-α, IL-1β, NO, COX-2, and PGE2 production, attenuated TLR4 expression and NF-κB.[95]

Dosage
Daily dose 2–6ml of 1:1.
Typical weekly dosage 15–40ml of 1:1.

Contraindicated: hypertension, sodium and water retention, hypokalemia, arising from the mineralocorticoid effect; consider *Taraxacum officinale* leaf alongside.

Hydrocotyle asiatica

Preclinical: *H. asiatica* and its triterpenoids show anti-inflammatory, anti-apoptotic effects, improve mitochondrial function, and are antioxidant, anti-proliferative.[96]

Asiatic acid: Reduction in the production of inflammatory factors (IL-1β, IL-6, TNF-α). Inhibition of the NF-κB signalling pathway, and thus provides alleviation of pelvic inflammation (in vitro). Promotes apoptosis and inhibits the growth of ovarian cancer cells.[97-99]

Madecassoside is shown in vivo to facilitate collagen synthesis and angiogenesis.[100]

Dosage
Daily dose 3–6ml of 1:2.
Typical weekly dosage 20–40ml of 1:2.

Viburnum prunifolium

From the Eclectics: acts promptly in spasmodic dysmenorrhoea, especially with excessive flow, and was prescribed for menstrual irregularities in previously sterile females, stating that pregnancy had promptly occurred, suggesting it affects and restores normal functional ovarian activity.[101-103] This picture looks similar to that of endometriosis.

Preclinical studies: ethanolic extracts have uterine sedative, relaxant,[104] and spasmolytic activity.[105-107] Experiments with human uterine tissue show a relaxant activity in isolated uterine tissue in vitro.[108,109]

Viburnum opulus, a related species is often used interchangeably with *Viburnum prunifolium*; studies with *Vib. op.* showed decreased adhesion scores of endometriotic implants, endometriotic foci areas, reduced endometriotic volumes and reduced TNF-α, VEGF and IL-6.[110]

Dosage: higher ethanol percentages do not always confer higher activity. French researchers found that *Viburnum prunifolium* bark extracted in 30% ethanol was five times more spasmolytic than a 60% extract.[111]
Daily dose 1.5–4.5ml of 1:2.
Typical weekly dose: 10–30ml of 1:2.

Vitex agnus-castus (see also book 1)

Preclinical studies: dopaminergic, anti-inflammatory, lipoxygenase inhibition,[112] analgesic, immunomodulatory, opioidergic, anti-angiogenic, antioxidant activity and increases melatonin levels.[113]

Dopaminergic effect of *Vitex*: dopamine and its agonists are decreased in active endometriotic lesions in experimental models.[114] Dopamine agonists in experimental endometriosis have anti-angiogenic effects acting through VEGFR-2 activation.[115] This may be one of the many reasons why *Vitex agnus-castus* and *Actaea racemosa* might be helpful in endometriosis.

Vitex is known to increase melatonin secretion:[116] endometriosis is associated with low levels of melatonin and can be influenced by treatment with melatonin in experimental models.[117,118] It causes regression of endometriotic implants in vivo by modulating angiogenesis, tissue levels of antioxidants and MMPs. Melatonin also leads to reduction of plasma levels of LH and oestradiol, and has an influence on oestrogen, progesterone and androgen receptors.[119] Melatonin receptors have been observed in vivo in the uterine endometrium.[120,121] A combination of curcumin and melatonin decreased COX-2 expression and repressed the NF-kappaB pathway, also inhibiting MMP-2, MMP-9 and TIMP-2 expression.[122]

Clinical trials: not specific to endometriosis but shown to be of benefit in menorrhagia, regulated menstrual cycle, aiding conception.[123–126]

Dosage: Many herbalists would prescribe relatively high doses of *Vitex* in endometriosis; this would make sense in relation to its effect on melatonin levels and dopaminergic action.

Typical daily dose for endometriosis 7.5–15ml of 1:3.
Typical weekly dose 10–30ml of 1:3.

Zingiber officinale

Preclinical study in endometriosis: reduced and atrophied endometriosis foci, antioxidant,[127,128] inhibits prostaglandin[129] and leukotriene biosynthesis, inhibited synthesis of pro-inflammatory cytokines (IL-1, TNF-α, and IL-8) in macrophages. Downregulated inflammatory iNOS and COX-2 gene expression[130–132] reduced the elevated expression of NFκB, inhibited proliferation,[133] induced apoptosis, diminished the secretion of VEGF,[134] inhibited angiogenesis and cell adhesion invasion motility.[135–138]

Clinical studies in dysmenorrhoea: ginger found to be as effective as NSAIDs in giving pain relief.[139,140]

Dosage
Typical daily dosage 2.5–6ml of 1:3.
Typical weekly dosage 5–10ml of 1:3.

Table 8.3: Clinical studies: natural compounds, endometriosis

Compound	Clinical studies
Pycnogenol, a patented compound of procyanidins isolated from French maritime pine (*Pinus pinaster*)	**Preclinical studies** suggest that Pycnogenol selectively inhibits MMP and inhibits cyclooxygenases 1 and 2. **Clinical study:** women with endometriosis: compared to gonadotropin-releasing hormone agonist (Gn-RHa), reduced symptom scores. Researchers concluded that Pycnogenol is a valuable alternative to Gn-RHa in the treatment of endometriosis.[141]
Resveratrol rich in polyphenols	**Preclinical studies:** endometriosis model halts progression of the illness through its anti-angiogenic and anti-inflammatory properties.[142,143] Inhibited angiogenesis,[144,145] decreased endometrial cell proliferation and apoptosis.[146,147] Anti-inflammatory: inhibited the release of cytokines (TNF-α, IL-6, IL-8, VEGF and MCP-1)[148] and production of reactive oxygen species in monocytes, macrophages and lymphocytes. Reduced the expression of MMP-2, MMP-9.[149] Agonist and antagonist of oestrogen; reduced human endometrial proliferation through oestrogen receptor-α (ESRα).[150] **Clinical studies:** addition of resveratrol to contraceptive treatment potentiated the effect of oral contraceptives in relieving dysmenorrhea by inhibiting the expression of aromatase and COX-2 in the endometrium, resulting in reduction in pain scores, with 82% of patients reporting complete resolution of dysmenorrhoea and pelvic pain after 2 months of use.[151] Reduced pain scores and the level of carcinoembryonic antigen (CA125) in the treatment of dysmenorrhea patients.[152]
Ginsenosides (Panax ginseng)	**Preclinical studies:** Ginseng saponins reduce production of pro-inflammatory cytokines (TNF-α, interleukin (IL)-1β and IL-6).[153]

(*Continued*)

Table 8.3: (Continued)

Compound	Clinical studies
	Protopanaxadiol (PPD) and protopanaxatriol (PPT), metabolites of ginsenoside decrease the viability of ectopic endometrial stromal cells. PPD promoted the expression of progesterone receptor (PR), downregulated the expression of estrogen receptor α (ERα) in ectopic endometrial stromal cells, enhanced the cytotoxic activity of NK cells, suppressed the growth of ectopic lesions, enhanced the immune surveillance of ectopic lesions. Ginsenosides showed ability for binding to the active sites of steroid receptors (estrogen receptor α),[154] inhibited angiogenesis in endometrial models by blocking VEGF[155-158] and altering the fibrotic properties of endometriosis cells.[159] Clinical study: ginsenoside Rg3 given with gestrinone, volume of endometriotic lesions reduced compared to Rx gestrinone group on its own.[160]

Other herbs with preclinical research

Herb	Preclinical studies on endometriosis
Andrographis paniculata	**Preclinical:** reduced endometriotic lesions, analgesic, a NF-κB inhibitor, anti-tumour activity, inhibits angiogenesis. Inhibits COX-2 and TF expression in endometriotic stromal cells, modulates in uterine contractility.[161-163] Reduced lesion size, suppressed the growth of ectopic endometrium.[164-170] Adenomyosis model: inhibited proinflammatory and angiogenic mediators of cyclooxygenase-2 (COX-2), VEGF and NF-κB, suppressed the expression of oxytocin receptor and modulated in uterine contractility.[171-174] **Clinical trials:** no clinical trials on endometriosis, however, there were positive results in rheumatoid arthritis, which is also an inflammatory and autoimmune condition.[175] One pilot study using andrographolide had positive results in patients with symptomatic adenomyosis.[176]

(Continued)

(Continued)

Herb	Preclinical studies on endometriosis
Camellia sinensis High doses are required.[177]	**Preclinical:** most studies relate to epigallocatechin gallate, a polyphenol found in many foods, but predominantly in green tea. Inhibits E2-stimulated activation, proliferation and VEGF expression in endometrial cells. Reduces angiogenesis, inhibits adhesion and reduces the size and growth of the endometriotic lesions, upregulates NF-κB, increasing apoptosis.[178–191]
Citrus fruits studies on Naringenin only	Oestrogen and antioestrogenic activity, suppresses proliferation and increases apoptosis in human endometriosis cell lines,[192] inhibits angiogenesis.[193]
Curcuma longa: studies on curcumin only	In endometriosis acts on invasion, adhesion, apoptosis and angiogenesis in endometrial lesions.[194] **Anti-inflammatory:** inhibits cyclooxygenase-2 and lipoxygenase enzymes, TNF-alpha, IFN gamma, IL 1 and 6 by supressing NF-kB activation.[195–197] **Angiogenesis:** reduced the number of microvessels and protein expression of VEGF in the ectopic endometrium in vivo. **Invasion and adhesion:** inhibited the expression and activities of MMP-2, MMP-3, MMP-9[198–204] and VEGF protein in endometriosis models; endometriotic lesions were reduced.[205,206] **Apoptosis:** caused cell apoptosis, inhibited cell proliferation in endometrial tumour cells and reduced implant size and cell proliferation in an endometriosis model.[207–210] **Antioxidant:** reduces reactive oxygen species (ROS), microvessel density (MVD) and lipid peroxidation, inhibited cell proliferation.[211–214] **Anti-oestrogenic:** reduces estradiol production in the ectopic endometrium.[215] In vivo and in vitro show beneficial effects via altering the pericellular and extracellular matrix.[216]

(*Continued*)

(Continued)

Herb	Preclinical studies on endometriosis
Humulus lupulus (see book 1) studies on xanthohumol only	**Xanthohumol:** anti-proliferative, anti-inflammatory, anti-angiogenic properties. In vivo model of endometriosis: reduced the size of lesions and decreased microvessel density.[217]
Hypericum perforatum with *Hippophae rhamnoides*	*Preclinical:* oral combination of Hippophae rhamnoides and Hypericum perforatum oils decreased the volumes of endometriotic foci areas and reduced the levels of TNF-α, vascular VEGF and IL-6 in peritoneal fluids in vivo.[218]
Paeonia lactiflora	**Preclinical studies** with glucosides of paeony (TGP); anti-inflammatory; inhibiting the production of PGE2. Downregulated the level of pro-inflammatory cytokine IL-2 and upregulated the levels of IL-4 and TGF-β1.[219] Suppresses overactivated immune responses by inhibiting the proliferation of lymphocytes, balancing the function of Th1 cells and Th2 cells and inducing the apoptosis of lymphocytes.[220] **Clinical trials in autoimmune diseases:** beneficial for rheumatoid arthritis,[221] systemic lupus erythematosus,[222] Sjögren's syndrome, ankylosing spondylitis and chronic urticaria.[223]
Scutellaria baicalensis: studies on baicalein only	Baicalein may suppress the viability of human endometrial stromal cells through the NF-κB signalling pathway *in vitro*.[224]
Salvia miltiorrhiza	**In vivo:** reduces the serum levels of CA125 and the levels of IL-18 and TNF-α by significantly increasing the levels of IL-13 in peritoneal fluid.[225] Inhibits ectopic stromal cell proliferation by inhibiting MMP-9 mRNA and protein expression.[226]

(Continued)

(Continued)

Herb	Preclinical studies on endometriosis
Soya (see book 1) **studies on genistein only**	Isoflavones show anti-angiogenic activity,[227] decreased the expression of estrogen receptor α, VEGF and HIF-1α in peritoneal tissues and increased the expression of estrogen receptor β in vivo. Genistein also regulated angiogenesis by inhibiting the estrogen receptor in a murine model of peritoneal endometriosis.[228]
Tanacetum parthenium	**Preclinical studies:** inhibits serotonin release from platelets and leukocyte, which could explain its use for migraines and arthritis.[229,230] Inhibits production of inflammatory prostaglandins,[231–235] Inhibits mast cell degranulation and subsequent release of histamine, serotonin and other inflammatory cytokines (TNF-α, IL-1, NF-κB, and interferon-γ)[236–238] and cyclooxygenase.[239] Inhibits activity of enzymes 5-lipoxygenase, release of nitric oxide, PGE(2), IL-2 and IL-4 in vitro.[240–245] Spasmolytic effect from fresh leaf extracts (higher in parthenolide): inhibits smooth muscle spasm by blocking open potassium channels.[246]
Uncaria tomentosa[247]	**Preclinical studies:** reduction in the growth endometrial tissue, inhibits PGE2 and change cell cycle progression by inducing apoptosis, inhibits the production of TNF-α. Controls the expression of several pro-inflammatory cytokines; IL-1, IL-2, IL-6, and IL-8.[248–250]

8.4 Dietary recommendations

A range of diets have been recommended for endometriosis. The most commonly followed diets are gluten-reducing/eliminating, dairy-reducing/eliminating and FODMAP diet (low-fermentable oligosaccharides, disaccharides, monosaccharides and polyols).[251,252] Patients who had changed their diets reported various subjective effects of the dietary interventions.[253,254] However, no single diet appeared to provide greater benefit than others.

Mediterranean diet: found to reduce pain related to endometriosis.[255] It is generally seen as an anti-inflammatory diet and is associated with a lower risk of developing endometriosis.[256]

Diet rich in fruits and vegetables: there is evidence of a reduced risk of endometriosis in women who ate large amounts of green vegetables and fresh fruits.[257,258] Consumption of food rich in folic acid, vitamin A, C & E, zinc, selenium and copper is inversely proportional to the risk of developing endometriosis,[259] the relief of pain postoperatively associated with endometriosis and improvement of quality of life.[260,261]

Supplementation had no influence on the occurrence of endometriosis, which shows that the foods really supply much more than just those vitamins.[262,263]

Dairy-rich diet: unlike the common recommendations to exclude dairy, consumption of milk and other low-fat dairy products was linked to a lower risk of developing endometriosis, specifically yogurt and ice cream intake in adolescence may reduce the risk of subsequent endometriosis diagnosis.[264,265] The link was strongest for those taking more than three portions of dairy products per day, compared to women who consumed two or fewer portions. Good news also for those who enjoy butter, as no connection was found between the consumption of butter and the development of endometriosis.[266]

Soya foods and flaxseeds: in a Japanese study, higher levels of urinary genistein and daidzein, associated with diet rich in soya, was related to reduced advanced endometriosis risk.[267] Phytoestrogens, such as the isoflavones in soy and the lignans in flaxseed, competitively inhibit endogenous oestrogens. Isoflavones have anti-mutagenic, antioxidant qualities,[268] decrease the expression of VEGF peritoneal tissue, and regulate inflammation and angiogenesis of peritoneal endometriosis.[269] The use of isolated isoflavones is not advised. Isolated isoflavones were shown to maintain endometriosis and were linked to conversion of the disease to the malignant form.[270]

Table 8.4: Nutrients and their clinical effects: endometriosis

Nutrient	Clinical
Vitamin D: helps to regulate the immune system; a lack leads to increase of inflammatory mediators.	Women with the highest concentration of vitamin D had 24% less risk of developing endometriosis than the women with the lowest concentrations.[271]
Vitamin E	Reduces inflammation, inhibits proliferation of endometroid tissue in vitro; women with endometriosis were found to have lower levels of vitamin E prior to and after ovulation.
Narigenin from citrus fruits	Preclinical: naringenin has anti-angiogenic, anti-inflammatory properties,[272,273] suppresses proliferation, increases apoptosis in human endometriosis cell lines, inhibits angiogenesis by regulating VEGF.[274,275]
Omega 3	Omega 3 fatty acid consumption decreased the risk of endometriosis,[276] by reducing production of pro-inflammatory prostaglandins of the PGE2 pathway.

See Appendix for food sources.

Reduce intake

Avoid red meat: ham, beef and other kinds of red meat were connected with considerably higher endometriosis risk. These are inflammation-provoking foods as they are rich in arachidonic acid.[277] Animal fats and red meat cause higher levels of beta glucuronidase in the colon, thus increasing the recirculation of endogenous oestrogens.

Coffee and caffeine avoidance (lack of evidence): a meta-analysis has found that evidence for the demonisation of caffeine is insufficient.[278] However, one study indicated that products rich in caffeine increased concentrations of oestrogen and oestrone. Conversely, large amounts of caffeine, daily, are associated with an increase in the concentration of SHBG,[279] which would make the oestrogen less available. Overall, the negative associations in the past with coffee consumption might be exaggerated and moderate coffee consumption should not present an issue.

Gluten-free diet: in patients with endometriosis who are also suffering from coeliac disease, a gluten-free diet is recommended.[280]

Low FODMAP diet (not good long term health-wise): FODMAPs (fermentable oligosaccharides, disaccharides, monosaccharides and polyols) are short-chain carbohydrates (sugars) that the small intestine absorbs poorly, and are common in many fruits, vegetables, cereals, dairy products and legumes. For those with irritable bowel syndrome (IBS), a low-FODMAP diet has been shown to be effective in relieving the symptoms.[281] Women with endometriosis are frequently misdiagnosed with IBS, and many with endometriosis do also have IBS.[282,283] If IBS is present, a low FODMAP diet appears to be effective in relieving both gut symptoms and endometriosis.[284] Long term, the concern is that this diet might affect the microbiome, causing constipation and leading to nutritional deficiencies.

Reduce alcohol consumption: a higher percentage of women with endometriosis consumed alcohol than in the control group.[285–287] However, other studies have found no connections between the occurrence of endometriosis and alcohol consumption.[288–290]

Lifestyle

Weight loss: obesity leads to more conversion of androgen to oestrogen by fat cells. Reducing the number of fat cells reduces the androgen to oestrogen conversion, with a positive effect on liver oestrogen metabolism, and increases SHBG.

Exercise: aids oestrogen clearance, increases SHBG, increases cell sensitivity to insulin. Lack of exercise increases the level of circulating oestrogens.

CHAPTER 9

Uterine fibroids (uterine leiomyomas)

9.1 Presentation/symptoms, differential diagnosis and investigations

Uterine fibroids are benign fibrous tumours in the smooth muscle layer of the uterus and range in size from a few millimetres to massive growths of 20cm diameter and more.

There is a higher incidence of fibroids in black women, and these tend to develop at an earlier age.[1]

Symptoms and complications

Some 15–30% of women have symptoms, and these depend partly on location and size of the fibroids.

Submucosal (intrauterine): these can interfere with fertility issues as the endometrium around the fibroid does not undergo normal hormonal changes, affecting implantation. Pre-term birth and miscarriage rates are often higher.[2]

Intramural fibroids (within the muscle layer).

Subserousal fibroids (extra uterine), under the serous outer lining: if these are pedunculated there is the risk of torsion causing extreme pain; surgery may be needed.

Symptoms

- Anaemia (due to menorrhagia).
- Dysmenorrhoea: sensation 'as though everything might fall out' before or during the period.
- Heaviness in the lower abdomen.
- Menorrhagia.
- Pelvic discomfort, and if the fibroids are large this can lead to pressure symptoms such as urinary incontinence and constipation.[3]

Investigations

Once large enough, fibroids can be felt on abdominal examination. Diagnosis is by transabdominal or transvaginal ultrasound. An MRI may be used to delineate the number, size and location of fibroids, and hysteroscopy may be used to distinguish between sub-endometrial fibroids and large endometrial polyps.

Conventional treatment

If there are no symptoms the fibroids only need monitoring. As with cysts, large fibroids can be pedunculated and grow rapidly. In the latter case there is an increased risk of uterine sarcoma.

- Symptomatic treatment of pain and bleeding.
- Gonadotropin-releasing hormone (GnRH) analogues.
- Selective progesterone receptor modulators—effects fibroid shrinkage, in most patients. SPRM treatment leads to control of heavy menstrual bleeding and correction of anaemia.
- Hysterectomy or myomectomy.
- Uterine artery embolisation.
- High-frequency magnetic resonance-guided focused ultrasound surgery.

9.2 Pathophysiology of uterine fibroids

Uterine fibroids are benign fibrous tumours in the smooth muscle layer of the uterus.[4]

These fibroids are the result of increased proliferation of smooth muscle cells and a disorganised extracellular matrix (ECM) deposition such as collagens, fibronectin and proteoglycans.[5] Fibroids have relatively few blood vessels within the structure.[6,7]

Women tend to have multiple fibroids that can range in size from a few millimetres to massive growths of 20cm diameter and more.

The aetiology is unclear but many mechanisms play a role, including the influence of the sex steroid hormones,[8] growth factors, cytokines and chemokine concentrations. All have been implicated in the development and growth of fibroids.

The influence of the sex hormones: an increased concentration of oestrogen receptors is found in fibroids.[9] The enzyme aromatase, which governs the conversion of androstenedione into oestrone and testosterone into oestradiol, is increased in fibroid tissue.[10]

The effect of oestrogen on the growth and development of fibroids is complex and still a mystery. It is possible that oestrogens have an effect via influence on cytokines, growth or apoptosis factors.[11] Oestrogen is known to upregulate platelet-derived growth factor (PDGF) expression and downregulate activin, myostatin, epidermal growth factor (EGF) expression, and may stimulate the proliferation of fibroid cells by activating ATP-sensitive potassium channels.[12] Oestrogen influences the number of progesterone receptors, and it has been suggested that progesterone itself may promote fibroid growth.[13]

Progesterone has an influence on several mechanisms, including the downregulation of IGF-I expression. Different progesterone receptors can stimulate or inhibit.[14] It has also been suggested that progesterone could stimulate fibroid cell growth by downregulating tumour necrosis factor-α (TNF-α) expression.[15]

Abnormal response to injury hypothesis

Infection as injury: a case-control study showed the incidence of uterine fibroids was positively correlated with a history of pelvic infection. Thus, a history of chlamydia or PID, especially recurrent, may be relevant.[16]

Hypertension as injury: fibroid incidence, as well as risk of fibroid growth, increases with high blood pressure. For every diastolic increase of 10mmHG, the risk of fibroid growth increases by 8–10%.[17,18] The ECM responds to stretch, elevated hydrostatic pressure and increased osmotic forces.

Hypertension damages the smooth muscle lining of the arteries. Atherosclerosis is in part a proliferative condition of blood vessel walls,[19] elevated blood pressure causing smooth muscle injury and/or the secretion of cytokines (as in the pathogenesis of atherosclerosis). High-density lipids (HDLs), protective of atherosclerotic changes, are lower in women with fibroids, and thicker carotid intima-media have been shown to be positively associated with uterine fibroids.[20] Atherosclerosis and uterine fibroids are both smooth muscle monoclonal growths, which may in part explain this association.[21–23]

Menstruation as injury: vasoconstriction and hypoxia during menstruation causes the release of vasoconstrictive substances. This repeated 'injury' leads the smooth muscle cells to respond by synthesising extracellular fibrous matrix,[24–26] and causes excess inflammation with upregulation of MMPs and excessive concentrations of inflammatory cytokines such as interleukin-1 and TNF-α and transforming growth factor β (TGF-β).[27]

Growth factors, cytokines and chemokines: frequent mucosal injury with stromal repair reactions may release growth factors, and the whole range are shown to be involved, such as vascular endothelial growth factor (VEGF), EGF, heparin binding epidermal growth factor, PDGF, IGF, TGF-α, TGF-β, acidic fibroblast growth factor, prolactin, erythropoietin, interleukin-1 (IL-1) and IL-6.[28–30]

Genetic predisposition and epigenetic mechanisms: several tumour suppressor genes have been shown to be abnormally hypermethylated in fibroids compared to adjacent myometrium.[31,32] There is a higher prevalence and a significantly younger age at diagnosis, along with more severe pain, in black women compared with others. The underlying cause for the discrepancy is not well understood.[33]

Risk factors

Age: early 40s (although can be asymptomatic earlier), increasing incidence with age up to the menopause, then usually decreasing in size, which may be related to reduced oestrogen exposure.[34]

Early menarche[35]

Hypertension (see above)

Nulliparity: multiple pregnancies reduce the time of exposure to unopposed oestrogens relative to the number of live births.[36]

Obesity: correlates with an increased incidence of uterine fibroids.[37,38]

- Elevated BMI and obesity correlate with patients who have both fibroids and hypertension.[39-43]
- Obese premenopausal: decreased metabolism of oestradiol by the 2-hydroxylation route reduces the conversion of oestradiol to inactive metabolites, which could result in a relatively hyperoestrogenic state. 17 betahydroxysteroid dehydrogenase (17beta-HSD), which converts oestrone into oestradiol, is overexpressed.[44]

Oestrogen excess (including relative oestrogen excess): a higher incidence is found in those suffering from other oestrogen excess conditions such as endometrial hyperplasia and endometriosis.

- **Hormone-disrupting chemicals** such as phthalates and DDE have been linked to fibroids.
- **Oral contraceptives:** there is an elevated risk among women who use oral contraceptives in their early teenage years (13–16 years of age) compared with those who have never used them, although the link is not clear-cut and may depend on exactly which formulation is taken.
- **Tamoxifen** (anti-oestrogenic in breast tissue): has oestrogenic effects on the uterus and has been linked to fibroid growth in several clinical studies.

Smoking: reduced risk (but not previous smoking history), possibly related to anti-oestrogenic effect of cigarette smoking.

Chronic stress: Fluctuations in oestrogen and progesterone levels are caused by the activation of the HPA axis and the subsequent release of cortisol.[45] A study showed a positive association between the number of stressful events and the prevalence of fibroids.[46]

9.3 Herbal management of uterine fibroids

From clinical experience we can say that reducing the size of fibroids is difficult. Although occasionally one can effect change, success may be related to size and menopausal status.

There are a few herbs that have been shown in clinical studies to assist with shrinking fibroids such as *Camellia sinensis* and *Actaea racemosa*.

There is also research on individual compounds, in vitro and in vivo, in experimental fibroids, which might confirm the use of some herbs traditionally used for fibroids, indicating the possible pathways of activity.

Aims

In perimenopausal women, controlling the symptoms is the main aim as, post menopause, the fibroids will often shrink without intervention.[47] Even without attempting to reduce fibroid size, herbs can make an appreciable difference.

Broadly realistic aims include:

Reducing symptoms, especially menorrhagia, dependent on fibroid location (see relevant chapters)
Hormonal modulation
Inhibit cell proliferation: to prevent/slow growth
Address the impact of stress

Herbal management

Hormonal modulation

- <u>Reduce relative excess oestrogen</u>: phenolic phytoestrogens.
- <u>Address oestrogen clearance</u> by hepatics such as *Curcuma longa, Schisandra chinensis, Taraxacum officinale radix*: treat other issues related to oestrogen clearance such as diet and microbiome health.
- <u>Dopaminergic herbs</u>, to indirectly increase progesterone as well as lower prolactin levels: fibroids produce prolactin,[48] which is a growth promoter for vascular smooth muscle.[49] *Actaea racemosa, Paeonia lactiflora & Glycyrrhiza glabra, Vitex agnus-castus*.

Prevent/slow growth

- <u>Inhibit cell proliferation</u> and inhibit angiogenesis by activation of the apoptotic pathway and cell cycle arrest and inhibition of growth factors and/or their receptors. *Actaea racemosa, Camellia sinensis, Curcuma longa, Hydrastis canadensis, Paeonia lactiflora & Glycyrrhiza glabra*, resveratrol, *Vitex agnus-castus*.

- Inhibit inflammatory mediators: anti-inflammatory herbs such *Actaea racemosa*, bioflavonoids, *Camellia sinensis, Curcuma longa, Capsella bursa-pastoris, Paeonia lactiflora & Glycyrrhiza glabra*.
- Inhibit fibrosis by decreasing ECM deposition, profibrotic growth factor expression, and inactivation of activated cell types (responsible for myofibroblastic transformation): *Curcuma longa, Glycyrrhiza glabra*.
- Proteoglycan dermatopontin (DPT), an organiser of collagens, is decreased in fibroids as well as in keloids, which are a similar fibrous lesion.[50] Speculatively, *Hydrocotyle asiatica*, shown to prevent keloid scarring, might be helpful.
- Herbs that have been traditionally used to control benign growths: *Chelidonium majus, Echinacea angustifolia & purpurea* mix and *Thuja occidentalis*.

Manage any associated symptoms: menorrhagia and/or dysmenorrhoea.

Anti-haemorrhagic herbs: *Alchemilla vulgaris, Achillea millefolium, Capsella bursa-pastoris, Hydrastis canadensis, Vitex agnus-castus*.

Dysmenorrhoea: *Actaea racemosa, Anemone pulsatilla, Viburnum prunifolium*.

Improve pelvic circulation: emmenagogues, uterine tonics.

Actaea racemosa, Achillea millefolium, Alchemilla vulgaris.

Reduce the impact of stress: It is important to address the negative impacts of stress with herbs (e.g. adaptogens and nervines).

Herbs used in clinical practice

Achillea millefolium

Traditionally used for menorrhagia, going back to Dioscorides in AD40–90.

Preclinical studies

Anti-proliferative activities of extracts of *Achillea millefolium* on human tumour cell lines.[51] *Achillea's* hypotensive and vasoprotective effects[52,53] may be utilised here with reference to the injury hypothesis mentioned earlier.

Clinical study: effective in minimising the pain severity in primary dysmenorrhea.[54]

Dosage
Daily dose 3–12ml of 1:3.
 Typical weekly dose 15–40ml of 1:3.

Actaea racemosa

Preclinical studies
Dopaminergic activity: dopamine inhibits prolactin secretion and is anti-angiogenic, decreasing proliferation of MCF-7 cells. Prolactin is also produced by uterine tissues and is a growth promoter for vascular smooth muscle.[55-57]

Shown to induce apoptosis in endometriosis models: suppressed E2-induced cell proliferation in endometrial adenocarcinoma cells.[58] It is also known to be an anti-inflammatory, antioxidant,[59] anti-proliferative.[60]

Clinical studies: provided relief from menopausal symptoms and decreased fibroid volume compared with tibolone (a form of HRT). Fibroid size only decreased in the *Actaea* group. The study concluded that *Actaea* provides relief from menopausal symptoms and inhibits growth of fibroids.[61]

Dosage: note that 60% alcohol is needed to extract the triterpene glycosides.
 Daily dose: clinical trials used 80mg per day, which translates to 0.25ml of 1:3.
 Typical weekly dose 5–10ml of 1:3.

Alchemilla vulgaris

Preclinical studies
In vitro found to have hormone-dependent anticancer activity (breast and ovarian).[62-64]

Clinical study
An open study related to menorrhagia in teenage girls, using FE 50–60 gtt 3–5 times per day, 10–15 days before the period, found the volume of flow reduced and the cycle shortened. Premenstrual administration prevented menorrhagia from recurring.[65]

Dosage
Daily dose 6–12ml of 1:3.
Typical weekly dose 15–30ml of 1:3.

Capsella bursa-pastoris

In 1901 Boericke suggested its use for haemorrhage from uterine fibroids with aching in back and uterine haemorrhage with cramps and expulsion of clots.[66]

Preclinical studies (general)
Reduced coagulation time,[67,68] anti-inflammatory activity,[69] antineoplastic effects,[70] uterotonic effect.[71,72] The effect on menorrhagia and metrorrhagia may be a result of the increased contraction of smooth muscles. The hepatoprotective effects may be an added benefit, to aid elimination of oestrogen.[73,74] Antioxidant, preventing free radical damage.[75]

Indole-3-carbinol, a constituent also found in cruciferous vegetables: preclinical studies have shown these to have anti-inflammatory,[76-80] anti-fibrotic,[81] anti-proliferative,[82] and anti-angiogenic effects.[83]

Clinical studies
Two clinical studies for treatment of menorrhagia used *Capsella* alongside the orthodox treatment of mefenamic acid and oxytocin. The combination was more effective than orthodox treatment alone.[84,85]

Dosage
Daily dose 9–36ml of 1:3.
Typical weekly dosage 20–30ml of 1:3.
Dr Weiss states the maximum activity is reached 3 months after the manufacture date, as active principles form through the conversion of other principles and are lost again on extended storage.
The Eclectics suggested that 'fresh is best'.

Camellia sinensis

Preclinical studies with EGCG
In vitro: inhibited proliferation and induced apoptosis in fibroid cells.[86] Suppressed catechol-O-methyltransferase, which is involved with oestrogen metabolism and overexpressed in uterine fibroids.[87] Inhibited angiogenesis and MMP.[88]

In vivo reduced the volume and weight of fibroids,[89] as well as the incidence and size of fibroids.[90]

Clinical studies

800mg of green tea extract per day, given for 4 months, reduced uterine fibroid volume,[91] blood loss decreased; 14% developed amenorrhea in spite of normal serum FSH levels.

A combination of 25μg vitamin D, 150mg EGCG, 5mg vitamin B6 was used BID for 4 months, and fibroid volume decreased.[92]

Dosage: on average a single serving of green tea contains roughly 150mg of EGCG. The dose used in the study quoted was 800mg green tea extract, giving 360mg of EGCG per day.

Glycyrrhiza glabra

Preclinical studies with isoliquiritigenin (a phenolic compound) related to fibroids:

In vitro studies on human uterine fibroid cells reduced cell proliferation and induced apoptosis,[93] arrested cell cycle and nucleus condensation only in uterine fibroid and not myometrial cells.

Other relevant preclinical research

<u>Isoliquiritigenin</u> in vivo inhibited the activation of NF-κB[94] and suppressed TNF-α-induced activation,[95] has an anti-fibrotic effect and inhibited the expression ECM proteins and MMPs.[96]

<u>Triterpenes and flavonoids</u> have anti-inflammatory and antioxidant properties, as well as decreasing cell proliferation, angiogenesis and inducing apoptosis.[97–100]

Dosage

Daily dose 2–6ml of 1:1.

Typical weekly dosage 15–40ml of 1:1.

Contraindicated: hypertension, sodium and water retention, hypokalemia, arising from its mineralocorticoid effects; consider *Taraxacum officinale* leaf alongside.

Hydrastis canadensis

This is traditionally used by the Eclectics for submucosal myoma, haemorrhagic endometriosis and heavy menstrual bleeding. It was suggested that it acts upon the uterine mucous membrane, exciting vascular contractions through which mechanism it diminishes congestion of the genital organs.[101]

Ellingwood suggests that it produces contraction of the unstriped muscular fibres, slowly but permanently stimulating the removal of excess of growth "in the incipient stage of the development of tumours within the uterine structure, or fibroid growths".[102]

Preclinical studies on berberine
In vitro: in uterine fibroid cells it inhibited intracellular aromatase, blocked oestrogen- and progesterone-induced proliferation, induced apoptosis without affecting normal uterine smooth muscle cells.[103]

In vivo: reduced fibroids.[104–107]

Dosage
Daily dose 3–6ml of 1:5.
Typical weekly dose 10–20ml of 1:5.

Paeonia lactiflora & *Glycyrrhiza glabra*

Preclinical research
Affects modulation of the dopaminergic system, reducing prolactin levels and normalising progesterone levels.[108]

Clinical trial
Reduced dysmenorrhea in women with uterine fibroids.[109] Alleviated antipsychotic drug-induced hyperprolactinemia.[110–113]

Dosage: Japanese clinical trials used a Paeonia and licorice combination equivalent to 8–12g/day, equal parts of each. However aqueous ethanol is a more effective solvent than water for many of the constituents.
Typical weekly dose 20–30ml of 1:1 of each herb.

Discussion point: paeony and licorice reduce testosterone levels via stimulation of aromatase activity, thereby increasing oestrogen, which is often given as a reason why they are useful in the treatment of PCOS.[114] However, does this negatively affect fibroids? A higher concentration of aromatase is found in fibroid tissue, leading to increased localised conversion of androstenedione into oestrone and testosterone into oestradiol.[115] Herbs are more complex than one single action so it is probable that other activities override the increased effects of aromatase; we also know it is a dopaminergic herb, which indirectly influences progesterone levels.

Thuja occidentalis

The Eclectics used *Thuja* internally as well as externally for abnormal growths, and tissue degeneration in the mucous and cutaneous tissues, including cancer, and found it retarded growth and prolonged the life of the patient.[116] Ellingwood describes the use of douches for carcinomatous growths in the vagina, alongside internal drops of *Thuja* every four hours.[117] It was used in combination with *Echinacea* for this purpose.[118] Many present-day herbalists use *Thuja* for the treatment of fibroids.

Preclinical studies: *In vitro* and *in vivo* test models it stimulated the cell-mediated immune system and decreased pro-inflammatory cytokines, thereby inhibiting metastasis.[119]

The anti-mitotic effect of individual constituents α/β-thujone demonstrated in vitro, in vivo: diminishes cell viability, is anti-proliferative, proapoptotic and antiangiogenic,[120] stimulates cell-mediated and humoral immune response and production of IL-2 and IFN-γ, anti-metastatic.[121,122]

Dosage
Daily dose 1.5–3ml of 1:5.
Typical weekly dosage 10–20ml of 1:5.

Vitex agnus-castus

There is no research on *Vitex agnus-castus* and fibroids, but some of the following factors might explain why herbalists find *Vitex* useful in fibroids and may also explain the tendency to use *Vitex* in higher doses for fibroids.

Dopaminergic activity: dopamine inhibits prolactin secretion. Prolactin is also produced by uterine tissues and is a growth promoter for vascular smooth muscle.[123] Dopamine and dopamine-agonist medications have anti-angiogenic effects[124] and reduce proliferation of MCF-7 cells (breast cancer cell line).[125] Might *Vitex*, with its dopaminergic action, be having a similar effect?

Indirectly progesteronic by reducing prolactin secretion.[126]

Increases melatonin secretion when taken in relatively high doses.[127,128] Melatonin reduced cell proliferation in vivo, reducing the extracellular matrix of fibroid growths.[129]

Dosage: for fibroids, higher doses are used
Daily dose for fibroids: 7.5–15ml of 1:3,

Typical weekly dose for fibroids 20–35ml of 1:3.

External

Ricinus communis: Castor oil packs

Castor oil is a fixed oil expressed from the seed of *Ricinus communis*, refined to remove ricin, which is toxic.

Herbalists commonly recommend the use of castor oil packs for fibroids. It is said to have been made popular by the healer Edgar Cayce (1877–1945), although the use of castor oil dates to ancient Egypt.

Constituents include ricinoleic acid (80% to 90% of the total fatty acids), and other fatty acids include oleic acid and linoleic acid.[130]

Preclinical study: ricinoleic acid, compared to capsaicin, was shown to have antinociceptive and anti-inflammatory effects, depleting substance P in the presence of neurogenic inflammation, in an action similar to capsaicin.[131]

Clinical research with castor oil externally: comparing this to ultrasound gel and vaseline for their effect on surface pain caused by extracorporeal shock waves, assessing the intensity of pain, castor oil came out best as a contact medium.[132]

Immune system and liver function: castor oil packs were applied over the liver and abdomen for 2 hours with heat, in healthy adults. An increase in T11 cells was seen, contributing to an overall increase in lymphocytes. At the 24-hour mark, total lymphocytes declined, remaining within normal limits.

People with "fatigue" applied castor oil packs over the liver area for 1½ hours per day, 5 days per week for 2 weeks. Total lymphocyte counts normalised and were lower at the end of treatment vs baseline, and those with initially elevated liver enzymes and cholesterol levels normalised.[133]

Chronic constipation: castor oil packs on nursing home residents. Applied to the abdomen for 60 minutes on 3 consecutive days, this resulted in improved faecal consistency, a reduction in straining and improvement in evacuation. No change to the frequency of bowel movements nor the amount of faeces evacuated.[134]

Castor oil packs may have antinociceptive and anti-inflammatory effects, modulate white blood cell count and have a positive effect on liver function and cholesterol levels. It has been speculated that castor oil exerts its effects through the activation of prostaglandins as well as through local depletion of substance P.[135] Topical application of castor oil has been shown to reduce the pain of neurogenic inflammation and improve symptoms of constipation.

A castor oil pack is made by soaking a cloth or cotton wool in warm castor oil and placing it on the abdomen, sometimes using heat packs.

Table 9.1: Studies: herb combinations and isolates

Herb/constituent	Studies
Combination *Cinnamomum cassia*, *Prunus persica* **seed**, *Poria cocos* **and** *Paeonia suffruticosa*	Premenopausal women 27 to 52 years, 22.5g per day of dried herb was found to shrink uterine fibroids (less than 10cm in diameter at the outset). Menorrhagia and dysmenorrhea improved. Shrinkage of the fibroids was found in about 60% of patients.[136,137]
Curcumin	**Preclinical** Anti-proliferative and anti-fibrotic effects on fibroid cells via regulation of apoptotic pathway,[138] inhibited TGF-β-related endothelial-to-mesenchymal transition and attenuated endothelial cell fibrosis.[139] Decreased uterine fibroid cell proliferation,[140] anti-inflammatory[141,142] anti-adhesion,[143] reduced oestradiol production in the ectopic endometrium,[144] affected serum lipid levels.[145]
Resveratrol	**Preclinical studies related to fibroids** Anti-proliferative and anti-fibrotic effects, induced apoptosis and cell cycle arrest in human uterine fibroid cells.[146] **Clinical trial** in endometriosis: the expression of both aromatase and cyclooxygenase-2 were inhibited significantly more in the eutopic (normally situated) endometrium of patients using OCP and resveratrol therapy, compared with the results for patients using oral contraceptives alone.[147]

9.4 Dietary and lifestyle recommendations

Dairy: in a prospective study consumption was correlated to reduced risk.[148] Investigators suggested that calcium in dairy products may reduce fat-induced cell proliferation by maintaining intracellular calcium concentrations; additionally the butyric acid in milk fat is antineoplastic, inducing differentiation and apoptosis, and inhibiting proliferation and angiogenesis.

High vegetable and fruit intake: The beneficial effects are plentiful, including the anti-proliferative effect of flavonoids. A case-control study showed that the risk of uterine fibroids was inversely associated with the intake of green vegetables and fruit. Another study found that a high intake of fruit, particularly citrus fruit, was inversely associated with uterine fibroids risk.[149] The association was stronger when served two or more times per day.[150]

Lignan-rich diet: a clinical study found that urinary excretion of lignans (flaxseed) was inversely associated with uterine fibroid risk.[151] As a phenolic phytoestrogen it displaces endogenous oestrogen, exerting an influence on an oestrogen dominant environment (see book 1).[152]

Fermented foods: to ensure healthy gut flora and enable breakdown and utilisation of ingested phytoestrogens (see book 1).

Weight control: long-term weight gain correlates with the incidence of uterine fibroids.[153]

Lifestyle aspects: as mentioned in previous chapters, stress has a profound effect on hormones, as well as having important contributory factors to hypertension and atherosclerosis, all of which are implicated in fibroid growth.[154] It is important to address the impact of stress with herbs (e.g. adaptogens and nervines) as well as lifestyle recommendations, such as meditation, yoga, being outside in nature, hobbies, etc.

Other

Beer: A beer a day or more increased the risk of developing uterine fibroids by more than 50%.[155]

Table 9.2: Individual compounds of vegetables and fruit

Constituent	Studies
Anthocyanins	In vitro study related to fibroids: anthocyanin-rich strawberries induced apoptosis and suppressed glycolysis and fibrosis in uterine fibroid cells, reduced fibronectin, collagens and versican mRNA expression in UF cells.[156,157]
Epigallocatechin-3-gallate (EGCG)	Clinical trial with EGCG reduced the volume of uterine fibroids and improved symptoms of anaemia and blood loss.[158]
	The effect was thought to be due to the inhibitory action of EGCG on catechol-O-methyltransferase (COMT), elevated in uterine fibroids and involved in their pathogenesis.[159] COMT is also implicated in cardiovascular disease and high blood pressure; it reduced atherosclerotic lesions induced by COMT in vivo.[160]
Genistein	In vitro genistein inhibits the proliferation of cultured uterine fibroid cells,[161] stimulates fibroid cell proliferation at low concentration[162] and inhibits fibroid cell proliferation at high concentration, induces apoptosis in fibroid cells.[163] Downregulates activin A, Smad3, and other TGF-β pathway genes in human uterine fibroid cells.[164]
	In vivo reduces the incidence and size of spontaneously occurring fibroids.[165]
Lycopene	Preclinical study related to fibroids (in vivo): Lycopene as well as tomato powder supplementation reduces the incidence and size of spontaneously occurring fibroids.[166,167] There is an inverse correlation between tomato intake and risks for various tumours and epithelial cancers (prostatic, lung, pancreatic, gastric, cervical and ovarian).[168]

(*Continued*)

Table 9.2: (Continued)

Constituent	Studies
Omega 3	Anti-inflammatory and immunomodulatory effects, through decreasing the levels of C-reactive protein, IL-6, and TNF-α, which are involved in the formation of uterine fibroids.[169] Preclinical study: in vitro, omega 3 fatty acids remodelled membrane architecture and downregulated the expression of genes involved in mechanical signalling and lipid accumulation in fibroid cells.[170]
Quercitin	In vitro studies related to fibroids: quercetin and indole-3-carbinol decreased collagen and fibronectin mRNA expression (inhibit extracellular matrix expression) and the migration pattern in uterine fibroid cells.[171]
Sulforaphane	Preclinical study (in vitro): sulforaphane reduces proliferation and inflammation of uterine fibroid cells.[172]
Vitamin A	Clinical study: a large observational study of 22,583 pre-menopausal women showed a dose-dependent relationship between vitamin A and the formation of uterine fibroids.[173] It is possible that vitamin A deficiency increases uterine fibroid occurrence.[174] Animal sources of vitamin A appear to be primarily responsible. Vitamin A influences cellular differentiation, gene expression, immunity and has antineoplastic activity. Retinoic acid (an active metabolite of vitamin A) mediates growth-related functions, shown to have an anti-proliferative effect,[175] regulating cell proliferation and apoptosis.[176,177]

(Continued)

Table 9.2: (Continued)

Constituent	Studies
Vitamin D	**Serum vitamin D levels** correlated with fibroid size, more so in women of colour.[178] Women of colour have a higher risk of serum vitamin D deficiency compared to white women and are 3–4 times more likely to have UF.[179,180] Preclinical studies: in vitro, inhibits the growth of uterine fibroid cells through the downregulation of kinases and Bcl2, and suppresses catechol-O-methyltransferase (COMT) expression and activity.[181] In vivo, high doses of vitamin D3 shrank uterine fibroids by as much as 75%.[182] Clinical trials: vitamin D treatment inhibited growth of fibroid.[183,184] Vitamin D (plus EGCG and vitamin B6) decreased volume by 34.7%.[185]

See Appendix for food sources.

CHAPTER 10

Cervical dysplasia

10.1 Presentation/symptoms, differential diagnosis and investigations

In a normal healthy cervix, the bottom layer of squamous cells, the basal cells, are large and round with big nuclei. Closer up to the surface the cells are smaller, flatter and lose their nuclei before moving to the top. Overall, from the basal layer to the superficial layer, these cells undergo an increase in size and a reduction in nuclear size.

Cervical dysplasia is the abnormal growth of the cells that line the surface of the cervix, usually caused by the human papillomavirus (HPV). The affected area is the squamocolumnar junction of the mucous membrane of the cervix—these cells are the most susceptible to premalignant transformation. Those affected are typically 25 to 35 years old but the condition can occur at any age. When mild cervical dysplasia is present the majority (65–70%) will regress by themselves and only a small percentage will go on to develop cervical cancer.[1] The possibility of progression to cervical cancer increases with the severity of the dysplasia and HPV subtype. On average this will take 10–15 years to progress if untreated.

Categories of dysplasia

- Mild dysplasia: the basal cell layer is thicker, up to one-third the total thickness.
- Moderate dysplasia: the abnormal cell layer extends into the middle third layers.
- Severe dysplasia: extending into the top third.
- Carcinoma "in situ": not invasive. Risk of progression to cancer but remains treatable.

Human papillomavirus (HPV) is the usual cause of cervical dysplasia, spread through skin contact and sexual transmission. A high percentage of the adult population is thought to be exposed (75% in the U.S.).[2-4]

Most women with HPV never get dysplasia at all. HPV infection alone is not sufficient to cause invasive cervical cancer, and only about 10 women per 100,000 get cervical cancer.[5] Other factors play a role, environmental and host immune responses to HPV infection suggesting either inherited susceptibility or resistance to the transforming properties of oncogenic papillomaviruses.

A hundred HPV subtypes have been identified. Some are much more likely to cause cellular abnormalities. Depending on HPV subtype, some are more aggressive, such as HPV 16 (50–60% of cervical cancer) and HPV 18 (10–12%), and can develop into cancer within 18 months. But these are the exceptions rather than the norm.

Risk factors for cervical dysplasia and cervical cancer

- Age: rarely in those under 20, the highest incidence at midlife, under the age of 50. In women over 65 the incidence tends to be related to those who do not have regular Pap screening.
- Chlamydia infection: a possible cofactor to HPV in the development of cervical cancer, possibly by affecting the host's immunity or causing chronic inflammation. *C. trachomatis* infection increases the expression of HPV 16, suggesting that *C. trachomatis* has the ability to modify HPV activity.[6]
- Diethylstilbestrol exposure: daughters of women who took diethylstilbestrol (DES) during pregnancy, which was Rx for miscarriage, premature labour and complications in pregnancy in the 1940s and 1971.

- Diet: low in fruits and vegetables.[7]
- Family history of cervical cancer, although the evidence is not clear.[8]
- HPV infection.
- Immunosuppression: HIV.
- Non-condom use: condoms provide prevention as well as increased regression of cervical dysplasia, even of CIN II or higher.[9]
- Oral contraceptives: the risk of cervical cancer increased with longer duration of use, returning to normal 10 years after use, although not all papers are conclusive. OCP has been linked to an increase in the incidence of adenocarcinoma. Steroid hormones are thought to increase the expression of HPV 16 oncogenes, which in turn bind to and degrade tumour suppressor gene product, leading to carcinogenesis.
- CIN 2 and 3 are associated with higher 16-alpha hydroxyestrone and fewer 2-hydroxyestrogen metabolites.
- Obesity: although this was said to be due to lower uptake of cervical screening.[10]
- Pregnancy: the mechanism is not fully understood. Three or more full-term pregnancies seem to increase the risk of developing cervical cancer, as well as giving birth before age of 22.[11]
- Sexual history: multiple partners.
- Smoking: Nicotine concentrates in the glands of the cervix; smoking alters immune function and affects the levels and distribution of ascorbic acid; ascorbic acid in the plasma as well as in the cells of the cervix and the vagina is reduced in smokers. Smoking also plays a role in the early stages of carcinogenesis, from the acquisition of HPV infection to the development cervical cancer. Smoking worsens all the processes of cervical cancer.[12]
- Chronic stress and diurnal cortisol are related to the presence of HPV infection and may play a role in HPV-associated cervical carcinogenesis.[13]

Symptoms

Asymptomatic.

Occasionally can cause menorrhagia, abnormal bleeding (typically after intercourse), spotting, or watery vaginal discharge.

Advanced cervical cancer: pelvic pain, difficulty with urination and oedema, along with signs of advanced malignancy.

Investigations

Papanicolaou (Pap) test: the test can detect changes in the cervix before cancer develops or in the early stages.

Pap smears are screening tests and not diagnostic. Colposcopy and cervical biopsies are diagnostic methods for an accurate diagnosis.

Those with hysterectomies may still have their cervix intact and need to be checked.

For abnormal Pap results, two systems are used for reporting and are overlapping, so it is important to be aware of the terminology involved.

CIN: Cervical intraepithelial neoplasia, cellular abnormalities before cancer:

- CIN I (mild dysplasia)
- CIN II (moderate dysplasia)
- CIN III (severe dysplasia to carcinoma in situ)

SIL: squamous intraepithelial lesion, Bethesda system. Changes are classified on a scale of low grade to high grade.

- ASC (Atypical Squamous Cells): not quite abnormal, but not normal either. Pap tests are usually repeated and if atypia persists, the woman should be evaluated as greater risk of cervical cancer.
  - ASC-H Atypical Squamous Cells: cannot rule out high-grade (precancerous) lesions and the women can be at greater risk for CIN 2 or CIN 3. Colposcopy and biopsies are required.
  - AGC-US (Atypical Glandular Cells of Undetermined Significance): borderline, some abnormal cells, low-grade squamous intraepithelial lesions. More than 50% of women with AGC-US are found to be 'clear'. These findings can also indicate chronic endocervicitis, microglandular hyperplasia of the endocervix, ciliated cell metaplasia of the endocervix and those with IUDs. AGC-US cells could have come from tubal or ovarian cells or even metastasis from the pelvis. Significant cervical lesions can be present, such as high-grade CIN or adenoma carcinoma.
    With both findings, ASC-US and ASC-H, HPV testing is recommended, and further evaluation is needed.

- LSIL (Low-grade Squamous Intraepithelial Lesions): mild dysplasia (previous called CIN I) and cellular changes associated with HPV, early changes in the size, shape and number of abnormal cells. Intraepithelial indicates that abnormal cells are present in the surface layer of cells, not the deeper glandular layer. Colposcopy and biopsies are recommended.
- HSIL (High-grade Squamous Intraepithelial Lesions): moderate to severe dysplasia, precancerous lesions and carcinoma in situ (preinvasive cancer that involves only the epithelium), usually treated aggressively as it has a higher likelihood of progressing to cervical cancer. Colposcopy and biopsies are recommended. Women with a histological diagnosis of HSIL (CIN 3) need to be treated to reduce the risk of developing invasive cervical carcinoma.

CIN I and CIN II: 40–50% of abnormal smear tests spontaneously revert to normal.[14] In mild dysplasia the reversion can be within two years.

CIN III or HSIL: in severe dysplasia or carcinoma in situ that affects the full thickness of the epidermis, spontaneous regression is unlikely if untreated and may become invasive and penetrate the basement membrane.

Prevention

Vaccination offers 90% protection against HPV infection, cervical dysplasia and cancer.[15]

- Cervarix against HPV 16, 18
- Gardasil (Silgard) against HPV 16, 18, 6, 11
- Gardasil 9 against nine HPV types—6, 11, 16, 18, 31, 33, 45, 52, 58—supposed to protect against 90% of cervical cancer cases[16]

Conventional treatment

Manage moderate and severe dysplasia by removal. There is some ongoing debate about the treatment of mild dysplasia.

- Wait and monitor: for mild dysplasia, as most will revert to normal tissue. Mild dysplasia can be observed for longer, as long as close follow-ups are in place.

- Cryotherapy: reserved for mild dysplasia (CIN 1), and devitalised tissue is sloughed as a watery discharge over the next 10 to 14 days. The cervix usually heals within a month.
- Conisation: remove a cone-shaped piece of cervix and cervical canal, which can occasionally lead to 'incompetent cervix' during pregnancy.
- Laser ablation: allows for precise management of lesions where biopsy is not possible; tissue taken as in conisation.
- LEEP (Loop Electrosurgical Excision Procedure), LETZ (Loop Excision of the Transformation Zone), LLETZ (Large Loop Excision of the Transformation Zone): all used in moderate-to-severe degree dysplasia. Can lead to reduced cervical mucus, bleeding and has the risk of incomplete removal of the lesion. Scarring can affect fertility by obstruction of the endocervical canal, as well as damaging the cervical crypts needed for formation of cervical mucus and the collection and storage of sperm. Scarring can also potentially affect cervical dilatation in labour.

Recurrences of dysplasia can occur due to new infection, reactivation of the virus due to immune system changes or inadequate prior treatment with residual cells that then persist and regrow.

10.2 Herbal management of cervical dysplasia

There is a long list of herbs that has been shown to impact on cervical cancer cells in vitro, inhibiting carcinogenesis through various mechanisms including antioxidant, cytotoxic and anti-angiogenic actions, and reducing HPV replication. This suppresses different stages of carcinogenesis: initiation, promotion and progression.

We cannot directly extrapolate from these studies that these will all be of use in cervical dysplasia although, applied topically, they may have a direct effect on cancer cells.

Aims

Prevent the progression and/or reverse cervical dysplasia with local as well as internal treatment

Internal treatment focused on immunity to aid resistance to viral exposure, dampen inflammation, restore mucous membrane health, regulate hormones, support the nervous system

Local topical treatment: herbal suppositories with antiviral, antimicrobial, anti-mitotic, anti-inflammatory activity, local tissue health and repair, support mucous membrane health

Herbal management

Internal treatment

Adaptogens, nervines: as mentioned elsewhere, mental well-being will affect the immune and endocrine system, and there will often be additional stress related to the diagnosis and treatment:[17] *Astragalus membranaceus, Eleutherococcus senticosus, Panax ginseng, Withania somnifera.*

Anti-inflammatory: *Achillea millefolium, Camellia sinensis, Curcuma longa, Zingiber officinale.*

Antineoplastic and prevention of proliferation: *Actaea racemosa, Astragalus membranaceus, Camellia sinensis, Curcuma longa, Echinacea ang/purp, Ganoderma lucidum, Silybum marianum, Thuja occidentalis.*

Antiviral: *Thuja occidentalis*, internally and topically.

Bitters: to improve nutrient absorption, improve microbiome and to reduce enteropathic oestrogen recycling: *Achillea millefolium, Artemisia absinthum, Berberis vulgaris, Salvia rosmarinus (Rosmarinus officinalis).*

Hepatics: *Curcuma longa, Salvia rosmarinus (Rosmarinus officinalis), Silybum marianum, Taraxacum radix.*

Immune-enhancing: *Astragalus membranaceus, Baptisia tinctora, Echinacea ang/purp, Eleutherococcus senticosus, Thuja occidentalis.*

Lymphatics: *Calendula officinalis, Phytolacca decandra, Thuja occidentalis.*

Mucous membrane restorative: *Hydrastis canadensis, Plantago lanceolata.*

Treat relative oestrogen excess: polyphenolic phytoestrogenic herbs (*Linum sativum*, soya, *Trifolium repens*) to displace endogenous oestrogen and reduce relative excess, as oestrogen is one of the risk factors for dysplasia.

Dopaminergic herbs: to increase progesterone levels indirectly and lower prolactin levels. *Actaea racemosa, Vitex agnus-castus.*

Uterine tonic herbs/emmenagogues (increase pelvic circulation): *Achillea millefolium, Actaea racemosa, Alchemilla vulgaris, Angelica sinensis, Artemisia absinthium, Artemisia vulgaris, Calendula officinalis*.

Topical local treatment, as pessaries

Antiviral and anti-mitotic: *Camellia sinensis, Filipendula ulmaria, Hydrastis canadensis, Myrtus communis, Thuja occidentalis*.

Healing and/or restoring mucous membranes: *Aloe vera* gel, *Calendula officinalis, Hydrocotyle asiatica*.

Improve vaginal pH and microbiome: *Berberis vulgaris, Hydrastis canadensis, Lactobacillus* (yogurt).

Herbs used in clinical practice

Typical herbalists' approach to mild dysplasia would be to use *Calendula* (possibly with EO) pessaries and general internal systemic support.

Internal treatment

Astragalus membranaceus

Clinical studies: an *Astragalus*-containing Chinese herbal medicine combined with chemotherapy for the treatment of cervical cancer enhanced the efficacy and reduced toxicity of chemotherapy.[18]

Dosage
Daily dose 2.25–4.25ml of 1:1.
 Typical weekly dose 20–30ml of 1:1.

Camellia sinensis

Preclinical studies: in vitro showed regression of cervical dysplasia and prohibited the growth of HPV-positive cervical cancer cells. The mechanisms are thought to be apoptosis, cell cycle arrest, modification of gene expression and antitumour effects.[19–21]

Clinical studies

<u>HPV-infected cervical lesions</u>: using green tea topically and or orally, the topical treatment groups improved the most significantly compared to oral alone.[22,23]

<u>Women diagnosed with CIN II, III, or cervical cancer</u>: using green tea intake of several cups per week, over a two-year period, was associated with 40% reduced odds of cervical cancer.[24]

Dosage used in trials
300mg per day orally.

Curcuma longa

Preclinical studies: curcumin in vitro on cervical cancer cells, downregulation of viral oncogenes in HPV-associated cells, downregulation of HPV 18 transcription. Inhibits carcinogenesis through various mechanisms including antioxidant, anti-inflammatory, proapoptotic, antiangiogenic and immunomodulatory properties.[25] Curcumin is involved in the suppression of all three stages of carcinogenesis: initiation, promotion and progression.[26]

Clinical study: curcumin in patients with different cancers, including uterine cervical intraepithelial neoplasm. The starting dose was 500mg/day, over time increased to 12,000mg/day. Histologic improvement of precancerous cells was noted in one out of the four patients.[27]

Dosage
Turmeric powder contains about 3.14% curcumin.[28] If we round up very generously to 4% curcumin, we have 0.2g of curcumin in one 5g teaspoon of turmeric powder.

Dosages in trials have varied from 0.5 to 12g of curcumin per day, which would translate to 2.5–60 teaspoons of turmeric per day to achieve these levels of curcumin. This is obviously not practically possible, hence the use of extracts.

It is possible that lower quantities may be required if the whole root is used instead of isolated curcumin, as it is not unusual in plants to find that one constituent enhances the absorption of another. When using turmeric in food the bioavailability of curcumin is enhanced by the presence of black pepper, oils and lecithin. While there is evidence that warrants supplementing high doses of curcumin, it is most likely worthwhile to top this up with the whole extract, e.g. as 'golden milk'.

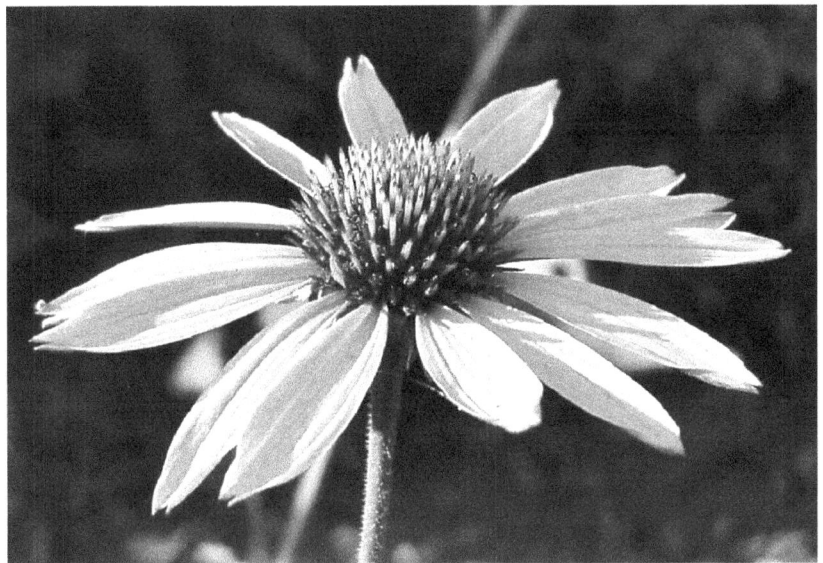

Echinacea pupurea

Echinacea purpurea and angustifolia

Preclinical: tincture 1:10, looking at cytotoxic effects on different cervical tumour lines, both *E. angustifolia* and *Thuja occidentalis* found to be effective, *E. angustifolia* showing more activity than *T. occidentalis*.[29]

Clinical studies:
Echinacea purpurea and *angustifolia* (taken orally) on patients with HPV infection, with post treatment CO_2 Laser treatment to investigate relapse rates, was successful in reducing relapse incidence of lesions in patients treated for genital condylomatosis.[30]

Dosage
Echinacea angustifolia/purpurea radix mix: daily dose 4.5–9ml of 1:3 60%. Typical weekly dose 20–50ml of 1:3.

Ganoderma lucidum

Preclinical studies: in vitro, shown to block the cell cycle and promote apoptosis of cervical cancer cells.[31] *Ganoderma lucidum* extracts in melanoma and triple-negative breast cancer cells inhibited the release of IL-8, IL-6, MMP-2 and MMP-9 in cancer cells under pro-inflammatory conditions, decreased the viability of cancer cells and reduced cell migration.[32]

In vivo: cervical carcinoma model, suppressed the growth through the regulation of the apoptotic process.[33]

Clinical studies: in breast cancer patients alongside chemotherapy, *Ganoderma* showed an increase of IFN-γ (marker for immune stimulation effect) and a decrease in the levels of TNF-a (a marker for anti-inflammation), compared to chemotherapy by itself.[34]

Dosage
Daily dose 2–20g, the higher end dose for cancer/pre-cancer.
The majority of practitioners use 1–6g daily.

Panax ginseng

Preclinical studies: different types of ginsenoside induce apoptosis through a variety of signalling cascades. Ginsenoside-Rg5, a constituent of steamed ginseng, induced increases in apoptosis, genotoxic effects in cervical cancer cells and chemotherapeutic activity in human cervical cancer cells.[35,36]

Dosage
Daily dose 1.5–9ml of 1:3.
Typical weekly dose 10–25ml of 1:3.

Thuja occidentalis

The Eclectics used the herb internally, as well as externally, for tissue degeneration in the mucous membrane and recommended *Thuja* for abnormal growths, including cancer, indicating that it retards growth and prolongs life. Ellingwood describes the use of douches for carcinomatous growth in the vagina, alongside internally 15 drops of *Thuja* with *Echinacea angustifolia* every four hours. The Eclectics used it for viral infections such as epithelioma, papilloma (warts) and condylomata (warts around the anus or genitals), although they reported mixed effectiveness.

Preclinical research
Homeopathic medicine, including the mother tincture 1:10: looking at cytotoxic effects on different cervical tumour lines, both *E. angustifolia*

and *T. occidentalis* were found to be effective. *E. angustifolia* showed more activity than *T. occidentalis*.³⁷

In HPV 16-infected cervical cancer cells *Thuja* mother tincture (1:10) showed significant anti-proliferative and anti-migratory actions induced via dual apoptosis and autophagy. Thujone, taken orally, showed greater anti-proliferative and anti-migratory potential. The study concluded that the 'multi-targeting' anticancer activity of *Thuja* drug and thujone for HPV-infected cervical cancer shows potential for therapeutic efficacy for HPV infections.³⁸

Dosage
Daily dose 1.5–3ml of 1:5 60%.
Typical weekly dose 10–15ml of 1:3 60%.

Topical treatment

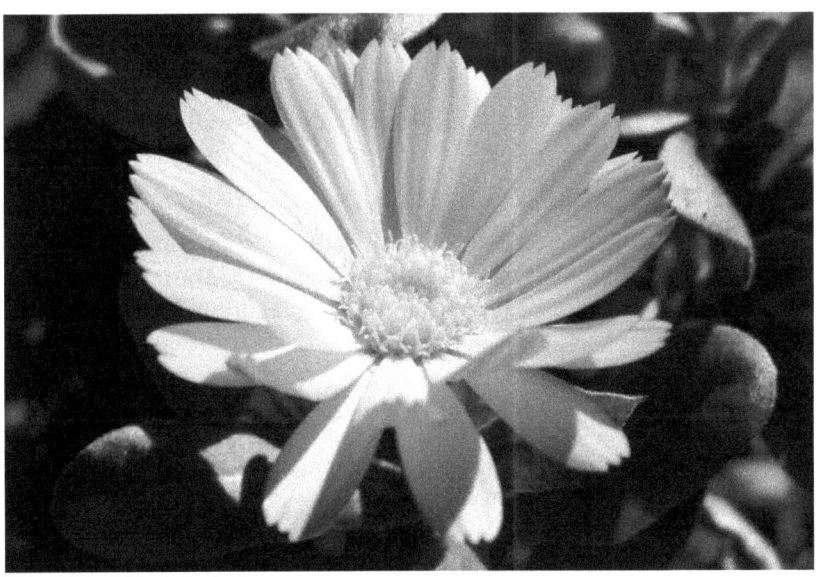

Calendula officinalis

Preclinical studies: cytotoxic activity toward different cancer cell lines, including cervical cancer cells. In vivo, oral administration confirmed anti-genotoxic/protective, antitumour and antimetastatic effects.³⁹

Filipendula ulmaria

Traditionally used for its anti-ulcerogenic,[40] anti-inflammatory activities, which could all contribute to its positive effects in cervical dysplasia.[41] In vitro, shown to inhibit T-cell proliferation and complement cascade activation; is also an antioxidant and decreases vascular/capillary permeability, which all play a role in the inflammatory response.[42]

Salicylates, in *Filipendula ulmaria*,[43] are often used externally to treat warts, another action that can be of help in HPV-related conditions.

Preclinical studies: local administration in vivo of the decoction resulted in a 39% drop in the frequency of squamous-cell carcinoma of the cervix and vagina.[44]

Clinical study: decoction applied intravaginally: a positive response was recorded in a majority of the patients and half had complete regression. However, the level of dysplasia was not stated.[45]

Myrtus communis

Preclinical studies: in vitro anticarcinogenic potential, cytoprotective and anti-inflammatory.

Clinical study: patients with cervical lesions and HPV infection, comparing the efficacy of herbal vaginal suppository (10% of myrtle aqueous extract and 0.5% of myrtle essential oil) and placebo. The interventional group benefited significantly with an HPV clearance rate of 92.6% and the change in cervical lesion size was 71.4%.[46]

Table 10.1: Preclinical studies (in vitro) on cervical cancer cells

Achillea millefolium	Cytotoxic activities against cervical cancer cells, leading to apoptosis and cell growth arrest.[47]
Berberine	Decreased cell viability and induced growth inhibition in cervical cancer cells.[48]
Salvia rosmarinus (*Rosmarinus officinalis*)	Inhibited cell proliferation.[49]

(Continued)

Table 10.1: (Continued)

Silybum marianum	Silymarin: suppressed the survival, migration and invasion of cervical cancer cells. Silymarin induced human cervical cancer cell death through both apoptotic and necrotic pathways. Prevented cancer cells from dividing and reproducing, shortened the lifespan of cancer cells. Reduced blood supply to tumours. Studies suggest milk thistle can act synergistically with chemotherapy.[50]
Taraxacum radix	Antitumour effect, affected proliferation, survival and cell migration. Leads to apoptosis.[51]
Zingiber officinale	Methanolic extract of *Zingiber officinale* rhizome for anticancer activity against human cervical cancer cells, inhibitory effects on cell proliferation and induction of apoptosis.[52] 6-gingerol: anti-tumourigenic and pro-apoptotic activities against cervical cancer cells in vitro and in vivo.[53] 6-shogaol: anticancer properties, via various pathways involved in cell death.[54]

Other herbs and individual constituents that have been shown to have effect on cervical cancer cell lines are: *Commiphora molmol*,[55] *Salvia miltiorrhiza*,[56] baicalein,[57] emodin, a constituent of *Rheum palmatum*,[58,59] and quercetin.[60]

Pessary recipe
2 parts cocoa butter
1 part beeswax or other hard vegetable wax (candelilla, carnauba)
4% infused oil
1% essential oil (if using)
Melt together and pour into moulds.

10.3 Dietary and lifestyle recommendations

Clinical Research

Dairy: a diet high in milk, yogurt, tofu and fish, with green vegetables, had a moderately decreased risk for cervical dysplasia/carcinoma.[61]

Cruciferous vegetables: contain sulforaphane and indole-3-carbinol known to reduce the incidence of cancer.

Lignans: found in flaxseeds, may also play a role in lowering pre-malignancies of the cervix: plasma levels of equol and enterodiol are positively associated with a lower cervical dysplasia risk (see book 1 for more detail).[62]

Mediterranean diet: a diet rich in vegetables, legumes, fruits and nuts, cereals, fish, and a high ratio of unsaturated to saturated lipids, lowered the risk of HPV infection.[63]

Papaya: rich in lycopene, a study found that HPV-positive women with higher consumption of papaya reduced the SIL risk.[64]

Probiotics: Lactobacillus spp. is protective by maintaining the "cervical epithelial barrier" function.[65] Women with unhealthy cervicovaginal microbiota are more likely to acquire infections including HPV. Clinical studies in women with HPV-positive and cervical lesion, found that probiotics increased the clearance of cervical cellular abnormalities and HPV infection.[66,67,68]

Vegetable and fruit consumption: associated with lowered risk of HPV persistence, and reduced risk of developing cervical dysplasia.[69,70,71,72,73,74] This is most likely a result of their richness in vitamins and minerals, as well as other constituents of plant based foods that are known to prevent and clear cervical dysplasia and HPV infections (see below under individual nutrients and clinical research).

Other: intake of red, processed meats, dipping sauces and chips are associated with a higher risk of HPV infection.[75]

Individual nutrients

Nutrients	Studies
Carotenoids (alpha carotene, beta carotene, and beta cryptoxanthin, lutein, zeaxanthin, and lycopene	Clinical: associated with regression of cervical dysplasia, prevention of cancer, as well as offering protection against persistent HPV.[76,77] Lycopene: higher serum concentrations associated with decreased risk of CIN I, CIN III, and cervical cancer.[78,79] Papaya: a case-control study of 265 HPV-positive women, higher consumption of papaya reduced the SIL risk.[80]
CoQ10	Plasma CoQ10 levels lower in those with CIN and cervical cancer.[81]

(*Continued*)

(Continued)

Nutrients	Studies
Indole-3-carbinol converted in the stomach to multiple compounds including diindolylmethane	Preclinical study: in vivo prevented progression from cervical dysplasia to cervical cancer and increased immune response.[82] Clinical study: indole-3-carbinol (I-3-C) orally, 200 or 400mg/day, led to reduction CIN, 2/16 alpha-hydroxyestrone ratio changed to healthier outlook, with a positive effect in women with vulvar intraepithelial neoplasia, often caused by HPV.[83]
Multivitamin including A, C, D, E, folate, lycopene, calcium	Protective against cervical dysplasia and reduction of HPV persistence.[84,85,86] Low serum levels A, E, folate, lycopene, vitamin E has been associated with increased risk of developing cervical dysplasia.[87,88]
Omega-3-fatty acids, particularly DHA	In vitro prevention of HPV malignant conversion.[89]
Polyphenols: includes broad range of flavonoids	Clinical trials; shown to have antitumoral, chemo- and radiosensitizer effects.[90] Polyphenols inhibit the proliferation of HPV cells, through induction of apoptosis, growth arrest, inhibition of DNA synthesis and modulation of signal transduction pathways.[91] In vitro: quercetin helps to sensitize cervical cancer cells to apoptosis caused by cisplatin,[92] and showed a radiosensitizing enhancement.[93] In vitro: apigenin sensitised cervical cancer cells to paclitaxel and induced apoptosis.[94] Isoflavones: 7,3',4'-trihydroxyisoflavone and formononetin increased the cytotoxicity of epirubicin.[95] Genistein enhanced the radiosensitivity human cervical cancer cell line.[96] Clinical study: green tea[97,98] with curcumin, both rich in polyphenols found to benefit (see under herbal treatment).[99]

(Continued)

(Continued)

Nutrients	Studies
Selenium and zinc	Lower selenium[100] and zinc levels[101] is associated with an increased risk of cervical dysplasia and cervical cancer.
Sulforaphane, stored as the precursor, glucosinolate converted to sulforaphane by myrosinase, e.g. chewing or chopping	In vitro: delays development of malignancy by arresting cell growth.[102] Sulforaphane may increase glutathione and glutathione-related enzymes (needed in liver as protective and for phase 2).
Vitamin A[103]	Higher intake and higher serum levels associated with a lower risk of cervical cancer.[104] Lower intake associated with higher cervical cancer risk.[105]
Vitamin B9 (folate), vitamin B12	Low serum concentrations of B9[106,107] and B12[108] are associated with cervical cancer. Serum homocysteine is predictive of invasive cervical cancer risk.[109] Methylation of DNA is lower in women with invasive cervical cancer[110] and associated with HPV infection, folate and B12 are also involved in this process.[111,112]
Vitamin C	Lower intake and lower plasma levels of vitamin C found in women with cervical dysplasia.[113]
Vitamin D	Vitamin D3 intake reduced cervical dysplasia.[114]
Vitamin E (tocopherol), fat soluble	Found to be protective against non-oncogenic HPV persistence.[115] Plasma levels in patients with cervical dysplasia and cancer were lower.[116] It is suggested that it may enhance the immunological functions and modulate the inflammatory response to infection.[117]

CHAPTER 11

Benign breast disorders

11.1 Presentation/symptoms, differential diagnosis and investigations

Non-proliferative lesions in the breast tissue usually present as lumpy or rope-like and more generally as painful breasts. The most common are fibrocystic breast changes (formerly called fibrocystic breast disease) and fibroadenomas. Histological fibrocystic changes are common and normal, and do not always lead to symptoms.[1,2] Most breast lumps are not cancerous but will often cause concern and raise the fear of breast cancer. It is reassuring to note that pain is not a typical presenting complaint for breast cancer.[3]

Cyclic mastalgia: cyclic breast pain and tenderness is the most common symptom of fibrocystic breast changes alongside swelling and lumpiness.[4] The tenderness is often a dull, heavy, bilateral ache around the upper outer breast area, radiating to the upper arm and axilla.

Cyclic mastalgia is experienced alongside other premenstrual symptoms, such as anxiety and depression.[5-8] Relief of depression was noted in women whose pain was treated successfully.[9] Symptoms can also appear in early pregnancy or in those taking oestrogen and progesterone, due to breast tissue proliferation.

Noncyclic mastalgia is less common: usually occurring in the 40s and 50s and postmenopausal.[10] The pain is constant or intermittent, unilateral and localised.[11] There is often no underlying cause, but consider the possibility of pregnancy, mastitis, trauma, thrombophlebitis, macrocysts, benign tumours or cancer.[12]

Key information to obtain from the case history

- Age: fibrocystic breast changes usually occurs in the 30s–40s and disappears during pregnancy or menopause[13,14]
- Family history of breast cancer or breast conditions
- Onset and breast changes: are they associated with the cycle?
- Oral contraceptive and HRT use, past and present
- PMH of breast cancer
- Pregnancy
- Presence of nipple discharge
- Skin changes
- Similar presentation in the past, as well as outcome
- Systemic symptoms: weight loss, malaise, bone pain
- Unilateral or symmetrical

Physical examination

This should be performed after menses, particularly in those with painful breasts, otherwise a thorough examination may not be possible.

Observation:
Symmetry is important and should be checked in several positions, with hands on hips and palms in front of forehead, to aid comparison. Note that size difference between breasts is common, a mirror-image thickening in the opposite breast indicating a normal condition.

Check for any nipple abnormalities: inversion, retraction, discharge, crusting, or skin changes such as dimpling, retraction, oedema, erythema, scaling, ulceration.

Palpation:
Palpate breasts in a circular pattern from the nipple outwards. In normal breasts, one can feel the irregularly textured mix of glands, fat and connective tissue. All breasts feel different.

A lump merging with the surrounding tissue is most likely normal as it reflects a higher density. However, in women over the age of 30 it warrants further investigation.

Ensure that the chest wall and underlying muscle are examined to determine whether any pain is related to these structures. Be sure to also palpate lymph glands in the axilla.

It is worthwhile to encourage women to perform self-examination, to become familiar with the variation typically occurring in a cycle and what is normal for them.

Red flag

A non-cyclical, unilateral, irregular palpable mass, stony hard, usually (but not always) without pain, feeling different to the other breast tissue, fixed to the skin or chest wall, with dimpling of the skin, which looks like orange peel (*peau d'orange*) and nipple discharge.[15] Axillary lymph nodes may be matted or fixed.

Investigations

Mammogram

Ultrasound: this is better for evaluating younger women's dense breast tissue, which is tightly packed with lobules, ducts and connective tissue (stroma). An ultrasound can help distinguish between fluid-filled cysts and solid masses.

Fine-needle aspiration: this is used to drain fluid from a cyst and can resolve discomfort.

Breast biopsy
Pregnancy testing if pain is unexplained and has lasted less than several months.

Table 11.1: Differential diagnosis

Condition	Lump description	Pain	Nipple discharge	Other
Cyst (cystic mastitis) Often after menopause	Smooth, mobile swelling, rubber-like, upper outer quadrants and in the central margins of the breast, localised.	Mild discomfort or no pain unless inflamed.		
Duct ectasia		Tender retro areolar area	Green, yellow, or clear discharge[16]	Erythema Nipple retraction
Fat necrosis	Unilateral, hard, irregular swelling. May be overlaying bruising of the skin or 'teeth' marks.			History of trauma
Fibroadenoma Between ages 20–40, enlarge during pregnancy, reduce in size as patients age.	Multiple or single, smooth, solid, firm, rubbery, rounded/oval, well defined, darting around.[17]	Usually not painful	No	Adolescents: tend to grow and are usually removed.

BENIGN BREAST DISORDERS

Fibrocystic breast Between ages 30–50, subsides after the menopause.[18] Worse with HRT.	Mobile, symmetrical, nodular, lumpy, rope-like, or areas of thickening which blend into the surrounding tissue, typically in upper outer part of the breast.	Cyclical tenderness, heavy, not always tender	Green or dark brown non-bloody, leak without pressure	History of similar findings
Galactocele Occurring in lactating breast and can occur up to 6 to 10 months after lactation stops.	Unilateral, round smooth, mobile swelling			Resolves after aspiration, occasionally become infected.
Intraductal papilloma	Small nodule in the retro areolar region		Bloody, sudden discharge	
Large breasts		Diffuse, bilateral breast pain		Due to stretching of cooper's ligaments
Lipoma: rare	Soft, lobulated swelling			'Pseudolipoma' is a bunching of fat between retracted suspensory ligaments of the breast, associated with malignancy.

(Continued)

Table 11.1: (Continued)

Condition	Lump description	Pain	Nipple discharge	Other
Malignant carcinoma majority occurs in women over age 60	Asymmetric, hard irregular swelling, fixed to the skin, or fixed deeply.	No pain	Rare: nipple discharge	Nipple retraction. *Peau d'orange*, axillary and/or supraclavicular lymphadenopathy. Hepatomegaly. Painless in 85% of cases. FH of breast cancer risk factors, early menarche, and late or no first pregnancy.
Mastitis	Swelling, erythema	Pain, severe		
Phyllodes tumour (malignant)	Mobile, may become very large, and increase in size just in a few weeks.			
Sebaceous cyst	Small, mobile swelling fixed to the skin.			May be infected, discharge, redness.

Other

<u>Generalised swelling</u>: may occur in pregnancy, lactation and puberty. May also occur with mastitis.

<u>Costochondritis</u>: pain and tenderness of the costochondral or chondrosternal joints, with involvement of the second through fifth costal cartilages.

<u>Tietze syndrome</u>: similar symptoms but also has swelling of the cartilaginous articulations and with involvement of the second and third costochondral junctions.

Conventional treatment

Breast pain: nonsteroidal anti-inflammatory drugs (NSAIDs), ibuprofen, paracetemol.

Stop or change of oral contraceptives, occasionally short-term use of danazol (a synthetic male hormone) or tamoxifen (which blocks the effects of oestrogen).

Breast cysts: fine-needle aspiration. Occasionally surgical removal.

11.2 Pathophysiology of benign breast disorders

Hormonal

Mammary gland development, maturation and differentiation respond to the cyclical changes of the hormones.[19] Initially proliferation of breast tissue is influenced by oestrogen, and after ovulation, alveolar secretory activity is influenced by progesterone, ending with a period of involution.[20]

There is a clear cyclical association, but consistent hormonal abnormalities have not been identified, although increased thyrotropin-induced prolactin secretion has been observed. Symptoms may be related to increased tissue sensitivity to oestrogen with related fluid retention. Other potential drivers are excess oestrogen, progesterone deficiency, a decreased progesterone–oestrogen ratio, as well as thyroid hormone abnormality.

Studies have suggested that excess oestrogen and anovulation were associated with benign breast conditions.[21] An increased prevalence of benign breast lesions is seen in postmenopausal women taking oestrogens and progestins, and reduced in those on anti-oestrogen medication.[22] Oestrogen, both endogenous and exogenous (HRT, oral contraceptive pill), causes an increase in prolactin secretion.

Fluid–electrolyte balance

Shifts in the water–electrolyte balance in nonlactating breasts related to prolactin levels lead to cyclic painful swelling of breast microcysts.[23] Breast volume can increase during the luteal phase.[24]

Lipid profile aberrations

Cyclical aberrations are observed in lipid metabolism, a finding that led to low-fat dietary recommendations. Diets containing 15% fat intake were associated with a decrease in symptoms compared to a general diet.[25-27] It could be that reducing lipids affects circulating oestrogen (oestradiol, oestrone) levels.[28]

Neuroendocrine

Perceived stress was associated with mastalgia. Fibrocystic breasts appear more responsive to adrenaline, the presence of which increases adenylate cyclase activity and cAMP production.[29]

11.3 Herbal management of benign breast disorders

Fibrocystic breast changes, fibroadenoma and cyclic mastalgia.

Aims

Reduce pain, local congestion and fluid retention
Reduce excess oestrogen, prolactin
Address the impact of stress

Herbal management

<u>Aid digestion and the microbiome</u>: to improve overall absorption of nutrients, bitter herbs.

<u>Ease fluid retention</u>: diuretics (*Taraxacum officinale folia, Galium aparine*).

<u>Reduce local congestion</u>: improving lymphatic clearance (*Calendula officinalis, Galium aparine, Phytolacca decandra, Thuja occidentalis*) as well as improving circulation (*Ginkgo biloba*).

<u>Reduce excess oestrogen</u>: oestrogen-promoting herbs, those with steroidal saponins, are best avoided. Use of phenolic phytoestrogens to

diminish the effect of endogenous oestrogen by competitively binding to oestrogen receptors (soya and flaxseeds). Support the clearance of oestrogen via liver (*Taraxacum officinale radix, Silybum marianum*).

Ensure regular bowel movements (*Taraxacum officinale radix*) and a healthy gut flora (*Tarax rad, Berberis vulgaris,* garlic) to reduce the enterohepatic recirculation of oestrogen.

Reduce prolactin: correct relative progesterone deficiency, *Actaea racemosa, Paeonia lactiflora & Glycyrrhiza glabra, Vitex agnus-castus.*

Reduce the impact of stress: addressing the hypothalamic-pituitary-ovarian axis with adaptogens (*Hydrocotyle asiatica, Schisandra chinensis*) and nervines (*Leonurus cardiaca, Melissa offinalis, Verbena officinalis*).

Key herbs used in clinical practice

Calendula officinalis

Traditionally used as a lymphatic internally.[30]

Dosage
Daily dosage for internal 2–7ml per day of 1:3 25%.
 Typical weekly dosage 15–30ml 1:3 per week.

Ginkgo biloba

Clinical study: patients with congestive symptoms of premenstrual syndrome received either 160mg/day of *Ginkgo* extract or placebo from day 16 of the menstrual cycle to day 5 of the following cycle. *Ginkgo* improved breast tenderness as well as other symptoms such as oedema, anxiety, depression and headache.

Dosage
Needs to be used for at least 6 weeks for any benefit.
 Daily dosage 3–4ml of standardised 2:1.
 Typical week dosage 15–30ml of standardised 2:1.

Phytolacca decandra

One of the herbs favoured by herbalists for treatment of fibrocystic breasts, it has anti-inflammatory, lymphatic, alterative, and immune-stimulating properties.

The American Eclectics saw this as a herb that acts upon the glandular structures, specifically upon the mammary glands, and recommended

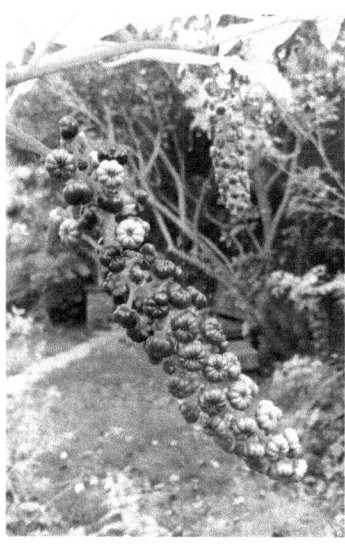

its use for mastitis, soreness and swelling associated with the menstrual cycle.[31] They would also use it for cancerous growths, internally as well as externally.

Phytolacca is a powerful herb and warrants some caution, and only small doses are needed. In the UK we tend to use only the dried herb as the fresh root contains pokeweed mitogens, which can cause poisoning. Small traces can still be present in the dry root but are unlikely to be absorbed through the gut wall, as they are too large; note that saponins in *Phytolacca* could irritate the gut wall and increase the absorption of the mitogens.

There are no clinical trials on *Phytolacca*, but it has been used extensively by herbalists and found to be beneficial for fibrocystic breast changes.

Dosage
Daily dosage 0.15–0.7ml of 1:5.

Typical weekly dosages 5ml of 1:5 per week; some would say not to use long term, and not over 6 months.

Vitex agnus-castus

This herb has been well researched in cyclical mastalgia and fibrocystic breast changes. It is a dopaminergic herb, reducing levels of prolactin, and has an effect via the opioid receptors. Typically used for PMS that includes symptoms of cyclic mastalgia, it relieves the intensity of the symptoms as well as lowering the associated increased serum prolactin level.[32-35] In trials it is shown to be as effective as dopamine agonists, nonsteroidal anti-inflammatory drugs, serotonin reuptake inhibitors and hormonal contraceptives.[36-39]

Dosage
Daily dose 0.6–1.5ml of 1:3.
　　Typical weekly dose 5–10ml of 1:3.

Table 11.2: Clinical trials: herbs and herbal constituents

Herb	Clinical trial
Cinnamomun zeylanicum	Reduced the intensity of mastalgia.[40]
Curcumin	Reduced mastalgia when taken for 7 days before menstruation and 3 days during menstruation.[41]
Hypericum perforatum	Reduce severity of mastalgia when used for PMS.[42]
Isoflavones from red clover	Benefit in mastalgia, 40mg more effective than 80mg of isoflavone per day.[43]
Linum usitatissimum: daily flaxseed powder (25g)	Helpful and more effective than omega 3 for cyclical mastalgia.[44-46]
Matricaria chamomilla	Effective for mild to moderate mastalgia.[47]
Nigella sativa (Ranunculaceae) same family as *Actaea racemosa* and *Anemone pulsatilla*[48]	Nigella sativa oil made into a syrup shown to be of benefit in cyclic mastalgia.[49-51]
Soy: daily soy protein consumption	Showed both objective and subjective reduction in both breast tenderness and fibrocystic changes.[52] Another study showed that soy led to a reduction of pain.[53] Isoflavone exposure was inversely associated with fibrocystic breast conditions and breast cancer, and the results suggest that effects on cancer risk occur early in carcinogenesis.[54]

11.4 Dietary and lifestyle recommendations

A diet rich in fruit, vegetables, nuts and seeds: a high intake of fresh fruits and vegetables is associated with a reduced risk of proliferative and atypical lesions in the breasts, and reduces risk of breast cancer.[55]

Diets high in nuts and fibre: a high intake by adolescents was associated with lower risk of benign fibrocystic breasts, as well as lower risk of breast cancer later on in life.[56]

Oils in the diet: women in the highest quartile of eicosapentaenoic acid concentrations in erythrocytes were less likely to have a non-proliferative fibrocystic condition.[57,58] Comparison trials with fish oil, evening primrose oil, wheatgerm and corn oils all appear to have similar effect.[59,60] It was suggested that either all have the same effect, no effect, or the effect was due to the vitamin E used to prevent oxidation.

In the past Evening Primrose, containing linoleic acid and gamma linoleic acid, was frequently used for breast tenderness.[61] Studies indicated that women with mastalgia have increased levels of saturated fatty acids and reduced proportions of essential fatty acids, especially of gamma-linolenic acid (GLA), and it was thought that this caused hypersensitivity of the breast tissue to hormones.[62] GLA was thought to restore the saturated/unsaturated fatty acid balance and decrease sensitivity to the sex hormones. Low levels of the GLA metabolite dihomogamma-linolenic acid may affect breast sensitivity to prolactin.[63] However, not all studies have a positive outcome, a few indicated it was modestly better than placebo,[64] and other studies show no effect.[65,66]

Foods to ensure a healthy gut flora: to reduce the hepato-recycling of oestrogen, and ensure the absorption of the phenolic phytoestrogens.

A diet rich in fruits, vegetables, fibre, fermented foods and low in sugar are all important to maintain the health of the colon microflora. *Lactobacillus acidophilus* supplementation has been shown to lower faecal beta-glucuronidase involved with recycling of oestrogen.[67]

Iodine and breast tissue

Breast tissue has a high concentration of iodine, especially during pregnancy and lactation.[68] Iodine is found in the terminal and interlobular duct cells in the breast, the areas involved in cystic changes, and is also used in the production of thyroid hormones. The exact mechanism by which iodine is involved with fibrocystic breast changes is not well understood. It has been suggested that a low or deficient amount of iodine causes the epithelium to be more sensitive to oestrogen stimulation.

In those with fibrocystic breast changes, thyroxin reduced mastodynia, serum prolactin levels and breast nodules in patients who have normal thyroid levels.[69] There could be an element of subclinical hypothyroidism present, and/or iodine deficiency.

The daily recommended intake (NHS) for adults is 140 micrograms (μg) per day, more for those who are pregnant and breastfeeding (the latter up to 260μg). In the past, iodine deficiency was endemic in certain areas, leading to goitre. However, international efforts since the early 1990s have reduced the incidence of iodine deficiency worldwide, although some groups are still affected.[70] Those that are at higher risk of having low iodine intake are vegans and those with lactose intolerance and food allergies.[71] Deficiencies of iron, selenium, vitamin A may interact with iodine and thyroid function.[72] One research paper does suggest that intake of iodine should be increased in adults to at least 1mg/day in specific pathologies, due to its extrathyroidal actions such as possible antioxidant, anti-inflammatory, activation of apoptotic pathways and immune modulator activities.[73]

Up to 1mg/day is considered safe for most people. However, ingestion of over 1.1mg/day might be problematic for those that are sensitive, as it can cause subclinical or overt thyroid dysfunction in patients with pre-existing thyroid disease. Excess iodine inhibits thyroid hormone synthesis, increasing TSH stimulation, leading to goitre formation and hypothyroidism. For those with autoimmune thyroid disease extra iodine intake can cause adverse effects including thyroiditis, hypothyroidism, hyperthyroidism and thyroid papillary cancer.[74]

To avoid an excess of iodine it would seem best to stick to food sources for iodine, such as seaweed (kelp,[75] nori, kombu and wakame), seafood/fish, eggs and dairy products (although this may depend on whether cows have an iodine feed supplement).

Isoflavone phytoestrogen-rich foods

Soya: daily soy protein reduced symptoms of breast tenderness and fibrocystic disease.[76,77] Isoflavone intake was inversely associated with fibrocystic breast conditions and breast cancer, and thus protective.[78]

Linum usitatissimum: the powder was found to be of benefit in mastalgia[79] and premenstrual syndrome.[80,81]

Clinical studies of interest (but not necessarily recommended)

Low-fat diets show benefits to symptoms but they are not recommended in the long term: clinical studies suggest reducing the dietary fat intake to 20% of total calories results in decreases in circulating oestrogens[82] and reducing elevated prolactin levels.[83] A clinical study comparing a diet containing 15% fat intake to 36% fat intake showed reduced body weight and cholesterol levels and reduced mastalgia in the low-fat diet.[84,85] A modest reduction in fat intake alongside an increase in fruit, vegetables and grain intake did not alter the risk of benign proliferative breast disease.[86] Low-fat diets may have been popular in the past but they are not considered healthy overall.

Limiting or eliminating caffeine (methylxanthine) intake (coffee, tea, cola, chocolate and caffeinated medications): this is regularly recommended for fibrocystic breast changes, although results from clinical studies are not conclusive. Some clinical studies suggest that a reduction of caffeine intake decreased pain or provided complete relief.[87] No association found with fibroadenoma or other forms of benign breast disease.[88] Why it might be of benefit is that methylxanthines cause elevated 3′,5′-cyclic adenosine monophosphate (cAMP) in the fibrocystic tissue and circulating catecholamines, causing the overproduction of fibrous tissue and cyst fluid.[89]

It is possible that the conflicting outcomes shown in studies might be related to individual thresholds of response to methylxanthines in women. As it might be relatively simple to cut out caffeine it might be worth a try. However, do remember a sudden withdrawal will cause headaches.

Table 11.3: Clinical trials, specific foods and nutrients

Nutrient	Clinical trials
A combination product containing garlic, beta-carotene, vitamin E and vitamin C	Reduced the severity of mastalgia, premenstrual syndrome and caused regression of palpable symptoms of breast fibromatosis.[90]
Cysteine, cysteine-rich foods: NAC is made by the human liver by altering the amino acid cysteine. Cystine is made up of two cysteine molecules bonded together and is nutritionally equivalent to cysteine.	N-acetyl cysteine (no food sources exist for this form): decreased cyclical mastalgia, lowered plasma level of C-reactive protein, increased total plasma glutathione and is effective as antioxidant. NAC impacts both the production and release of progesterone from ovarian granulosa cells,[91] as well as reducing inflammation.[92]
Iodine	Reduction of nodules and resolution of fibrosis and pain relief using high amounts of iodine.[93] Typical range used was 1 to 6mg/day had beneficial actions in fibrocystic breast disease.[94] Combination of GLA, iodine and selenium (selenium was added to reduce the adverse effects of increased iodine intake on the thyroid[95]) reduced nodularity and the need for painkillers for breast pain.[96] Combination of omega 3, iodine and chlorophyll derivatives, reduced mastalgia, premenopausal syndrome and breast cyst regression.[97]
Vitamin A/beta-carotene	There are specific retinoid receptors present in breast tissue. A small trial, with intake 150,000 IU of vitamin A daily led to clearance of symptoms and pain reduction of benign breast disease.[98]

(*Continued*)

Table 11.3: (Continued)

Nutrient	Clinical trials
Vitamin B6	Reduced the prevalence and pain severity in periodic and non-periodic mastalgia,[99] although other trials suggested no benefit.[100]
Vitamin E	Small studies suggested a potential beneficial effect,[101] other studies indicated no effect.[102–104] Vitamin E may inhibit ER-positive cell growth by altering the cellular response to oestrogen.[105]
Wheatgerm	Reduced mastalgia when taken from 16th day of menstrual cycle to the 5th day of the next.[106]

See Appendix for food sources.

Lifestyle advice

<u>Comfortable, supportive bra</u>: A fitted sports bra provided superior support resulting in perceived pain reduction.[107]

<u>Exercise</u>: swimming or breaststroke movements to aid movement and relieve congestion, application of alternating hot and cold water to affected area.

<u>Stress</u>: perceived stress was associated with mastalgia.[108] Fibrocystic breasts appear more responsive to epinephrine, the presence of which increases adenylate cyclase activity and cAMP production. Subjects who performed relaxation techniques had substantially more pain-free days and less anxiety than controls.[109]

<u>Smoking</u>: a risk factor for breast cancer, the nicotine in cigarette smoke has also been associated with fibrotic changes in the breast.[110]

CHAPTER 12

Lichen sclerosus

12.1 Presentation/symptoms, differential diagnosis and investigations

Lichen sclerosus is an anogenital chronic inflammatory skin condition causing scarring of the skin, which can lead to narrowing of the affected areas. It can appear at any age but is most often seen in post-menopausal women.

This condition is under-recognised and misdiagnosed, partly due to the reluctance to seek help. Early on the presentation can be confused with eczema, non-specific vulvitis or thrush.[1] The overall incidence of lichen sclerosus seems to be rising.[2]

Symptoms

Sclerotic plaques starting as small patchy, thin, white, shiny, smooth spots on the labia, perineum, and perianally with persistent pruritus.

When severe, the scarring can cause dyspareunia, difficulty with urination and, if the anal area is affected, constipation. Splitting of the vulval skin can cause stinging and pain.

A small percentage (3%) can develop malignancy, so there is need to take note of unusual lumps, abnormal bleeding or changes in the skin texture.

Investigation

The clinical features are usually enough to diagnose,[3] however a specialist might take a vulval biopsy if diagnosis is uncertain. Lichen sclerosus commonly coexists with thyroid disease, so it is worthwhile to screen for thyroid conditions.

Differential diagnosis: eczema, psoriasis, lichen planus, precancerous lesions (vulval intraepithelial neoplasia) and rarely, vulval cancer.

Pathophysiology

This is an inflammatory condition,[4] and over time there are changes in vasculature as well as loss of elastic fibres.

The pathogenesis is unknown, but several mechanisms may be involved:

- There is a higher incidence among pre-menarche and post-menopausal females, the times when oestrogen levels are reduced: oestrogen affects collagen content and glycosaminoglycan concentrations, therefore affecting skin hydration and texture.[5]
- Serum levels of dihydrotestosterone were found to be decreased in patients with untreated vulvar lichen sclerosis. However treatment with topical testosterone did not provide any benefit.[6] It has been suggested that past disturbances of the androgen-dependent growth of the vulvar skin by OCPs, especially those with antiandrogenic properties, may trigger the early onset of lichen sclerosis in susceptible women.[7]
- Genetic elements: a positive family history.[8]
- Another suggestion is that an autoimmune reaction causes sclerotic tissue formation. Thyroid disease, vitiligo, and other autoimmune diseases (1 in 4) are commonly found in those with lichen sclerosus,[9] with thyroid disease being the most common.[10]
- Infections: Epstein-Barr Virus DNA was found in 26.5% of 34 vulvar biopsies of patients with lichen sclerosus compared with none in controls.[11]
- Flare-ups can occur if under stress, after sex or long walks. This is probably due to friction.

Conventional treatment

Lichen sclerosus should be treated as soon as the disease is recognised or suspected, to reduce the exposure to and damaging effects of oxidative stress, which can potentially lead to malignancy. Early treatment favours better outcomes and is important to prevent scarring. In some cases, the condition can disappear on its own, in the younger age group, but more often the condition is chronic.

Typically, topical corticosteroids are the first-line treatment. Once the condition is stabilised there are effective herbal alternatives to keep the condition contained and reduce flare-ups.

12.2 Herbal management of lichen sclerosus (LS)

Lichen sclerosus should be treated as soon as the condition is suspected or recognised, to reduce the damaging effects, which could potentially lead to malignancy. Early treatment favours a better outcome overall and is important to prevent scarring. In some cases, the condition can disappear on its own, but more commonly the condition is chronic.

Topical application of vitamin E oil or olive oil are associated with a reduction in topical corticosteroid use in those with lichen sclerosus, with over half of women studied being able to eliminate the use of corticosteroids altogether.[12] Long-term maintenance with emollients or moisturisers has been shown to control lichen sclerosus, and these measures are of use after the condition has been stabilised with topical steroids.

Herbs macerated in oils will have an emollient effect by virtue of the oil used. Additional benefits could be extrapolated from traditional use, such as reducing inflammation and prevention of scarring. It would be good sense to utilise herbs with these known effects in our emollient/moisturising oil preparations.

Aims

To control lichen sclerosus and prevent scar formation
Reduce inflammation and the need for use of corticosteroids
Ensure local tissue hydration with oestrogenic herbs and by increasing pelvic circulation

Herbal management

Internal

Anti-inflammatory: *Actaea racemosa, Glycyrrhiza glabra, Vaccinium myrtillus.*

Ensure tissue hydration: internally hydration can be influenced by phenolic, steroidal and triterpenoid oestrogenic herbs in perimenopausal women: *Actaea racemosa, Asparagus racemosus,* soy, flaxseed.

Pelvic circulation support: *Achillea millefolium, Alchemilla vulgaris, Vaccinium myrtillus.*

GIT health: as with other autoimmune conditions, ensure health of the gut flora and the GIT more widely, including checking for food triggers: bitters, fibre-rich food etc.

Immune response, support as with other autoimmune conditions: *Echinacea angustifolia* and *purpurea*, adaptogens *Hydrocotyle asiatica* (and see above).

Nervines and adaptogens, if stress is an exacerbating factor: *Actaea racemosa, Melissa officinalis, Withania somnifera.*

Topical

Anti-inflammatory
Preparation in oils: *Calendula officinalis, Chamomilla recutica, Hydrocotyle asiatica.*

Emmolients, antipruritics: *Hydrocotyle asiatica* in sesame oil, *Stellaria media,* Vitamin E oil, olive oil.

Anti-inflammatories and anti-cicatrisation to prevent scar formation: *Calendula officinalis, Hydrocotyle asiatica* oil.

Prevent progression to malignancy: *Camellia sinensis, Curcuma longa* (topically as well as internally). Flavonoid-rich herbs.

Herbs used in clinical practice

In our clinical experience, two herbs that have worked extremely well topically are *Hydrocotyle asiatica* and *Calophyllum inophyllum*.

Hydrocotyle asiatica synonym *Centella asiatica*

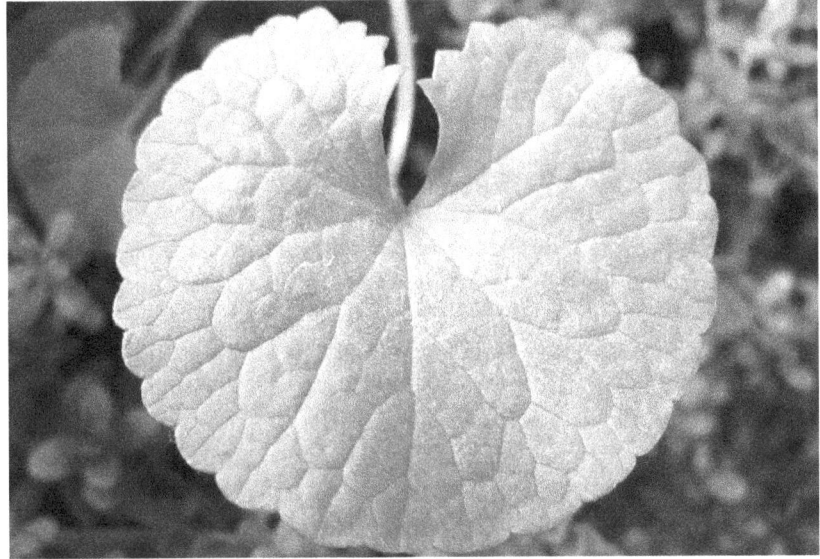

Centella asiatica

We have found *Hydrocotyle* infused in sesame oil (*Sesamum indicum*) to be especially effective. The topical use of sesame oil may be adding to the beneficial effect as it has antioxidant and anti-inflammatory properties. It has also showed a chemopreventive effect in a vivo model of skin cancer, suggesting the potential for prevention of malignancy.[13]

Usually, *Hydrocotyle* oil by itself is effective. If not enough, one could add Tamanu oil (see below), which is effective but expensive.

Hydrocotyle is traditionally used for the treatment of a variety of skin lesions including burns, hypertrophic scars, scleroderma lesions, lupus, leprosy, eczema, psoriasis,[14] varicose ulcers.[15]

The constituents considered to be important are the pentacyclic triterpenes, mainly asiaticoside, madecassoside, asiatic and madecassic acids.

Preclinical studies
Wound-healing effects: stimulation of fibronectin synthesis.[16]

Asiatic acid had an influence on collagen synthesis and matrix remodelling,[17] and was found to have a beneficial effect in the maintenance of connective tissue[18] as well as strengthening of weakened veins.[19]

The triterpene fraction also has an impact on extracellular matrix protein deposition, stimulates fibroblast proliferation, decreases the activity of metalloproteinases,[20,21] plus proangiogenic, antioxidative effects and inhibited the inflammatory phase of hypertrophic scars and keloids.[22–25]

All this might explain why *Hydrocotyle* is effective for scar management.[26,27]

Clinical study in patients with scleroderma

Scleroderma is an autoimmune condition that affects skin and connectives tissues as well as internal organs. With this condition, the body makes too much collagen, causing the skin to tighten and thicken, leading to scarring. A beneficial effect is seen in topical as well as internal use of *Hydrocotyle* in scleroderma, both in localised and systemic scleroderma. A decrease was seen in vascular disorders, hard lesions, hyperpigmentation and improvement in the patients' general condition. A beneficial effect was also seen with topical application on finger ulcers due to scleroderma.[28]

Although scleroderma is a different condition, there are similarities in the underlying processes.

Calophyllum inophyllum (Tamanu oil)

Preclinical studies

In vitro, on isolated human fibroblasts from the vagina, showed healing properties, increasing the proliferation of cells and collagen III. It also has anti-inflammatory and analgesic properties.[29]

Vaginal pessaries could be based on *Hydrocotyle* and *Calophyllum* oils with the addition of *Foeniculum vulgare* and *Lavandula angustifolia* EO. This would also help with vaginal atrophy, especially useful in postmenopausal women.

Table 12.1: Clinical studies (only a few clinical studies have been run on patients with lichen sclerosus)

Cream content used	Outcome
Two sisters: a case report using cream containing thyme extract EO (less than 0.1%) in a cream base.	Case report: successful outcome.[30]

(Continued)

Table 12.1: (Continued)

Cream content used	Outcome
Cream containing avocado oil, soybean extracts, vitamin E, used topically, as well as a supplement, anti-inflammatory, anti-fibrotic and emollient actions. Avocado extracts in vitro showed preventative effect on oral cancer cell lines.[31]	Clinical study: improvement in subjective and objective global scores.[32] Preclinical: Avocado oil: research on wound models led to faster re-epitheliasation, higher hydroxyproline content of the repaired wound, increased collagen synthesis and a decrease in the numbers of inflammatory cells.[33]
Vitamin E ointment compared with an emollient, after the condition was stabilised with topical corticosteroids.	Clinical study: both vitamin E and emollient were helpful in maintaining LS remission, reducing the risk of LS relapse over a 52-week maintenance treatment.[34]

Other oils for topical use

Coconut oil: anti-inflammatory effects, including in chronic inflammation, reducing granuloma formation and serum alkaline phosphatase activity.[35]

Lavender EO: promoted wound healing by promoting collagen synthesis and differentiation of fibroblasts, accompanied by upregulation of TGF-β in vivo.[36,37]

Chamomile EO: anti-inflammatory, the constituent azulene increases moisture in the skin. Chamomile is also an antioxidant, found to reduce stretch marks and reduce itching.[38]

12.3 Dietary and lifestyle recommendations

Eat an anti-inflammatory/antioxidant diet rich in vegetables and fruit. Incorporate a range of colours in the daily diet, as well as healthy oils (omega 3), nuts, seeds and legumes. All these are rich in antioxidants, preventing malignancy and may prevent lichen sclerosus development.

Individual compounds have shown to be malignancy preventatives such as proanthocyanidins in berries,[39] lycopene found in tomatoes, melons,[40] lignans, quercetin, resveratrol[41] and curcumin.[42]

Table 12.2: Clinical studies: specific nutrients

Nutrient study	Outcome lichen sclerosus
Carotenoids	Intake of carotenoids was inversely and strongly associated with vulvar lichen sclerosus.[43]
Epidemiological study[44]	Worsening with specific food, 26%, especially pork. Use a food diary.
Small study with Vitamin A + Vitamin E orally for 12 months without any topical treatment.[45]	Clinical improvement was seen in 91% after 6 months of treatment. On follow-up nine patients had no relapse after 1 year of treatment, in one pruritus recurred after 6 months.
Vitamin D: case study with calcitriol 0.5 microgram oral daily intake.	Case study: LS resistant to different therapeutics. Lesions improved and the improvement persisted after discontinuation of therapy.[46]

See Appendix for food sources.

Lifestyle advice

Lubricants during sex to reduce friction, especially if it is painful.

Use non-soap-based washes, avoid bubble baths and soaps in the genital area, which can increase dryness by removing natural body oils as well as affecting the beneficial bacteria.

Urinary incontinence and the consequent use of absorbent underwear are more commonly present in those with lichen scerosus[47] Consider using natural, unbleached materials for sanitary ware and pantyliners, soft unbleached or non-chlorine bleached toilet paper and soft towels.

Wearing silk underwear has been shown to reduce symptoms, possibly as it avoids irritation by friction.[48] Avoid tight clothes which can make the area hot and itchy.

CHAPTER 13

Premenstrual syndrome (PMS)

(brief recap from book 1)[1]

Introduction

PMS consists of a wide array of physiological symptoms that regularly attend the luteal phase of the menstrual cycle, affecting over 10% of women of reproductive age.

PMS is poorly understood and, as is common in most conditions, is multi-factorial with many proposed mechanisms.

Proposed contributing factors include: progesterone to oestrogen balance, neurotransmitters, endorphins, melatonin, thyroid hormones, aldosterone and prolactin, as well as chronic inflammation, etc.

Predisposing factors include being overweight, stress and exogenous hormones. Other risks include alcohol, recreational drug use and smoking, along with family history and unhealthy or unbalanced eating habits.

Endogenous contributory factors include metabolic syndrome and changes in hormonal balance, as seen for example in menarche and perimenopause.

Symptoms commonly include headaches, bloating, breast tenderness, poor sleep, irritability and water retention.

- During the late luteal phase, levels of both oestrogen and progesterone fall. The change in oestrogen levels, or in the ratio oestrogen/progesterone of the hormones, is implicated in PMS.
- High densities of oestrogen and progesterone receptors are present in brain regions that regulate emotions, drives and perceptions. This may explain the range of emotional and psychological effects of PMS.
- The symptoms of PMS are also closely tied to serotonin and dopamine levels (monoamines with a strong influence on mood) in the brain as well as the opioid and GABA pathways.

Some women suffer extreme anxiety and agitation, known as PMDD. This is typically present in the early luteal phase as progesterone rises. Many of these women have experienced trauma earlier in their lives.

Herbal management, initial focus

- Treat the symptoms: sleep, anxiety, bloating, breast tenderness and so on.
- Address the predisposing factors: diet and exercise, particularly to reduce inflammation.
- Support elimination, liver function and healthy gut flora.

Subsequent treatment focus

- Treatment of any underlying health conditions, particularly digestive.
- Providing support for neuroendocrine function.
- Adequate nutrition to ensure balanced production of neurotransmitters and anti-inflammatory prostaglandins.

Table: Herbal management

Issue to address	Herbal treatment
Intestinal health	Gentle laxatives: *Taraxacum radix, Rumex crispus* and flax seeds, to aid elimination and to re-establish a healthy microflora. A healthy gut flora is crucial for the absorption of some of plant constituents, especially the phenolic phytoestrogens. Herbs with lipotrophic factors (choline): *Taraxacum radix*, which helps with removal of fat and bile in the liver, aiding elimination of oestrogen, avoiding recirculation/recycling of oestrogens. Bitter herbs: to aid the absorption crucial nutrients involved in metabolism of the hormones: *Achillea millefolium, Artemisia absinthium, Matricaria chamomilla, Taraxacum officinale*, etc. Herbs to encourage healthy gut flora: *Artemisia absinthium, Berberis vulgaris*, garlic, *Ulmus fulva*.
Endocrine function: herbs traditionally listed as nervines and hormonal tonics, targeted towards particular dysfunctions in PMS.	Prolactin-lowering: dopaminergic herbs such as *Actaea racemosa, Paeonia lactiflora* with *Glycyrrhiza glabra, Vitex agnus-castus*—these also indirectly affect progesterone production. Phenolic phytoestrogens, steroidal saponin and triterpene-rich herbs for low-oestrogen environment in perimenopause: *Actaea racemosa, Dioscorea villosa*, soya, flaxseed, *Trifolium pratense*. Adaptogens, hypothalamic-pituitary-adrenal (HPA) axis: *Eleutherococcus senticosus, Rhodiola rosea, Schisandra chinensis, Withania somnifera*.[2] Thyroid support: *Avena sativa, Capsicum minimum, Eleutherococcus senticosus, Glycyrrhiza glabra, Nigella sativa*,[3] *Panax ginseng, Turnera diffusa*.
Nervines, as neurotransmitters interplay with the endocrine system.	Nervine support for symptoms of anxiety and/or depression: *Hypericum perforatum, Lavandula officinalis, Matricaria chamomilla, Melissa officinalis, Scutellaria lateriflora, Stachys betonica, Valeriana officinalis, Verbena officinalis, Withania somnifera*.

(*Continued*)

Table: (Continued)

Issue to address	Herbal treatment
Specific symptoms	Fluid retention and bloating, diuretics and circulatories: *Ginkgo biloba*, *Taraxacum officinale fol*, *Vitex agnus-castus*.
	Treatment of mastalgia: *Ginkgo biloba*, *Paeonia lactiflora* and *Glycyrrhiza glabra*, *Ruscus aculeatus*, *Taraxacum officinale fol*, *Vitex agnus-castus*.
	Preventative treatment for migraines related to cycle, avoid trigger foods: *Actaea racemosa* (careful as in high doses will give frontal headache), *Ginkgo biloba*, *Stachys betonica*, *Tanacetum parthenium*, *Vitex agnus-castus*.

Dietary recommendations

A diet rich in complex carbohydrates, vegetables, fruit, nuts, seeds, fish, legumes and fermented foods including yogurt, to aid and maintain a healthy blood sugar, observing regular mealtimes.

PMS risk is associated with fast food consumption and irregular breakfasts.[4]

Reduce alcohol intake (a moderate association with PMS risk).[5,6] Reduce caffeine if symptoms of anxiety are present.

Avoid environmental oestrogens (pesticides on food, plastics, air fresheners and cosmetics): eat organic and use non-industrial household products.

- Include plant foods for oestrogen excess or deficiency: nuts, seeds and legumes, such as soy foods.
- Tryptophan-rich foods to support serotonin and melatonin production: nuts, seeds, tofu, cheese, red meat, chicken, turkey, fish, oats, beans, lentils and eggs.
- Support healthy gut flora: probiotics, lactofermented vegetables, beans, pulses and root vegetables to establish normal intestinal flora. Support using bitter and perhaps warming, carminative herbs.

CHAPTER 14

Menopause

(brief recap from book 1[1])

Menopause has been covered in great detail in the first book, which focuses on it as an example of oestrogen deficiency and discusses a range of hormonal herbs in detail.

During the perimenopause and menopause, the decrease in oestrogen leads to symptoms such as hot flushes and night sweats, cognitive instability, sleep disturbances and vaginal atrophy. However, there is more than just the reduction of oestrogen, there is cross talk between dopamine, serotonin, progesterone, adrenalin and the thyroid, oestrogen, epidermal growth factors, insulin and so on.

Hormones are complicated: 1 plus 1 is not always 2.

Perimenopause

- The lead-up to the menopause can begin from age 40–51.
- Actual menopause typically begins around ages 45–55.
- Irregular ovulation occurs as there are fewer ovarian eggs left, from 1–2 million at birth to just a few thousand. The length of the follicular phase shortens; there is an increased incidence of anovulatory cycles with an implied lack of progesterone, hence heavy bleeding.

- Hormonal tests: the first sign can be increased FSH, although one can have normal levels as blood tests detect only a certain percentage of FSH peptides.
- Lower levels of oestrogens are found 6 months to 1 year before true menopause. Progesterone declines before oestrogen, which leads to abnormal menstruation (excessive blood loss, absent period, persistent and more frequent menstruation) and worsens PMS symptoms.
- Oestrogen affects the nervous system and central neurotransmitters: lower levels affect mood, memory and cognition, and temperature regulation.
- Menopausal symptoms reflect the adaptation of the body to oestrogen deprivation.

Postmenopause

- Postmenopausal LH and FSH stimulate the secretion of androgens and oestrogen.
- Almost all oestrogens (as oestrone) are derived from the aromatisation of androgen, which are, in turn, derived from adrenals and the ovaries. The adrenals become the most important source of the sex hormones. The ovaries still play an important role post-menopausally; women with oophorectomies have reduced formation by the adrenals.
- SHBG decreases due to relative increase in testosterone (also reduced in hypothyroidism, obesity, hyperprolactinaemia).
- Oestrogen low, no build-up of the uterine lining, no menses.

Herbal management: summary

- Assist with adjustment to the change, supporting the body to produce the required sex hormones by ovaries, adrenals and other parts of the body. The ideal outcome is to eventually withdraw herbal treatment, as this is not replacement therapy!
- Ensure and promote healthy GIT and liver function, which are crucial for the metabolism of the hormones. Work on creating and sustaining healthy bacterial flora to make phytoestrogens bioavailable. Use probiotics and prebiotics to establish normal intestinal flora, such as slippery elm, plus lots of vegetables and fruit for the fibre content. Alongside this, consider the use of bitters and antimicrobials, when appropriate.

- Promote a healthy weight.
- Encourage exercise as this will help with metabolism, thyroid function and bone density.

Table 14.1: Herbal management

Issues to address	Herbal treatment
Adrenal support	Adaptogens: *Actaea racemosa, Astragalus membranaceus, Eleutherococcus senticosus, Panax ginseng, Salvia officinalis*
Anxiety, depression	Nervines: *Avena sativa, Hypericum perforatum, Leonurus cardiaca, Melissa officinalis, Verbena officinalis*
Circulatory herbs to aid mood, fatigue, and support CVS	*Achillea millefolium, Angelica sinensis* (this is not an oestrogenic herb!), *Crataegus laevigata, Ginkgo biloba* Cardioprotective, lipid metabolism modulation: *Allium sativum, Curcuma longa, Cynara scolymus, Trigonella foenum-graecum*
Digestive system support, aiding assimilation and gut flora to make phytoestrogenic herbs bioavailable	Bitters: *Artemisia absinthum* (bitters are cooling), *Berberis vulgaris, Taraxacum officinale radix, Verbena officinalis*
Dry vagina and other mucous membranes, protect and moisten the mucous membranes	*Actaea racemosa, Althaea officinalis folia, Asparagus racemosus, Chamaelirium luteum, Glycyrrhiza glabra, Plantago lanceolata, Zea mays*
Elimination	*Schisandra chinensis, Silybum marianum, Taraxacum officinale radix*
Hormonal	*Actaea racemosa, Asparagus racemosus, Dioscorea villosa, Glycyrrhiza glabra, Humulus lupulus, Linum sativa, Paeonia lactiflora* plus *Glycyrrhiza glabra, Salvia officinalis*, soy, *Trifolium pratense, Trillium erectum, Vitex agnus-castus*

(Continued)

Table 14.1: (Continued)

Issues to address	Herbal treatment
Hot flushes, night sweats	*Astragalus membranaceus, Eleutherococcus senticosus, Panax ginseng, Salvia officinalis*
Maintaining bone density	*Actaea racemosa, Astragalus membranaceus, Camellia sinensis, Equisetum arvense, Humulus lupulus, Panax ginseng, Salvia officinalis,* soy, *Trifolium pratense*

SECTION TWO

MONOGRAPHS OF HERBS FREQUENTLY USED IN WOMEN'S HEALTH, WITHOUT A HORMONAL REPUTATION

Achillea millefolium

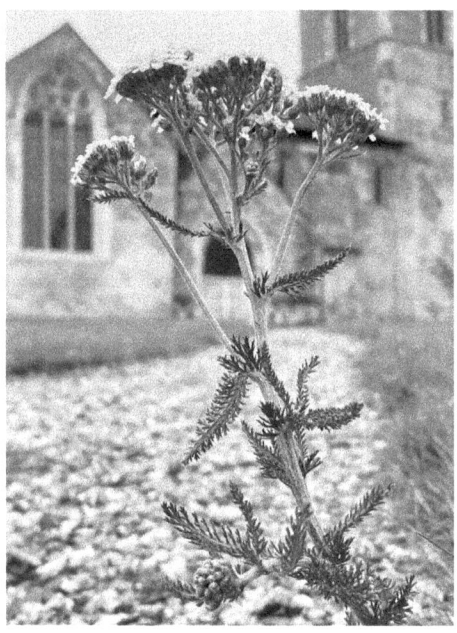

Yarrow: from the Anglo-Saxon *gearwe*. In Dutch it is named *yerw*.

Pliny (AD 23/24–79): states that Achillea was named for Achilles, a physician who was one of the first to use a species of this plant as a vulnerary.[1]

Millefolium: refers to its foliage.

East Anglia: place the leaf inside the nose and recite:

Yarroway, yarroway, bear a white blow,
if my love love me,
my nose will bleed now. (Bleed = an omen of success)

Yarrow put inside a flannel and placed under the pillow before bed, having repeated the following words, brought a vision of the future husband or wife:

Thou pretty herb of Venus' tree,
Thy true name it is Yarrow;
Now who my bosom friend must be,
Pray tell thou me tomorrow.

Commonly used in traditional medicine world-wide as a cure-all.

Yarrow pollen was found in a *Homo neanderthalensis* grave at Shanidar in Iraq dated to 60,000 B.P.[2,3] It has been suggested that these plants were chosen because of the symbolism of their therapeutic potential.[4]

Pliny the elder (AD23/24–79): indicated it for *looseness of the bowels*, bleeding, excessive menstruation (sometimes given as a sitz bath) and earache.[5]

Dioscorides (AD40–90): says it stops bleeding, including from wounds and abnormal menstrual bleeding, and reduces inflammation. A decoction could be used as a douche for menstrual bleeding and be drunk for dysentery.[6]

John Parkinson (1567–1650): notes a decoction could be drunk warm for ague. *If it be put into the nose, assuredly it will stay the bleeding of it.* Although it is also suggested that a leaf being rolled up and applied to the nostrils causes a nose bleed, thus affording relief from headache.

Nicholas Culpeper (1616–1654): describes it as drying, using it for wounds, for toothache and to stop *the bloody flux*, and as an ointment for the scalp *to stay the shedding off of hair.*

Linnaeus the Dalecarlians (1707–1778): mentions its use as a substitute for hops in the making of ale, believing it to impart intoxicating qualities.[7]

In Europe it was known as *Herba militaris*, the military herb. An ointment made from *Achillea* was used by army surgeons over centuries as a vulnerary for battle wounds.

In the Orkneys milfoil tea is used for dispelling melancholy.

The Eclectics: describe it as a diffusive vasostimulant, for peripheral circulation, especially pelvic organs with a tonic influence upon the venous system and mucous membranes. They used yarrow for a range of conditions such as:

Urinary system: chronic diseases of the urinary system, deficient renal action, in acute or chronic Bright's disease in its incipient stage (Bright's disease is an historical classification of kidney diseases now known as acute or chronic nephritis: oedema, proteinuria, frequently accompanied by hypertension and heart disease).[8]

Bleeding: haemoptysis, haematuria and other forms of haemorrhage where the bleeding is small in amount.

Gynaecology: atonic amenorrhoea, menorrhagia and vaginal leucorrhoea thought of as one of the best agents for the relief of menorrhagia.[9] Best in strong infusion and its use must be persisted with.[10]

Actions

Astringent, antidiarrhoeal, vulnerary
Antihaemorrhagic, haemostyptic, including for internal bleeding (haemoptysis, haematuria, menorrhagia)
Anti-inflammatory
Antimicrobial
Antipyretic
Antispasmodic
Bitter, cholagogue and choleretic
Diffuse vasostimulant, peripheral vasodilator, diaphoretic, hypotensive
Diuretic
Uterine tonic, emmenagogue

Indications

Amenorrhoea (esp. atonic), dysmenorrhoea, menorrhagia (esp. atonic)
Diarrhoea, dysentery
Fever
GIT spasm, dyspepsia
Haemorrhoids
Hypertension, (especially for raised diastolic)[11]
Internal bleeding, haematuria, etc.
Pelvic congestion
Urinary irritation
Topically for slow-healing wounds and skin conditions.
Insect repellent.[12]

Constituents

Monoterpenes: borneol, camphor, 1.8-cineole, eucalyptol, limonene, terpineol and α-thujone.
  Sesquiterpenes and sesquiterpene lactones: achillicin, achillin, milefin and millefolide, derivatives azulene and chamazulene[13] formed during steam distillation of the oil from proazulenes, e.g. achillin and achillicin.
  Flavonoids: kaempferol, luteolin, apigenin.[14,15]
  Other: coumarins, phenolic acids (salicylic and caffeic acid), sterols, N-alkylamides.[16]
  The diversity and complexity of the constituents provide the broad spectrum of activity.

Preclinical studies

A wide range of activities are shown in these in vitro and in vivo studies, many of them lending support to the rationale behind the traditional uses, some suggest intriguing new areas of thought.[17]

Analgesic and antipyretic: the whole extract was antipyretic. The salicylic acid derivatives (eugenol and menthol) showed local analgesia and antipyretic activity.

Anticancer: *Achillea* was found to be a selective inhibitor of prostate cancer cells.[18-20] Three sesquiterpenoids (achimillic acids A, B and C) were active against leukaemia cells.[21]

Anti-inflammatory: the aqueous extract showed anti-inflammatory activity in vivo.[22] Using the extract had activity similar to, or greater than, that of indomethacin (a NSAID).[23] A gel containing 6% yarrow extract was equal to a diclofenac sodium gel.[24] The anti-inflammatory action partly mediated by inhibition of MMP-2 and -9.[25] Proazulenic sesquiterpene lactones were shown to inhibit COX-2.[26]

Antimicrobial (in vitro): against *Helicobacter pylori* (methanol extract) at concentrations easily obtained in the stomach after oral dosing,[27] also active against *Shigella dysenteriae*,[28] the water extract effective against *Salmonella typhimurium*.[29]

Essential oil: against *Streptococcus pneumoniae, Clostridium perfringens, Candida albicans, Mycobacterium smegmatis, Acinetobacter lwoffii* and *Candida krusei*.[30]

Antiparasitic (in vitro): aqueous extracts showed antimalarial and antibabesial activity.[31]

Antioxidant[32]

Antispasmodic: an antispasmodic effect on isolated jejunum and ileum.[33] The flavonoid aglycones quercetin, luteolin and apigenin showed potent individual antispasmodic action, and concentrations of these flavonoids in tea would be high enough to produce the effect. The mechanism is due in part to a calcium-channel blocking activity and in part to mediator-antagonistic effects.[34]

Anxiolytic: an aqueous extract in vivo.[35]

Autoimmune encephalomyelitis: treatment with aqueous preparation attenuated disease severity, inflammatory responses and demyelinating lesions. In addition, following treatment with *A. millefolium*, serum levels of TGF-β were increased in EAE-induced models.[36]

Choleretic effect: in 20% methanolic extract.[37]

Gastric emptying, stimulation: a water extract of *Achillea* had a spasmogenic effect on the gastric antrum.[38]

Gastroprotective, (in vivo): an aqueous yarrow extract had non-significant organ-specific effects on glutathione formation.[39,40] The hydroalcoholic extract prevented the reduction of glutathione (GSH) levels and superoxide dismutase (SOD) activity after induced gastric lesions and inhibited induced gastric ulcers.[41]

Haemostyptic: shown to accelerate the coagulation of blood, in vitro and in vivo. An infusion shortened recalcification time in human blood plasma.[42]

Hepatoprotective, (in vivo): a 70% aqueous-methanol extract improved liver enzyme levels and reduced histopathology.[43]

Hypotensive, negative inotropic and chronotropic effect, vasodilator and bronchodilator activities: possibly mediated through Ca2+ antagonism and an endothelium-dependent relaxant component (in vivo).[44]

Mosquito bite prevention, topical use: a study found that use of yarrow leaf extract reduces biting by *Aedes* mosquitoes.[45]

Oestrogenic, non-significant: apigenin and luteolin, which occur in many other plants, are 4000 to 4 million times less potent than the active pharmaceutical control, 17β-estradiol.[46] The relevance to human consumers is therefore questionable.[47]

Skin rejuvenation: receptors for ACTH and β-endorphin decrease with ageing in the human epidermis. *Achillea* extract upregulated ACTH and β-endorphin receptor expressions, improved expression profile of cytokeratin 10, transglutaminase-1 and filaggrin, increased epidermal thickness, and improved the appearance of wrinkles and pores.[48]

Vasoprotective: flavonoids and dicaffeolylquinic acid derivatives reduced vascular inflammation.[49]

Clinical studies

Episiotomy: *Achillea millefolium* ointment reduced perineal pain levels, redness, oedema and ecchymosis of episiotomy wound.[50]

Chronic kidney disease: 1.5g of powdered *A. millefolium* flower was given 3 days a week for 2 months. Plasma nitrite and nitrate concentrations decreased slightly after 2 months, the authors suggesting that higher doses or a longer duration of administration may make these changes more significant. An increased plasma nitric oxide concentration is a possible mechanism of bleed tendency in patients who suffer chronic kidney disease.[51]

Gastric secretions increased: a study from 1926 using *Achillea* tincture (70%) increased the secretion of gastric juice in healthy volunteers.[52]

Multiple sclerosis: a water extract (500mg), decreased the annual relapse rate in MS. Lesions decreased, the time to first relapse increased, showed improvement on several MS testing scores and improved performance in word-pair learning.[53]

Oral mucositis as side-effect of chemotherapy: *A. millefolium* distillate healed oral mucositis better than the routine solution.[54]

Primary dysmenorrhea: *A millefolium* as a tea taken during menstruation minimised pain severity in primary dysmenorrhoea.[55]

Combination products including *Achillea millefolium*:

IBS symptoms: *Boswellia carterii, Zingiber officinale* and *Achillea millefolium* combination was effective in eliminating IBS symptoms and its related symptoms of depression and anxiety.[56]

Osteoarthritis: *Tanacetum parthenium, Populus tremulides* and *Achillea millefolium* showed similar reduction of subjective symptoms compared to ibuprofen.[57]

Venous leg ulcers: a topical preparation including *Achillea, Symphytum, Salvia* and *Calendula* healed surface and venous leg ulcers, outperforming a topical antibiotic.[58]

Cautions, contraindications

Contact dermatitis which may be connected to sesquiterpenes.

Summary of use in gynaecology

- Uterine and pelvic circulation affects, clears pelvic congestion, reducing uterine flooding and pain due to engorged pelvic veins.
- Menstrual irregularities (amenorrhoea, menorrhagia and metrorrhagia), improves uterine tone, which may correct bleeding due to uterine atony.
- Atony and relaxation of tissue, discharges, leucorrhea.
- Dysmenorrhoea.
- Endometriosis, fibroids, perimenopausal bleeding.

Dosage

Daily dose 3–12ml of 1:3.
  Typical weekly dose 15–40ml of 1:3.

Alchemilla vulgaris

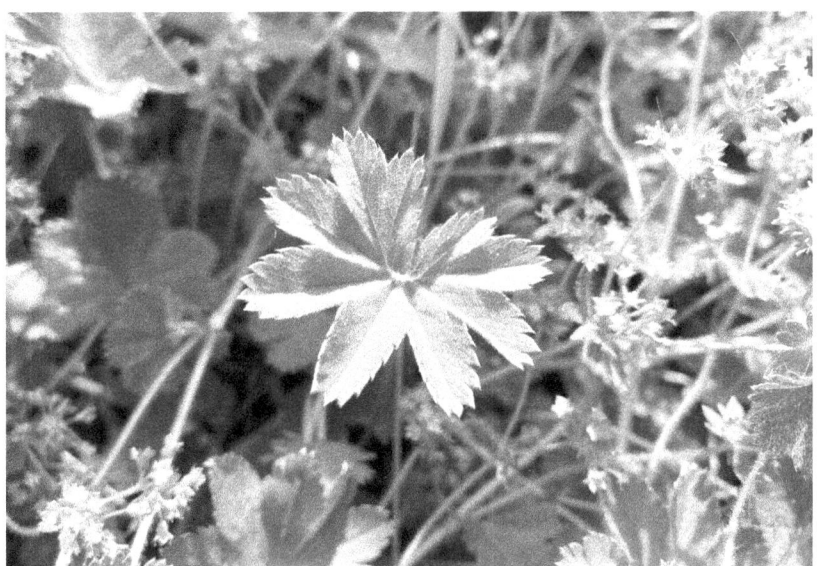

Lady's mantle

Its name comes from the Arabic word *Alkemelych*, meaning alchemy.

Alchemical virtues are ascribed to the dewdrops found in the foliage, used in tonics for longevity and other mystic potions.

The plant was highly respected by the ancient German tribes and was devoted to Frigg, the goddess of nature and fertility.

In the Middle Ages it was associated with the Virgin Mary (Lady's Mantle) as supposedly the leaves resemble a mantle, or cloak.

Used traditionally and in folk medicine across Europe for centuries for women's complaints. Also used for wound healing internally and externally, as an astringent for vomiting and excessive discharge of fluid from the body, including diarrhoea.[1]

Several sources suggest that it will reduce the size of large and or sagging breasts and for use when the womb is too cold, moist and slippery, and allows the foetus to slip out.

Hildegard von Bingen (1098–1179): recommended it for throat ulcers as an astringent, as an emmenagogue, diuretic, and for use in mouthwashes, baths, poultices.

Andrés Laguna de Segovia (1499–1559): *Astringes parts for those who want to appear virginal.*

John Parkinson (1567–1650): called it a most singular wound herb and said it will make the body more fit and able to retain conception.

Nicholas Culpeper (1616–1654): *It is one of the most singular wound herbs and used in all wounds inward and outward, to drink a decoction thereof and wash the wounds therewith, externally wonderfully drieth up all humidity of the sores and abateth all inflammations thereof. It quickly healeth green wounds, cureth old sores, though fistulous and hollow.*

Matthiolus (1626): *Alchemilla* juice placed on the breast with linen cloths does not make it grow larger.[2]

John Hill (1716–1775): uses the root for *overflowings of the menses and bloody fluxes*, and also talks about firming of the breasts; *apply the leaves to breast to make them recover their form after they have been swelled with milk*. He says this is where the name lady's mantle comes from.

Elizabeth Blackwell (1737): *great Force to stop inward Bleeding, the immoderate Flux of the Menses, and the Fluor albus. The Leaves applyed outwardly are accounted good for lank flagging Breasts, to bring them to a greater Firmness and smaller Compass.*[3]

Father Künzle (1928) a Swiss herbalist: *A woman in Glarnerland, who had already had 10 births, with the last three putting her between life and death, the doctors prophesied that the 11th birth would bring her certain death. This 11th birth did come, but it was not fatal at all, nor was it a miscarriage, but the easiest and best of all eleven, and the child was the loveliest and strongest of all; how did this come about? On the advice of a herbalist, the good woman had been drinking a cup of lady's mantle every day from the third month.*[4]

Madaus wrote in 1938: as well as for use in menorrhagia, to ensure a good delivery and complete expulsion of the afterbirth a cup of the tea is drunk three times a day, four weeks before delivery. Interestingly, he prescribed it for obesity as a result of ovarian dysfunction and generally for pathological pain in the abdomen.[5]

Actions

Astringent, anti-haemorrhagic, anti-inflammatory.

Indications

Diarrhoea, dysentery, endometriosis, fibroids, passive haemorrhage, menorrhagia, and to aid fertility.

Constituents

Kaempferol glycosides

Polyphenols: apigenin, caffeic acid, catechin, chlorogenic acid, ellagic acid, ferulic acid, gallic acid, hyperoside, isoquercetin, kaempferol, luteolin, morin, quercetin, rutin and tiliroside.[6]

Tannins: ellagitannins.

Triterpenes: oleanolic acid, ursolic acid, tormentic acid, euscopic acid.

Modes of extraction: methanolic, ethanolic (EtOH), ethyl acetate and water extracts have shown different quantities. The highest yields of gallic acid, caffeic acid, catchin, quercetin[7] were found in ethyl-acetate (EA) extract, the highest of chlorogenic acid in the EtOH extract.

Note of interest: has many of the same constituents as *Camellia sinensis*.

Hormones: very little preclinical research has pointed towards any specific hormonal effect. Despite this many herbalists suggest it is progesteronic and an LH inhibitor.[8] Tradition points toward its use in menorrhagia, and although in such cases progesterone might be prescribed, this does not translate to the herb being progesteronic.

One study assessed 150 herbs, which were tested for their capacity to compete with oestradiol and progesterone binding to receptors, in vitro. The six highest progesterone-receptor-binding herbs (which did not include *Alchemilla*) underwent further specific testing, and were found to be neutral or antagonist.[9] This suggests that these herbs have very little, if any, direct progesteronic activity.

When considering the worth of in vitro studies of herbs and receptor binding, it is important to note the shortcomings: for example, pre-clinical studies show polysaccharides and tannins interact non-specifically with many receptors including progesterone, however these constituents are unable to enter the blood stream to physically reach those receptors.

Testing on isolated cells may not transfer to real-body situations.

There do appear to be plants that contain tiny amounts of progesterone, although too low to have any hormonal effect. Herbs that are thought to be progesteronic have either no appreciable quantities of those compounds or none at all.[10] Their activity is not due to progesterone content.

Precursors of progesterone contained within plants such as diosgenin (see book 1) are widely accepted to be a myth as lab modifications are needed to produce this.

Herbs that have been shown to improve progesterone levels in human studies are *Actaea racemosa*, *Paeonia lactiflora* & *Glycyrrhiza glabra*,[11] and *Vitex agnus-castus*,[12,13] which rely on the function of the corpus luteum; post menopausally they will have no effect on progesterone levels.

Having said all this, there is one thesis that looked at the effect of high $ZnSO_4$ concentrations in drinking water on the liver, spleen and ovaries in vivo and the protective effect of *Alchemilla vulgaris*. The study concluded that *Alchemilla* did have protective effects on ovary, liver and spleen, and it was also noted that those on *Alchemilla* (six subjects) not subject to a zinc overdose showed an increase in progesterone.[14]

Preclinical studies

There is a mine of information on in vitro and some in vivo studies but very little data outside this. It would be presumptuous to assume all these actions translate directly to the therapeutic use of *Alchemilla*. However, they do give some intriguing windows into possible activity.

Angioprotective[15]

Antibacterial, antifungal properties[16]

Anticoagulant activity[17]

Anti-inflammatory: a methanolic extract inhibited the activity of COX-1 and COX-2 enzyme.[18]

Antioxidant activity[19]

Antiviral activity, aqueous solutions:[20] antiviral (orthopoxviruses).

Anxiolytic, intra-peritoneal: non-sedating, modulating anxiety states.[21,22]

Endometriosis: *Alchemilla mollis* and *A. persica* in endometriosis model reduced endometriosis and inflammatory markers; both herbs thought to be of benefit in the treatment of endometriosis.[23]

Gastroprotective activity: against *Helicobacter pylori*.[24]

Hepatoprotective and renal protective:[25,26] showed a protective role in cisplatin-induced toxicity, decreased the levels of serum parameters of the liver (total bilirubin and ALP), kidneys (urea and creatinine), and improved enzyme antioxidant activity.[27]

Hypotensive: methanolic extracts showed microvascular and blood pressure lowering effects via a vasodilatory effect.[28]

Lipase and amylase inhibitory activity: leading to a decrease in caloric yield and weight loss. Suggested to be of benefit in obesity and type 2 diabetes.[29,30]

Neuroprotective activity: suppressed neuroinflammation, the inhibitory effect on acetylcholinesterase and tyrosinase suggests a use in the prevention and treatment of neurodegenerative diseases.[31]

Skin aging: an inhibiton of elastase, the level of inhibition is associated with tannin concentration,[32] the kaempferol glycosides inhibited elastase and trypsin in vitro, with angioprotective effects.[33]

Suppression of tumour development: showed cytotoxic effects against several cancer cell lines, including oestrogen-dependent tumours. Prevents tumourigenesis as well as suppressing tumour cell growth.[34-36]

Wound healing effects: topically induced epithelial cell growth, promitotic activity in epithelial cells and myofibroblasts.[37]

Clinical studies

On aphthous ulcers: highly effective, shown to accelerate healing when used in combination with glycerine.[38]

Menorrhagia, in teenage girls: the volume of flow reduced when used 10–15 days before period. The cycle also shortened and premenstrual administration prevented menorrhagia from recurring.[39]

Anti-obesity: a combination of *Alchemilla vulgaris*, *Olea europaea*, *Mentha longifolia* and seeds of *Cuminum cyminum*. Researchers speculated the combination increased both satiety and thermogenesis in brown fat cells.[40]

Summary of use in gynaecology

- Menorrhagia, leucorrhoea, endometriosis, fibroids, incompetent cervix.
- Pointers from Madaus and research related to obesity and diabetes is suggestive of a role in PCOS.
- Partus preparator.
- Conception aid (according to the old herbalists).

Dosage

Daily dose 6–12ml of 1:3.
Typical weekly dose 15–30ml of 1:3.

Anemone pulsatilla

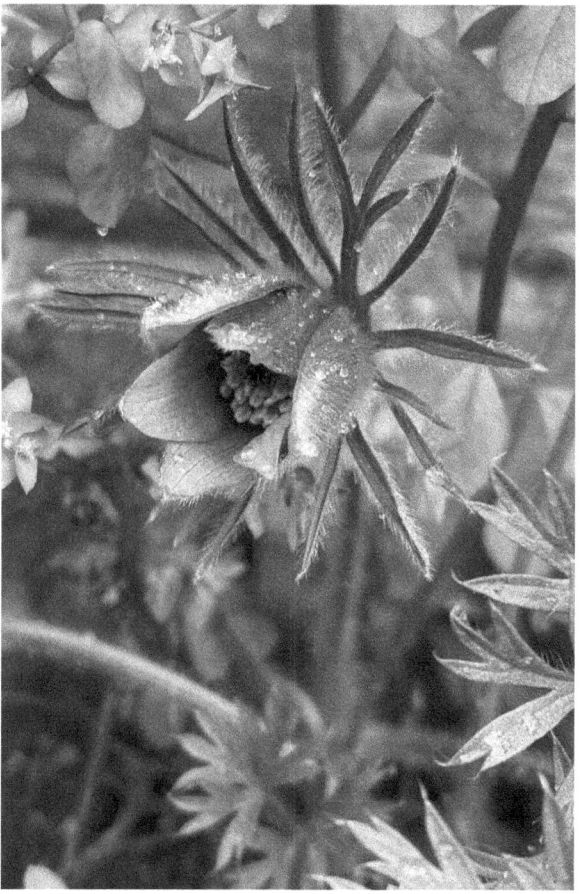

Pasque flower, *Pulsatilla vulgaris*.

Anemone comes from the Greek νεμος (ánemos), meaning wind flower.

Culpeper suggests that the flowers never open when the wind blows and the seed also flies away with the wind; he says this he got from Pliny and added "if not, blame him".[1]

The name Pasque flower most likely arises because they bloom at late Easter. The juice of the purple sepals gives a green stain to paper and linen, used to colour the Paschal, or Easter, eggs in some countries.

Various *Anemone* species are used in the ethnomedicine of India, Korea, Mongolia, Tibet, America, Europe and traditional Chinese medicine.

Dioscorides (AD50–70): *the juice of root into the nostrils helps in purging the head. Boiled in raisin wine and applied it cures inflammation of the eyes, and mends scars in the eyes and moisture in the eyes and cleans filthiness of ulcers. And in pessary it encourages the menstrual flow, rubbed on it takes away leprosy.*[2]

The external use for eyes has repeated by herbalists over the centuries, for example, from John Gerard (1633): *it was more used amongst Greek physicians, who much commend the juice of them of taking away the scales which grow on the eyes.*[3]

Nicholas Culpeper (1653): repeats the same words from Dioscorides.[4] Used over centuries for eye diseases (cataracts).[5]

The Native Americans used it for muscular aches and headaches and other unspecified illness.[6]

In the latter half of the 19th century it became a favourite of the Eclectics and homoeopaths. They said that only the fresh herb is effective and should not be kept longer than 1 year, and they gave very small doses of the plant.[7] A specific picture of an 'Anemone type' was given: fair, blue-eyed, tearful, weepy women. It was used as an emmenagogue for amenorrhoea, or menstruation that is suppressed, tardy or scanty as a consequence of cold, or from emotional causes. It was also used as an analgesic and spasmolytic for dysmenorrhoea,[8] for *ovaritis and ovaralgia with tensive, tearing pain*, and for epididymitis and orchitis due to gonorrhoeal infection or to metastasis from mumps.[9]

Prof. Chandler: *in painful menstruation, especially that form called neuralgic, common in the unmarried, commencing often at puberty.* He suggested moderate doses, three times a day during the menstrual interval, and up to every hour, according to the severity of the pain during the menstrual time. He claimed that permanent cures follow in many cases and marked beneficial results in most others: *It is impossible to lay down rules for specific differentiation between the remedies pulsatilla and cimicifuga. As a rule, for dysmenorrhea of the virgin or the unmarried, I give the choice to pulsatilla; while to the married, before pregnancy or after its occurrence, I have preferred cimicifuga.*[10]

Anemone pulsatilla and *Gelsemium sempervirens* were among the ten most-often prescribed herbs by the Eclectics in the 1920s. These herbs were given in small doses for very specific symptomatic indications. A common method was to put from 10 to 30 drops in 4 ounces (120ml) of water, prescribed by the teaspoon.

Actions

Analgesic, sedative, spasmolytic.

Indications

Specifically used for painful conditions of the female or male reproductive systems. Dysmenorrhea, primary as well as secondary, such as endometriosis, pelvic inflammatory disease, orchitis, epididymitis.

Other: insomnia, migraine or tension headaches, neuralgia, for earache used as drops in the ear.

Traditionally indicated if any of the above are related to or accompanied by anxiety.

Weiss: internally to treat the inner eye conditions such as iritis, scleritis, diseases of the retina and glaucoma.[11]

Constituents

Alkaloids, coumarins, flavonoids, phenolic compounds, saponins, tannins, triterpenoids, volatile oil.[12-14]

A lactonic glucoside (ranunculin) is found in the fresh intact aerial parts. This degrades in the presence of water, by enzymatic process upon crushing the plant or in freeze drying, to form protoanemonin which is toxic and unstable. Protoanemonin dimerises to form anenomin, which is non-toxic. Drying and ethanol promotes dimerisation with a consequent reduction of toxicity. However, overdose of dried extracts has been reported as leading to violent gastritis and irritation of the kidneys and urinary tract. This seems to suggest that some of the protoanemonin is retained in dried preparations.

Preclinical studies

There is little research on *Anemone pulsatilla* itself. It is a part of the Ranunculaceae family, which contains herbs such as *Petasites hybridis*, *Aconitum napellus* and *Actaea racemosa*, some better researched, which have similar actions upon the nervous system and which have been used as anodynes and anti inflammatories.[15] *Anenome pulsatilla* also has anodyne and anti inflammatory activities. Locally applied it produces numbness and tingling and may even *excite violent inflammation*s. This is due to *anemonin* and strongly resembles the action of *Aconite*.[16]

Pharmacological studies, in vivo: pulsatilla and anemonin produce a hypnotic state with reduced sensitivity, followed by a state of paralysis that is progressive, affecting the extremities and respiratory muscles. At the same time, it decreased the intensity of heartbeats without a change in blood pressure.[17]

1916 ex vivo: shown to reduce uterine contraction.[18]

1938 studies by Madaus (in vivo): the emmenagogic effects were confirmed. It was also noted that the anemonin could still be detected in highly dilute homeopathic tincture (D4).[19]

1998 study (in vitro): reduces smooth muscle spasm.[20]

Preclinical studies of other anemone species

Pulsatilla chinensis and *Pulsatilla koreana* have similar constituents, shown to have antitumour, antimicrobial, anti-inflammatory, sedative, analgesic, anti-convulsant and anti-histamine activity.[21]

Individual constituents preclinical research

Anemonin

- Anticancer compounds[22,23]
- Inhibits pigmentation synthesis in human melanocytes, inhibits melanin synthesis.[24]
- Anti-inflammatory against intestinal injury: improving mucosa restoration, alleviating intestinal inflammation (by reducing the production of nitric oxide, endothelin-1, soluble intercellular adhesion molecule)[25] and preventing intestinal microvascular dysfunction.[26]
- Alleviated nerve injury after cerebral ischaemia and reperfusion in vivo by improving antioxidant activities and inhibiting apoptosis pathway.[27]
- Sedative activity: in small doses it is a central nervous system depressant, lowering heart rate and respiration.[28] This depressant capacity may account for the herb's ability to treat anxiety and emotional hypersensitivity.

Cinnamic acid (cinnamate)

- Tyrosinase inhibitor. Tyrosinase is responsible for synthesising catecholamines and oxidising excess dopamine,[29] perhaps thus affecting dopamine synthesis in cells. Cinnamic acid was found to be a neuroprotective.

Triterpenoid saponins

- Anticancer activity via multiple pathways: cell cycle arrest and apoptosis induction.
- Anti-inflammatory and anti-hyperlipidemic immunomodulatory activity in vivo.
- Slight haemolytic effect.
- Immunomodulatory, enhanced the specific antibody and cellular responses.[30]
- Antioxidant and antimicrobial activities.[31]

Protoanemonin and anemonin

- Sedating
- Antipyretic[32]
- Induces a significant reduction in spontaneous motor activity (protoanemonin more potent than anemonin).[33]
- Central nervous system stimulant.[34]

Some of the volatile oils

- Antibacterial activity.[35]

Summary of use in gynaecology

Used for primary and secondary dysmenorrhoea, especially endometriosis, adenomyosis, and pelvic inflammatory disease.

Cautions and contraindications

Children, neurological disease, depression and psychosis, liver and kidney disease, history of allergy or anaphylactic reaction. Pregnancy.

Adverse reactions

No adverse reaction for dried preparations, if used at the recommended dosage.

Overdose of dried preparation can cause violent gastritis, irritation of the kidneys and urinary tract.

Fresh plant preparations can cause severe irritation of the skin and mucosa with itching, rashes, pustules, gastroenteritis, vomiting, purging, irritation of the kidneys.

It depresses heart action, lowering arterial tension and reducing the temperature and pulse rate, with a paralysing effect on both sensory and motor nerves. Coma and convulsions have resulted from very large doses.[36,37]

Dosage

The Eclectics suggest that only the fresh herb should be used.[38]

The United States Pharmacopoeia of 1890 states *it should be carefully preserved, and not kept longer than one year.*[39]

In the UK it is more common to use the dried preparation.[40]

Dried plant tincture

Daily dose 0.9–3ml of 1:10.

Weekly dose 6.3–21ml of 1:10.

In reproductive tract pain, toothache, insomnia or acute attacks of migraine or dysmenorrhoea doses of 0.75ml–2ml can be given half-hourly.

Angelica sinensis

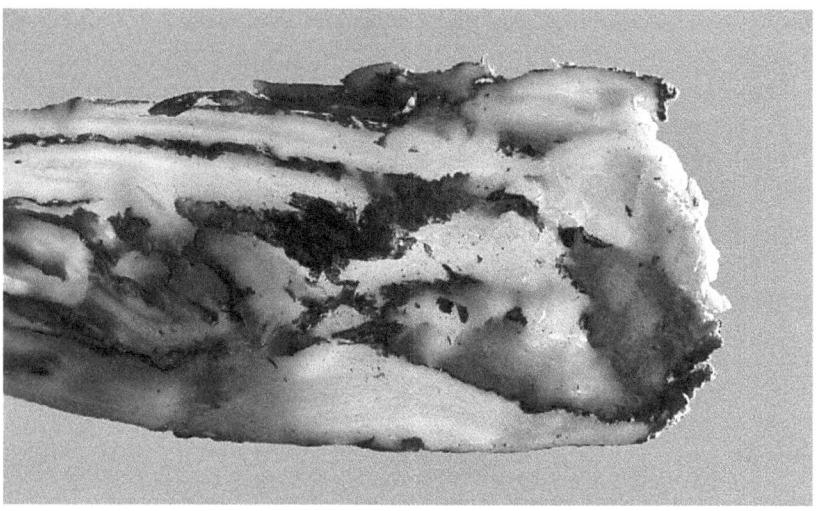

Pinyin name: *Dang Gui*: "state of return", "ought to return".

Shen Nong Ben Cao Jing, of the Han Dynasty (AD25–225): used for women's diseases, traditionally to enrich blood, promote blood circulation, for blood deficiency and menstrual disorders (dysmenorrhea and irregular menstrual cycle[1]), modulate the immune system, for chronic constipation (elderly) and the debilitated. The 'women's ginseng'.[2]

Used in trauma departments in hospitals in China along with other herbs for bruises, fractured or broken bones, swelling and injuries of the tendons.[3]

Tradititional Chinese Medicine categorises this herb as sweet, acrid, bitter and warm, suitable for cold-type blood-deficient patients.

- Tonifies blood, heart and liver blood deficiencies: symptoms include anaemia, pale complexion, brittle nails, dry hair, dizziness, blurred vision and palpitations.
- To nourish the blood and invigorate circulation, cold types of menstrual disorders, stagnation, regulation of menstruation.

Actions

Anti-arrhythmic, anti-anaemic, pelvic circulatory, anti-inflammatory, antiplatelet, female tonic, mild laxative.

Indications

Anaemia
Constipation, colic
Dysmenorrhoea, amenorrhoea
General tonic for fatigue
Impaired circulation, cardiovascular disorders

Major constituents[4]

<u>Benzenoids</u>: valerophenone-*o*-carboxylic acid and vanillic acid.
   <u>Coumarins</u>: angelol G, angelicone and umbelliferone.
   <u>Phenylpropanoids</u>: (*E*)-ferulic acid, 4-hydroxy-3-methoxycinnamic-acid, coniferyl ferulate.
   <u>Polysaccharides</u>
   <u>Terpenes</u>: β-cadinene, carvacrol and *cis*-β-ocimene.
   <u>Volatile oils</u>: ligustilide, which can account for over 5%.

Preclinical studies

Extensively studied, however mainly preclinical studies. When studied in vivo *Angelica* was given either intravenously or interperitoneally.
   Anti-atherosclerotic effects: relaxed isolated aorta and increased the production of vascular endothelial growth factor (VEGF).[5-8]
   Antiarrhythmic: prolonged the effective refractory period and action potentials of myocardium in vivo.[9-13]
   Antihepatotoxic activity.[14-16]
   Anti-inflammatory: inhibition of thromboxane A2 formation and prostaglandin E2 production.[17]
   Antineoplastic effects: stimulates macrophages, enhances phagocytosis, inhibits tumour growth, and inhibits metastasising of melanoma cells (furanocoumarins).[18-22]
   Antithrombotic activity/Antiplatelet effects: inhibited platelet aggregation and serotonin release. Showed a reduction in the concentration of plasma fibrinogen, changes in cell surface charge and a decrease in blood viscosity.[23-25]
   Antiulcer effects: showed enhanced gastric ulcer healing, promoted wound repair.[26] The polysaccharides demonstrated protective effects on gastrointestinal mucosal damage.[27]

Coronary blood flow increased: decreased myocardial oxygen consumption.[28] Provided protection against ischaemia- and reperfusion-induced myocardial dysfunction and injury.[29-31] Shown to have calcium channel blocking activity.[32]

Haematologic effects: this effect might be due to the polysaccharides, which may enhance hematopoiesis by stimulating macrophages, fibroblasts and muscle tissue to secrete haematopoietic growth factor.[33,34]

Hypotensive: ferulic acid reduced blood pressure and increased the number of opened capillaries as well as blood flow (improving microcirculation).[35]

Immunostimulant and immunosuppressant effects: protects against endotoxemia and experimental sepsis.[36-40]

Oestrogenic effects: none in vitro and in vivo.[41,42]

Pulmonary hypertension reduced: (coumarins) by antagonising calcium, may stimulate beta 2-receptors.[43]

Renoprotective effects: *Dong quai* and *Astragalus* in a ratio of 1:5 decoction (in vivo) orally alleviated hyperlipidaemia in nephrotic model, retarded the progression of renal fibrosis and deterioration of renal function.[44]

Smooth muscle activity: uterine effects. Some experiments on the whole root of *dong quai* have shown a stimulant activity in vivo,[45,46] while others have shown that it can relax or coordinate uterine contractions (make more rhythmic), depending on uterine tone. Volatile-oil components inhibit spontaneous uterine contractions in isolated uteri, whereas water/alcohol-soluble components stimulated uterine activity in vivo.[47] Ligustilide, butylidenephthalide and ferulic acid inhibited contractions of isolated uteri.[48-52] Ligustilide inhibited contractions in a concentration-dependent manner and possessed a non-specific antispasmodic activity.[53,54]

Clinical studies

Limited in number, these are mostly uncontrolled trials, some looking at individual constituents only. Many studies used intravenous or intramuscular modes of administration.

Gynaecological

Abnormal endometrium case report: a woman with atypical polypoid adenomyoma (an unusual form of precancerous endometrial proliferation) and infertility. Oral use for 4 months corrected her endometrium to normal and pregnancy followed. Her doctors suggested that *dong quai* may have acted as an ovulation inducer.[55]

Amenorrhoea and dysmenorrhoea: studies published in 1899 and 1910 on the treatment of amenorrhoea and dysmenorrhoea taken for 1 week before menstruation.[56–59] Relieved premenstrual pain and increased menstrual flow, decreased dysmenorrhoea, successfully treated amenorrhoea. Reduced severe bleeding in those chronic endometritis, decreasing menstrual pain.[60] No abortifacient activity observed in two pregnant women treated.[61]

Dysmenorrhoea: ligustilide at 450mg/day in an uncontrolled trial compared with aqueous extract. The effectiveness was much higher for ligustilide alone.[62] Essential oil orally relieved menstrual pain.[63]

Uterine smooth muscle stimulation: decoctions of the roots stimulated uterine smooth muscle in female patients (doses and conditions not stated).[64]

Menopause: clinical trials found no difference between placebo or *Angelica sinensis* for treatment of menopausal symptoms and indicated that is had no oestrogen-like responses in endometrial thickness or in vaginal maturation.[65]

Similarly, it did not relieve hot flushes in prostate cancer patients receiving androgen deprivation therapy.[66]

Menopause, hot flushes: a combination of 375mg *Angelica sinensis*, 150mg chamomile reduced the frequency and severity of hot flushes in menopausal women compared to placebo. There was no change in oestogen, FSH or LH, nor morphological changes on vaginal scan.[67]

Migraine, menstrual: a combination of soy isoflavones 60mg, *Angelica sinensis* 100mg and *Actaea racemosa* 50mg daily for 24 weeks reduced the frequency of menstrual-associated migraine attacks compared to placebo, with a reduction in severity score and dosage of triptan and analgesics.[68]

Tubal occlusion: uterine irrigation with extract, uncontrolled trial over 9 months, n=34; 79% regained tubal patency and 53% became pregnant.[69]

Other, oral use

Anaemia, chronic, case report: male with end stage renal disease. An improvement in anaemia and well-being, with once-weekly consumption of 12g *dong quai* and 52g paeony.

Blood viscosity: a decoction of the roots lowered whole blood viscosity after administration to six patients.[70]

Gastrointestinal bleeding: effective for patients with upper gastrointestinal bleeding, 4.5g powder, three times per day.[71,72]

Haematologic effects: case report of a haemodialysis patient with anaemia resistant to erythropoietin who had an improvement in haemoglobin and haematocrit after consuming *dong quai*.[73]

Other, intravenous or intramuscular injection

Ischaemic stroke: given IV reduced the size of cerebral infarction and improved neurological deficit scores.[74]

COPD: reduced pulmonary hypertension, improved forced expiratory volume and was beneficial.[75,76]

Hepatitis, cirrhosis: intramuscular injection. Improved the condition of patients with hepatitis, liver cirrhosis.[77]

Cautions and contraindications

Acute viral infections, children, diarrhoea caused by weak digestion (traditional), menorrhagia, haemorrhagic diseases, lactation.

Anticoagulant therapy: decreased prothrombin in vivo.[78] However, in one study where healthy volunteers took 1g daily for 3 weeks, arachidonic acid-induced platelet aggregation was inhibited in only 2 of 24 subjects. No effect was observed on platelet aggregation induced by ADP, collagen, epinephrine or ristocetin. Taking *dong quai* in combination with aspirin did not increase the antiplatelet effects of aspirin.[79]

Pregnancy: it has been suggested that it should not be used during the first trimester or in women with a tendency to spontaneous abortion.[80] However, in TCM several classic formulas specifically use *dong quai* to tonify blood and stabilise pregnancy.

Summary of use in gynaecology

A pelvic circulatory tonic, useful in secondary dysmenorrhoea, menorrhagia due to lack of tone, along with anaemia, and as a female tonic.

Dosage

The Chinese Pharmacopoeia: 9–15ml/day of 1:1.[81]
 Daily dose 6–12ml of 1:3.
 Typical weekly dose 15–25ml of 1:3.

Capsella bursa-pastoris

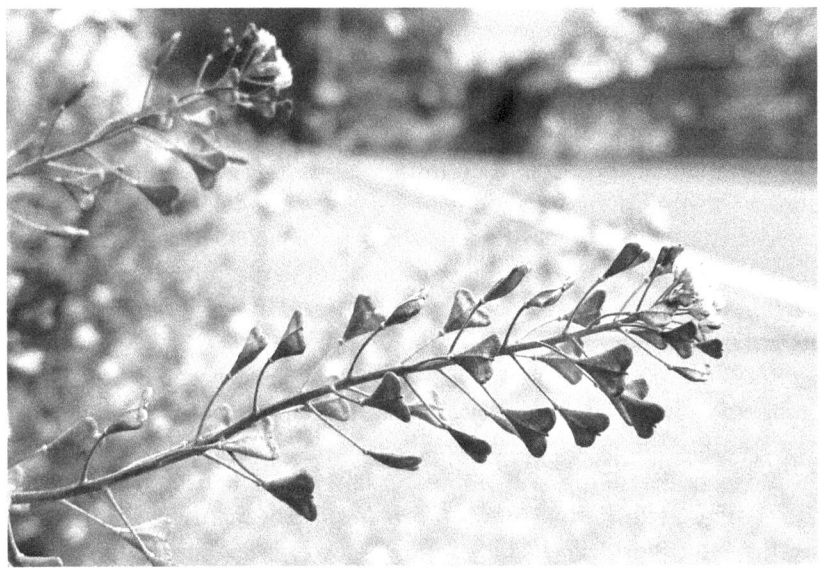

Shepherd's purse

Capsella = little box (the fruit). *Bursa pastoris* = purse of the shepherd, the flat seed-pouches of the plant thought to look like a leather purse. In France called *Bourse de pasteur*, and in Germany *Hirtentasche*.

The Irish name 'Clappedepouch' is an allusion to lepers, who stood at cross-roads with a bell or clapper, receiving their alms in a cup at the end of a long pole.[1]

Used on all continents.[2-4]

Dioscorides (AD40-90): says it induces the menstrual flow and is abortifacient.[5]

Nicholas Culpepper (English physician, 1652/3): it helps bleeding from wounds—inward or outward—and *if bound to the wrists, or the soles of the feet, it helps the jaundice. The herb made into poultices, helps inflammation and St. Anthony's fire. The juice dropped into ears, heals the pains, noise and matterings thereof. A good ointment may be made of it for all wounds, especially wounds in the head.*[6]

The Eclectics used shepherd's purse to treat haematuria, menorrhagia and benign abdominal tumours. Ellingwood says: *This agent has been noted for its influence in haematuria ... soothing irritation of the renal or vesical organs. In cases of uncomplicated chronic menorrhagia it has accomplished permanent cures, especially if the discharge be persistent.*[7]

From the *American Journal of Pharmacy* (1888): *For a long time it was employed, boiled in red wine, as a styptic in haemorrhages of various kind, a use which has recently been revived in Europe.* Among its constituents are little volatile oil, identical with that of black mustard.[8]

In 1897 Bombelon, a French chemist, suggested its *prompt use to arrest bleedings and flooding*—and these exact words are repeated over and over again in monographs from then until the present day. Bombelon mentions a Dr Von Ehrenwall who relates a case of female flooding, which had defied all the ordinary remedies and for which he tried an infusion of the shepherd's purse, with the result that the bleeding stopped after the first teacupful. He also says that it was used in former times to promote the regular monthly flow in women.[9]

Mrs Grieve's *A Modern Herbal* (1931): incorporated some of Bombelon's material, and she says that herbalists find this one of the best specifics for stopping haemorrhages of all kinds—of the stomach, the lungs, or the uterus, and more especially bleeding from the kidneys, and compared the herb to ergot and *Hydrastis*. She mentions its use during the First World War as a substitute for ergot in uterine bleeding, curative in various uterine haemorrhages, especially those associated with uterine cramp and colic, and in various passive haemorrhages from mucosal surfaces.[10,11]

Steinmetz (1954) put forward the idea that the herb's haemostatic action was due to the fungi *Cystopus candidus* and *Peronospora grisea*, found on *Capsella*.[12,13]

Dr Weiss (in *Herbal Medicine*): The haemostatic action may be owing to a peptide with oxytocin-like activity, but he says that its use for severe uterine bleeding is not recommended owing to unreliability. He mentions a study that noted that the maximum activity of shepherd's purse extract was attained only 3 months after the manufacture date. He stated that the haemostatic properties are inconsistent and that it is possible that the active principles only form in the herb after some time through the conversion of other principles that are lost as further conversions occur in storage. It is also possible that active principles are destroyed in the gastrointestinal canal and these points, taken together, may explain the different results reported by investigators. Weiss suggest the plant has only limited use, although he does reluctantly recommend it for uterine bleeding persisting over a period of time, particularly essential uterine haemorrhage and sometimes haemorrhage due to myoma: *The plant has the one advantage: it is perfectly safe.*[14]

In the *American Dispensatory* it is claimed that 'the fresh herb is decidedly more active than the dried'.[15]

Constituents

Flavonoids: quercitin, diosmetin, luteolin, hesperetin and theriglucosides (e.g. rutin, diosmin, hesperidin).

Aliphatic and phenolic acids: fumaric acid, citric acid, oxalic acid.

Glucosinolate (sinigrin): the glucosinolate breakdown product indole-3-carbinol.[16]

Actions

Anti-haemorrhagic, mild diuretic, urinary antiseptic.

Specific indications

Symptomatic treatment of menorrhagia, metrorrhagia, haemorrhage, haematuria, diarrhoea.

Topically for superficial skin wounds, bruising, nosebleeds.

Preclinical studies

Very little detail of the individual studies is available.

Anti-haemorrhagic: accelerated the rate of the coagulation of the blood markedly and rapidly. Comparing commercial oxalic acid in the same concentration as would be present in the herbal extract, they were found to possess the same power to reduce coagulation time in vivo.[17,18] Ex vivo tests also indicate that extracts accelerate coagulation of blood.[19]

Anti-inflammatory activity: anti-inflammatory effect demonstrated of the phenolic glycosides.[20]

Antimicrobial: antibacterial and antifungal activity.[21-23]

Antineoplastic: effects in vivo.[24]

Capillary permeability: isolated flavonoids showed a reduction in capillary permeability.[25]

Coronary blood flow, increased: coronary vasodilation, hypotensive, negative chronotropic and positive inotropic effects.[26]

Diuresis (orally and intraperitoneal administration): increased glomerular filtration rate.[27]

Gastroprotective: blocked the formation of stress-induced ulcers and reduced recovery time without affecting gastric secretion.[28]

Hepatoprotective[29,30]

Muscarine-like effects have been reported with dose-dependent lowering and elevation of blood pressure and increased uterine contraction, but no reference to the study is given in the Commision E monographs.[31,32]

Sedative: CNS-depressant action.[33]

Smooth muscle stimulant: in vitro studies showed it induced contraction of the small intestine and induced uteroactivity similar to oxytocin. Tracheal contractions induced in vivo were unaffected by adrenaline, which did inhibit acetylcholine-induced contractions.[34]

Uterotonic effect: extracts moderate acetyl cholinesterase inhibitors in vivo.[35,36] Extracts caused strong contractions of the small intestines and uterus in vivo and exerted contractile activity on the uterus, which was similar to that of oxytocin.[37,38] Water extracts (infusions) enhanced the uterine tonus of isolated uterine tissue.[39] It was speculated that the effect on menorrhagia and metrorrhagia seem to be mediated through an increased contraction of smooth muscles and a uteromimitic effect.

Clinical studies

Two clinical studies, using *Capsella* alongside orthodox treatment (mefenamic acid and oxytocin) found the combination more effective than orthodox treatment by itself.

Heavy menstrual bleeding: triple-blinded, randomised clinical trial looking at the effects of hydroalcoholic extracts of *Capsella* on menorrhagia, mefenamic acid plus *Capsella* in capsules. A significant decrease in the amount of menstrual bleeding in both groups. The mean decrease was significantly more in the *Capsella* group.[40]

Postpartum haemorrhage: single-blinded, randomised, clinical trial (n=100) using a hydroalcoholic extract of *Capsella bursa-pastoris* alongside oxytocin. Immediately after placental expulsion, the intervention group was given 10 sublingual drops of the combination extract and the control group was given 10 sublingual drops of the placebo plus oxytocin. Decrease in the amount of bleeding was significantly more in the *Capsella* group.[41]

Adverse effects

No adverse effects known, although it has been suggested to use with caution in breastfeeding, as glucosinolates excrete into breastmilk, and in people with a history of kidney stones due to the oxalate content.

Summary of use in gynaecology

Used for menorrhagia, in fibroids and endometriosis, along with other haemostyptic herbs.

Dosage

Daily dose 9–36ml of 1:3.
Typical weekly dose 15–30ml of 1:3.

Caulophyllum thalictriodes

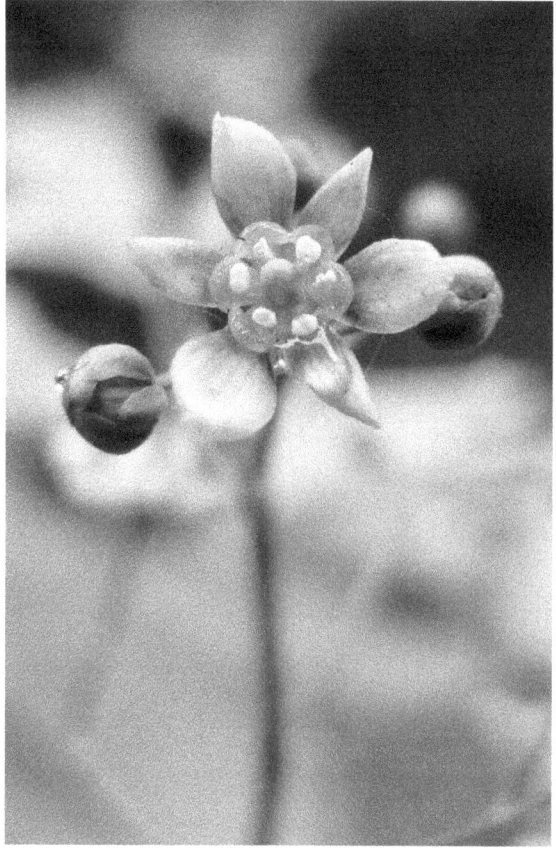

Blue cohosh, Papoose root, Blue ginseng, Yellow ginseng.

The name Blue cohosh comes from the dark blue berry-like structures and "cohosh" from the Algonquin name for the plant, coming from the word for "rough", which refers to the texture of the roots.[1]

The roasted seeds have been used as a coffee substitute.

Peter Smith (1813): Blue cohosh is first mentioned by him in a commercial pamphlet suggesting that Native American women made use of a decoction of the root, taking it regularly for a period of two to three weeks before the time for labour.[2] However, ethnobotanical studies suggest that Native Americans used the herb mainly for stalled labour.[3,4]

Constantine Samuel Rafinesque (c. 1828) mentions its use by Native Americans as a powerful emmenaogue, promoting delivery.[5,6]

Based on the recommendations by Smith and Rafinesque, the Eclectics used it in the 19th century, recommending it for amenorrhea, dysmenorrhea, menorrhagia, labour induction, to assure a prompt labour, to reduce the pain of childbirth and as partus preparator 2–3 weeks prior to the due date.[7]

It was commonly used as an alternative to ergot by the Eclectic physicians, who commented that it led to more effective natural contractions, whereas ergot led to continuous, spasmodic contractions.[8]

John King (1854): *My experience has been so uniform and conclusive on this point, that I do not hesitate to assert that it prevents not only a too painful labour, but it prevents those premature labours which are so common among the weakly women of this age.* It became the herb to be recommended for difficult labours,[9] rigidity of the os uteri (although King mentions that *Gelsemium* is more effective for this) and speedy labour.[10] Only small doses were used, typically a few drops of mother tincture.[11,12]

Ellingwood (1908): recommended 10 drops of the tincture of 1:10 *Caulophyllum* once every half-hour for delayed labour with rigid os and spasmodic pains, where the patient is worn out with fatigue.[13]

Blue cohosh was official in the *United States Pharmacopoeia* from 1882 to 1905 for labour induction and in the *National Formulary* from 1916 to 1950.[14]

Around the beginning of the twenty-first century *Caulophyllum* came back into vogue as midwives began using it regularly in America.[15] At that time it had become a more common practice to induce women who were over 40 weeks of pregnancy; one survey indicated that almost 50% of women had their labour induced.[16] Women were looking for alternatives since one of the common consequences of medical induction is that more interventions are needed.[17] In a survey of midwives in America, *Caulophyllum* was the most commonly prescribed herb for women past their due date to stimulate labour.[18]

This survey also included some adverse effects attributed to the use of *Caulophyllum* and *Actaea racemosa*, including nausea, increased meconium-stained fluid and transient foetal tachycardia.[19] The product, dose, duration and timing of use in pregnancy was not specified. It is difficult to suggest herbal causation given these particular complications are more common in pregnancies close to or post-term, for which these herbs were often being used.

Some herbal traditions warn that *Caulophyllum* can cause precipitous labour when used by itself and mention that it can affect foetal heart tone during delivery.

Case reports have suggested possible adverse effects, but on the available evidence it is difficult to establish causality between use of the herb and adverse events as a consequence of late-term and post-term pregnancy.[20]

Actions

Spasmolytic, uterine and ovarian tonic, emmenagogue, oxytocic.

Indications

Amenorrhea, dysmenorrhea, menorrhagia, uterine pain or inflammation, uterine prolapse or atony.

Other indications include spasmodic conditions of smooth muscle, including abdominal cramping, rheumatic conditions, muscular weakness and nervous debility.

Constituents

<u>Quinolizidine alkaloids</u>: taspine, N-methylcytisine, anagyrine
<u>Aporphine alkaloids</u>: magnoflorine
<u>Triterpene saponins</u>: caulosaponin and caulophyllosaponin

Preclinical studies

The actions of constituents are extrapolated from studies of isolates in vitro and in vivo and from studies with other plants.

Quinolizidine alkaloids:

- <u>Taspine, N-methylcytisine, anagyrine</u>: teratogenic.[21-23]
- <u>N-methylcytisine (caulophylline)</u>: a nicotinic agonist,[24] raises blood pressure (when injected), stimulating intestinal and respiratory motility.[25] Caulophylline's structure is similar to sparteine, and it has been suggested that this might explain its oxytocic activity. A small percentage of people are unable to metabolise sparteine by N-oxidation,[26,27] and it might be that, as in sparteine, a percentage of women are unable to metabolise caulophylline (and other alkaloids

in blue cohosh), resulting in adverse effects. This could explain why there are relatively few reports of negative effects.
- Aporphine alkaloid, magnoflorine: decreased arterial blood pressure, inducing hypothermia in vivo, induced contractions in the isolated pregnant rat uterus and stimulated isolated guinea pig ileal preparations.[28]

Triterpene saponins

Caulosaponin and caulophyllosaponins: had an oxytocic effect on isolated uterus, constricting coronary and carotid blood vessels and had a spasmogenic action on isolated intestines. Inhibited ovulation in vivo.[29,30]

The whole extract

Anti-inflammatory[31]
    Mild bradycardia: on hearts in situ.[32]
    Inhibition of ovulation: interruption of implantation.[33]
    Oxytocic, uterine stimulant: increased uterine tone but decreased rate and amplitude of contractions; in vivo studies demonstrated no uterine activity.[34] No effect on the uterus when administered in high doses.[35-40]
    Teratogenic[41]

Adverse effects

Blue cohosh berries are poisonous to children when consumed raw. The root can cause contact dermatitis.[42]

Case report: a 21-year-old woman using blue cohosh tincture (cited as 10 to 20 doses/day, strength not given) in an attempt to cause an abortion developed tachycardia, sweating, abdominal pain, vomiting and muscle weakness. The symptoms were consistent with nicotinic toxicity and resolved over 24 hours after discontinued use.[43]

Of the case reports suggesting toxicity and adverse effects, just one is plausible: The mother used blue cohosh tablets and the newborn had severe congestive heart failure and a myocardial infarction; at 2 years of age the child remained on digoxin therapy. The labour was precipitous, coming on suddenly and lasting one hour.[44]

A neonatal MI is extremely rare, and one main cause is maternal cocaine use. After the event the tablets were not analysed, nor the herb quantity specified. It has been put forward that using a crude form of blue cohosh in powders, capsules and tablets contains the greatest quantity of alkaloids and saponins.

Two further case reports related to *Caulophyllum* use disregarded by other papers:

Neonate's stroke: tests results indicated the need to consider cocaine as a possible cause.[45,46]

Severe multi-organ hypoxic injury on taking blue and black cohosh at 42 weeks' gestation; no information on product, dose, timing etc.[47] The adequacy of resuscitation training in the independent midwives was put forward as a possible factor.[48,49]

In these case reports direct causality cannot be established. Foetal complications, including intrauterine death, begin to increase after 40 weeks' gestation. Induction at 41 weeks is normally recommended as studies have demonstrated that induction is associated with lower perinatal mortality. Increased meconium, tachycardia, or need for resuscitation may occur as a result of a post-term pregnancy. The question we have to consider is which adverse effects are related to the herb and which can be attributed to a pregnancy requiring intervention. Given the widespread use that surveys noted above indicate, why are more adverse events not being reported?

We should also note that blue cohosh was traditionally used for stalled labour and not as partus preparator, nor for induction.

Analysis of blue cohosh products have been shown to have enormous variability in the constituent and depends on the type of product, i.e. dried herb, capsules, liquid extracts, data suggests the safest way to take blue cohosh is as a tincture.

Table: Estimated maximum daily intakes of blue cohosh alkaloids and saponins based on label information[50]

Form	Alkaloids estimated intake mg/day	Saponins estimated intake mg/day
Root, cut	75	420.3
Root, powder	20–36.4	61.5–83
Capsules	15.6–47.8	79.9–190.3
Liquid extract	0.9–17.3	9.3–79.1

Summary of use in gynaecology

Not commonly used but possibly of use in amenorrhoea, and cautiously in stalled labour.

Personal experience:

The use of 10ml of 1:5 in 100ml alongside *Mitchella, Rubus idaeus, Actaea racemosa, Viburnum opulus, Gelsemium sempervirens*, 5–10 drops between contractions during labour. All four labours were between 1 and 3 hours long.

Cautions, contraindications

Should not be used during pregnancy, as data regarding safety is limited.[51-53]

Due to doubt about teratogenic effects, avoid in women wishing to conceive and in pregnancy.

Dosage

Daily dose 1.4ml of 1:5 (max. 25 drops).

Maximum weekly dose 10ml of 1:5 60–65% alcohol, not to be used on its own.

Leonurus cardiaca

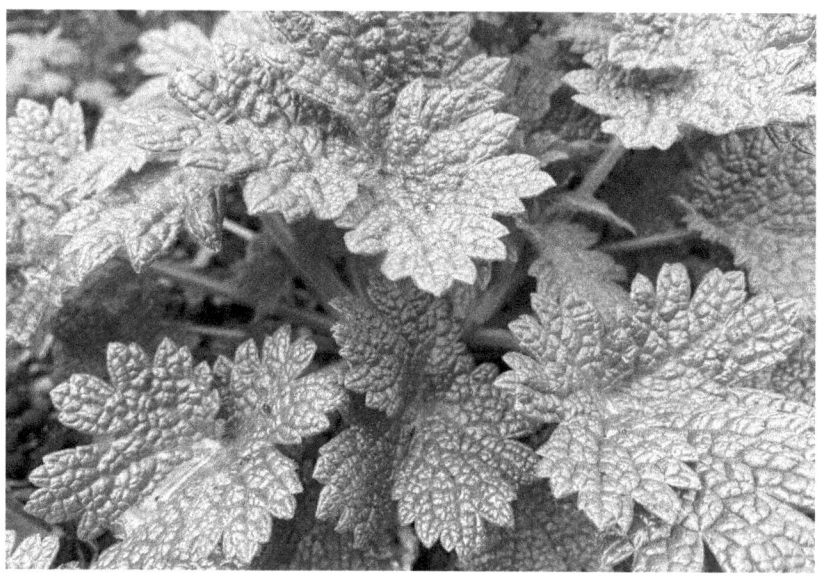

Motherwort

Leonurus: Greek for Lion's tail
Cardiaca: Latin for heart

Found and used all over the world,[1,2] called *Leonurus cardiaca* in the West; there is similar use of *Leonurus* species in Traditional Chinese Medicine.[3]

Used in some countries in soup alongside lentil or split peas, and as flavouring for beer and tea.[4]

John Gerard (1598): *The powder in wine provoketh not only urine and the monthly courses, but also is good for them that it is hard travail with child;*[5] he also described its use for cardiac weakness.

John Parkinson (1640): described its use for heart palpitations, and as a woman's tonic for difficult labour and promoting menstruation.[6]

Nicholas Culpeper (1652): *There is no better herb to take melancholy vapours from the heart, to strengthen it, and make a merry, cheerful, blithe soul than this herb. Besides, it makes women joyful mothers of children, and settles their wombs as they should be, therefore we call it Motherwort.*[7]

Native Americans used motherwort to treat gynecological disorders.[8]

The physiomedicalists and Eclectics used *Leonurus* in similar conditions: William Cook (1869): *a nervine tonic and antispasmodic*, used to stimulate *gentle outward circulation*, *appetite and digestion*, for the facilitation and increase of the menses, and relief of uterine pains associated with nervous conditions.[9] Felter similarly describes *Leonurus* in both *King's American Dispensatory* and *The Eclectic Materia Medica*, recommending a warm infusion for amenorrhea and the restoration of suppressed lochia (postpartum discharge).[10,11]

Actions

Cardiotonic, hypotensive, antiarrhythmic
Emmenagogue
Nervine tonic
Spasmolytic

Specific indications

Amenorrhoea, dysmenorrhoea, palpitations related to nervous cardiac disorder, coronary heart disease, anxiety.

It is speculated to be of use as an adjuvant for hyperthyroidism (preclinical studies, and symptom picture).

Constituents

Alkaloids: stachydrine, betonicine, leonurine (found in *Leonurus* species but disputed[12,13]), leonuridin, leonurinine.

Flavonoids: glycosides of apigenin, kaempferol and quercetin, e.g. hyperoside, kaempferol-3-D-glucoside, rutin.

Iridoids

Tannins and pseudotannins: e.g. pyrogallol, catechins.

Terpenoids: volatile oil, resin, wax, ursolic acid.

Possibly cardiac glycosides: bufadienolide/bufanolide type.

Citric acid, malic acid, oleic acid, bitter principles, choline and a phenolic glycoside (caffeic acid 4-rutinoside).[14,15]

Preclinical studies (in vitro and in vivo)

Analgesic effects: the ethanolic extract increases antinociceptive activity, supporting the analgesic properties of the extract, with the action mediated through peripheral and central inhibitory mechanisms.[16]

Anti-inflammatory and antioxidant
- Leonurine downregulated the levels of proinflammatory cytokines (TNF-α and IL-6), upregulated the level of anti-inflammatory cytokine IL-10, and inhibited the expression of nitric oxide synthase (iNOS) and COX-2.[17] Leonurine reduced inflammatory responses in endometritis models and suppressed the TNF-α and IL-1β mRNA levels in uterus tissues.[18]
- Ursolic acid: showed anti-inflammatory, antioxidative and cytotoxic activities.
- An acetone/water extract reduced platelet aggregation in the presence of arachidonic acid.[19]
- Polyphenolic compounds, mainly flavonoids, showed antioxidant activity in several in vitro studies.[20,21]

Antimicrobial: an acetone–water extract and its component, ursolic acid, were effective against *Staphylococcus aureus* and *E. coli*.

Anxiolytic and antidepressant: in vitro *Leonurus* shows an interaction with GABA type A receptor.[22]

Cardiotonic:
- Shows potential as an antianginal and antiarrhythmic agent: decreased blood pressure and heart rate, increased coronary blood flow. Also inhibited the inward calcium and potassium channels and lengthened Q-T, P-Q intervals.[23,24]
- Hypotensive activity (by injection) shown in normal and hypertensive states.[25]
- Ursolic acid: suppresses nuclear factor-kappa B signalling in cancer cells, improves insulin signalling in adipose tissues, reduces the expression of markers of cardiac damage, decreases inflammation in the brain, reduces apoptotic signalling in the liver, and reduces atrophy in skeletal muscles.[26] It was suggested that the cardioprotective mechanism of ursolic acid could involve the mitochondria as ursolic acid induced uncoupling of oxidative phosphorylation in the heart mitochondria; mild mitochondrial uncoupling has been proposed as one of the mechanisms of cardioprotection.
- Stachydrine: cardioprotective and vasoprotective activities.[27]
- Circulatory effect (injected): an undefined species of *Leonurus* decreased the development of acute ischaemic cerebral oedema and reduced disorders of monoamine metabolism and mortality.[28] Leonurine ameliorates cognitive dysfunction in vivo in chronic cerebral hypoperfusion.[29]

- Another species of motherwort (*Leorunus heterophyllus*) decreased blood viscosity and fibrinogen volume, and increased the deformability of red blood cells, enabling them to change shape and to flow into the microvessels, and had an antiplatelet aggregation effect.[30]

Nephroprotective: leonurine protected against kidney damage, reducing inflammation.[31,32]

TSH inhibition: showed a reduction of excess thyroid hormone production, attributed to the rosmarinic acid content.

Uterine tonic: an extract of leonurine showed uterotonic activity.[33,34]
Stachydrine shows oxytocic activity and anti-fibrotic properties (on various types of fibrosis), decreasing inflammatory and oxidative stress through multiple molecular mechanisms.[35]

Clinical studies

L. cardiaca oil extract showed positive effects on systolic blood pressure, diastolic blood pressure, heart rate and ECG in patients with stages 1 and 2 arterial hypertensions. There were also improvements in anxiety, emotional liability, headache and sleep disorders, especially visible for stage 1 patients.[36]

A motherwort injection combined with oxytocin prevented postpartum hemorrhage after caesarean section.[37]

Cautions, contraindications

Not to be used in pregnancy.

Summary of use in gynaecology

As an emmenagogue for amenorrhoea and oligomenorrhoea, other indictions dysmenorrhoea, anxiety and palpitations.

Dosage

Daily dose 4–10ml of 1:3.
    Typical weekly dose 15–25ml of 1:3.

Mitchella repens

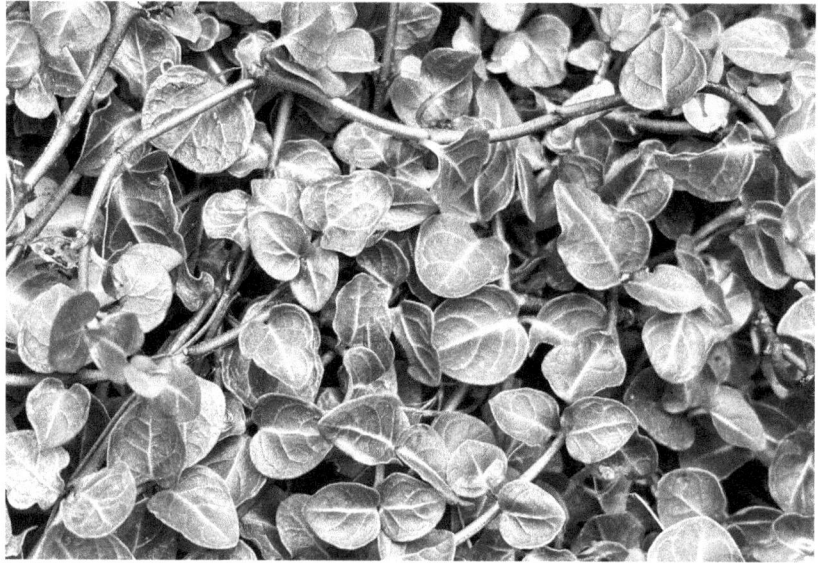

Known as Partridgeberry as it was thought that the berries were eaten by partridges.

Mitchella repens was named after John Mitchell, an 18th-century botanist and physician from Virginia, who worked with Carl Linnaeus on the flora of the New World.

The plant is native to the Eastern half of North America and is currently on the United Plant Savers' "To Watch" list.[1]

Native Americans used it as a partus preparatory to ease childbirth and prevent severe labour pain and complications. They also used it for insomnia, hives, fever, rheumatic pain, fluid retention, urological problems and disorders of the kidneys. Its use as a partus preparatory was adopted by the colonisers and was extensively written about in the Eclectic literature.

The Eclectics reported that *Mitchella* exerts a direct influence upon the female reproductive system, giving tone and improving functional activity. It was used as an uterine tonic, to promote menstruation, remove false pains and any unpleasant sensations in the latter months of pregnancy. Many writers commented on its effectiveness as a good preparative to labour *rendering the birth of the child easier, and less liable to accidents.*[2] Another commented: *There is no doubt that proper medication during pregnancy will often favor a mild and speedy delivery.*[3]

Ellingwood added that mothers, instead of dread and terror, looked forward to birth without anxiety or fear, and as *Labor approaches, those that have taken the herb are devoid of the irritating, aggravating complications, the preparatory stage is simple, the dilatation is completed quickly, the expulsive contractions are strong, unirritating, and effectual, and are much less painful than without the remedy.* Also recommended for preventing digestive troubles and albuminuria as well as auto-toxemia[4] and post-partum haemorrhages.[5,6]

Constituents

Alkaloids, glycosides, resin, tannins[7] and triterpenoid saponins.[8]

Action

Uterine tonic and partus preparator.

Specific indications

Partus preparator, dysmenorrhoa, relieves congestion in the pelvic organs, prevents spontaeneous abortion (can then be used throughout the pregnancy), recurrent miscarriage.[9–11]

Preclinical studies

Very little research has been done on this herb. *Mitchella repens* contracts uterine smooth muscle ex vivo, which provides some support for the empirical claim that *Mitchella* can augment labour contractions.[12]

Personal experience: I always took Mitchella for the last 6 weeks before due date, and while also having taken raspberry leaves from month 3 onwards. All four labours were quick (3.5–1 hours), very easy and, in the last labour, with little pain until the very end.

Summary of use in gynaecology

As a partus preparatory, uterine tonic, dysmenorrhoea, and for prevention of recurrent miscarriages.

Dosage

The Eclectics recommended it to be taken from the 2nd trimester to 6 weeks before due date and to increase dosages when getting closer to labour. If not taken as a partus preparator, it can also be helpful when taken during labour.

Daily dosage 6–12g, or 6–12ml of 1:3.

Typical weekly dosage 15–30ml of 1:3.

Rubus idaeus

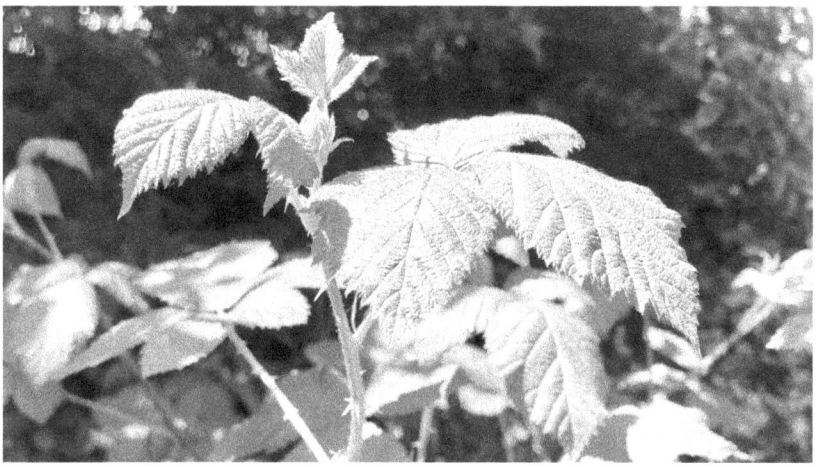

Raspberry leaf

Used all over the world for centuries, it is mentioned by Pliny in the first Century AD. Raspberry leaf is commonly seen as interchangeable with blackberry leaf when used as an astringent, to treat wounds, diarrhoea and colic pain.

John Gerard (1545–1612): refers to the use of the decoction in all cases of bleeding.[1]

Nicholas Culpeper (1616–1654): mentions it in *The Complete Herbal*, for *too much flowing of the women's courses*.

Native Americans used a strong infusion of red raspberry leaves for childbirth pains.[2] This use seem to have been taken on by the colonist.

Samuel Thompson (1769–1843): noted its use as a maternity aid to *regulate everything as nature requires, if pains are untimely it will make it all quiet, if timely but lingering give more alongside capsicum*.[3]

A.I. Coffin (1838): used the leaf for *obstruction of menses, premature labour pains, [to] promote progress of labour, for sickness in early pregnancy. During labour strong decoction was recommended, at the onset of pains, using at intervals, occasionally adding Capsicum annuum.*

Both Thomson and Coffin discuss the use of raspberry during labour rather than in preparation for labour.[4]

Many of the Eclectics would use it similarly:

King's Dispensatory (1898): *It is said that raspberry will, during labor, increase the activity of the uterine contractions when these are feeble, even in instances where ergot has failed, and that it has been found serviceable in after-pains.*[5]

Richard Lawrence Hool (1918): *The warm infusion, combined with composition powder, is a valuable medicine for women in labour, quieting untimely pains, but rendering them more efficient if labour has really commenced. Give one teacupful of the infusion every hour until labour is completed. It may be taken, with grateful results, for several months before the expected event. If this herb were generally used instead of ordinary tea haemorrhage would rarely occur after confinement and instruments would rarely be required.*[6]

Rubus also has a long history of use by UK herbalists. In 1942 Fletcher Hyde mentions its role in preparation for childbirth. The dosage he recommends is 3–4 pints per week in the last 3 months and a full pint of hot tea with 2 teaspoons of Composition Essence when labour begins.[7] Composition Essence contains *Hamamelis virginiana cortex, Capsicum frutescens, Lobelia inflata, Myrica cerifera, Zingiber officinalis, Cinnamon verum, Syzygium aromaticum,* Essential Oil blend (*Cassia, Cajeput, Peppermint, Clove Bud, Eucalyptus, Pimento*) and steviosides.

Rubus is at present one of the most frequently used herbs during pregnancy.[8,9] In Australia, Raspberry leaf was commonly prescribed by complementary and integrative medicine practitioners for use by pregnant women.[10–12] Australian midwives recommended raspberry leaf to women experiencing post-date pregnancy, and frequently used it during their own pregnancies.[13]

Actions

Astringent, partus preparator, anti-diarrhoeal.

Indications

Abnormal bleeding from the uterus, stomach or bowels as well as diarrhoea.

Ensuring healthy uterine function at childbirth (when taken during pregnancy).

Topically for tonsillitis, conjunctivitis, sore throat and mouth ulcers.

Constituents

Flavonoids (e.g. rutin, kaempferol, quercetin)
Minerals: calcium, chromium, iron, magnesium, manganese, potassium, selenium
Monoterpenes: geraniol, linalool

Polypeptides
Tannins: ellagic acid, gallotannins, ellagitannin

Preclinical studies

Laboratory studies have focused on the action of raspberry leaf on smooth muscle, including the uterus, ileum and rectum. The search was on after the initial clinical findings by Whitehouse in the 1940s, who described three cases in women a week after birth using an intrauterine bag to get an overview of the effect on uterine contractions. Contractions were diminished in force and frequency, and occurred at evenly spaced intervals, while secondary contractions were eliminated.[14]

J.H. Burn, professor of pharmacology at Oxford University (1941): in response to Whitehouse, who had asked if anything was known of the action of raspberry leaves, identified antispasmodic and uterine sedative properties in various extracts of raspberry leaf in vivo.[15]

Beckett and collegues (1954) conducted in vivo and in vitro studies with several extracts of raspberry leaf: some increased uterine contractions while other relaxed the uterus; *a principle is present which causes relaxation of the muscle of the uterus when this is tonically contracted, and which diminishes the force and frequency of rhythmic contractions [in labour].*[16]

Bamford (1970s): using uterine strips from pregnant as well as non-pregnant animals and humans showed it had little or no effect on uteri from the non-pregnant, but inhibited the contractions of the pregnant; intrinsic rhythm appeared to become more regular in most cases and contractions were less frequent. The authors discussed that one major problem in obstetrics is incoordination of uterine action, and speculated it may be that raspberry leaf extract is able to help the course of labour by producing more coordinated uterine contractions.[17]

Relaxant activity in vitro: two components of raspberry leaf extract exhibited relaxant activity in an ileum; the methanol extract exhibited the largest response.[18]

Uterotonic: in isolated uterine strips the leaf contracts or relaxes uterine smooth muscles. It is suggested that some constituents interact with components of the Beta-2 adrenoceptor.[19]

In vitro: tea and capsule caused weak contractions whereas an ethanol extract had little effect on contractility. Preparation as well as pregnancy status and animal used resulted in varied responses.[20]

CYP inhibitor in vitro: raspberry leaf, especially the ethanolic extract, was found to be a powerful CYP inhibitor.[21]

Clinical studies

Whitehouse (*BMJ*, 1941): contractions were diminished in force and frequency, and occurred at evenly spaced intervals; secondary contractions were eliminated, as outlined above. The main effect on the non-pregnant uterus is relaxation.[22]

Clinical trial with raspberry leaf tablets (2 × 1.2g per day) from 32 weeks gestation until labour showed a shortening of the second stage of labour and a lower rate of forceps deliveries. There was a non-significant increase in pregnancy-induced hypertension and pre-eclampsia. Overall, taking raspberry was not associated with any increase of adverse events in labour. Dosages used in this trial were lower than traditionally used dosages.[23]

A retrospective study: this study examined the safety and efficacy of raspberry leaf intake and found no identified side effects for the women or their babies. It also found that the length of the first stage was shorter, the mother was less likely to receive an artificial rupture of their membranes or require a caesarean section, forceps or vacuum birth than the women in the control group.[24]

Another retrospective study in Norway (n=34): focusing on the use of herbal drugs by pregnant women in Norway, noted an increase in caesarean section among the cohort taking raspberry leaf, but lack of information on dosage, duration, timing and form of raspberry leaf, small sample size, selection bias and lack of control of variables makes the result difficult to rely on.[25]

A case report: suggested a relationship between raspberry leaf and insulin. A 38-year-old nulliparous woman with gestational diabetes requiring insulin, developed hypoglycaemia after consuming raspberry leaf tea (2 cups per day for three days) at 32 weeks' gestation. Self-withdrawal and reintroduction suggested that raspberry leaf had led to the hypoglycaemic episodes.[26]

Adverse effects

Safety studies

- Toxicity is shown in animal studies when large amounts of raspberry leaf extract, as well as isolated components, were injected intravenously or intraperitoneally.[27,28]

- In vivo: high-dose ingestion resulted in a shorter length of gestation, smaller litter size, an increase in fluid consumption and a decrease in pup weights on postnatal day 4 and 5 with treatment.[29]
- Safety in vivo (N10): high oral dose of raspberry from conception onward, found a lengthening of gestation, a reduction in the number of live births in the raspberry group, and females in the next generation of offspring had a significantly earlier puberty.[30]
- Two studies looking at long-term alterations in the activity of cytochrome P450: in both studies raspberry leaf was used at much higher doses than a woman would normally consume.[31]

It is difficult to know what to extrapolate from these studies. As herbalists we may bear in mind that high doses or inappropriate methods of delivery were used, injection or intraperitoneally, which are not reflective of our real-world usage.

Retrospective study: this study examined the safety and efficacy of raspberry leaf intake and found no identified side effects for the women or their babies.[32]

Causes miscarriages and premature labour? Some suggest caution against using raspberry leaf during pregnancy. The rationale given is that *Rubus* can stimulate uterine tissue. This originated from one reference from the 1970s of an experiment where contractions were initiated in strips of human uteri of 10–16 weeks of pregnancy, removed from the body and injected with raspberry leaf extract.[33]

Summary of use in gynaecology:

Given all the research, the long history of raspberry leaf use, and the large proportion of women that currently use it in pregnancy, we can conclude it is useful and safe as partus preparatory.

Also for menorrhagia, dysmenorrhoea and as a uterine tonic.

Dosage

Tea 10–15g/day.
    Daily dose 15ml of 1:3.
    Typical weekly dosage 15–25ml of 1:3.

Thuja occidentalis

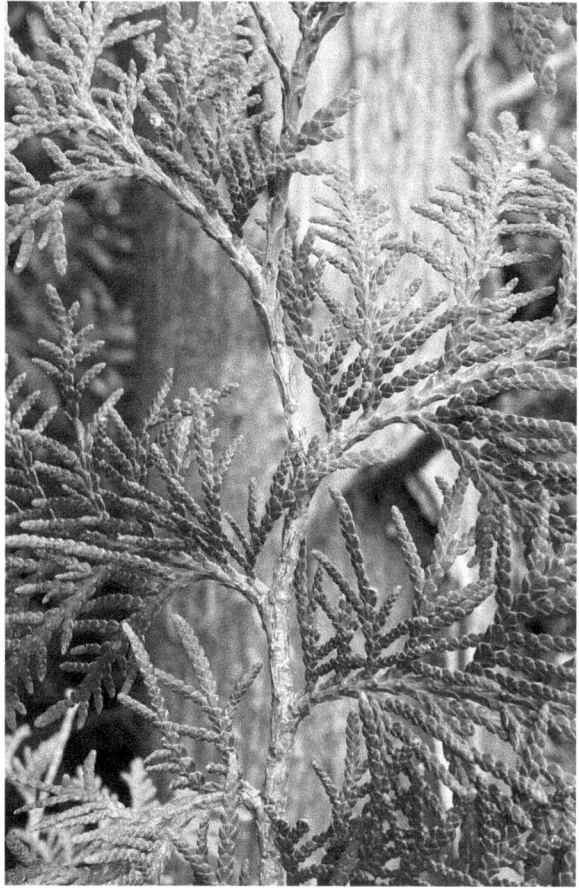

Arbor vitae, Tree of life, Yellow cedar, False white cedar, Eastern white cedar.

Derived from the Greek word "thuo", which means to sacrifice: the fragrant camphoraceous wood was burnt with sacrifices.

Named 'arbor vitae' by Clusius in the 16th century.

John Parkinson (1640): mentions the use for those *long time troubled with a purulentous cough, and shortness of breath, use of the leaves taken with bread and butter, thereby expectorating the phlegm stuffing the lungs and to clearing the passages.*[1]

John Gerard (1597): classifies it as hot and dry, an excellent cordial and of a very pleasant smell.

The Eclectics: used the herb internally as well as externally for abnormal growths, tissue degeneration in the mucous and cutaneous tissues, including cancer, and found it retards growth and prolongs the life of the patient. It was also said to have an affinity with the broncho-pulmonic and genito-urinary mucous tracts.[2-5]

Ellingwood (1908): describes the use of douches for carcinomatous growth in the vagina, *In the described case report the growth cleared, and made the patient made full recovery. For this it was used in combination with Echinacea.*[6]

Specific indications from the Eclectics:

Epithelioma, papilloma (i.e. warts), condylomata (around the anus or genitals), although they reported mixed effectiveness.

Nasal polypi, also beneficial for catarrhal discharges and post-nasal catarrh, used internally four or five times daily, with *Hydrastis* as a spray.

Chancroids (a sexually transmitted disease): eases pain, reduces discharge and odour, prevents lymphatic engorgement, promotes healing.

Catarrhal granulation of the cervix uteri: used locally, an aqueous solution used per tampon.

Granular ophthalmia or simple trachoma, a chronic, contagious infection of the conjunctiva and cornea caused by the bacterium *Chlamydia trachomatis*.

Indolent or gangrenous ulcers, bed sores and other open ulcers.

Chronic skin diseases

Atonic amenorrhea

Thuja became known for its use in vaccination, especially by homeopaths, who would use the mother tincture. This use was first mentioned by Wizenmann in 1930, where *thuja* was used for acquired constitutional damage from smallpox and vaccinations.[7] Dr Madaus in 1938 described its use for vaccine damage.[8]

Thuja was listed in the *US Pharmacopoeia* from 1882 to 1894 as a uterine stimulant and diuretic.

Actions

Antimicrobial: antiviral and antifungal
Anti-mitotic: this effect might be related to its immunostimulant activity.

Diuretic
Emmenagogue
Expectorant
Immunomodulation: influencing the first phase of phagocytosis, increases the activity of white blood cells.
Stimulating depurative/alterative

Indications

Internally

Atonic amenorrhoea.
　Arthritis including osteo-, rheumatoid and psoriatic arthritis, and psoriasis.
　Cystitis and enuresis.
　Respiratory infections, bronchial catarrh, bronchitis, acute respiratory tract infections and the common cold (combined with *Echinacea purpurea, Echinaceae pallida* and *Baptisia tinctoria*).
　Immunomodulation combined with *Baptisia* and *Echinacea*. This combination can be used in acute infections or for prophylaxis in lower doses for up to two months.
　Uterine fibroids as well as carcinoma, breast and lung carcinomas, alongside external use.

Externally

Arthritis, psoriasis, fresh *Thuja* tops boiled in lard as a salve in arthritic joints pain.
　Cervical dysplasia, external alongside internal use.
　Nasal polyps, especially if the fresh plant tincture is used.
　Warts, papillomas and condylomas caused by HPV.[9]

Constituents

Coumarins: umbelliferone.
　Flavonoids: kaempferol, myricetin, myricitrin, quercetin and quercitrin.
　Tannins: catechins, gallocatechin and proanthocyanidines.[10]
　Volatile oil (1.4–4%): thujone (0.76–2.4%), borneol, camphene, limonene, myricene, α-terpine, terpinolene.

Preclinical studies

The polysaccharides from *Thuja* have been intensively studied, but as the tincture will have very little polysaccharides we have referenced below only studies using methanolic extracts, which reflect the modern herbal use.

Polysaccharides broadly show antiviral and immunostimulating effects, with the ability to inhibit HIV-1[11] and influenza A,[12] and have an anti-tumour activity.[13]

Anti-inflammatory:[14] in an ulcerative colitis model inhibited the inflammatory process and normalised the structure of the intestinal mucosa.[15] *Artemisia absinthum*, another herb that contains thujone, has also been shown to be effective for inflammatory bowel disease.

Hydroalcoholic extracts of *Thuja occidentalis* corrected the levels of inflammatory markers and oxidative stress in diabetic models, alongside restoration of neuronal functions, indicating a use in treating diabetic neuropathy.[16]

Antimicrobial: antiviral, antibacterial[17,18] and antifungal[19] activities.[20]

Anti-mitotic effect: α/β-thujone, in vitro, in vivo: diminishes cell viability with anti-proliferative, proapoptotic, and antiangiogenic properties.[21]

Thujone (in vitro, in vivo): antitumoral, stimulated cell-mediated immune response and production of IL-2 and IFN-γ,[22] inhibiting metastasis in vivo.[23]

Antioxidant: demonstrated a protective activity against oxidative stress by increasing glutathione levels in blood.[24]

Antipyretic: methanolic extracts of the whole plant were comparable to paracetamol and aspirin.[25]

Anti-atherosclerotic: improved lipid profiles, the anti-atherosclerotic activity was marked by the increase in HDL-cholesterol and a reduction in the atherogenic index.[26]

Antiviral: shown to have activity against influenza in cell culture.[27]

Gastroprotective comparable to omeprazole: reduced gastric acid production and regenerated the gastric epithelium.[28] Interestingly, the Eclectics describe the use of *Thuja* in drop doses for ulcerated stomachs. Ellingwood describes a patient with chronic diarrhoea and ulceration of the bowels using an enema daily with successful results.[29]

Hepato-protective: ethanol fractions used in acute and chronic induced liver damage.[30,31]

Hypoglycemic: in vivo.[32]

Immune modulator: the aerial parts in methanolic extract and isolated polysaccharides both stimulated the cell-mediated immune system and decreased pro-inflammatory cytokines, thereby inhibiting metastasis of tumour cells.[33] The extract stimulated phagocytosis, the most prominent effect being noted on the first phase of phagocytosis.[34]

Radiation protective (in vivo): given intraperitoneally, the methanolic extract had protective effects against gamma-induced toxicity.[35]

Preclinical studies with Esberitox®, a proprietary formulation containing *Thuja occidentalis, Echinacea purpurea, Echinacea pallida* and *Baptisia tinctoria*.

Enhances antibody response and did not induce any systemic increase in cytokine titers, probably causes a local activation of cytokine-producing cells for 'priming'.[36,37]

Influenza A models: prolonged mean survival time, and reduced lung consolidation and virus titers. Effective as preventative due to immunostimulation rather than antiviral activity.[38]

Clinical studies

There are no clinical trials with *Thuja*, although there are some recent case reports.

Case report: in a case of verruca vulgaris, which led to cutaneous squamous cell carcinoma in a young renal allograft recipient, treatment with *T. occidentalis* helped to eradicate the remaining lesions without compromising graft function.[39]

Case report: positive effect on laryngeal papilloma, reported in the *BMJ*.[40] Ellingwood also wrote about the use in papilloma of the larynx where *Thuja* was used topically alongside small, often drop doses, given internally.

Clinical studies with Esberitox®

Common cold: enhancement of the immune response was observed in recall antigens, with decreased duration of the cold.[41] It was more effective when treatment was begun immediately on the appearance of symptoms.[42,43]

Adjuvant to antibiotic treatment in bacterial upper respiratory infection,[44] and in treatment of acute exacerbation of chronic bronchitis; a better result was seen with the combination.[45]

Chemo-radiation: diminished the side effects of combined chemo-radiation in women with advanced breast cancer, promoted the recuperation of the haemapoietic system.[46,47]

Oral immunity in children affected by dental caries: increase of lysozyme as well as s-IgA was seen in children from prophylactic groups, and prevention of dental caries in children with moderate and high caries.[48]

Cautions and contraindications

Thujone-containing plants in normal doses do not have abortive effects.[49] *Artemisia absinthium* has concentrations of thujone higher than in *Thuja*, and has only been reported to have toxic effects when used long term, over years.

Decoctions of *Thuja* have traditionally been used for their abortive properties, usually combined with other herbs.[50] The abortifacient effect suggested in the literature is most likely related to the gastrointestinal pain and violent intestinal spasms caused by high doses, which would often also result in lethal toxicity.[51] A 1938 report describes a case where a 22-year-old girl who had drunk *Thuja* twig infusion for a few weeks in order to induce abortion at the end of the first trimester. She then made herself a vaginal rinse with the tea, which led to loss of consciousness, convulsions and, after two days, to death. No abortion occurred.[52]

However, it still would be prudent to avoid using in pregnancy and lactation.

Safe in treatments for acute viral respiratory tract infections.[53–55]

Esberitox® has been used in clinical trials with good safety data, although one study reported mild nausea.[56,57]

Summary of use in gynaecology

For vaginal infections combined with *Echinacea angustifolia* and *purpurea* plus *Baptisia tinctora*.

For growths, such as fibroids.

For cervical dysplasia and human papillomavirus-related infections.

Dosage

Daily dose 1.5–3ml of 1:5.

Typical weekly dose 10–20ml of 1:5.

Viburnum prunifolium

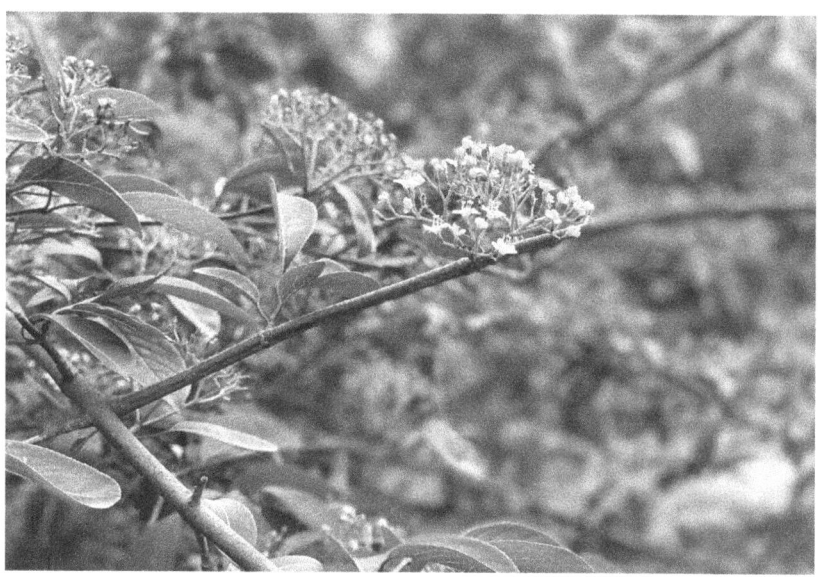

Black haw

Traditionally used for dysmenorrhoea, false labour pains, threatened miscarriage and asthma. It was common practice among planters to make their slaves drink an infusion of *Viburnum* daily while pregnant, to prevent abortion from taking the abortifacient Cottonroot.[1]

Viburnum prunifolium was seen by the Eclectics as one of the most important uterine tonics.[2] The Eclectics would use it in amenorrhea, metrorrhagia, as partus preparatory and for morning sickness; it was given for menstrual irregularities, and it was claimed that in *previously sterile females pregnancy has promptly occurred, proving the influence of the agent in restoring normal functional ovarian activity.*[3,4]

Many of the Eclectics extol its virtues in use for threatened or recurrent miscarriage.

Ellingwood describes a case where *Viburnum prunifolium* caused the womb to suspend expulsive action and to retain a dead foetus for months. It had been given in large doses after the first trimester, and no return of the expulsive effort occurred until after use was discontinued in the seventh month, after which a 4-month-old mummified foetus was expelled without detriment to the health of the patient.

Theodore Shennon (1896): quotes many physicians of his time, and all mention frequent use for prevention of recurrent miscarriage, including in cases where there were pains and haemorrhage with dilated external os.[5]

R.L. Payne (1888): describes a patient who had had six miscarriages. *Viburnum* was given for the last 3 months of the seventh pregnancy, which went to term. The eighth pregnancy was similar, but the ninth ended at the 7th or 8th month; it seems that *Viburnum* had been given up on the assumption that it had had nothing to do with the previous results.[6]

The British Pharmaceutical Codex (1911): writes that Black haw depresses the medulla and spinal cord without affecting the higher cerebral centres, and therefore depresses respiration and induces a large fall in blood pressure. It has sedative effects on the uterus, to prevent threatened abortion and to control haemorrhage. It is also claimed to give good results in asthma, dysmenorrhoea and spasmodic affections of plain muscle.[7]

Constituents

Arbutin, salicin, salicylic acid, scopoletin (a coumarin), flavonoids (amentoflavone), iridoid glycosides (iridoids play a significant role in the biological activity),[8] triterpenes and triterpenic acids.[9]

Scopoletin is thought to be important in relation to smooth muscle antispasmodic activity.[10]

Actions

Spasmolytic, uterine tonic and sedative.

Indications

Dysmenorrhoea, endometriosis, threatened miscarriage, recurrent miscarriage.

Preclinical studies

In vitro: ethanolic extracts have uterine sedative, relaxant, spasmolytic activity.[11–13]

<u>In vivo</u>: both species (*Vib. op.* and *Vib. prun.*) have antispasmodic effects on the uterus.[14,15]

<u>Experiments with human uterine tissue</u>: a relaxant activity in isolated uterine tissue in vitro.[16]

There are no clinical studies with *Viburnum prunifolium*.

Summary of use in gynaecology

Primary and secondary dysmenorrhoea, and for the prevention of miscarriage. Some traditional uses also point to it as an ovarian tonic and for use in amenorrhoea.

Adverse effects

Nausea and vomiting may occur with large doses.

There is a suggestion of caution in those with history of kidney stones due to the presence of oxalate and oxalic acid. Oxalate is unlikely to be present in an aqueous ethanolic liquid extract in sufficient quantities to justify a precaution.

Dosage

Higher ethanol percentages do not always confer higher activity. French researchers found that *Viburnum prunifolium* bark extracted at 30% ethanol was five times more spasmolytic than a 60% extract.[17]

Daily dosage 1–3ml of 1:3.

Typical weekly dosage 20–45ml of 1:3.

For dysmenorrhoea in acute treatment: daily dose 2–7ml of 1:3.

In dysmenorrhoea it must be taken for at least 3 to 4 days, before and after the menstrual period.

APPENDIX

Vitamins, minerals and other important nutrients

Vitamin/mineral	Food source
Arginine: a precursor of nitric oxide synthesis, it is required for angiogenesis, embryogenesis, hormone secretion and fertility in general	Nuts (walnuts, hazelnuts, pecans, peanuts, almonds, cashews, and brazil nuts), seeds (sesame and sunflower), oats, corn, cereals, buckwheat, brown rice, dairy products, meat and chocolate
Betaine: can also be obtained by endogenous synthesis from choline	Bran and wheatgerm, goji berries, spinach, beets, whole grain, seafood (especially marine invertebrates), quinoa
Boron	Leafy greens (spinach, kale), broccoli, nuts, apples, dried fruit especially raisins
Calcium	Leafy greens, nuts, seeds, dairy produce

(*Continued*)

(Continued)

Vitamin/mineral	Food source
Carotenoids	**Carotenoids** (alpha carotene, beta carotene, beta cryptoxanthin, lutein, zeaxanthin and lycopene are fat-soluble pigments giving the variety of colour in many fruits and vegetables). Foods contain different carotenoids in different levels, so a variety should be used to obtain appropriate levels of the major health-promoting dietary carotenoids Dark green leafy vegetables (kale, spinach, broccoli), orange and yellow vegetables (carrots, sweet potatoes, pumpkin, butternut squash, peppers), tomatoes, eggs **Lycopene** in red and pink foods: apricots, guava, papaya, pink grapefruit, red pepper, tomatoes, watermelon. Lycopene bioavailability in cooked tomato products is higher than in unprocessed fresh tomatoes, and when eaten alongside fat, will be better absorbed
Choline: another nutrient crucial for liver function[1]	Almonds, dairy, eggs, fish, fruits, shiitake mushrooms, soybeans, vegetables especially the cruciferous family, whole grains, quinoa
Chromium	Many whole grains, fruits and vegetables, lean meats, nuts, poultry and eggs, spices, brewer's yeast, beer, wine. Ascorbic acid increases chromium absorption
Coenzyme Q10: the concentration of CoQ10 decreases in many diseases as well as in ageing	Rich sources: mainly meat (especially organ meats), poultry and oily fish (trout, mackerel, salmon and tuna)

(Continued)

(Continued)

Vitamin/mineral	Food source
Synthesised in most human tissues using pantothenic acid (B5) and pyridoxine (B6)	Other good sources whole grains, soybean products (tofu, soy milk, soy yogurt), corn, olive and canola oils, nuts and seeds. Fruit, vegetables, eggs and dairy products are moderate sources of CoQ10
Flavonoids	Vegetables and fruit with a variety of colours, berries, grapes, red wine (anthocyanins), green and black tea, cocoa, citrus fruit, parsley, thyme, chili pepper, onions, peppers, broccoli, spinach, apples, many herbs (rosemary, peppermint, chamomile, oregano, parsley, turmeric, etc.) **Quercitin:** apples, cherries, citrus fruits, raspberries, red grapes, green leafy vegetables, onions, especially red onions **Anthocyanins:** blueberries, raspberries, strawberries, fruit and vegetables **Epigallocatechin-3-gallate (EGCG):** *Camellia sinensis* and pomegranate seeds
Glutathione: a tripeptide needed for numerous processes including maintaining redox balance, enhancing metabolic detoxification, regulating the immune system, and oestrogen metabolism Vitamin C is needed to convert oxidised glutathione back to its active form[2] Cysteine: an important amino acid involved in glutathione synthesis—see NAC below	Dietary sources of glutathione: spinach, avocados, asparagus and okra;[6] however, these are poorly absorbed, and cooking and storage conditions also have an effect on levels Cruciferous/sulfur-rich vegetables such as broccoli, Brussels sprouts, cauliflower, kale, watercress and mustard greens, garlic, shallots and onions are helpful for many reasons, one being that they increase glutathione levels[7,8] Herbs that increase glutathione levels (in vitro and in vivo studies): *Silybum marinanum*,[9] *Curcuma longa* (curcumin)[10]

(*Continued*)

(Continued)

Vitamin/mineral	Food source
Selenium, needed for glutathione activity Exercise: although overtraining without adequate nutrition and rest decreased glutathione production[3,4] A good night's sleep: glutathione peroxidase activity was significantly lower in those with insomnia[5]	
Indole-3-carbinol converted in the stomach to multiple compounds, including diindolylmethane	Cruciferous vegetables: broccoli, cabbage, Brussels sprouts, cauliflower and kale, *Capsella bursa-pastoris* Daily dose of 350–500mg: equivalent to 300–500g of cruciferous vegetables. 400mg is size of one-third of a head of cabbage
Iodine	Seaweed (kelp, nori, kombu and wakame), seafood/fish and eggs, dairy products (although depends if cows have iodine feed supplement)
Iron (Fe) Vitamin C enhances iron absorption; it captures non-heme iron and stores it in a form that is more easily absorbed	Heme iron is more readily absorbed: red meat, seafood, poultry Non-heme iron: blackstrap molasses, legumes (red kidney beans, chickpeas, soya), nuts and seeds, dried fruit (apricots), dark chocolate, leafy green vegetables
Isoflavones	Soya beans, tofu, soya milk, edamame, chickpeas, fava beans, lentils, peas, pistachios, peanuts and other fruits and nuts Lignans: flaxseeds, sesame seeds, legumes, whole grains, nuts and seeds A healthy gut flora is needed to be able to benefit from the isoflavones in the diet

(*Continued*)

(Continued)

Vitamin/mineral	Food source
L-carnitine	Mainly found in animal products such as meat, fish, poultry, milk and dairy products (whey)
Melatonin (produced by the pineal gland): found in the follicular fluid; reduced levels are found in those with unexplained infertility	Tart cherries or tart cherry juice (also used to help with sleep), Goji berries, eggs, milk (typically used as sleep aid), fish, and nuts, especially pistachios and almonds
Magnesium (Mg)	Dark leafy green vegetables, whole grain, legumes, seeds, nuts, fish
Methionine: for metabolism of oestrogen	Brazil nuts, cashew nuts, dairy, garlic, legumes, onions, quinoa, firm tofu, sunflower seeds
N-acetylcysteine (NAC) or cysteine or cystine, the acetylated form of cysteine, a rate-limiting nutrient in glutathione synthesis Cysteine, cystine-rich foods: NAC is made by the human liver by altering the amino acid cysteine. Cystine is made up of two cysteine molecules bonded together and is nutritionally equivalent to cysteine	Cystine is two cysteine molecules bonded together, found in high-protein foods; also needed are adequate amounts of folate, vitamin B6 and vitamin B12: spinach, bananas, salmon, tuna, white meat, yogurt, cheese, eggs, sunflower seeds, legumes (beans and lentils), broccoli and onions; wholemeal products such as oatmeal As a supplement it is not well absorbed
Omega 3: eicosapentaenoic acid [EPA] and docosahexaenoic acid [DHA]) 2 and 4g per day	Fish especially cold-water fatty fish (salmon, mackerel, tuna, herring and sardines), algae, seaweed. Nuts and seeds: flaxseed, chia seeds, hemp seeds, walnuts, edamame beans, kidney beans. Eggs, meats and dairy products from grass-fed animals. Plant oils (flaxseed oil, soybean oil, canola oil)
Probiotics	Yogurt, kefir, sauerkraut, tempeh, miso

(Continued)

(Continued)

Vitamin/mineral	Food source
Selenium (Se)	Brazil nuts (selenium per 5g:96mg), dairy products such as yogurt, cottage cheese, fish (tuna, sardines, halibut), shrimps, oats, wholemeal foods, eggs, turkey, chicken, spinach, lentils, sunflower seeds, mushrooms
Sulforaphane stored as precursor, glucosinolate Converted to sulforaphane by myrosinase, e.g. chewing or chopping	Cruciferous vegetables, bok choy, broccoli and broccoli sprouts, Brussels sprouts, cabbage, cauliflower, Chinese cabbage, collard greens, kale, kohlrabi, mustard, rutabaga, turnips. The highest levels are found in raw vegetables. The isothiocyanates are not present in the cells but are produced following cell wall destruction (cutting, crushing, chewing)
Vitamin A	Oily fish (mackerel, salmon, tuna), liver (beef, lamb, cod liver oil), cheese, butter, eggs, milk, yogurt Betacarotene-rich foods, which the body can convert into retinol; see carotenoids above
Vitamin B1	Yeast, nuts, whole grains, legumes, blackstrap molasses, cauliflower, kale, asparagus, potatoes, oranges, fish, beef, pork, eggs
Vitamin B6	Legumes (chickpeas), dark leafy greens. Fruits: avocados, bananas, papayas, oranges, cantaloupe; beef liver, chicken, tuna, salmon; sweet potatoes, potatoes, nuts (pistachio, walnuts), seeds (sunflower seeds, roasted chestnuts)

(*Continued*)

(Continued)

Vitamin/mineral	Food source
Vitamin B9, folate	Dark green leafy vegetables (turnip greens, spinach, romaine lettuce, asparagus, Brussels sprouts, cabbages, kale, broccoli); legumes (lentils), nuts (peanuts), seeds (sunflower seeds), fruits (oranges), whole grains, seafood, eggs, bananas, asparagus, spinach, (avocado), beet, wheat bran. It is water-soluble, so steaming is best
Vitamin B12	Fish, meat, poultry, eggs and dairy products
Vitamin B complex	Milk, cheese, eggs, chicken and red meat, liver and kidneys; tuna, mackerel and salmon, shellfish, dark green vegetables, beets, avocados, whole grains, legumes, nuts and seeds
Vitamin C	Fruits and vegetables, particularly citrus fruits, kiwi, tomatoes, dark green leafy vegetables, melons and strawberries, peppers, cruciferous vegetables (broccoli, Brussels sprouts, cabbage, cauliflower), potatoes
Vitamin D	In summertime at midday the UVB rays are most intense and efficient at making vitamin D
	Skin exposure of 35% provides sufficient but suboptimal vitamin D, at midday in summer, 3 times a week for ½ hour
	Sources of D3: fatty fish (herring, salmon, tuna, sardines) and fish liver oils, egg yolks, cheese and liver. Some foods are fortified with vitamin D. Mushrooms exposed to 20 minutes of sunshine contain vitamin D2

(*Continued*)

(Continued)

Vitamin/mineral	Food source
	Winter sun levels are 10 to 100% lower than the summer levels so in many high latitudes (>40 degrees) the sun provides no vitamin D in winter. Darker-skinned people have more melanin, need longer exposure (30 min–3 hours) and are at higher risk of deficiency Vitamin D supplementation is likely to be needed for most people
Vitamin E	Plant-based oils, e.g. wheatgerm and wheatgerm oil, safflower and soybean oil Nuts and seeds: sunflower seeds, pine nuts, almonds, peanuts, pumpkin seeds Also: avocado, kiwi, mango, peppers, leafy greens, spinach, asparagus, fish
Vitamin K	Two types of vitamin K: phylloquinone, found in green leafy vegetables, soyabean, canola oil, and menaquinones found in some animal foods, e.g. meat, cheese and eggs, fermented foods, e.g. fermented soya beans Intestinal bacteria produce Vitamin K; a healthy gut flora is also needed, but antibiotics will interfere with the gut flora
Zinc (Zn)	Oats, shiitake mushrooms, spinach, legumes (lentils, chickpeas, green peas, tofu and other soy products), nuts and seeds (almonds, cashew, pumpkin seeds), dairy (yogurt), seafood, eggs, lean meats and poultry

Summary of dietary suggestions

- Brassica family vegetables, such as kale, broccoli, cauliflower, are rich in indole-3 carbinol, helpful for oestrogen metabolism.
- Choline-rich foods: another nutrient crucial for liver function[11] found in fish, dairy, eggs, fruits, vegetables, whole grains.
- Colourful fruit and vegetables are full of flavonoids, with anti-inflammatory and anti-proliferative activities.
- Dairy (full fat): rich in B vitamins (B12, niacin and riboflavin), calcium, Vitamin A, D, phosphorus, potassium.
- Fats including extra virgin olive oil, avocados, coconut.
- Fatty fish, including salmon, tuna, sardines, mackerel.
- Fibre-rich foods such as wholemeal flour, vegetables and fruit will help with a healthy microbiome and reduce constipation.
- Garlic, onions and legumes are rich in methionine for the metabolism of oestrogen.
- Live yogurt, fermented foods, to maintain healthy gut flora, as lactobacillus reduces recirculation of endogenous oestrogen and is needed for the absorption of phytoestrogens.
- Nuts and seeds: Brazil, cashews, pine nuts, walnuts, almonds, pistachios, sunflower seeds.
- Organic foods if possible, avoiding xeno-oestrogens from pesticides in the environment (see book 1).
- Spices: turmeric, ginger: the list could be extensive.
- Wholemeal foods: rich in B vitamins, needed for metabolism of oestrogen in the liver.

NOTES

Section One: Specific Conditions
Chapter 1: Dysmenorrhoea

1. Proctor M, Farquhar C. (2006). Diagnosis and management of dysmenorrhoea. *BMJ (Clinical Research Ed.).* 332(7550):1134–1138.
2. Kural M, Noor NN, Pandit D, Joshi T, Patil A. (2015). Menstrual characteristics and prevalence of dysmenorrhea in college going girls. *J Fam Med Prim Care.* 4(3):426–431.
3. Kural M, Noor NN, Pandit D, Joshi T, Patil A. (2015). Menstrual characteristics and prevalence of dysmenorrhea in college going girls. *J Fam Med Prim Care.* 4(3):426–431.
4. Stoelting-Gettelfinger W. (2010). A case study and comprehensive differential diagnosis and care plan for the three Ds of women's health: Primary dysmenorrhea, secondary dysmenorrhea, and dyspareunia. *J Am Acad Nurse Pract.* 22(10):513–522.
5. Bernardi M, Lazzeri L, Perelli F, Reis FM, Petraglia F. (2017). Dysmenorrhea and related disorders. *F1000 Research.* 6:1645.
6. Kural M, Noor NN, Pandit D, Joshi T, Patil A. (2015). Menstrual characteristics and prevalence of dysmenorrhea in college going girls. *J Fam Med Prim Care.* 4(3):426–431.

7. Hopcroft K, Forte V. (2014). *Symptom Sorter*. Radcliffe Publishing Ltd, 18 Marcham Rd, Abingdon OX14 1AA, UK.
8. Kural M, Noor NN, Pandit D, Joshi T, Patil A. (2015). Menstrual characteristics and prevalence of dysmenorrhea in college going girls. *J Fam Med Prim Care*. 4(3):426–431.
9. Proctor M, Farquhar C. (2006). Diagnosis and management of dysmenorrhoea. *BMJ (Clinical Research Ed.)*. 332(7550):1134–1138.
10. Beatty MN, Blumenthal PD. (2009). The levonorgestrel-releasing intrauterine system: Safety, efficacy, and patient acceptability. *Therap Clin Risk Man*. 5(3):561–574.
11. Breech LL, Laufer MR. (1999). Obstructive anomalies of the female reproductive tract. *J Rep. Med*. 44(3):233–240.
12. Dawood MY. (2006). Primary dysmenorrhea: Advances in pathogenesis and management. *Obstet Gynecol*. 108(2):428–441.
13. Dawood MY. (2006). Primary dysmenorrhea: Advances in pathogenesis and management. *Obstet Gynecol*. 108(2):428–441.
14. Lien HC, Sun WM, Chen YH, et al. (2003). Effects of ginger on motion sickness and gastric slow-wave dysrhythmias induced by circular vaction. *Am J Physiol Gastrointest Liver Physiol*. 284(3):481–489.
15. Granger I, Serradeil-le Gal C, Augereau JM, Gleye J. (1992). Benzophenanthridine alkaloids isolated from *Eschscholzia californica* cell suspension cultures interact with vasopressin (V1) receptors. *Planta Med*. 58(1):35–38.
16. Oladosu FA, Tu FF, Hellman KM. (2018). Nonsteroidal antiinflammatory drug resistance in dysmenorrhea: Epidemiology, causes, and treatment. *Am J Obstet Gynecol*. 218(4):390–400.
17. Yaeesh S, Jamal Q, Khan AU, Gilani AH. (2006). Studies on hepatoprotective, antispasmodic and calcium antagonist activities of the aqueousmethanol extract of *Achillea millefolium*. *Phyto Res*. 20:546–551.
18. Gharib Naseri MK, Mard SA, Farboud Y. (2005). Effect of *Anethum graveolens* extract on rat uterus contractions. *Iran J Basic Med Sci*. 8:263–270.
19. Mehmood MH, Munir S, Khalid UA, Asrar M, Anwarul, Gilani AH. (2015). Antidiarrhoeal, antisecretory and antispasmodic activities of *Matricaria chamomilla* are mediated predominantly through K^+-channels activation. *BMC Comp Altern Med*. 15:75.
20. Mirabi P, Dolatian M, Mojab F, Majd HA. (2011). Effects of valerian on the severity and systemic manifestations of dysmenorrhea. *Int J Gynaecol Obstet*. 115:285–288.

21. Fedele L, Marchini M, Acaia B, Garagiola U, Tiengo M. (1989). Dynamics and significance of placebo response in primary dysmenorrhea. *Pain*. 36(1):43–47.
22. Smith ID, Temple DM, Shearman RP. (1975). The antagonism by antiinflammatory analgesics of prostaglandin f 2 alpha-induced contractions of human and rabbit myometrium in vitro. *Prostaglandins*. 10(1):41–57.
23. Kudolo GB, Dorsey S, Blodgett J. (2002). Effect of the ingestion of *Ginkgo biloba* extract on platelet aggregation and urinary prostanoid excretion in healthy and Type 2 diabetic subjects. *Thromb Res*. 108(2–3):153–160.
24. Gencel VB, Benjamin MM, Bahou SN, Khalil RA. (2012). Vascular effects of phytoestrogens and alternative menopausal hormone therapy in cardiovascular disease. *Mini Rev Med Chem*. 12(2):149–174.
25. Lien HC, Sun WM, Chen YH, et al. (2003). *Am J Physiol Gastrointest Liver Physiol*. 284(3):481–489.
26. Lemmens-Gruber R, Marchart E, Rawnduzi P, Engel N, Benedek B, Kopp, B. (2006). Investigation of the spasmolytic activity of the flavonoid fraction of *Achillea millefolium* s.l. on isolated guinea-pig ilea. *Arzneimittelforschung*. 56:582–588.
27. Yaeesh S, Jamal Q, Khan AU, Gilani AH. (2006). Studies on hepatoprotective, antispasmodic and calcium antagonist activities of the aqueous-methanol extract of *Achillea millefolium*. *Phyto Res*. 20:546–551.
28. Mehmood MH, Munir S, Khalid UA, Asrar M, Anwarul, Gilani AH. (2015). Antidiarrhoeal, antisecretory and antispasmodic activities of Matricaria chamomilla are mediated predominantly through K^+-channels activation. *BMC Comp Altern Med*. 15:75.
29. Zeng J, Zhao DS, Wu B. (2002). A study on chemical constituents in the herb of *Mentha spicata*. *J Zhongguo Zhong. Yaoza Zhi*. 27:749–751.
30. Fennerty M. (2001). NSAID-related gastrointestinal injury: Evidence-based approach to preventable complication. *Postgrad Med*. 110:87–92.
31. Hawthorn M, Ferrante J, Luchowski E, Rutledge A, Wei XY, Triggle DJ. (1988). The action of peppermint oil and menthol on calcium channel dependent processes in intestinal, neuronal and cardiac preparation. *J Aliment Pharmacol Ther*. 2(2):101–118.
32. Gharib Naseri MK, Mard SA, Farboud Y. (2005). Effect of *Anethum graveolens* extract on rat uterus contractions. *Iran J Basic Med Sci*. 8:263–270.
33. Scudder JM. (1898). *The American Eclectic Materia Medica and Therapeutics*.
34. Palmer CD. (1919). The Clinical Use of a Selection of Vegetable Remedies.

35. Potter SOL. (1902). *A Compend of Materia Medica, Therapeutics, and Prescription.*
36. Mirabi P, Dolatian M, Mojab F, Majd HA. (2011). Effects of valerian on the severity and systemic manifestations of dysmenorrhea. *Int J Gynaecol Obstet.* 115:285–288.
37. Jenabi E, Asle Toghiri M, Hejrati P. (2012). The comparison of the effects of antiplain of *Valeriana officinalis* risom and mefenamic acid in relief of primary dismenorrhea. *Iran J Obstet Gynecol Infertil.* 5:44–48.
38. Kazemian A, Parvin N, Delaram M, Deris F. (2017). Comparison of analgesic effect of *Valeriana officinalis* and mefenamic acid on primary dysmenorrhea. *J Med Plant.* 4:153–159.
39. Mirabe P, Dolatian M, Mojab F, Alavimajd H. (2011). Effects of valerian on the systemic manifestations of dysmenorrhea. *Int J Gynecol Obstet.* 115:285–288.
40. Dolatian M, Mirabe P, Mojab F, Alavimajd H. (2010). Effects of *Valeriana officinalis* on the severity of dysmenorrheal symptoms. *J Reprod Infertil.* 10:253–259.
41. Scudder JM. (1870). *Specific Medication and Specific Medicines.*
42. Pharmaceutical Society of Great Britain. (1911). *The British Pharmaceutical Codex: An Imperial Dispensatory for the Use of Medical Practitioners and Pharmacists.*
43. Jarboe CH, Schmidt CM, Nicholson JA, Zirvi KA. (1966). Uterine relaxant properties of *Viburnum*. *Nature.* 212:837.
44. Cometa MF, Parisi L, Palmery M, Meneguz A, Tomassini L. (2009). In vitro relaxant and spasmolytic effects of constituents from *Viburnum prunifolium* and HPLC quantification of the bioactive isolated iridoids. *J Ethnopharmacol.* 123:201–207.
45. Jarboe CH, Zirvi KA, Nicholson JA, Schmidt CM. (1967). Scopoletin an antispasmodic component of *Viburnum opulus* and *prunifolium*. *J Med Chem.* 10:488–489.
46. Balansard G, Chausse D, Boukef K. et al. (1983). Selection criteria for a Viburnum extract, *Viburnum prunifolium* L., as a function of its veinotonic and spasmolytic action. *Plantes Med Phytother.* 17(3):123–132.
47. Grzanna R, Lindmark L, Frondoza CG. (2005). Ginger: An herbal medicinal product with broad anti-inflammatory actions. *J Med Food.* 8:125–132.
48. Mustafa T, Srivastava KC, Jensen KB. (1993). Drug development: Report 9. Pharmacology of ginger, *Zingiber officinale*. *J Drug Dev.* 6:25–89.

49. Kiuchi F, Iwakami S, Shibuya M, Hanaoka F, Sankawa U. (1992). Inhibition of prostaglandin and leukotriene biosynthesis by gingeroles and diarylhepatanoids. *Chem Pharmacol Bull.* (Tokyo). 40(2):387–391.
50. Ozgoli G, Goli M, Moattar F. (2009). Comparison of effects of ginger, mefenamic acid, and ibuprofen on pain in women with primary dysmenorrhea. *J Altern Comp Med.* 15:129–132.
51. Jenabi E. (2013). The effect of ginger for relieving of primary dysmenorrhoea. *J Pak Med Assoc.* 63(1):8–10.
52. Daily JW, Zhang X, Kim DS, Park S. (2015). Efficacy of ginger for alleviating the symptoms of primary dysmenorrhea: A systematic review and meta-analysis of randomized clinical trials. *Pain Med.* 16(12):2243–2255.
53. Rahnama P, Montazeri A, Huseini HF, Kianbakht S, Naseri M. (2012). *Effect of Zingiber officinale* R. rhizomes (ginger) on pain relief in primary dysmenorrhea: A placebo randomized trial. *BMC Comp Altern Med.* 12:92.
54. Ozgoli G, Goli M, Moattar F. (2009). Comparison of effects of ginger, mefenamic acid, and ibuprofen on pain in women with primary dysmenorrhea. *J Altern Comp Med.* 15(2):129–132.
55. Pakniat H, Chegini V, Ranjkesh F, Hosseini MA. (2019). Comparison of the effect of vitamin E, vitamin D and ginger on the severity of primary dysmenorrhea: A single-blind clinical trial. *Obstet Gynecol Sci.* 62(6):462–468.
56. Halder A. (2012). Effect of progressive muscle relaxation versus intake of ginger powder on dysmenorrhoea amongst the nursing students in Pune. *Nurs J India.* 103(4):152–156.
57. Shirvani MA, Motahari-Tabari N, Alipour A. (2015). The effect of mefenamic acid and ginger on pain relief in primary dysmenorrhea: A randomized clinical trial. *Arch Gynecol Obstet.* 291(6):1277–1281.
58. Halder A. (2012). Effect of progressive muscle relaxation versus intake of ginger powder on dysmenorrhoea amongst the nursing students in Pune. *Nurs J India.* 103(4):152–156.
59. Kashefi F, Khajehei M, Tabatabaeichehr M, Alavinia M, Asili J. (2014). Comparison of the effect of ginger and zinc sulfate on primary dysmenorrhea: A placebo-controlled randomized trial. *Pain Manag Nurs.* 15(4):826–833.
60. Daily JW, Zhang X, Kim DS, Park S. (2015). Efficacy of ginger for alleviating the symptoms of primary dysmenorrhea: A systematic review and meta-analysis of randomized clinical trials. *Pain Med.* 16(12):2243–2255.

61. Rahnama P, Montazeri A, Huseini HF, Kianbakht S, Naseri M. (2012). Effect of *Zingiber officinale* R. rhizomes (ginger) on pain relief in primary dysmenorrhea: A placebo randomized trial. *BMC Comp Altern Med.* 12:92.
62. Ozgoli G, Goli M, Moattar F. (2009). Comparison of effects of ginger, mefenamic acid, and ibuprofen on pain in women with primary dysmenorrhea. *J Altern Comp Med.* 15(2):129–132.
63. Pakniat H, Chegini V, Ranjkesh F, Hosseini MA. (2019). Comparison of the effect of vitamin E, vitamin D and ginger on the severity of primary dysmenorrhea: A single-blind clinical trial. *Obstet Gynecol Sci.* 62(6):462–468.
64. Halder A. (2012). Effect of progressive muscle relaxation versus intake of ginger powder on dysmenorrhoea amongst the nursing students in Pune. *Nurs J India.* 103(4):152–156.
65. Shirvani MA, Motahari-Tabari N, Alipour A. (2015). The effect of mefenamic acid and ginger on pain relief in primary dysmenorrhea: A randomized clinical trial. *Arch Gyecol Obstet.* 291(6):1277–1281.
66. Halder A. (2012). Effect of progressive muscle relaxation versus intake of ginger powder on dysmenorrhoea amongst the nursing students in Pune. *Nurs J India.* 103(4):152–156.
67. Halder A. (2012). Effect of progressive muscle relaxation versus intake of ginger powder on dysmenorrhoea amongst the nursing students in Pune. *Nurs J India.* 103(4):152–156.
68. Daily JW, Zhang X, Kim DS, Park S. (2015). Efficacy of ginger for alleviating the symptoms of primary dysmenorrhea: A systematic review and meta-analysis of randomized clinical trials. *Pain Med.* 16(12):2243–2255.
69. Rahnama P, Falah-Hosseini H, Mohamadi K, Modares M, Khajavi Shojaei K, Askari M, Shahriari AR, Mozayeni P. (2011). Effects of *Zingiber officinale* on primary dysmenorrhea. *J Med Plants.* 9:81–86.
70. Felter HW, Lloyd JU. (1898). *King's American Dispensatory.*
71. Weiss RF. (1988). *Weiss's Herbal Medicine: Classic Edition.*
72. National Research Council (US) Panel on Anticholinesterase Chemicals; National Research Council (US) Panel on Anticholinergic Chemicals. (1982). *Possible Long-Term Health Effects of Short-Term Exposure to Chemical Agents:* Volume 1, *Anticholinesterases and Anticholinergics.* Appendix I, Digest Report Anticholinergic Chemicals. Washington DC: National Academies Press.
73. Felter HW, Lloyd JU. (1898). *King's American Dispensatory.*

74. Ramadan M, Goeters S, Watzer B, Krause E, Lohmann K, Bauer R, Hempel B, Imming P. (2006). Chamazulene carboxylic acid and matricin: A natural profen and its natura prodrug, identified through similarity to synthetic drug substances. *J Nat Prod.* 69:1041–1045.
75. Yaeesh S, Jamal Q, Khan AU, Gilani, AH. (2006). Studies on hepatoprotective, antispasmodic and calcium antagonist activities of the aqueous-methanol extract of *Achillea millefolium*. *Phyto Res.* 20:546–551.
76. Yaeesh S, Jamal Q, Khan AU, Gilani, AH. (2006). Studies on hepatoprotective, antispasmodic and calcium antagonist activities of the aqueous-methanol extract of *Achillea millefolium*. *Phyto Res.* 20:546–551.
77. Lemmens-Gruber R, Marchart E, Rawnduzi P, Engel N, Benedek B, Kopp B. (2006). Investigation of the spasmolytic activity of the flavonoid fraction of *Achillea millefolium* s.l. on isolated guinea-pig ilea. *Arzneimittelforschung.* 56:582–588.
78. Jenabi E, Fereodoony B. (2015). Effect of *Achillea millefolium* on relief of primary dysmenorrhea: A double-blind randomized clinical trial. *J Pediatr Adolesc Gynecol.* 28(5):402–404.
79. Radfar S, Shahoie R, Noori B, Jalilian F, Nasab, LH. (2018). Comparative study on the effect of *Matricaria chamomile* and *Achillea millefolium* capsules on Primary Dysmenorrhea Intensity of dormitory students of Kurdistan University of Medical Sciences. *J Pharmacol Res Int.* 25(3):1–7.
80. Wuttke W, Jarry H, Seidlová-Wuttke D. (2006). *Cimicifuga* extract for the treatment of climacteric complaints. *J Endocrinol Reprod.* 10(2):106–110.
81. Reame NE, Lukacs JL, Padmanabhan V, Eyvazzadeh AD, Smith YR, Zubieta JK. (2008). Black cohosh has central opioid activity in postmenopausal women: Evidence from naloxone blockade and positron emission tomography neuroimaging. *Menopause.* 15(5):832–840.
82. Brice-Ytsma H, McDermott A. (2020). *Herbal Medicine in Treating Gynaecological Conditions: Herbs, Hormones, Pre-Menstrual Syndrome and Menopause.* London: Aeon.
83. Brice-Ytsma H, McDermott A. (2020). *Herbal Medicine in Treating Gynaecological Conditions: Herbs, Hormones, Pre-Menstrual Syndrome and Menopause.* London: Aeon.
84. Lima CM, Lima AK, Melo MG, Serafini MR, Oliveira DL, de Almeida EB. et al. (2013). Bioassay-guided evaluation of *Dioscorea villosa*—an acute and subchronic toxicity, antinociceptive and anti-inflammatory approach. *BMC Comp Altern Med.* 28(13):195.
85. Ellingwood F. (1919). *The American Materia Medica, Therapeutics and Pharmacognosy.*

86. McKay DL, Blumberg JB. (2006). A review of the bioactivity and potential health benefits of chamomile tea (*Matricaria recutita* L.). *Phyto Res.* 20(7):519–530.
87. Shipochliev T, Dimitrov A, Aleksandrova E. (1981). Anti-inflammatory action of a group of plant extracts. *Preventive Vet Med.* 18(6):87–94.
88. Al-Hindawi MK, Al-Deen IH, Nabi MH, Ismail MA. (1989). Anti-inflammatory activity of some Iraqi plants using intact rats. *J Ethnopharmacol.* 26(2):163–168.
89. Braga PC, Dal Sasso M, Fonti E, Culici M. (2009). Antioxidant activity of bisabolol: Inhibitory effects on chemiluminescence of human neutrophil bursts and cell-free systems. *Pharmacol.* 83(2):110–115.
90. Safayhi H, Sabieraj J, Sailer ER, Ammon HP. (1994). Chamazulene: An antioxidant-type inhibitor of leukotriene B4 formation. *Planta Med.* 60(5):410–413.
91. Srivastava JK, Pandey M, Gupta S. (2009). Chamomile, a novel and selective COX-2 inhibitor with anti-inflammatory activity. *Life Sci.* 85(19–20):663–669.
92. Miguel FG, Cavalheiro AH, Spinola NF, Ribeiro DL, Barcelos GR, Antunes LM. et al. (2015). Validation of a RP-HPLC-DAD method for chamomile (*Matricaria recutita*) preparations and assessment of the marker, apigenin-7-glucoside, safety and anti-inflammatory effect. *Evid Based Comp Alter Med.* 828437.
93. Taniguchi F, Tagashira Y, Suou K, Iwabe T, Harada T. (2009). Apigenin inhibits TNFa-induced cell proliferation in endometriotic stromal cells. Obstet & Gynecol, Tottori University Faculty of Medicine, Yonago, Japan. *Oral Presentation Endometriosis Special Interest Group.* 92:3 S11.
94. Rekka EA, Kourounakis AP, Kourounakis PN. (1996). Investigation of the effect of chamazulene on lipid peroxidation and free radical processes. *Res Commun Mol Pathol Pharmacol.* 92(3):361–364.
95. McKay DL, Blumberg JB. (2006). A review of the bioactivity and potential health benefits of chamomile tea (*Matricaria recutita* L.). *Phyto Res.* 20(7):519–530.
96. Maschi O, Cero ED, Galli GV, Caruso D, Bosisio E, Dell'Agli M. (2008). Inhibition of human cAMP-phosphodiesterase as a mechanism of the spasmolytic effect of *Matricaria recutita* L. *J Agric Food Chem.* 56(13):5015–5020.
97. Mehmood MH, Munir S, Khalid UA, Asrar M, Anwarul, Gilani AH. (2015). Antidiarrhoeal, antisecretory and antispasmodic activities of *Matricaria chamomilla* are mediated predominantly through K^+-channels activation. *BMC Comp Altern Med.* 15:75.

98. Achterrath-Tuckermann U, Kunde R, Flaskamp E. et al. (1980). Pharmacological investigations with compounds of chamomile. V. Investigations on the spasmolytic effect of compounds of chamomile and Kamillosan on the isolated guinea pig ileum. *Planta Med.* 39:38–50.
99. Marder M, Paladini AC. (2002). GABA(A)-receptor ligands of flavonoid structure. *Curr Top Med Chem.* 2(8):853–867.
100. Lorenzo PS, Rubio MC, Medina JH, Adler-Graschinsky E. (1996). Involvement of monoamine oxidase and noradrenaline uptake in the positive chronotropic effects of apigenin in rat atria. *Eur J Pharmacol.* 312(2):203–207.
101. Reis LS, Pardo PE, Oba E, Kronka S, Frazatti-Gallina NM. (2006). *Matricaria chamomilla* CH12 decreases handling stress in Nelore calves. *J Vet Sci.* 7(2):189–192.
102. Awad R, Levac D, Cybulska P, Merali Z, Trudeau VL, Arnason JT. (2007). Effects of traditionally used anxiolytic botanicals on enzymes of the gamma-aminobutyric acid (GABA) system. *Can J Physiol Pharmacol.* 85(9):933–942.
103. Viola H, Wasowski C, Levi de Stein M. et al. (1995). Apigenin, a component of *Matricaria recutita* flowers, is a central benzodiazepine receptors-ligand with anxiolytic effects. *Planta Med.* 61(3):213–216.
104. Shinomiya K, Inoue T, Utsu Y. (2005). Hypnotic activities of chamomile and passiflora extracts in sleep-disturbed rats. *Biol Pharmacol Bull.* 28(5):808–810.
105. Karimian Z, Sadat Z, Abedzadeh M, Sarafraz N, Kafaei Atrian M, Bahrami N. (2013). Comparison of the effect of mefenamic acid and *Matricaria chamomilla* on primary dysmenorrhea in Kashan Medical University Students. *J Ardabil Uni Med Sci.* 13(4):413–420.
106. Jahanian M, Rakhshandeh H, Teimuri M. (1999). The effect of chamomile extract on dysmenorrhea. *Med J Mashad Uni Med Sci.* 42:33.
107. Modaress M, Mirmohhamad M, Oshireh Z, Mehran A. (2011). Comparison of the effect of mefenamic acid and *Matricaria chamomilla* capsules on primary dysmenorrhea. *J Babol Uni. Med. Sci.* 13:50–58.
108. Jenabi E, Ebrahimzadeh S. (2010). Chamomile tea for relief of dysmenorrhea. *Iran J Obstet Gynecol Infertil.* 13(1):39–42.
109. Jahanian M, Rakhshandeh H, Teimuri M. (1999). The effect of chamomile extract on dysmenorrhea. *Med J Mashad Uni Med Sci.* 42:33.
110. Yazdani M, Shahriary M, Hamedi B. (2005). Comparison of fennel and chamomile drops versus control in the treatment of primary dysmenorrhea. *J Hormozgan Uni Med Sci.* 8:57–61.

111. Felter HW, Lloyd JU. (1905). *King's American Dispensatory*, 18th ed., rev. 3, vol. 2. Portland: Eclectic Medical Publications, 1983, pp. 1246–1247.
112. Kimura M, Kimura I, Takahashi K, Muroi M, Yoshizaki M, Kanaoka M. et al. (1984). Blocking effects of blended paeoniflorin or its related compounds with glycyrrhizin on neuromuscular junctions in frogs and mice. *Jpn J Pharmacol*. 36:275–282.
113. Maeda T, Shinozuka K, Baba K, Hayashi M, Hayashi E. (1983). Effect of *shakuyaku-kanzoh-toh*, a prescription composed of *shakuyaku* (*Paeoniae* radix) and *kanzoh* (*Glycyrrhizae* radix) on guinea pig ileum. *J Pharmaco-bio-Dynamics*. 6(3):153–160.
114. Tsuji S, Yasuda K, Sumi G, Cho H, Tsuzuki T, Okada H, Kanzaki H. (2012). *Shakuyaku-kanzo-to* inhibits smooth muscle contractions of human pregnant uterine tissue in vitro. *J Obstet Gynaecol Res*. 38(7):1004–1010.
115. Wang D, Wang W, Zhou Y, Wang J, Jia D, Wong HK, Zhang, ZJ. (2015). Studies on the regulatory effect of peony-glycyrrhiza decoction on prolactin hyperactivity and underlying mechanism in hyperprolactinemia rat model. *Neurosci Lett*. 606:60–65.
116. Shibata T, Morimoto T, Suzuki A, Saito H, Yanaihara T. (1996). The effect of *Shakuyaku-kanzo-to* on prostaglandin production in human uterine myometrium. *Nihon Sanka Fujinka Gakkai Zasshi*. 48(5):321–327.
117. Sakamoto S, Mitamura T, Iwasawa M, Kitsunai H, Shindou K, Yagishita Y. et al. (1998). Conservative management for perimenopausal women with uterine leiomyomas using Chinese herbal medicines and synthetic analogs of gonadotropin-releasing hormone. *In Vivo*. 12:333–337.
118. Sumi G, Yasuda K, Tsuji S, Kanamori C, Tsuzuki T, Cho H, Nishigaki A. et al. (2015). Lipid-soluble fraction of *Shakuyaku-kanzo-to* inhibits myometrial contraction in pregnant women. *J Obstet Gynaecol Res*. 41(5):670–679.
119. Jarry H, Leonhardt S, Gorkow C, Wuttke W. (1994). In vitro prolactin but not LH and FSH release is inhibited by compounds in extracts of *Agnus castus*: Direct evidence for a dopaminergic principle by the dopamine receptor assay. *Exp Clin Endocrinol*. 102(6):448–454.
120. Webster DE, Lu J, Chen SN, Farnsworth NR, Wang ZJ. (2006). Activation of the mu-opiate receptor by *Vitex agnus-castus* methanol extracts: Implication for its use in PMS. *J Ethnopharmacol*. 106(2):216–221.
121. Webster DE, He Y, Chen SN, Pauli GF, Farnsworth NR, Wang ZJ. et al. (2011). Opioidergic mechanisms underlying the actions of *Vitex agnus-castus* L. *Biochem Pharmacol*. 81:170–177.

122. Webster DE, Lu J, Chen SN, Farnsworth NR, Wang ZJ. (2006). Activation of the mu-opiate receptor by *Vitex agnus-castus* methanol extracts: Implication for its use in PMS. *J Ethnopharmacol.* 106(2):216–221.
123. Choudhary MI, Azizuddin, Jalil S, Nawaz SA, Khan KM, Tareen RB. et al. (2009). Antiinflammatory and lipoxygenase inhibitory compounds from *Vitex agnus-castus. Phytother Res.* 23:1336–1339.
124. Chan EWC, Wong SK, Chan HT. (2018). Casticin from *Vitex* species: A short review on its anticancer and anti-inflammatory properties. *J Integr Med.* 16(3):147–152.
125. Dericks-Tan JS, Schwinn P, Hildt C. (2003). Dose-dependent stimulation of melatonin secretion after administration of *Agnus castus. Exp Clin Endocrinol Diabetes.* 111(1):44–46.
    Diaz BL, Llaneza PC. (2008). Endocrine regulation of the course of menopause by oral melatonin: First case report. *Menopause.* 15(2):388–392.
126. Shahhosseini Z, Amin GH, Salehi Sormaghi MH, Danesh M, Abedian K. (2006). The effect of *Vitex* drop on dysmenorrhea. *J Mazandaran Uni Med Sci.* 15:15–21.
127. Aksoy AN, Gözükara I, Kabil Kucur S. (2014). Evaluation of the efficacy of *Fructus agni casti* in women with severe primary dysmenorrhea: A prospective comparative Doppler study. *J Obstet Gynaecol Res.* 40(3):779–784.
128. Schwertner A, Conceição Dos Santos CC, Costa GD, Deitos A, de Souza A. et al. (2013). Efficacy of melatonin in the treatment of endometriosis: A phase II, randomized, double-blind, placebo-controlled trial. *Pain.* 154(6):874–881.
129. Brice-Ytsma H, McDermott A. (2020). *Herbal Medicine in Treating Gynaecological Conditions: Herbs, Hormones, Pre-Menstrual Syndrome and Menopause.* London: Aeon.
130. Gharib Naseri MK, Mard SA, Farboud Y. (2005). Effect of *Anethum graveolens* extract on rat uterus contractions. *Iran J Basic Med Sci.* 8:263–270.
131. Heidarifar R, Mehran N, Heidari A, Tehran HA, Koohbor M, Mansourabad MK. (2014). Effect of dill (*Anethum graveolens*) on the severity of primary dysmenorrhea in compared with mefenamic acid: A randomized, double-blind trial. *J Res Med Sci.* (Isfahan). 19(4):326–330.
132. Mueller A. (1899). Versuche über die Wirkungsweise des Extrakts des chinesischen Emmenagogon Tang-kui (Man-mu) oder Eumenol-Merek. *Münchener Medizinische Wochenschrift.* 46:796–798.

Langes H. (1901). Beobachtungen bei der Verwendung einiger neuer Medikamente. Eumenol, Dionin und Stypticin. *Therapeutische Monatshefte.* 7:363.

Palm R. (1910). Erfahrungen mit Eumenol. *Münchener Medizinische Wochenschrift.* 1:23–25.

133. Palm R. (1910). Erfahrungen mit Eumenol. *Münchener Medizinische Wochenschrift.* 1:23–25.

Buck P. (1899). Un nouveau remède spécifique contre la dysmenorrhée: l'eumenol. *Belgique médicale.* 2:363–365.

134. World Health Organization. (2001). *WHO Monographs on Selected Medicinal Plants*, vol. 2. Geneva: WHO.

135. Langes H. (1901). Beobachtungen bei der Verwendung einiger neuer Medikamente. Eumenol, Dionin und Stypticin. *Therapeutische Monatshefte.* 7:363.

136. Mueller A. (1899). Versuche über die Wirkungsweise des Extrakts des chinesischen Emmenagogon *Tang-kui (Man-mu)* oder Eumenol-Merek. *Münchener Medizinische Wochenschrift.* 46:796–798.

137. Keller K. (1992). Cinamomum species. In: De Smet PAGM, Keller K, Hansel R, Chandler RF. (eds). *Adverse Effects of Herbal Drugs.* Berlin: Springer-Verlag, vol. 1, pp. 105–114.

138. Akhavan Amjadi M, Mojab F, Shahbaz-Zadegan S. (2009). Effects of *Cinnamomum zeylanicum* on the severity and systemic manifestations of dysmenorrhea. *Med J Arak Uni.* 9:204–209.

139. Jahangirifar M, Taebi M, Dolatian M. (2018). The effect of cinnamon on primary dysmenorrhea: A randomized, double-blind clinical trial. *Com Ther Clin Pract.* 33:56–60.

140. Jaafarpour M, Hatefi M, Khani A, Khajavikhan J. (2015). Comparative effect of cinnamon and ibuprofen for treatment of primary dysmenorrhea: A randomized double-blind clinical trial. *J Clin Diagn Res.* 9(4):QC04–QC7.

141. Shams Ardakani MR, Hadjiakhoondi A, Jamshidi AH, Abdi Kh. (2005). The study of volatile oil of *Foeniculum vulgare* Miller, in their tissue culture and comparison with the whole plant. *J Med Plants.* 4(15):73–80.

142. Ostad SN, Soodi M, Shariffzadeh M, Khorshidi N, Marzban H. (2001). The effect of fennel essential oil on uterine contraction as a model for dysmenorrhea, pharmacology and toxicology study. *J Ethnopharmacol.* 76:299–304.

143. Zendehdel M, Taati M, Amoozad M, Hamidi F. (2012). Antinociceptive effect of the aqueous extract obtained from *Foeniculum vulgare* in mice: The role of histamine H1 and H2 receptors. *Iran J Vet Res.* 13:100–106.

144. Jahromi BN, Tartifizadeh A, Khabnadideh S. (2003). Comparison of fennel and mefenamic acid for the treatment of primary dysmenorrhea. *Int J Gynecol Obstet*. 80:153–157.
145. Delaram M, Forouzandeh N. (2011). The effect of fennel on the primary dysmenorrhea in students of Shahrekord University of Medical Sciences. *Jundishapur Sci Med J*. 10:81–88.
146. Khorshidi N, Ostad SN, Mosaddegh M, Soodi M. (2003). Clinical effects of fennel essential oil on primary dysmenorrhea. *Iran J Pharmacol Res*. 2:89–93.
147. Yazdani M, Shahriari M, Hamedi B. (2004). Comparison of fennel and chamomile extract and placebo in treatment of premenstrual syndrome and dysmenorrhea. *Med J Hormozgan Univ*. 8:57–61.
148. Moslemi L, Aghamohammadi A, Bekhradi R, Zafari M. (2012). Comparing the effects of vitamin E and fennel extract on intensity of primary dysmenorrhea. *J Mazandaran Univ Med Sci*. 22:103–107.
149. Mahboubi M. (2019). *Foeniculum vulgare* as valuable plant in management of women's health. *J Menopausal Med*. 25(1):1–14.
150. Salehi A, Marzban M, Amini F. (2019). Review article: Effect of *Foeniculum vulgare* on primary dysmenorrhea: A systematic review and meta-analysis. *Women's Health Bull*. 6(1):e74240.
151. Modaress Nejad V, Motamedi B, Asadi-pour M. (2006). Comparison between the pain-relief effect of fennel and mefenamic acid on primary dysmenorrhea. *J Rafsanjan Uni Med Sci*. 5(1):1–6.
152. Nazarpour S, Azimi H. (2007). Comparison of therapeutic effects of fennelin and mefenamic acid on primary dysmenorrhea. *J Mazandaran Uni Med Sci*. 17:54–61.
153. Namavar Jahromi B, Tartifizadeh A, Khabnadideh S. (2003). Comparison of fennel and mefenamic acid for the treatment of primary dysmenorrhea. *Int J Gynecol Obstet*. 80:153–157.
154. Namavar Jahromi B, Tartifizadeh A, Khabnadideh S. (2003). Comparison of fennel and mefenamic acid for the treatment of primary dysmenorrhea. *Int J Gynaecol Obstet*. 80:153–157.
155. Khourshidi N, Ostad SN, Mosaddegh M, Sooudi M. (2003). Clinical effects of fennel essential oil on primary dysmenorrhea. *Iran J Pharmacol Res*. 2:89–93.
Delaram M, Forozandeh N. (2001). Effects of *Foeniculum vulgare* extract on primary dysmenorrhea. *J Med. Sci*. 10:81–88.
156. Nazarpour S, Azimi H. (2007). Comparison of therapeutic effects of fennelin and mefenamic acid on primary dysmenorrhea. *J Mazandaran Uni Med Sci*. 17:54–61.

157. Namavar Jahromi B, Tartifizadeh A, Khabnadideh S. (2003). Comparison of fennel and mefenamic acid for the treatment of primary dysmenorrhea. *Int J Gynaecol Obstet.* 80:153–157.
158. Ghodsi Z, Asltoghiri M. (2014). The effect of fennel on pain quality, symptoms, and menstrual duration in primary dysmenorrhea. *J Pediatr Adolesc Gynecol.* 27(5):283–286.
159. Torkzahrani SH, Akhavan AM, Mojab F, Alavi-majd H. (2007). Clinical effects of *Foeniculum vulgare* extract on primary dysmenorrhea. *J Reproduct Infertil.* 1:45–51.
160. Fennerty M. (2001). NSAID-related gastrointestinal injury: Evidence-based approach to preventable complication. *Postgrad Med.* 110:87–92.
Zeng J, Zhao DS, Wu B. (2002). A study on chemical constituents in the herb of *Mentha spicata. J Zhongguo Zhong. Yaoza Zhi.* 27:749–751.
Hawthorn M, Ferrante J, Luchowski E. et al. (1988). The action of peppermint oil and menthol on calcium channel dependent processes in intestinal, neuronal and cardiac preparations. *J Aliment Pharmacol Ther.* 2:101–118.
161. Amoyi Rokn-Abad M, Sarfraz N. (2012). Comparison effect of supermint and Ibuprofen on dysmenorrhea. *J Ghom Uni Med Sci.* 5:37–41.
162. Boskabady MH, Shafei MN, Saberi Z, Amini S. (2011). Pharmacological effects of *Rosa damascena. Iran J Basic Med Sci.* 14(4):295–307.
163. Mahboubi M. (2015). *Rosa damascena* as holy ancient herb with novel applications. *J Trad Comp Med.* 6(1):10–16.
164. Boskabady MH, Kiani S, Rakhshandah H. (2006). Relaxant effects of *Rosa damascena* on guinea pig tracheal chains and its possible mechanism(s). *J Ethnopharmacol.* 106(3):377–382.
165. Rakhshandah H, Shakeri MT, Ghasemzadeh MR. (2007). Comparative hypnotic effect of *Rosa damascena* fractions and Diazepam in mice. *Iran J Pharmacol Res.* 6(3):193–197.
166. Tseng YF, Chen CH, Yang YH. (2005). Rose tea for relief of primary dysmenorrhea in adolescents: A randomized controlled trial in Taiwan. *J Midwifery Women's Health.* 50(5):e51–57.
167. Bani S, Hasanpour S, Mousavi Z, Mostafa Garehbaghi P, Gojazadeh M. (2014). The effect of *Rosa damascena* extract on primary dysmenorrhea: A double-blind cross-over clinical trial. *Iran Red Cresc Med J.* 16(1):e14643.
168. Hajhashemi V, Ghannadi A, Hajiloo M. (2010). Analgesic and anti-inflammatory effects of *Rosa damascena* hydroalcoholic extract and its essential oil in animal models. *Iran J Pharmacol Res.* 9(2):163–168.

Rakhshandah H, Hosseini M. (2006). Potentiation of pentobarbital hypnosis by *Rosa damascena* in mice. *Indian J Exp Biol*. 44(11):910–912.

Rakhshandeh H, Vahdati-Mashhadian N, Dolati K, Hosseini M. (2008). Antinociceptive effect of *Rosa damascena* in mice. *J Biol Sci*. 8(1):176–180.

169. Cook, W. (1869). *The Physiomedical Dispensatory*.
170. Mengoni ES, Vichera G, Rigano LA, Rodriguez-Puebla ML, Galliano SR, Cafferata EE. et al. (2011). Suppression of COX-2, IL-1β and TNF-α expression and leukocyte infiltration in inflamed skin by bioactive compounds from *Rosmarinus officinalis* L. *Fitoterapia*. 82:414–421.
171. Tahoonian-Golkhatmy F, Abedian Z, Emami SA, Esmaily H. (2019). Comparison of rosemary and mefenamic acid capsules on menstrual bleeding and primary dysmenorrhea: A clinical trial. *Iran J Nurs Midwifery Res*. 24(4):301–305.
172. Raisa Dehkordi Z, Rafieian-Kopaei M, Hosseini-Baharanchi F. (2019). A double-blind controlled crossover study to investigate the efficacy of *Salix* extract on primary dysmenorrhea. *Comp Ther Med*. 44:102–109.
173. Shara M, Stohs SJ. (2015). Efficacy and safety of white willow bark (*Salix alba*) extracts. *Phytother Res*. 29(8):1112–1116.
174. Salmalian H, Saghebi R, Moghadamnia AA, Bijani A, Faramarzi M. et al. (2014). Comparative effect of *Thymus vulgaris* and ibuprofen on primary dysmenorrhea: A triple-blind clinical study. *Caspian J Internal Med*. 5(2):82–88.
175. Direkvand-Moghadam A, Khosravi A. (2012). The impact of a novel herbal *Shirazi Thymus Vulgaris* on primary dysmenorrhea in comparison to the classical chemical ibuprofen. *J Res Med Sci*. (Isfahan). 17(7):668–670.
176. Iravani M. (2009). Clinical effects of *Zataria multiflora* essential oil on primary dysmenorrhea. *J Med Plants*. 8:54–60.
177. Iravani M. (2009). Clinical effects of *Zataria multiflora* essential oil on primary dysmenorrhea. *J Med Plants*. 8:54–60.
178. Yassin S. (2012). Herbal remedy used by rural adolescent girls with menstrual disorders. *J Am Sci*. 8(1):467–473.
179. Younesy S, Amiraliakbari S, Esmaeili S, Alavimajd H, Nouraei S. (2014). Effects of fenugreek seed on the severity and systemic symptoms of dysmenorrhea. *J Reprod Infertil*. 15(1):41–48.
180. Colombo D, Vescovini R. (1985). Controlled clinical study on the efficacy of the blueberry's cyanide antagonists [anticyanides] in the treatment of primary dysmenorrhea. *G Ital Ostet Ginecol*. 7(12):1033–1038.

181. Colombo D, Vescovini R. (1985). Controlled clinical study on the efficacy of the blueberry's cyanide antagonists [anticyanides] in the treatment of primary dysmenorrhea. *G Ital Ostet Ginecol.* 7(12):1033–1038.
182. Nikkhah S, Dolatian M, Naghii MR, Zaeri F, Taheri SM. (2015). Effects of boron supplementation on the severity and duration of pain in primary dysmenorrhea. *Comp Ther Clin Pract.* 21(2):79–83.
183. Zarei S, Mohammad-Alizadeh-Charandabi S, Mirghafourvand M, Javadzadeh Y, Effati-Daryani F. Effects of calcium-vitamin D and calcium-alone on pain intensity and menstrual blood loss in women with primary dysmenorrhea: A randomized controlled trial. *Pain Med.* 18(1):3–13.
184. Proctor ML, Murphy PA. (2001). Herbal and dietary therapies for primary and secondary dysmenorrhoea. *Cochrane Database Syst Rev.* (3):CD002124.
185. Deutch B, Jorgensen EB, Hansen JC. (2000). Menstrual discomfort in Danish women reduced by dietary supplements of omega-3 PUFA and B12 (fish oil or seal oil capsules). *Nutr Res.* 20(5):621–631.
186. Harel Z, Biro FM, Kottenhahn RK, Rosenthal SL. (1996). Supplementation with omega-3 polyunsaturated fatty acids in the management of dysmenorrhea in adolescents. *Am J Obstet Gynecol.* 174(4):1335–1338.
187. Gokhale LB. (1999). Curative treatment of primary (spasmodic) dysmenorrhoea. *Indian J Med Res.* 103:227–231.
188. Proctor ML, Murphy PA. (2001). Herbal and dietary therapies for primary and secondary dysmenorrhoea. *Cochrane Database Syst Rev.* (3):CD002124.
189. Moini A, Ebrahimi T, Shirzad N, Hosseini R, Radfar M, Bandarian F, Jafari-Adli S, Qorbani M, Hemmatabadi M. (2016). The effect of vitamin D on primary dysmenorrhea with vitamin D deficiency: A randomized double-blind controlled clinical trial. *Gynecol Endocrinol.* 32(6):502–505.
190. Saei Ghare Naz M, Kiani Z, Rashidi Fakari F, Ghasemi V, Abed M, Ozgoli G. (2020). The effect of micronutrients on pain management of primary dysmenorrhea: A systematic review and meta-analysis. *J Caring Sci.* 9(1):47–56.
191. Ziaei S, Faghihzadeh S, Sohrabvand F, Lamyian M, Emamgholy T. (2001). A randomized placebo-controlled trial to determine the effect of vitamin E in treatment of primary dysmenorrhoea. *Obstet Gynaecol.* 108:1181–1183.

192. Golomb L, Solidum A, Warren M. (1998). Primary dysmenorrhea and physical activity. *Med Sci Sports Exerc*. 30(6):906–909.
193. Choi P, Salmon P. (1995). Symptom changes across the menstrual cycle in competitive sportswomen, exercisers and sedentary women. *Br J Clin Psychol*. 34:447–460.
194. Metheny W, Smith R. (1989). The relationship among exercise, stress and primary dysmenorrhea. *J Behav Med*. 12(6):569–586.
195. Akin M, Weingand K, Hengehold D, Goodale MB, Hinkle R, Smith R. (2001). Continuous low-level topical heat in the treatment of dysmenorrhea. *Obstet Gynecol*. 97(3):343–349.
196. Bakhtshirin F, Abedi S, YusefiZoj P, Razmjooee D. (2015). The effect of aromatherapy massage with lavender oil on severity of primary dysmenorrhea in Arsanjan students. *Iran J Nurs Midwif Res*. 20(1):156–160.

Chapter 2: Menorrhagia

1. Hapangama DK, Bulmer JN. (2016). Pathophysiology of heavy menstrual bleeding. *Women's Health* (Lond). 12(1):3–13.
2. Royal College of Obstetricians and Gynaecologists. (2012). National menstrual heavy bleeding audit. Second Annual Report. London: Royal College of Obstetricians and Gynaecologists. www.rcog.org.uk.
3. Evans J, Salamonsen LA. (2012). Inflammation, leukocytes and menstruation. *Rev Endocr Metab Disord*. 13(4):277–288.
4. Henriet P, Gaide Chevronnay HP, Marbaix E. (2012). The endocrine and paracrine control of menstruation. *Mol Cell Endocrinol*. 358(2):197–207.
5. Garry R, Hart R, Karthigasu KA, Burke C. (2009). A re-appraisal of the morphological changes within the endometrium during menstruation: A hysteroscopic, histological and scanning electron microscopic study. *Hum Reprod*. 24(6):1393–1401.
6. Aguilar HN, Mitchell BF. (2010). Physiological pathways and molecular mechanisms regulating uterine contractility. *Hum Reprod Update*. 16(6):725–744.
7. Hapangama DK, Bulmer JN. (2016). Pathophysiology of heavy menstrual bleeding. *Women's Health* (Lond). 12(1):3–13.
8. Warner PE, Critchley HO, Lumsden MA, Campbell-Brown M, Douglas A, Murray GD. (2004). Menorrhagia II: Is the 80-mL blood loss criterion useful in management of complaint of menorrhagia? *Am J Obstet Gynecol*. 190(5):1224–1229.

9. Karlsson TS, Marions LB, Edlund MG. (2014). Heavy menstrual bleeding significantly affects quality of life. *Acta Obstet Gynecol Scand.* 93(1):52–57.
10. Jabbour HN, Kelly RW, Fraser HM, Critchley HO. (2006). Endocrine regulation of menstruation. *Endocr Rev.* 27(1):17–46.
11. Archer DF. (2012). Vascular dysfunction as a cause of endometrial bleeding. *Gynecol Endocrinol.* 28(9):688–693.
12. Karlsson TS, Marions LB, Edlund MG. (2014). Heavy menstrual bleeding significantly affects quality of life. *Acta Obstet Gynecol Scand.* 93(1):52–57.
13. Jabbour HN, Kelly RW, Fraser HM, Critchley HO. (2006). Endocrine regulation of menstruation. *Endocr Rev.* 27(1):17–46.
14. Bray GA. (2002). The underlying basis for obesity: Relationship to cancer. *J Nutr.* 132(Suppl. 11):S3451–S3455.
15. Nandi A, Chen Z, Patel R, Poretsky L. (2014). Polycystic ovary syndrome. *Endocrinol Metab Clin North Am.* 43(1):123–147.
16. Brice-Ytsma H, McDermott A. (2020). *Herbal Medicine in Treating Gynaecological Conditions: Herbs, Hormones, Pre-Menstrual Syndrome and Menopause.* London: Aeon.
17. Gargett CE, Rogers PA. (2001). Human endometrial angiogenesis. *Reproduction.* 121(2):181–186.
18. Shivhare S Biswas, Bulmer JN, Innes BA, Hapangama DK, Lash GE. (2014). Altered vascular smooth muscle cell differentiation in the endometrial vasculature in menorrhagia. *Hum Reprod.* 29(9):1884–1894.
19. Hapangama DK, Bulmer JN. (2016). Pathophysiology of heavy menstrual bleeding. *Women's Health* (Lond). 12(1):3–13.
20. Archer DF. (2012). Vascular dysfunction as a cause of endometrial bleeding. *Gynecol Endocrinol.* 28(9):688–693.
21. Abberton KM, Taylor NH, Healy DL, Rogers PA. (1999). Vascular smooth muscle cell proliferation in arterioles of the human endometrium. *Hum Reprod.* 14(4):1072–1079.
22. Hurskainen R, Teperi J, Paavonen J, Cacciatore B. (1999). Menorrhagia and uterine artery blood flow. *Hum Reprod.* 14(1):186–189.
23. Hurskainen R, Teperi J, Paavonen J, Cacciatore B. (1999). Menorrhagia and uterine artery blood flow. *Hum Reprod.* 14(1):186–189.
24. Kelly RW, Lumsden MA, Abel MH, Baird DT. (1984). The relationship between menstrual blood loss and prostaglandin production in the human: Evidence for increased availability of arachidonic acid in women suffering from menorrhagia. *Prostaglandins Leukot Med.* 16(1):69–78.

25. Critchley HOD, Maybin JA. (2011). Molecular and cellular causes of abnormal uterine bleeding of endometrial origin. *Semin Reprod Med*. 29(5):400–409.
26. Pelzer ES, Willner D, Buttini M, Huygens F. (2018). A role for the endometrial microbiome in dysfunctional menstrual bleeding. *Antonie Van Leeuwenhoek*. 111(6):933–943.
27. Gargett CE, Rogers PA. (2001). Human endometrial angiogenesis. *Reproduction*. 121(2):181–186.
28. Graubert MD, Ortega MA, Kessel B, Mortola JF, Iruela-Arispe ML. (2001). Vascular repair after menstruation involves regulation of vascular endothelial growth factor-receptor phosphorylation by sFLT-1. *Am J Path*. 158(4):1399–1410.
29. Jones WHS. (1956). [Pliny, the Elder] *Naturalis Historia. English and Latin*. Cambridge, MA: Harvard University Press.
30. Osbaldeston TA, Wood RPA (eds). (2000). *Dioscorides: De materia medica*. Johannesburg: Ibidis Press.
31. Felter HW, Lloyd JU. (1898). *King's American Dispensatory*.
32. Lloyd, JU, Ellingwood F. (1919). *American Materia Medica*.
33. Ramadan M, Goeters S, Watzer B, Krause E, Lohmann K, Bauer R, Hempel B, Imming P. (2006). Chamazulene carboxylic acid and matricin: A natural profen and its natura prodrug, identified through similarity to synthetic drug substances. *J Nat Prod*. 69:1041–1045.
34. Benedek B, Kopp B, Melzig MF. (2007). *Achillea millefolium* L. s.l.—is the anti-inflammatory activity mediated by protease inhibition? *J Ethnopharmacol*. 113(2):312–317.
35. Choudhary MI, Jalil S, Todorova M, Trendafilova A, Mikhova B, Duddeck H, Rahman AU. (2007). Inhibitory effect of lactone fractions and individual components from three species of the *Achillea millefolium* complex of Bulgarian origin on the human neutrophils respiratory burst activity. *Nat Prod Res*. 21:1032–1036.
36. Nemeth E, Bernath J. (2008). Biological activities of yarrow species (*Achillea* spp.). *Curr Pharmacol Des*. 14(29):3151–3167.
37. Sellerberg U, Glasl H. (2000). Pharmacognostical examination concerning the hemostyptic effect of *Achillea millefolium* aggregate. *Sci Pharmacol*. 68(2):201–206.
38. Yaeesh S, Jamal Q, Khan AU, Gilani AH. (2006). Studies on hepatoprotective, antispasmodic and calcium antagonist activities of the aqueous-methanol extract of *Achillea millefolium*. *Phyto Res*. 20:546–551.
39. Lemmens-Gruber R, Marchart E, Rawnduzi P, Engel N, Benedek B, Kopp B. (2006). Investigation of the spasmolytic activity of the

flavonoid fraction of *Achillea millefolium* s.l. on isolated guinea-pig ilea. *Arzneimittelforschung.* 56:582–588.
40. Dall'Acqua S, Bolego C, Cignarella A, Gaion RM, Innocenti G. (2011). Vasoprotective activity of standardized *Achillea millefolium* extract. *Phytomed.* 18(12):1031–1036.
41. Jenabi E, Fereidoony B. (2015). Effect of *Achillea millefolium* on relief of primary dysmenorrhea: A doubleblind randomized clinical trial. *J Pediatr Adolesc Gynecol.* 28:402–404.
42. De Laguna A. (1590). *Pedacio Dioscorides Anazarbeo, acerca de la material medicinal, y de los venenos mortiferos, traduzido de lengua griega en la vulgar castellana illustrado y con claras y substantiales annotations, y con las figures de innumeras plantas exquisitas y raras por el doctor Andres de laguna, medical de Julio III, Pont. Maxi.*
43. Trouillas P, Calliste C-A, Allais D-P. et al. (2003). Antioxidant, antiinflammatory and antiproliferative properties of sixteen water plant extracts used in the Limousin countryside as herbal teas. *Food Chem.* 80(3):399–407.
44. Hamad I, Erol Ö, Pekmez M, Onay-Uçar E. (2007). Free radical scavenging activity and protective effects of *Alchemilla vulgaris* (L.). *J Biotechnol.* 131(2):S40–S41.
45. Borodin IuI, Seliatitskaia VG, Obukhova LA. et al. (1999). [Effect of polyphenol fraction from *Alchemilla vulgaris* on the morphofunctional state of the thyroid in rats exposed to cold] [article in Russian]. *Biull Eksp Biol Med.* 127(6):697–699.
46. Filippova EI. (2017). Antiviral activity of lady's mantle (*Alchemilla vulgaris* L.) extracts against orthopoxviruses. *Bull Exp Biol Med.* 163(3):374–377.
47. Petcu P, Andronescu E. (1979). Treatment of juvenile meno-metrorrhagia with *Alchemilla vulgaris* fluid extract. *Clujul Med.* 52(3):266–270.
48. Bastien JW. (1983). Pharmacopeia of Qollahuaya Andeans. *J Enthonopharmacol.* 8(1):97–111.
49. Khare CP. (2007). *Indian Medicinal Plants, An Illustrated Dictionary.* New York: Springer, p. 119.
50. Ellingwood F, Lloyd JU. (1898). *American Materia Medica, Therapeutics and Pharmacognosy.*
51. Harste W. (1928). Die medizinische Wirkung der *Capsella Bursa pastoris* sowie der auf ihr lebenden Parasiten Cystopus candidus und Peronospora parasitica mit besonderer Berücksichtigung des Entwicklungsganges der beiden Pilze. *Archiv der Pharmazie.* 266(3):133–151.

52. Grieve M. (1971). *A Modern Herbal*. New York: Dover Publications.
53. Jurisson S. (1971). Determination of active substances of *Capsella bursa pastoris*. *Tartuu Riiliku Ulikooli Toim*. 270:71–79.
54. Shipochliev T. (1981). Uterotonic action of extracts from a group of medicinal plants. *Vet Med Nauki*. 18(4):94–98.
55. Kuroda K, Takagi K. (1968). Physiologically active substance in *Capsella bursa-pastoris*. *Nature*. 220(168):707–708.
56. Schumann E. (1939). Newer concepts of blood coagulation and control of haemorrhage. *Am J Obstet Gynecol*. 38:1002–1007.
Steinberg A. Segal HI, Parris HM. (1940). Role of oxalic acid and certain related dicarboxylic acids in the control of haemorrhage. *Ann Otol Rhinol Laryngol*. 49:1008–1021.
57. Vermathen M, Glasl H. (1993). Effect of the herb extract of *Capsella bursa-pastoris* on blood coagulation. *Planta Med*. 59(Suppl.): A670.
58. Cha JM, Suh WS, Lee TH, Subedi L, Kim SY, Lee KR. (2017). Phenolic glycosides from *Capsella bursa-pastoris* (L.) Medik and their anti-Inflammatory activity. *Molecules* (Basel). 22(6):1023.
59. Kuroda K, Takagi K. (1968). Physiologically active substance in *Capsella bursa-pastoris*. *Nature*. 220(168):707–708.
60. Shipochliev T. (1981). Uterotonic action of extracts from a group of medicinal plants [In Bulgarian]. *Vet Med Nauki*. 18:94–98.
61. Grosso C, Vinholes J, Silva LR, de Pinho BG, Gonçalves RF, Valentão P, Jäger AK, Andrade PB. (2011). Chemical composition and biological screening of *Capsella bursa-pastoris*. *Brazil J Pharmacog*. 21(4):635–644.
62. Naafe M, Kariman N, Keshavarz Z, Khademi N, Mojab F, Mohammadbeigi A. (2018). Effect of hydroalcoholic extracts of *Capsella bursa-pastoris* on heavy menstrual bleeding: A randomized clinical trial. *J Altern Complement Med*. 24(7):694–700.
63. Ghalandari S, Kariman N, Sheikhan Z, Mojab F, Mirzaei M, Shahrahmani H. (2017). Effect of hydroalcoholic extract of *Capsella bursa pastoris* on early postpartum hemorrhage: A clinical trial study. *J Altern Complement Med*. 23(10):794–799.
64. Weiss RF. (1988). *Herbal Medicine* [trans. by Meuss AR from the 6th German edn of *Lehrbuch der Phytotherapie*]. Gothenburg: AB Arcanum.
65. Jaafarpour M, Hatefi M, Khani A, Khajavikhan J. (2015). Comparative effect of cinnamon and ibuprofen for treatment of primary dysmenorrhea: A randomized double-blind clinical trial. *J Clin Diagn Res*. 9(4):QC04–C07.

66. Jaafarpour M, Hatefi M, Najafi F, Khajavikhan J, Khani A. (2015). The effect of cinnamon on menstrual bleeding and systemic symptoms with primary dysmenorrhea. *Iran Red Cresc Med J*. 17(4):e27032.
67. Milewicz A, Gejdel E, Sworen H, Sienkiewicz K, Jedrzejak J, Teucher T, Schmitz H. (1993). *Vitex agnus castus* extract in the treatment of luteal phase defects due to latent hyperprolactinemia. Results of a randomized placebo-controlled double-blind study. *Arzneimittelforschung*. 43(7):752–756.
68. Probst V, Roth OA. (1954). On a plant extract with a hormone-like effect. *Dtsch Med Wschr*. 79(35):1271–1274.
69. Kayser HW, Istanbullouglu S. (1954). Eine Behandlung von Menstruationsstörungen ohne Hormone. *Hippokrates*. 25:717–718.
70. Bleier W. (1959). Phytotherapy in irregular menstrual cycles or bleeding periods and other gynecological disorders of endocrine origin. *Zentralblatt Gynakol*. 81(18):701–709.
71. Yavarikia P, Shahnazi M, Hadavand Mirzaie S, Javadzadeh Y, Lutfi R. (2013). Comparing the effect of mefenamic acid and *Vitex agnus* on intrauterine device induced bleeding. *J Caring Sci*. 2(3):245–254.
72. Zamani M, Mansour Ghanaei M, Farimany M, Nasrollahie SH. (2007). Efficacy of mefenamic acid and *Vitex* in reduction of menstrual blood loss and Hb changes in patients with a complaint of menorrhagia. *Iran J Obstet Gynecol Infertil*. 10(1):79–86.
73. Eltbogen R, Litschgi M, Gasser UE, Flueeli A, Nebel S, Zahner C. (2014). *Vitex agnus-castus* extract (ZE440) improves symptoms in women with menstrual cycle irregularities. *Reprod Endocri*. 28:86–91.
74. van Breemen RB, Tao Y, Li W. (2011). Cyclooxygenase-2 inhibitors in ginger (*Zingiber officinale*). *Fitoterapia*. 82(1):38–43.
75. Kashefi F, Khajehei M, Alavinia M, Golmakani E, Asili J. (2015). Effect of ginger (*Zingiber officinale*) on heavy menstrual bleeding: A placebo-controlled, randomized clinical trial. *Phytother Res*. 29(1):114–119.
76. Mobli M, Qaraaty M, Amin G, Haririan I, Hajimahmoodi M, Rahimi R. (2015). Scientific evaluation of medicinal plants used for the treatment of abnormal uterine bleeding by Avicenna. *Arch Gynecol Obstet*. 292(1):21–35.
77. Goshtasebi A, Mazari Z, Behboudi Gandevani S, Naseri M. (2015). Anti-hemorrhagic activity of *Punica granatum* L. flower (Persian golnar) against heavy menstrual bleeding of endometrial origin: A double-blind, randomized controlled trial. *Med J Islam Repub Iran*. 29:199.

78. Memarzadeh H. Eftekhar T, Tansaz M. et al. (2015). Evaluation of efficacy of *Punica granatum* L. (Persian gulnar) on uterine leiomyoma related menorrhagia. *Int J Biosciences*. 6:18–25.
79. Morales-Borges RH. (2020). Flavonoids and ferrochel in women with iron deficiency anemia of abnormal uterine bleeding: Our experience in community based private hematology/oncology and integrative medicine practice. *Int J Comp Alt Med*. 13(5):197–198.
80. Alanwar A, Abbas AM, Hussain SH, Elhawwary G, Mansour DY, Faisal MM, Elshabrawy A, Eltaieb E. (2018). Oral micronised flavonoids versus tranexamic acid for treatment of heavy menstrual bleeding secondary to copper IUD use: A randomised double-blind clinical trial. *Eur J Contracept Reprod Health Care*. 23(5):365–370.
81. Mukherjee GG, Gajarai AJ, Mathias J, Marva D. (2005). Treatment of abnormal uterine bleeding with micronized flavonoids. *Int J Gynecol Obstet*. 89(2):156–157.
82. Canzi E, Ribelo Lopez A, Aquino A. et al. (2017). Citrustherapy: The Tahiti lemon juice effects on the menstrual flow. *Proceedings of 6th Brazilian Conference on Natural Products*. Anais eletrônicos. Campinas, Galoá.
83. Qaraaty M, Kamali SH, Dabaghian FH. et al. (2014). Effect of myrtle fruit syrup on abnormal uterine bleeding: A randomized double-blind, placebo-controlled pilot study. *Daru: J Fac Pharm, Tehran Univ Medical Sciences*. 22(1):45.
84. Mukherjee GG, Gajaraj AJ, Mathias J, Marya D. (2005). Treatment of abnormal uterine bleeding with micronized flavonoids. *Int J Gynaecol Obstet*. 89(2):156–157.
85. Cassidy A, Bingham, Setchell KD. (1994). Biological effects of a diet of soy protein rich in isoflavones on the menstrual cycle of premenopausal women. *Am J Clin Nutr*. 60(3):333–340.
86. Lithgow DM, Politzer WM. (1977). Vitamin A in the treatment of menorrhagia. *S Afr Med J*. 51(7):191–193.
87. Yassaee F, Hadadianpour S. (2020). The effects of cobalamin and B-complex on hypermenorrhea. *J Res Med Sci*. 25:30.
88. Hallberg L, Hulthén L. (2000). Prediction of dietary iron absorption: An algorithm for calculating absorption and bioavailability of dietary iron. *Am J Clin Nutr*. 71(5):1147–1160.
89. Abbaspour N, Hurrell R, Kelishadi R. (2014). Review on iron and its importance for human health. *J Res Med Sci*. (Isfahan). 19(2):164–174.
90. Hurrell R, Egli I. (2010). Iron bioavailability and dietary reference values. *Am J Clin Nutr*. 91(5):1461S–1467S.

91. Cohen JD, Rubin HW. (1960). Functional menorrhagia: Treatment with bioflavonoids and vitamin C. *Curr Ther Res Clin Exp.* 2:539–542.
92. Dasgupta PR, Dutta S, Banerjee P, Majumdar S. (1983). Vitamin E (alpha tocopherol) in the management of menorrhagia associated with the use of intrauterine contraceptive devices (IUCD). *Int J Fertil.* 28(1):55–56.
93. Zekavat OR, Fathpour G, Haghpanah S, Dehghani SJ, Zekavat M, Shakibazad N. (2017). Acquired vitamin K deficiency as unusual cause of bleeding tendency in adults: A case report of a nonhospitalized student presenting with severe menorrhagia. *Case Rep Obstet Gynecol.* 4239148.

Chapter 3: Amenorrhoea and oligomenorrhoea

1. Rebar R. (2000). Evaluation of amenorrhea, anovulation, and abnormal bleeding. [updated 2018 Feingold KR, Anawalt B, Blackman MR. et al. (eds)] *Endotext* [Internet]. MA: South Dartmouth: MDText.com, Inc.
2. Pinkerton JV. (2023). Amenorrhoea. *MSD Manual* [online].
3. Hopcroft K, Forte V. (2014). *Symptom Sorter*. Radcliffe Publishing Ltd, 18 Marcham Rd, Abingdon OX14 1AA, UK.
4. Pinkerton JV. (2023). Amenorrhoea. *MSD Manual* [online].
5. Hassan I, Ismail KM, O'Brien S. (2004). PMS in the perimenopause. *J Br Menopause Soc.* 10(4):151–156.
6. Rebar R. (2000). Evaluation of amenorrhea, anovulation, and abnormal bleeding. [updated 2018 Feingold KR, Anawalt B, Blackman MR. et al. (eds)] *Endotext* [Internet]. MA: South Dartmouth: MDText.com, Inc.
7. Meczekalski B, Katulski K, Czyzyk A, Podfigurna-Stopa A, Maciejewska-Jeske, M. (2014). Functional hypothalamic amenorrhea and its influence on women's health. *J Endocrin Invest.* 37(11):1049–1056.
8. Meczekalski B, Podfigurna-Stopa A, Warenik-Szymankiewicz A, Genazzani AR. (2008). Functional hypothalamic amenorrhea: Current view on neuroendocrine aberrations. *Gynecol Endocrinol.* 24:4–11.
9. De Souza MJ, Toombs RJ, Scheid JL. et al. (2009). High prevalence of subtle and severe menstrual disturbances in exercising women: Confirmation using daily hormone measures. *Hum Reprod.* 25:491–503.
10. Gordon MC. (2010). Functional hypothalamic amenorrhea. *N Engl J Med.* 363:365–371.
11. Harlow SD. (2000). Menstruation and menstrual disorders: The epidemiology of menstruation and menstrual dysfunction. In: Goldman MB,

Katch M. (eds). *Women and Health*. San Diego: Academic Press, pp. 99–113.
12. Gordon CM, Ackerman KE, Berga SL, Kaplan JR. et al. (2017). Functional hypothalamic amenorrhea: An Endocrine Society Clinical Practice Guideline. *J Clin Endocrinol. Metab.* 102:1413–1439.
13. Marshall LA. (1994). Clinical evaluation of amenorrhea in active and athletic women. *Clin Sports Med.* 13:371–387.
14. Gordon CM, Ackerman KE, Berga SL, Kaplan JR. et al. (2017). Functional hypothalamic amenorrhea: An Endocrine Society Clinical Practice Guideline. *J Clin Endocrinol. Metab.* 102:1413–1439.
15. Podfigurna A, Maciejewska-Jeske M, Meczekalski B, Genazzani AD. (2020). Kisspeptin and LH pulsatility in patients with functional hypothalamic amenorrhea. *Endocrine.* 70:635–643.
16. Valdes-Socin H, Rubio Almanza M, Tomé Fernández-Ladreda M, Debray FG, Bours V, Beckers A. (2014). Reproduction, smell, and neurodevelopmental disorders: Genetic defects in different hypogonadotropic hypogonadal syndromes. *Front Endocrinol.* (Lausanne). 5:109.
17. Rivier C, Brownstein M, Spiess J, Rivier J, Vale W. (1982). In vivo corticotropin-releasing factor-induced secretion of adrenocorticotropin, b-endorphin, and corticosterone. *Endocrinology.* 110:272–278.
18. Gordon MC. (2010). Functional hypothalamic amenorhea. *N Engl J Med.* 363:365–371.
19. Kalra SP, Crowley WR. (1992). Neuropeptide Y: A novel neuroendocrine peptide in the control of pituitary hormone secretion, and its relation to luteinizing hormone. *Front Neuroendocrinol.* 13:1–46.
20. Panossian A, Wikman G, Kaur P, Asea A. (2012). Adaptogens stimulate neuropeptide y and hsp72 expression and release in neuroglia cells. *Front Neuroscience.* 6:6.
21. Gerasimova H. (1970). Effect of *Rhodiola rosea* extract on ovarian functional activity. *Proc Scientific Conference on Endocrinology and Gynecology.* Sverdlovsk, Russia: Siberian Branch of the Russian Academy of Sciences, pp. 46–48.
22. Xiong J, Tian Y, Ling A, Liu Z, Li Zhao, Cheng G. (2022). Genistein affects gonadotrophin-releasing hormone secretion in GT1–7 cells via modulating kisspeptin receptor and key regulators. *Syst Biol Reprod Med.* 68(2):138–150.
23. Xia N, Li J, Wang H, Wang J, Wang Y. (2015). *Schisandra chinensis* and *Rhodiola rosea* exert an anti-stress effect on the HPA axis and reduce

hypothalamic c-Fos expression in rats subjected to repeated stress. *Exp Ther Med.* 11(1):353–359.
24. Ryterska K, Kordek A, Załęska P. (2021). Has menstruation disappeared? Functional hypothalamic amenorrhea—what is this story about? *Nutrients.* 13(8):2827.
25. Schaal K, Van Loan MD, Casazza GA. (2011). Reduced catecholamine response to exercise in amenorrheic athletes. *Med Sci Sports Exerc.* 43:34–43.
26. Ryterska K, Kordek A, Załęska P. (2021). Has menstruation disappeared? Functional hypothalamic amenorrhea—what is this story about? *Nutrients.* 13(8):2827.
27. Tranoulis A, Georgiou D, Soldatou A, Triantafyllidi V, Loutradis D, Michala L. (2019). Poor sleep and high anxiety levels in women with functional hypothalamic amenorrhoea: A wake-up call for physicians? *Eur J Obstet Gynecol Reprod Biol. X.* 3:100035.
28. Chung FF, Yao CC, Wan GH. (2005). The associations between menstrual function and life style/working conditions among nurses in Taiwan. *J Occup Health.* 47:149–156.
29. Baumgartner A, Dietzel M, Saletu B. et al. (1993). Influence of partial sleep deprivation on the secretion of thyrotropin, thyroid hormones, growth hormones, prolactin, luteinizing hormone, follicle stimulating hormone, and estradiol in healthy young women. *Psychiatry Res.* 48:153–178.
30. Brzezinski A, Lynch HJ, Seibel MM. et al. (1988). The circadian rhythm of plasma melatonin during the normal menstrual cycle and in amenorrheic women. *J Clin Endocrinol Metab.* 66:891–895.
31. Hall JE, Sullivan JP, Richardson GS. (2005). Brief wake episodes modulate sleep-inhibited luteinizing hormone secretion in the early follicular phase. *J Clin Endocrinol Metab.* 90:2050–2055.
32. Lawson CC, Whelan EA, Lividoti Hibert EN, Spiegelman D, Schernhammer ES, Rich-Edwards JW. (2011). Rotating shift work and menstrual cycle characteristics. *Epidemiology* (Cambridge, MA). 22(3):305–312.
33. Hakimi O, Cameron LC. (2017). Effect of exercise on ovulation: A systematic review. *Sports Med.* 47:1555–1567.
34. Sanders KM, Kawwass JF, Loucks T, Berga SL. (2018). Heightened cortisol response to exercise challenge in women with functional hypothalamic amenorrhea. *Am J Obstet Gynecol.* 218:230.e1–230.e6.
35. Borba VV, Zandman-Goddard G, Shoenfeld Y. (2018). Prolactin and autoimmunity. *Front Immunol.* 9:73.

36. Ryterska K, Kordek A, Załęska P. (2021). Has menstruation disappeared? Functional hypothalamic amenorrhea—what is this story about? *Nutrients*. 13(8):2827.
37. Bomba M, Corbetta F, Bonini L, Gambera A, Tremolizzo L, Neri F, Nacinovich R. (2014). Psychopathological traits of adolescents with functional hypothalamic amenorrhea: A comparison with anorexia nervosa. *Eat Weight Disord*. 19:41–48.
38. Tabakova P, Dimitrov M, Tashkov B. (1984). *Clinical Studies on the Preparation Tribestan in Women with Endocrine Infertility or Menopausal Syndrome*. Sofia, Bulgaria: 1st Obstetrical and Gynecological Hospital.
39. Xiong J, Tian Y, Ling A, Liu Z, Li Zhao, Cheng G. (2022). Genistein affects gonadotrophin-releasing hormone secretion in GT1–7 cells via modulating kisspeptin receptor and key regulators. *Syst Biol Reprod Med*. 68(2):138–150.
40. Ellingwood F. (1908). *Ellingwood's Therapeutist*, vol. 2.
41. Lloyd JU, Lloyd CG. (1884–1887). *Drugs and Medicines of North America*.
42. Palm R. (1910). Erfahrungen mit Eumenol. *Münchener Medizinische Wochenschrift*. 1:23–25.
43. Mueller A. (1899). Versuche über die Wirkungsweise des Extrakts des chinesischen Emmenagogon *Tang-kui* (*Man-mu*) oder Eumenol-Merek. *Münchener Medizinische Wochenschrift*. 46:796–798.
44. World Health Organization. (2001). *WHO Monographs on Selected Medicinal Plants*, vol. 2. Geneva: WHO.
45. Langes H. (1901). Beobachtungen bei der Verwendung einiger neuer Medikamente. Eumenol, Dionin und Stypticin. *Therapeutische Monatshefte*. 7:363.
46. Wong AY, Chan KS, Lau WL. (2007). Pregnancy outcome of a patient with atypical polypoid adenomyoma. *Fertil Steril*. 88:1438.e7–e9.
47. Darbinyan V, Kteyan A, Panossian A, Gabrielian E, Wikman G, Wagner H. (2000). *Rhodiola rosea* in stress induced fatigue—a double blind cross-over study of a standardized extract SHR-5 with a repeated low-dose regimen on the mental performance of healthy physicians during night duty. *Phytomed*. 7(5):365–371.
48. Punja S, Shamseer L, Olson K, Vohra S. (2014). *Rhodiola rosea* for mental and physical fatigue in nursing students: A randomized controlled trial. *PloS One*. 9(9):e108416.
49. Xia N, Li J, Wang H, Wang J, Wang Y. (2015). *Schisandra chinensis* and *Rhodiola rosea* exert an anti-stress effect on the HPA axis and reduce

hypothalamic c-Fos expression in rats subjected to repeated stress. *Exp Ther Med.* 11(1):353–359.
50. Gerasimova H. (1970). Effect of *Rhodiola rosea* extract on ovarian functional activity. *Proc Scientific Conference on Endocrinology and Gynecology.* Sverdlovsk, Russia: Siberian Branch of the Russian Academy of Sciences, pp. 46–48.
51. Kalra SP, Crowley WR. (1992). Neuropeptide Y: A novel neuroendocrine peptide in the control of pituitary hormone secretion, and its relation to luteinizing hormone. *Front Neuroendocrinol.* 13:1–46.
52. Panossian A, Wikman G, Kaur P, Asea, A. (2012). Adaptogens stimulate neuropeptide y and hsp72 expression and release in neuroglia cells. *Front Neuroscience.* 6:6.
53. Xia N, Li J, Wang H, Wang J, Wang Y. (2015). *Schisandra chinensis* and *Rhodiola rosea* exert an anti-stress effect on the HPA axis and reduce hypothalamic c-Fos expression in rats subjected to repeated stress. *Exp Ther Med.* 11(1):353–359.
54. Kalra SP, Crowley WR. (1992). Neuropeptide Y: A novel neuroendocrine peptide in the control of pituitary hormone secretion, and its relation to luteinizing hormone. *Front Neuroendocrinol.* 13:1–46.
55. Panossian A, Wikman G, Kaur P, Asea, A. (2012). Adaptogens stimulate neuropeptide y and hsp72 expression and release in neuroglia cells. *Front Neuroscience.* 6:6.
56. Gerhard I I, Patek A, Monga B, Blank A, Gorkow C. (1998). Mastodynon(R) bei weiblicher Sterilität. *Forsch Komplementarmed.* 5(6):272–278.
57. Eltbogen R, Litschgi M, Gasser UE, Flueeli A, Nebel S, Zahner C. (2014). *Vitex agnus-castus* extract (ZE440) improves symptoms in women with menstrual cycle irregularities. *Reprod Endocrinol.* 28:86–91.
58. Milewicz A, Gejdel E, Sworen H, Sienkiewicz K, Jedrzejak J, Teucher T, Schmitz H. (1993). *Vitex agnus castus* extract in the treatment of luteal phase defects due to latent hyperprolactinemia. Results of a randomized placebo-controlled double-blind study. *Arzneimittelforschung.* 43(7):752–756.
59. Bergmann J, Luft B, Boehmann S, Runnebaum B, Gerhard I. (2000). Die wirksamkeit des komplexmittels Phyto-Hypophyson L bei weiblicher, hormonell bedingter sterilität [The efficacy of the complex medication Phyto-Hypophyson L in female, hormone-related sterility. A randomized, placebo-controlled clinical double-blind study]. *Forsch Komplementarmed Klass Naturheilkd.* 7(4):190–199.

60. Ellingwood F. (1908). *Ellingwood's Therapeutist*, vol. 2.
61. Ellingwood F. (1919). *The American Materia Medica, Therapeutics and Pharmacognosy.*
62. Sher G, Barnard PG. (1976). The alleviation of uterocornual spasm of the Fallopian tubes during hysterosalpingography by intravenous administration of orciprenaline. *S Afr Med J.* 50(30):1164–1165.
63. Kort DH, Lobo RA. (2014). Preliminary evidence that cinnamon improves menstrual cyclicity in women with polycystic ovary syndrome: A randomized controlled trial. *Am J Obstet Gynecol.* 211(5):487.e1–487.e6.
64. Allen RW, Schwartzman E, Baker WL. et al. (2014). Cinnamon use in type 2 diabetes: An updated systematic review and meta-analysis. *Ann Fam Med.* 11(5):452–459.
65. Wiweko B, Susanto CA. (2017). The effect of metformin and cinnamon on serum anti-mullerian hormone in women having PCOS: A double-blind, randomized, controlled trial. *J Hum Reprod Sci.* 10(1):31–36.
66. Hajimonfarednejad M, Nimrouzi M, Heydari M, Zarshenas MM, Raee MJ, Jahromi BN. (2018). Insulin resistance improvement by cinnamon powder in polycystic ovary syndrome: A randomized double-blind placebo controlled clinical trial. *Phytother Res.* 32(2):276–283.
67. Wang JG, Anderson RA, Graham GM III, Chu MC. et al. (2007). The effect of cinnamon extract on insulin resistance parameters in polycystic ovary syndrome: A pilot study. *Fertil Steril.* 88(1):240–243.
68. Xu J, Bishop CV, Lawson MS, Park BS, Xu F. (2016). Anti-Müllerian hormone promotes pre-antral follicle growth, but inhibits antral follicle maturation and dominant follicle selection in primates. *Hum Reprod.* 31(7):1522–1530.
69. Mohebbi-Kian E, Mohammad-Alizadeh-Charandabi S, Bekhradi R. (2014). Efficacy of fennel and combined oral contraceptive on depot medroxyprogesterone acetate-induced amenorrhea: A randomized placebo-controlled trial. *Contraception.* 90(4):440–446.
70. Phipps W, Martini M, Lampe J. et al. (1993). Effect of flax seed ingestion on the menstrual cycle. *J Clin Endocrinol Metab.* 77:1215–1219.
71. Mokaberinejad R, Zafarghandi N, Bioos S, Dabaghian FH. et al. (2012). *Mentha longifolia* syrup in secondary amenorrhea: A double-blind, placebo-controlled, randomized trial. *Daru: J Fac Pharm, Tehran Univ Medical Sciences.* 20(1):97.
72. Mokaberinejad R, Akhtari E, Tansaz M. et al. (2014). Effect of *Mentha longifolia* on FSH serum level in premature ovarian failure. *Open J Obstet and Gynecol.* 4(7):356–360.

73. Ushiroyama T, Ikeda A, Higashio S, Hosotani T. et al. *Unkei-to* for correcting luteal phase defects. *J Reprod Med.* 48(9):729–734.
74. Yang P, Li L, Yang D, Wang C, Peng H, Huang H. et al. (2017). Effect of peony-glycyrrhiza decoction on amisulpride-induced hyperprolactinemia in women with schizophrenia: A preliminary study. *Evid Based Complement Alternat Med.* 7901670.
75. Yuan HN, Wang CY, Sze CW, Tong Y, Tan QR, Feng XJ. et al. (2008). A randomized, crossover comparison of herbal medicine and bromocriptine against risperidone-induced hyperprolactinemia in patients with schizophrenia. *J Clin Psychopharmacol.* 28(3):264–370.
76. Yamada K, Kanba S, Yagi G, Asai M. (1999). Herbal medicine (*skakuyaku-kanzo-to*) in the treatment of risperidone-induced amenorrhea. *J Clin Psychopharmacol.* 19:380–381.
77. Man SC, Li XB, Wang HH, Yuan HN, Wang HN, Zhang RG. et al. (2016). Peony-glycyrrhiza decoction for antipsychotic-related hyperprolactinemia in women with schizophrenia: A randomized controlled trial. *J Clin Psychopharmacol.* 36(6):572–579.
78. Aboraya A, Fullen JE, Ponieman BL, Makela EH, Latocha M. (2004). Hyperprolactinemia associated with risperidone. A case report and review of literature. *Psychiatry* (Edgmont). 1(3):29–31.
79. Fahrenholtz IL, Sjödin A, Benardot D, Tornberg ÅB. et al. (2018). Within-day energy deficiency and reproductive function in female endurance athletes. *Scand J Med Sci Sports.* 28(3):1139–1146.
80. Ryterska K, Kordek A, Załęska P. (2021). Has menstruation disappeared? Functional hypothalamic amenorrhea—what is this story about? *Nutrients.* 13(8):2827.
81. Xiong J, Tian Y, Ling A, Liu Z, Li Zhao, Cheng G. (2022). Genistein affects gonadotrophin-releasing hormone secretion in GT1-7 cells via modulating kisspeptin receptor and key regulators. *Syst Biol Reprod Med.* 68(2):138–150.
82. Yavari M, Rouholamin S, Tansaz M, Bioos S, Esmaeili S. (2014). Sesame a treatment of menstrual bleeding cessation in Iranian traditional medicine: Results from a pilot study. *Shiraz E Med J.* 15(3):e21893.
83. Ryterska K, Kordek A, Załęska P. (2021). Has menstruation disappeared? Functional hypothalamic amenorrhea—what is this story about? *Nutrients.* 13(8):2827.
84. Lopresti AL. (2020). The effects of psychological and environmental stress on micronutrient concentrations in the body: A review of the evidence. *Adv Nutr.* 11(1):103–112.

85. Hecht S, Pavlik R, Lohse P, Noss U, Friese K, Thaler CJ. (2009). Common 677C→T mutation of the 5,10-methylenetetrahydrofolate reductase gene affects follicular estradiol synthesis. *Fertil Steril*. 91(1):56–61.
86. McClung JP, Gaffney-Stomberg E, Lee JJ. (2014). Female athletes: A population at risk of vitamin and mineral deficiencies affecting health and performance. *J Trace Elem Med Biol*. 28(4):388–392.
87. Seelig MS. (1993). Interrelationship of magnesium and estrogen in cardiovascular and bone disorders, eclampsia, migraine and premenstrual syndrome. *J Am Coll Nutr*. 12(4):442–458.
88. Gaskins AJ, Chavarro JE. (2018). Diet and fertility: A review. *Am J Obstet Gynecol*. 218:379–389.
89. Jukic AMZ, Wilcox AJ, McConnaughey DR, Weinberg CR, Steiner AZ. (2018). 25-hydroxyvitamin D and long menstrual cycles in a prospective cohort study. *Epidemiol*. 29(3):388–396.
90. Magrone T, Russo MA, Jirillo E. (2017). Cocoa and dark chocolate polyphenols: From biology to clinical applications. *Front Immunol*. 9(8):677.
91. Koletzko B, Lehner F. (2000). Beer and breastfeeding. *Adv Exp Med Biol*. 478:23–28.
92. Michopoulos V, Mancini F, Loucks TL, Berga SL. (2013). Neuroendocrine recovery Initiated by Cognitive Behavioral Therapy in women with functional hypothalamic amenorrhea: A randomized controlled trial. *Fertil Steril*. 99:2084–2091.

Chapter 4: Infertility

1. Chua SJ, Danhof NA, Mochtar MH, van Wely M, McLernon DJ. et al. (2020). Age-related natural fertility outcomes in women over 35 years: A systematic review and individual participant data meta-analysis. *Hum Reprod*. 35(8):1808–1820.
2. Boivin J, Bunting L, Collins JA, Nygren KG. (2007). International estimates of infertility prevalence and treatment-seeking: Potential need and demand for infertility medical care. *Hum Reprod*. 22:1506–1512.
3. Deshpande PS, Gupta AS. (2019). Causes and prevalence of factors causing infertility in a public health facility. *J Hum Reprod Sci*. 12(4):287–293.
4. Fritz MA, Speroff L. (2011). *Clinical Gynaecologic Endocrinology and Infertility*, 8th ed. New Delhi: Wolters Kluwer Health—Lippincott Williams & Wilkins, Induction of eovulation, pp. 1293–1330.
5. Deshpande PS, Gupta AS. (2019). Causes and prevalence of factors causing infertility in a public health facility. *J Hum Reprod Sci*. 12(4):287–293.

6. Sharma R, Harlev A, Agarwal A, Esteves SC. (2016). Cigarette smoking and semen quality: A new meta-analysis examining the effect of the 2010 World Health Organization laboratory methods for the examination of human semen. *Eur Urol.* 70:635–645.
7. Locke, T. Blood type O linked fertility problems. Web MD. http://www.webmd.com/infertility-and-reproduction/news/20101025/bloodtype-o-linked-fertility-problems. Accessed 10 November 2011.
8. Grodstein F, Goldman M, Ryan L. et al. (1993). Relation of female infertility to consumption of caffeinated beverages. *Am J Epidemiol.* 137:1353–1360.
9. Axmon A, Rylander L, Stromberg U, Hagmar L. (2000). Time to pregnancy and infertility among women with a high intake of fish contaminated with persistent organochlorine compounds. *Scand J Work Environ Health.* 26(3):199–206.
10. Mahalingaiah S, Hart JE, Laden F. et al. (2016). Adult air pollution exposure and risk of infertility in the Nurses' Health Study II. *Hum Reprod.* 31(3):638–647.
11. Wilcox AJ, Weinberg CR, Baird DD. (1995). Timing of sexual intercourse in relation to ovulation. Effects on the probability of conception, survival of the pregnancy, and sex of the baby. *N Engl J Med.* 333(23):1517–1521.
12. Bigelow JL, Dunson DB, Stanford JB, Ecochard R, Gnoth C, Colombo B. (2004). Mucus observations in the fertile window: A better predictor of conception than timing of intercourse. *Hum Reprod.* 19(4):889–892.
13. Tabakova P, Dimitrov M, Tashkov B. (1984). *Clinical Studies on the Preparation Tribestan in Women with Endocrine Infertility or Menopausal Syndrome.* Sofia, Bulgaria: 1st Obstetrical and Gynecological Hospital.
14. Segal TR, Kim K, Mumford SL, Goldfarb JM, Weinerman RS. (2018). How much does the uterus matter? Perinatal outcomes are improved when donor oocyte embryos are transferred to gestational carriers compared to intended parent recipients. *Fertil Steril.* 110(5):888–895.
15. Unfer V, Casini L. et al. (2004). Phytoestrogens may improve the pregnancy rate in in vitro fertilization–embryo transfer cycles: A prospective, controlled, randomized trial. *Fertil Steril.* 82(6):1509–1513.
16. Unfer V, Casini M. et al. (2004). High dose of phytoestrogens can reverse the anti-estrogenic effects of clomiphene citrate on the endometrium in patients undergoing intrauterine insemination: A randomized trial. *J Soc Gynecol Investig.* 11(5):323–328.
17. Ellingwood F. (1908). *Ellingwood's Therapeutist*, vol. 2.
18. Lloyd JU, Lloyd CG. (1884–1887). *Drugs and Medicines of North America.*

19. Felter HW, Lloyd JU. (1898). *King's American Dispensatory*.
20. Fan CW, Cieri-Hutcherson NE, Hutcherson TC. (2021). Systematic review of black cohosh (*Cimicifuga racemosa*) for management of polycystic ovary syndrome-related infertility. *J Pharmacol Pract*. 35(6):991–999.
21. Shahin AY, Ismail AM, Zahran KM, Makhlouf AM. (2008). Adding phytoestrogens to clomiphene induction in unexplained infertility patients—a randomized trial. *Reprod Biomed Online*. 16(4):580–588.
22. Shahin AY, Ismail AM, Shaaban OM. (2009). Supplementation of clomiphene citrate cycles with *Cimicifuga racemosa* or ethinyl oestradiol—a randomized trial. *Reprod Biomed Online*. 19(4):501–507.
23. Shahin AY, Mohammed SA. (2014). Adding the phytoestrogen *Cimicifugae racemosae* to clomiphene induction cycles with timed intercourse in polycystic ovary syndrome improves cycle outcomes and pregnancy rates—a randomized trial. *Gynecol Endocrinol*. 30(7):505–510.
24. Kamel HH. (2013). Role of phyto-oestrogens in ovulation induction in women with polycystic ovarian syndrome. *Eur J Obstet Gynecol Reprod Biol*. 168(1):60–63.
25. Parkinson J. (1640). *Theatrum Botanicum*.
26. Langes H. (1901). Beobachtungen bei der Verwendung einiger neuer Medikamente. Eumenol, Dionin und Stypticin. *Therapeutische Monatshefte*. 7:363.
27. Palm R. (1910). Erfahrungen mit Eumenol. *Münchener Medizinische Wochenschrift*. 1:23–25.
    Buck P. (1899). Un nouveau remède spécifique contre la dysmenorrhée: l'eumenol. *Belgique médicale*. 2:363–365.
28. Mueller A. (1899). Versuche über die Wirkungsweise des Extrakts des chinesischen Emmenagogon *Tang-kui* (*Man-mu*) oder Eumenol-Merek. *Münchener Medizinische Wochenschrift*. 46:796–798.
29. Wong AY, Chan KS, Lau WL. et al. (2007). Pregnancy outcome of a patient with atypical polypoid adenomyoma. *Fertil Steril*. 88(1438).e7–e9.
30. Bone K. (2003). *A Clinical Guide to Blending Liquid Herbs*. London: Churchill Livingstone.
31. Phipps W, Martini M, Lampe J. et al. (1993). Effect of flax seed ingestion on the menstrual cycle. *J Clin Endocrinol Metab*. 77:1215–1219.
32. Farzana F, Sulaiman A, Ruckmani A, Vijayalakshmi K, Karunya Lakshmi G, Shri RS. (2015). Effects of flax seeds supplementation in polycystic ovarian syndrome. *J Res Med Sci*. 31(1):113–119.
33. Gerhard I, Patek A, Monga B, Blank A, Gorkow C. (1998). Mastodynon(R) bei weiblicher Sterilität. *Forsch Komplementarmed*. 5(6):272–278.

34. Eltbogen R, Litschgi M, Gasser UE, Flueeli A, Nebel S, Zahner C. (2014). *Vitex agnus-castus* extract (ZE440) improves symptoms in women with menstrual cycle irregularities. *Rep Endocrinol.* 28:86–91.
35. Milewicz A, Gejdel E, Sworen H, Sienkiewicz K, Jedrzejak J, Teucher T, Schmitz H. (1993). *Vitex agnus castus* extract in the treatment of luteal phase defects due to latent hyperprolactinemia. Results of a randomized placebo-controlled double-blind study. *Arzneimittelforschung.* 43(7):752–756.
36. Bergmann J, Luft B, Boehmann S, Runnebaum B, Gerhard I. (2000). Die wirksamkeit des komplexmittels Phyto-Hypophyson L bei weiblicher, hormonell bedingter sterilität [The efficacy of the complex medication Phyto-Hypophyson L in female, hormone-related sterility. A randomized, placebo-controlled clinical double-blind study]. *Forsch Komplementarmed Klass Naturheilkd.* 7(4):190–199.
37. Ghahremaninasab P, Shahnazi M, Khalili AF, Hamdi K. (2016). The effects of combined low-dose oral contraceptives and *Vitex agnus* on the improvement of clinical and paraclinical parameters of polycystic ovarian syndrome: A triple-blind, randomized, controlled clinical trial. *Iran Red Cresc Med J.* (in press):e37510.
38. Shayan A, Masoumi SZ, Shobeiri F, Tohidi S, Khalili, A. (2016). Comparing the effects of agnugol and metformin on oligomenorrhea in patients with polycystic ovary syndrome: A randomized clinical trial. *J Clin Diag Res.* 10(12):QC13–QC16.
39. Wiweko B, Susanto CA. (2017). The effect of metformin and cinnamon on serum anti-Mullerian hormone in women having PCOS: A double-blind, randomized, controlled trial. *J Hum Reprod Sci.* 10(1):31–36.
40. Shahin AY, Ismail AM, Zahran KM, Makhlouf AM. (2008). Adding phytoestrogens to clomiphene induction in unexplained infertility patients—a randomized trial. *Reprod Biomed Online.* 16(4):580–588.
41. Kumarapeli M, Karunagoda K, Perera PK. (2018). A randomized clinical trial to evaluate the efficacy of *Satapushpashatavari* powered drug with *Satapushpa-shatavari grita* for the management of polycystic ovary syndrome (PCOS). *Int J Pharmacol Sci Res.* 9(6):2494–2499.
42. Kamel HH. (2013). Role of phyto-oestrogens in ovulation induction in women with polycystic ovarian syndrome. *Eur J Obstet Gynecol Reprod Biol.* 168(1):60–63.
43. Moini Jazani A, Nazemiyeh H, Tansaz M. et al. (2018). Celery plus anise versus metformin for the treatment of oligomenorrhea in polycystic ovary syndrome: A triple-blind randomized clinical trial. *Iran Red Cresc Med J.* 20(5):e67181.

44. Ghavi F, Shakeri F. (2015). Effects of fennel on serum hormone levels in students with polycystic ovary syndrome. *Avicenna J Phytomed*. 5:42–43.
45. Takahashi K, Kitao M. (1994). Effect of TJ-68 (*shakuyaku-kanzo-to*) on polycystic ovarian disease. *Int J Fertil Menopausal Stud*. 39(2):69–76.
46. Ushiroyama T, Ikeda A, Sakai M, Hosotani T, Suzuki Y, Tsubokura S, Ueki M. (2001). Effects of *unkei-to*, an herbal medicine, on endocrine function and ovulation in women with high basal levels of luteinizing hormone secretion. *J Reprod Med*. 46(5):451–456.
47. Forouhari S, Heidari Z, Tavana Z, Salehi M, Sayadi M. (2013). The effect of soya on some hormone levels in women with polycystic ovary syndrome (balance diet): A crossover randomized clinical trial. *Bull Env Pharmacol Life Sci*. 3(1):246–250.
48. Swaroop A, Sarkari Jaipuriar A, Gupta SK, Manashi Bagchi M, Kumar P, Preuss HG, Bagchi D. (2015). Efficacy of a novel fenugreek seed extract (*Trigonella foenum-graecum*, Furocyst) in polycystic ovary syndrome (PCOS). *Int J Med Sci*. 12(10):825–831.
49. Fan CW, Cieri-Hutcherson NE, Hutcherson TC. (2021). Systematic review of black cohosh (*Cimicifuga racemosa*) for management of polycystic ovary syndrome-related infertility. *J Pharmacol Pract*. 8971900211012244.
50. Ushiroyama T, Ikeda A, Sakai M, Hosotani T, Suzuki Y, Tsubokura S, Ueki M. (2001). Effects of *unkei-to*, an herbal medicine, on endocrine function and ovulation in women with high basal levels of luteinizing hormone secretion. *J Reprod Med*. 46(5):451–456.
51. Arentz S, Smith CA, Abbott J, Fahey P, Cheema BS, Bensoussan A. (2017). Combined lifestyle and herbal medicine in overweight women with polycystic ovary syndrome (PCOS): A randomized controlled trial. *Phytotherapy Res*. 31(9):1330–1340.
52. Phipps W, Martini M, Lampe J. et al. (1993). Effect of flax seed ingestion on the menstrual cycle. *J Clin Endocrinol Metab*. 77:1215–1219.
53. Yuan HN, Wang CY, Sze CW, Tong Y, Tan QR, Feng XJ. et al. (2008). A randomized, crossover comparison of herbal medicine and bromocriptine against risperidone-induced hyperprolactinemia in patients with schizophrenia. *J Clin Psychopharmacol*. 28(3):264–370.
54. Milewicz A, Gejdel E, Sworen H, Sienkiewicz K, Jedrzejak J, Teucher T, Schmitz H. (1993). *Vitex agnus castus* extract in the treatment of luteal phase defects due to latent hyperprolactinemia. Results of a randomized placebo-controlled double-blind study. *Arzneimittelforschung*. 43(7):752–756.

55. Gerhard I, Patek A, Monga B, Blank A, Gorkow C. (1998). Mastodynon(R) bei weiblicher Sterilität. *Forsch Komplementarmed.* 5(6):272–278.
56. Eltbogen R, Litschgi M, Gasser UE, Flueeli A, Nebel S, Zahner C. (2014). *Vitex agnus-castus* extract (ZE440) improves symptoms in women with menstrual cycle irregularities. *Reprod Endocrinol.* 28:86–91.
57. Bergmann J, Luft B, Boehmann S, Runnebaum B, Gerhard I. (2000). Die wirksamkeit des komplexmittels Phyto-Hypophyson L bei weiblicher, hormonell bedingter sterilität [The efficacy of the complex medication Phyto-Hypophyson L in female, hormone-related sterility. A randomized, placebo-controlled clinical double-blind study]. *Forsch Komplementarmed Klass Naturheilkd.* 7(4):190–199.
58. Fan CW, Cieri-Hutcherson NE, Hutcherson TC. (2021). Systematic review of black cohosh (*Cimicifuga racemosa*) for management of polycystic ovary syndrome-related Infertility. *J Pharmacol Pract.* 8971900211012244.
59. Kumarapeli M, Karunagoda K, Perera PK. (2018). A randomized clinical trial to evaluate the efficacy of *Satapushpashatavari* powered drug with *Satapushpa-shatavari grita* for the management of polycystic ovary syndrome (PCOS). *Int J Pharmacol Sci Res.* 9(6):2494–2499.
60. Moini Jazani A, Nazemiyeh H, Tansaz M. et al. (2018). Celery plus anise versus metformin for the treatment of oligomenorrhea in polycystic ovary syndrome: A triple-blind randomized clinical trial. *Iran Red Cresc Med J.* 20(5):e67181.
61. Kort DH, Lobo RA. (2014). Preliminary evidence that cinnamon improves menstrual cyclicity in women with polycystic ovary syndrome: A randomized controlled trial. *Am J Obstet Gynecol.* 211(5):487.e1–487.e6.
62. Wiweko B, Susanto CA. (2017). The effect of metformin and cinnamon on serum anti-Mullerian hormone in women having PCOS: A double-blind, randomized, controlled trial. *J Hum Reprod Sci.* 10(1):31–36.
63. Hajimonfarednejad M, Nimrouzi M, Heydari M, Zarshenas MM, Raee MJ, Jahromi BN. (2018). Insulin resistance improvement by cinnamon powder in polycystic ovary syndrome: A randomized double-blind placebo controlled clinical trial. *Phytother Res.* 32(2):276–283.
64. Wang JG, Anderson RA, Graham GM III, Chu MC, Sauer MV, Guarnaccia MM. et al. (2007). The effect of cinnamon extract on insulin resistance parameters in polycystic ovary syndrome: A pilot study. *Fertil Steril.* 88(1):240–243.
65. Mokaberinejad R, Rampisheh Z, Aliasl J, Akhtari E. (2019). The comparison of fennel infusion plus dry cupping versus metformin in

management of oligomenorrhoea in patients with polycystic ovary syndrome: A randomised clinical trial. *J Obstet Gynaecol.* 39(5):652–658.
66. Mohebbi-Kian E, Mohammad-Alizadeh-Charandabi S, Bekhradi R. (2014). Efficacy of fennel and combined oral contraceptive on depot medroxyprogesterone acetate-induced amenorrhea: A randomized placebo-controlled trial. *Contraception.* 90:440–446.
67. Chen JT, Tominaga K, Sato Y, Anzai H, Matsuoka R. (2010). Maitake mushroom (*Grifola frondosa*) extract induces ovulation in patients with polycystic ovary syndrome: A possible monotherapy and a combination therapy after failure with first-line clomiphene citrate. *J Altern Comp Med.* 16(12):1295–1299.
68. Naeimi SA, Tansaz M, Sohrabvand F, Hajimehdipoor H, Nabimeybodi R, Saber S. et al. (2018). Assessing the effect of processed *Nigella sativa* on oligomenorrhea and amenorrhea in patients with polycystic ovarian syndrome: A pilot study. *Int J Pharmacol Sci Res.* 9(11):4716–4722.
69. Ushiroyama T, Ikeda A, Sakai M, Hosotani T, Suzuki Y, Tsubokura S, Ueki M. (2001). Effects of *unkei-to*, an herbal medicine, on endocrine function and ovulation in women with high basal levels of luteinizing hormone secretion. *J Reprod Med.* 46(5):451–456.
70. Ushiroyama T, Ikeda A, Higashio S, Hosotani T, Yamashita H, Yamashita Y, Suzuki Y, Ueki M. (2003). *Unkei-to* for correcting luteal phase defects. *J Reprod Med.* 48(9):729–734.
71. Yaginuma T, Isumi R, Yasui H, Arai T, Kawabata M. (1982). Effect of traditional herbal medicine on serum testosterone levels and its induction of regular ovulation in hyperandrogenic and oligomenorrheic women. *Nihon Sanka Fujinka Gakkai Zasshi.* 34(7):939–944.
72. Takahashi K, Yoshino K, Shirai T, Nishigaki A, Araki Y, Kitao M. (1988). Effect of a traditional herbal medicine (*shakuyaku-kanzo-to*) on testosterone secretion in patients with polycystic ovary syndrome detected by ultrasound. *Nihon Sanka Fujinka Gakkai Zasshi.* 40(6):789–792.
73. Tabakova P, Dimitrov M, Tashkov B. (1984). *Clinical Studies on the Preparation Tribestan in Women with Endocrine Infertility or Menopausal Syndrome.* Sofia, Bulgaria: 1st Obstetrical and Gynecological Hospital.
74. Swaroop A, Jaipuriar AS, Gupta SK, Bagchi M, Kumar P, Preuss HG, Bagchi D. (2015). Efficacy of a novel fenugreek seed extract (*Trigonella foenum-graecum*, FurocystTM) in polycystic ovary syndrome (PCOS). *Int J Med Sci.* 12(10):825–831.
75. Ghahremaninasab P, Shahnazi M, Khalili AF, Hamdi K. (2016). The effects of combined low-dose oral contraceptives and *Vitex agnus* on the

improvement of clinical and paraclinical parameters of polycystic ovarian syndrome: A triple-blind, randomized, controlled clinical trial. *Iran Red Cresc Med J*. (in press):e37510.
76. Shayan A, Masoumi SZ, Shobeiri F, Tohidi S, Khalili, A. (2016). Comparing the effects of agnugol and metformin on oligomenorrhea in patients with polycystic ovary syndrome: A randomized clinical trial. *J Clin Diag Res*. 10(12):QC13–QC16.
77. Milewicz A, Gejdel E, Sworen H, Sienkiewicz K, Jedrzejak J, Teucher T, Schmitz H. (1993). *Vitex agnus castus* extract in the treatment of luteal phase defects due to latent hyperprolactinemia. Results of a randomized placebo-controlled double-blind study. *Arzneimittelforschung*. 43(7):752–756.
78. Gerhard I, Patek A, Monga B, Blank A, Gorkow C. (1998). Mastodynon(R) bei weiblicher Sterilität. *Forsch Komplementarmed*. 5(6):272–278.
79. Eltbogen R, Litschgi M, Gasser UE, Flueeli A, Nebel S, Zahner C. (2014). *Vitex agnus-castus* extract (ZE440) improves symptoms in women with menstrual cycle irregularities. *Rep Endocrinol*. 28:86–91.
80. Bergmann J, Luft B, Boehmann S, Runnebaum B, Gerhard I. (2000). Die wirksamkeit des komplexmittels Phyto-Hypophyson L bei weiblicher, hormonell bedingter sterilität [The efficacy of the complex medication Phyto-Hypophyson L in female, hormone-related sterility. A randomized, placebo-controlled clinical double-blind study]. *Forsch Komplementarmed Klass Naturheilkd*. 7(4):190–199.
81. Arentz S, Smith CA, Abbott J, Fahey P, Cheema BS, Bensoussan A. (2017). Combined lifestyle and herbal medicine in overweight women with polycystic ovary syndrome (PCOS): A randomized controlled trial. *Phytother Res*. 31(9):1330–1340.
82. Farzana F, Sulaiman A, Ruckmani A, Vijayalakshmi K, Karunya Lakshmi G, Shri RS. (2015). Effects of flax seeds supplementation in polycystic ovarian syndrome. *J Res Med Sci*. 31(1):113–119.
83. Yaginuma T, Isumi R, Yasui H, Arai T, Kawabata M. (1982). Effect of traditional herbal medicine on serum testosterone levels and its induction of regular ovulation in hyperandrogenic and oligomenorrheic women. *Nihon Sanka Fujinka Gakkai Zasshi*. 34(7):939–944.
84. Takahashi K, Kitao M. (1994). Effect of TJ-68 (*shakuyaku-kanzo-to*) on polycystic ovarian disease. *Int J Fertil Menopausal Stud*. 39(2):69–76.
85. Abbasian Z, Jafari Barmak M, Barazesh F, Ghavamizadeh M, Mirzaei A. (2020). Therapeutic efficacy of *Trifolium pratense* L. on letrozole induced polycystic ovary syndrome in rats. *Plant Sci Today*. 7(3):501–507.

86. Maharjan R, Nagar PS, Nampoothiri L. (2010). Effect of *Aloe barbadensis* Mill. formulation on letrozole induced polycystic ovarian syndrome rat model. *J Ayurveda Integ Med*. 1(4):273–279.
87. Lee JC, Pak SC, Lee SH, Lim SC, Bai YH, Jin CS, Kim JS, Na CS, Bae CS, Oh KS. (2003). The effect of herbal medicine on nerve growth factor in estradiol valerate-induced polycystic ovaries in rats. *Am J Chin Med*. 31(6):885–895.
88. Stracquadanio M, Ciotta L, Palumbo MA. (2018). Effects of myo-inositol, gymnemic acid, and L-methylfolate in polycystic ovary syndrome patients. *Gynecol Endocrinol*. 34(6):495–501.
89. Ellingwood F. (1919). *The American Materia Medica, Therapeutics and Pharmacognosy*.
90. Ellingwood F. (1919). *The American Materia Medica, Therapeutics and Pharmacognosy*.
91. Sher G, Barnard PG. (1976). The alleviation of uterocornual spasm of the fallopian tubes during hysterosalpingography by intravenous administration of orciprenaline. *S Afr Med J*. 50(30):1164–1165.
92. Moini Jazani A, Nazemiyeh H, Tansaz M. et al. (2018). Celery plus anise versus metformin for the treatment of oligomenorrhea in polycystic ovary syndrome: A triple-blind randomized clinical trial. *Iran Red Cresc Med J*. 20(5):e67181.
93. Kumarapeli M, Karunagoda K, Perera PK. (2018). A randomized clinical trial to evaluate the efficacy of *Satapushpashatavari* powered drug with *Satapushpa-shatavari grita* for the management of polycystic ovary syndrome (PCOS). *Int J Pharmacol Sci Res*. 9(6):2494–2499.
94. Wei W, Zhao H, Wang A, Sui M, Liang K, Deng H, Ma Y, Zhang Y, Zhang H, Guan Y. (2012). A clinical study on the short-term effect of berberine in comparison to metformin on the metabolic characteristics of women with polycystic ovary syndrome. *Eur J Endocrinol*. 166(1):99–105.
95. Mokaberinejad R, Rampisheh Z, Aliasl J, Akhtari E. (2019). The comparison of fennel infusion plus dry cupping versus metformin in management of oligomenorrhoea in patients with polycystic ovary syndrome: A randomised clinical trial. *J Obstet Gynaecol*. 39(5):652–658.
96. Mohebbi-Kian E, Mohammad-Alizadeh-Charandabi S, Bekhradi R. (2014). Efficacy of fennel and combined oral contraceptive on depot medroxyprogesterone acetate-induced amenorrhea: A randomized placebo-controlled trial. *Contraception*. 90:440–446.
97. Kort DH, Lobo RA. (2014). Preliminary evidence that cinnamon improves menstrual cyclicity in women with polycystic ovary syndrome: A randomized controlled trial. *Am J Obstet Gynecol*. 211(5):487.e1–487.e6.

98. Allen RW, Schwartzman E, Baker WL. et al. (2013). Cinnamon use in type 2 diabetes: An updated systematic review and meta-analysis. *Ann Fam Med.* 11(5):452–459.
99. Wiweko B, Susanto CA. (2017). The effect of metformin and cinnamon on serum anti-Mullerian hormone in women having PCOS: A double-blind, randomized, controlled trial. *J Hum Reprod Sci.* 10(1):31–36.
100. Hajimonfarednejad M, Nimrouzi M, Heydari M, Zarshenas MM, Raee MJ, Jahromi BN. (2018). Insulin resistance improvement by cinnamon powder in polycystic ovary syndrome: A randomized double-blind placebo controlled clinical trial. *Phytother Res.* 32(2):276–283.
101. Wang JG, Anderson RA, Graham GM III, Chu MC, Sauer MV, Guarnaccia MM. et al. (2007). The effect of cinnamon extract on insulin resistance parameters in polycystic ovary syndrome: A pilot study. *Fertil Steril.* 88(1):240–243.
102. Xu J, Bishop CV, Lawson MS, Park BS, Xu F. (2016). Anti-Müllerian hormone promotes pre-antral follicle growth, but inhibits antral follicle maturation and dominant follicle selection in primates. *Hum Reprod.* 31(7):1522–1530.
103. Ushiroyama T, Ikeda A, Higashio S, Hosotani T, Yamashita H, Yamashita Y, Suzuki Y, Ueki M. (2003). *Unkei-to* for correcting luteal phase defects. *J Reprod Med.* 48(9):729–734.
104. Ushiroyama T, Ikeda A, Sakai M, Hosotani T, Suzuki Y, Tsubokura S, Ueki M. (2001). Effects of *unkei-to*, an herbal medicine, on endocrine function and ovulation in women with high basal levels of luteinizing hormone secretion. *J Reprod Med.* 46(5):451–456.
105. Yuan HN, Wang CY, Sze CW, Tong Y, Tan QR, Feng XJ. et al. (2008). A randomized, crossover comparison of herbal medicine and bromocriptine against risperidone-induced hyperprolactinemia in patients with schizophrenia. *J Clin Psychopharmacol.* 28(3):264–370.
106. Yamada K, Kanba S, Yagi G, Asai M. (1999). Herbal medicine (*skakuyaku-kanzo-to*) in the treatment of risperidone-induced amenorrhea. *J Clin Psychopharmacol.* 19:380–381.
107. Man SC, Li XB, Wang HH, Yuan HN, Wang HN, Zhang RG. et al. (2016). Peony-glycyrrhiza decoction for antipsychotic-related hyperprolactinemia in women with schizophrenia: A randomized controlled trial. *J Clin Psychopharmacol.* 36(6):572–579.
108. Aboraya A, Fullen JE, Ponieman BL, Makela EH, Latocha M. (2004). Hyperprolactinemia associated with risperidone. A case report and review of literature. *Psychiatry* (Edgmont). 1(3):29–31.

109. Yang P, Li L, Yang D, Wang C, Peng H, Huang H. et al. (2017). Effect of peony-glycyrrhiza decoction on amisulpride-induced hyperprolactinemia in women with schizophrenia: A preliminary study. *Evid Based Comp Alternat Med*. 7901670.
110. Yaginuma T, Izumi R, Yasui H, Arai T, Kawabata M. (1982). Effect of traditional herbal medicine on serum testosterone levels and its induction of regular ovulation in hyperandrogenic and oligomenorrheic women. *Nihon Sanka Fujinka Gakkai Zasshi*. 34(7):939–944.
111. Takahashi K, Yoshino K, Shirai T, Nishigaki A, Araki Y, Kitao M. (1988). Effects of traditional medicine (*Shakuyaku-kanzo-to*) on testosterone secretion in patients with polycystic ovarian syndrome detected by ultrasound. *Nihon Sanka Fujinka Gakkai Zasshi*. 40(6):789–792.
112. Takahashi K, Kitao M. (1994). Effect of TJ-68 (*shakuyaku-kanzo-to*) on polycystic ovarian disease. *Int J Fertil Menopausal Stud*. 39(2):69.
113. Chen JT, Tominaga K, Sato Y, Anzai H, Matsuoka R. (2010). Maitake mushroom (*Grifola frondosa*) extract induces ovulation in patients with polycystic ovary syndrome: A possible monotherapy and a combination therapy after failure with first-line clomiphene citrate. *J Altern Comp Med*. 16(12):1295–1299.
114. Elgoly AHM, Wahman LF, Yousef MH. (2018). Can *Panax ginseng* protect against fertility disorders in hypothyroid female albino rats? *Cell Mol Biol* (Noisy-le-grand). 64(13):97–102.
115. Bo Hyon Y, Young Sik C, SiHyun C, Byung Seok L, Si Kwan K, Seok Kyo S. (2018). Effects of ginseng on fertility. *Biomed J Sci &Tech Res*. 11(1).
116. Brown RP, Gerbarg PL, Ramazanov Z. (2002), *Rhodiola rosea*: A phytomedicinal overview. *Herbalgram* 56:40–52.
117. Gerasimova H. (1970). Effect of *Rhodiola rosea* extract on ovarian functional activity. *Proc Scientific Conference on Endocrinology and Gynecology*, Sverdlovsk, Russia: Siberian Branch of the Russian Academy of Sciences, pp. 46–48.
118. Taher MA, Atia YA, Amin MK. (2012). Improving an ovulation rate in women with polycystic ovary syndrome by using silymarin. *J Res Med Sci*. 12:1–8.
119. Tabakova P, Dimitrov M, Tashkov B. (1984). *Clinical Studies on the Preparation Tribestan in Women with Endocrine Infertility or Menopausal Syndrome*. Sofia, Bulgaria: 1st Obstetrical and Gynecological Hospital.
120. Milanov S, Maleeva A, Tashkov M. (1981). Tribestan effect on the concentration of some hormones in the serum of healthy subjects. *Chemical Pharmaceutical Research Institute*. Sofia, Bulgaria.

121. Arentz S, Smith CA, Abbott J, Fahey P, Cheema BS, Bensoussan A. (2017). Combined lifestyle and herbal medicine in overweight women with polycystic ovary syndrome (PCOS): A randomized controlled trial. *Phytother Res.* 31(9):1330–1340.
122. Swaroop A, Sarkari Jaipuriar A, Gupta SK, Manashi Bagchi M, Kumar P, Preuss HG, Bagchi D. (2015). Efficacy of a novel fenugreek seed extract (*Trigonella foenum-graecum*, Furocyst) in polycystic ovary syndrome (PCOS). *Int J Med Sci.* 12(10):825–831.
123. Bashtian MH, Emami SA, Mousavifar N, Esmaily HA, Mahmoudi M, Poor AHM. (2013). Evaluation of fenugreek (*Trigonella foenum-graceum* L.), effects seeds extract on insulin resistance in women with polycystic ovarian syndrome. *Iran J Pharm Res.* 12(2):475–481.
124. Mastroiacovo P, Leoncini E. (2011). More folic acid, the five questions: Why, who, when, how much, and how. *Biofactors.* 37(4):272–279.
125. Stephenson J, Heslehurst N, Hall J, Schoenaker DAJM. et al. (2018). Before the beginning: Nutrition and lifestyle in the preconception period and its importance for future health. *Lancet.* 391(10132):1830–1841.
126. Jauniaux E, Watson AL, Hempstock J, Bao Y, Skepper JN, Burton GJ. (2000). Onset of maternal arterial blood flow and placental oxidative stress: A possible factor in human early pregnancy failure. *Am J Pathol.* 157:2111–2122.
127. Turcksin R, Bel S, Galjaard S, Devlieger R. (2014). Maternal obesity and breastfeeding intention, initiation, intensity and duration: A systematic review. *Matern Child Nutr.* 10(2):166–183.
128. Kort HI, Massey JB, Elsner CW, Mitchell-Leef D. et al. (2006). Impact of body mass index values on sperm quantity and quality. *J Androl.* 27(3):450–452.
129. Schummers L, Hutcheon JA, Bodnar LM, Lieberman E, Himes KP. (2015). Risk of adverse pregnancy outcomes by prepregnancy body mass index: A population-based study to inform prepregnancy weight loss counseling. *Obstet Gynecol.* 125(1):133–143.
130. Zhang C, Solomon CG, Manson JE, Hu FB. (2006). A prospective study of pregravid physical activity and sedentary behaviors in relation to the risk for gestational diabetes mellitus. *Arch Intern Med.* 166(5):543–548.
131. Gaskins AJ, Chavarro JE. (2018). Diet and fertility: A review. *Am J Obstet Gynecol.* 218(4):379–389.
132. Chavarro JE, Rich-Edwards JW, Rosner BA, Willett WC. (2008). Protein intake and ovulatory infertility. *Am J Obstet Gynecol.* 198(2):210.e1–210.e2107.

133. Vujkovic M, de Vries JH, Lindemans J, Macklon NS. et al. (2010). The preconception Mediterranean dietary pattern in couples undergoing in vitro fertilization/intracytoplasmic sperm injection treatment increases the chance of pregnancy. *Fertil Steril*. 94(6):2096–2101.
134. Toledo E, Lopez-del Burgo C, Ruiz-Zambrana A, Donazar M. et al. (2011). Dietary patterns and difficulty conceiving: A nested case-control study. *Fertil Steril*. 96(5):1149–1153.
135. Twigt JM, Bolhuis ME, Steegers EA. et al. (2012). The preconception diet is associated with the chance of ongoing pregnancy in women undergoing IVF/ICSI treatment. *Hum Reprod*. 27:2526–2531.
136. Chavarro JE, Rich-Edwards JW, Rosner BA, Willett WC. (2007). A prospective study of dairy foods intake and anovulatory infertility. *Human Reprod*. 22(5):1340–1347.
137. Chavarro JE, Rich-Edwards JW, Rosner BA, Willett WC. (2008). Use of multivitamins, intake of B vitamins, and risk of ovulatory infertility. *Fertil Steril*. 89(3):668–676.
138. Westphal LM, Polan ML, Trant AS, Mooney SB. (2004). A nutritional supplement for improving fertility in women: A pilot study. *J Reprod Med*. 49:289–293.
139. Rumiris D, Purwosunu Y, Wibowo N, Farina A, Sekizawa A. (2006). Lower rate of preeclampsia after antioxidant supplementation in pregnant women with low antioxidant status. *Hypertens Pregnancy*. 25:241–253.
140. Fares S, Sethom MM, Khouaja-Mokrani C, Jabnoun S, Feki M, Kaabachi N. (2014). Vitamin A, E, and D deficiencies in Tunisian very low birth weight neonates: Prevalence and risk factors. *Pediatr Neonatol*. 55:196–201.
141. Mumford SL, Sundaram R, Schisterman EF. et al. (2014). Higher urinary lignan concentrations in women but not men are positively associated with shorter time to pregnancy. *J Nutr*. 144:352–358.
142. Unfer V, Casini ML, Gerli S, Costabile L, Mignosa M, Di Renzo GC. (2004). Phytoestrogens may improve the pregnancy rate in in vitro fertilization-embryo transfer cycles: A prospective, controlled, randomized trial. *Fertil Steril*. 82:1509–1513.
143. Al-Gubory KH. (2014). Environmental pollutants and lifestyle factors induce oxidative stress and poor prenatal development. *Reprod Biomed Online*. 29:17–31.
144. Wigle DT, Arbuckle TE, Turner MC, Bérubé A, Yang Q, Liu S, Krewski D. (2008). Epidemiologic evidence of relationships between

reproductive and child health outcomes and environmental chemical contaminants. *J Toxicol Environ Health B Crit Rev.* 11:373–517.
145. Abadia L, Chiu YH, Williams PL, Toth TL. et al. (2017). The association between pre-treatment maternal alcohol and caffeine intake and outcomes of assisted reproduction in a prospectively followed cohort. *Hum Reprod.* 32(9):1846–1854.
146. Greenwood DC, Thatcher NJ, Ye J, Garrard L. et al. Caffeine intake during pregnancy and adverse birth outcomes: A systematic review and dose-response meta-analysis. *Eur J Epidemiol.* 29(10):725–734.
147. Sharma R, Biedenharn KR, Fedor JM, Agarwal A. (2013). Lifestyle factors and reproductive health: Taking control of your fertility. *Reprod Biol Endocrinol.* 11:66.
148. Mohd Mutalip SS, Ab-Rahim S, Rajikin MH. (2018). Vitamin E as an antioxidant in female reproductive health. *Antioxidants* (Basel). 7(2):22.
149. Rostami K, Steegers EA, Wong WY, Braat DD, Steegers-Theunissen RP. (2001). Coeliac disease and reproductive disorders: A neglected association. *Eur J Obstet Gynecol Reprod Biol.* 96:146–149.
150. Kuscu NK, Akcali S, Kucukmetin NT. (2002). Celiac disease and polycystic ovary syndrome. *Int J Gynaecol Obstet.* 79:149–150.
Stephansson O, Falconer H, Ludvigsson JF. (2011). Risk of endometriosis in 11,000 women with celiac disease. *Hum Reprod.* 26:2896–2901.
151. Lasa JS, Zubiaurre I, Soifer LO. (2014). Risk of infertility in patients with celiac disease: A meta-analysis of observational studies. *Arq Gastroenterol.* 51(2):144–150.
152. Chavarro JE, Rich-Edwards JW, Rosner BA, Willett WC. (2007). Diet and lifestyle in the prevention of ovulatory disorder infertility. *Obstet Gynecol.* 110:1050–1058.
153. Battaglia C, Salvatori M, Maxia N, Petraglia F, Facchinetti F, Volpe A. (1999). Adjuvant L-arginine treatment for in-vitro fertilization in poor responder patients. *Hum Reprod.* 14(7):1690–1697.
154. Hofmeyr GJ, Manyame S, Medley N, Williams MJ. (2019). Calcium supplementation commencing before or early in pregnancy, for preventing hypertensive disorders of pregnancy. *Cochrane Database Syst Rev.* 9(9):CD011192.
155. Pravst I, Zmitek K, Zmitek J. (2010). Coenzyme Q10 contents in foods and fortification strategies. *Crit Rev Food Sci Nutr.* 50(4):269–280.
156. Xu Y, Nisenblat V, Lu C, Li R, Qiao J, Zhen X, Wang S. (2018). Pre-treatment with coenzyme Q10 improves ovarian response and embryo

quality in low-prognosis young women with decreased ovarian reserve: A randomized controlled trial. *Reprod Biol Endocrinol.* 16(1):29.
157. Haggarty P, McCallum H, McBain H, Andrews K. et al. (2006). Effect of B vitamins and genetics on success of in-vitro fertilisation: Prospective cohort study. *Lancet.* 367(9521):1513–1519.
158. He Y, Pan A, Hu FB, Ma X. (2016). Folic acid supplementation, birth defects, and adverse pregnancy outcomes in Chinese women: A population-based mega-cohort study. *Lancet.* 388:S91.
159. Hahn KA, Wesselink AK, Wise LA, Mikkelsen EM. et al. (2019). Iron consumption Is not consistently associated with fecundability among North American and Danish pregnancy planners. *J Nutr.* 149(9):1585–1595.
160. Agarwal A, Sengupta P, Durairajanayagam D. (2018). Role of L-carnitine in female infertility. *Reprod Biol Endocrinol.* 16(1):5.
161. Zarean E, Tarjan A. (2017). Effect of magnesium supplement on pregnancy outcomes: A randomized control trial. *Adv Biomed Res.* 6:109.
162. Espino J, Macedo M, Lozano G, Ortiz Á. et al. (2019). Impact of melatonin supplementation in women with unexplained infertility undergoing fertility treatment. *Antioxidants* (Basel). 8(9):338.
163. Younis M, Mahasneh A. (2020). Probiotics and the envisaged role in treating human infertility. *Middle East Fert Soc J.* 25(33).
164. Sirota I, Zarek SM, Segars JH. (2014). Potential influence of the microbiome on infertility and assisted reproductive technology. *Semin Reprod Med.* 32(1):35–42.
165. Mistry HD, Broughton Pipkin F, Redman CW, Poston L. (2012). Selenium in reproductive health. *Am J Obstet Gynecol.* 206(1):21–30.
166. Pieczyńska J, Grajeta H. (2015). The role of selenium in human conception and pregnancy. *J Trace Elem Med Biol.* 29:31–38.
167. Clagett-Dame M, Knutson D. (2011). Vitamin A in reproduction and development. *Nutrients.* 3(4):385–428.

Chapter 5: Vaginal discharge

1. Nasioudis D, Beghini J, Bongiovanni AM, Giraldo PC, Linhares IM, Witkin SS. (2015). α-amylase in vaginal fluid: Association with conditions favorable to dominance of lactobacillus. *Reprod Sci.* 22(11):1393–1398.
2. Al-Ghazzewi FH, Tester RF. (2016). Biotherapeutic agents and vaginal health. *J Appl Microbiol.* 121(1):18–27.
3. Allsworth JE. (2010). Bacterial vaginosis-race and sexual transmission: Issues of causation. *Sex Transm Dis.* 37(3):137–139.

4. Verstraelen H, Verhelst R. (2009). Bacterial vaginosis: An update on diagnosis and treatment. *Expert Rev Anti Infect Ther.* 7(9):1109–1124.
5. Stapleton A.E, Au-Yeung M, Hooton TM, Fredricks DN. et al. (2011). Randomized, placebo-controlled phase 2 trial of a *Lactobacillus crispatus* probiotic given intravaginally for prevention of recurrent urinary tract infection. *Clin Infec Dis.* 52:1212–1217.
6. Koumans EH, Sternberg M, Bruce C, McQuillan G, Kendrick J, Sutton M. et al. (2007). The prevalence of bacterial vaginosis in the United States, 2001–2004; associations with symptoms, sexual behaviors, and reproductive health. *Sex Transm Dis.* 34(11):864–869.
7. Al-Aali KY. (2015). Prevalence of vaginal candidiasis among pregnant women attending Al-Hada Military Hospital, Western Region, Taif, Saudi Arabia. *Int J Sci Res.* 4(5):1736–1743.
8. Berman S, Markowitz L. (2007). The prevalence of *Trichomonas vaginalis* infection among reproductive-age women in the United States, 2001–2004. *Clin Infect Dis.* 45(10):1319–1326.
9. Centers for Disease Control and Prevention. (2010). *Bacterial Vaginosis Statistics.* Available from: http://www.cdc.gov/std/bv/stats.htm.
10. Allsworth JE. (2010). Bacterial vaginosis-race and sexual transmission: Issues of causation. *Sex Transm Dis.* 37(3):137–139.
11. Verstraelen H, Verhelst R. (2009). Bacterial vaginosis: An update on diagnosis and treatment. *Expert Rev Anti Infect Ther.* 7(9):1109–1124.
12. Swidsinski A, Verstraelen H, Loening-Baucke V, Swidsinski S, Mendling W, Halwani Z. (2013). Presence of a polymicrobial endometrial biofilm in patients with bacterial vaginosis. *PLoS One.* 8(1):e53997.
13. Masoudi M, Kopaei MR, Miraj S. (2016). Comparison between the efficacy of metronidazole vaginal gel and Berberis vulgaris (*Berberis vulgaris*) combined with metronidazole gel alone in the treatment of bacterial vaginosis. *Electron Physician.* 8:2818–2827.
14. Masoudi M, Kopaei MR, Miraj S. (2016). Comparison between the efficacy of metronidazole vaginal gel and Berberis vulgaris (*Berberis vulgaris*) combined with metronidazole gel alone in the treatment of bacterial vaginosis. *Electron Physician.* 8:2818–2827.
15. Sabbatini S, Monari C, Ballet N, Mosci P. et al. (2018). Saccharomyces cerevisiae-based probiotic as novel anti-microbial agent for therapy of bacterial vaginosis. *Virulence.* 9:954–966.
16. Allsworth JE. (2010). Bacterial vaginosis-race and sexual transmission: Issues of causation. *Sex Transm Dis.* 37(3):137–139.

17. DeCherney AH, Nathan L, Goodwin TM, Laufer N. (2013). *Current Diagnosis & Treatment Obstetrics & Gynecology*. Boston: McGraw-Hill Education, p. 398.
18. Verstraelen H, Verhelst R, Roelens K, Temmerman M. (2012). Antiseptics and disinfectants for the treatment of bacterial vaginosis: A systematic review. *BMC Infect Dis*. 12:148.
19. Baery N, Ghasemi Nejad A, Amin M, Mahroozade S. et al. (2018). Effect of vaginal suppository on bacterial vaginitis based on Persian medicine (Iranian traditional medicine): A randomised double blind clinical study. *J Obstet Gynaecol*. 38(8):1110–1114.
20. Riggs M, Klebanoff M, Nansel T, Zhang J, Schwebke J, Andrews W. (2007). Longitudinal association between hormonal contraceptives and bacterial vaginosis in women of reproductive age. *Sex Transm Dis*. 34(12):954–959.
21. Bradshaw CS, Pirotta M, De Guingand D, Hocking JS. et al. (2012). Efficacy of oral metronidazole with vaginal clindamycin or vaginal probiotic for bacterial vaginosis: Randomised placebo-controlled double-blind trial. *PLoS One*. 7(4):e34540.
22. McDonald HM, Brocklehurst P, Gordon A. (2007). Antibiotics for treating bacterial vaginosis in pregnancy. *Cochrane Database Syst Rev*. (1):CD000262.
23. Roberts CL, Richard K, Kotsiou G, Morris JM. (2011). Treatment of asymptomatic vaginal candidiasis in pregnancy to prevent preterm birth: An open-label pilot randomized controlled trial. *BMC Pregnancy and Childbirth*. 11:18.
24. Van Gerwen OT, Camino AF, Sharma J, Kissinger PJ, Muzny CA. (2021). Epidemiology, natural history, diagnosis, and treatment of *Trichomonas vaginalis* in men. *Clin Infect Dis*. 73(6):1119–1124.
25. Krieger J, Alderete M. (1999). *Trichomonas vaginalis* and trichomonaiasis. In: Holmes K, Sparling F, Lemon S. et al. (eds), *Sexually Transmitted Diseases*, 3rd ed. New York: McGraw-Hill, pp. 587–604.
26. El-Sherbiny GM, El Sherbiny ET. (2011). The effect of *Commiphora molmol* (myrrh) in treatment of *Trichomoniasis vaginalis* infection. *Iran Red Cresc Med J*. 13(7):480–486.
27. el-Shazly AM, Morsy TA, Dawoud HA. (2004). Human *Monisziasis expansa*: The first Egyptian parasitic zoonosis. *J Egypt Soc Parasitol*. 34(2):515–518.
28. Schwebke JR. (2002). Cost effective screening for trichomoniasis. *Emerg Infect Dis*. 8:749; author reply 749–750.

29. Silver BJ, Guy RJ, Kaldor JM, Jamil MS, Rumbold AR. (2014). *Trichomonas vaginalis* as a cause of perinatal morbidity: A systematic review and meta-analysis. *Sex Transm Dis.* 41(6):369–376.
30. Meri T, Jokiranta TS, Suhonen L, Meri S. (2000). Resistance of *Trichomonas vaginalis* to metronidazole: Report of the first three cases from Finland and optimization of in vitro susceptibility testing under various oxygen concentrations. *J Clin Microbiol.* 38(2):763–767.
31. Gülmezoglu AM, Azhar M. (2011). Interventions for trichomoniasis in pregnancy. *Cochrane Database Syst Rev.* (5):CD000220.
32. Klebanoff MA, Carey JC, Hauth JC, Hillier SL. et al. (2001). National Institute of Child Health and Human Development Network of Maternal-Fetal Medicine Units. Failure of metronidazole to prevent preterm delivery among pregnant women with asymptomatic *Trichomonas vaginalis* infection. *N Engl J Med.* 345(7):487–493.
33. Wang Y, Zhang Y, Zhang Q, Chen H, Feng Y. (2018). Characterization of pelvic and cervical microbiotas from patients with pelvic inflammatory disease. *J Med Microbiol.* 67(10):1519–1526.
34. Ross J, Guaschino S, Cusini M, Jensen J. (2018). 2017 European guideline for the management of pelvic inflammatory disease. *Int J STD AIDS.* 29(2):108–114.
35. Jin BB, Gong YZ, Ma Y, He ZH. (2018). Gynecological emergency ultrasound in daytime and at night: Differences that cannot be ignored. *Ther Clin Risk Manag.* 14:1141–1147.
36. Das BB, Ronda J, Trent M. (2016). Pelvic inflammatory disease: Improving awareness, prevention, and treatment. *Infect Drug Resist.* 9:191–197.
37. Brotman RM, Klebanoff MA, Nansel TR, Andrews WW. et al. (2008). A longitudinal study of vaginal douching and bacterial vaginosis—a marginal structural modeling analysis. *Am J Epidemiol.* 168(2):188–196.
38. Brotman RM, Klebanoff MA, Nansel TR, Andrews WW. et al. (2008). A longitudinal study of vaginal douching and bacterial vaginosis—a marginal structural modeling analysis. *Am J Epidemiol.* 168(2):188–196.
39. Ibrahim AN. (2013). Comparison of in vitro activity of metronidazole and garlic-based product (Tomex(R)) on *Trichomonas vaginalis*. *Parasitol Res.* 112(5):2063–2067.
40. Joe MM, Jayachitra J, Vijayapriya M. (2009). Antimicrobial activity of some common spices against certain human pathogens. *J Med Plant Res.* 3(11):1134–1136.
41. Arbabi M, Delavari M, Fakhrieh Kashan Z, Taghizadeh M, Hooshyar H. (2016). Ginger (*Zingiber officinale*) induces apoptosis in *Trichomonas vaginalis* in vitro. *Int J Reprod Biomed.* 14(11):691–698.

42. Ibrahim AN. (2013). Comparison of in vitro activity of metronidazole and garlic-based product (Tomex(R)) on *Trichomonas vaginalis*. *Parasitol Res.* 112(5):2063–2067.
43. Hafizi MM, Doulatian M, Naghash A, Moatar F, Alavimajd H. (2010). The comparison of the effects of micosin vaginal cream (made of garlic) and metroniazole vaginal gel on treatment of bacterial vaginosis. *Arak Med Uni J.* 13(3):35–44.
44. Kordi M, Jahangiri N, Rakhshandeh H, Gholami H. (2005). Comparison of the effect of garlic extract vaginal douche and clotrimazol vaginal cream in the treatment of women with vaginal candidiasis. *Iran J Obestet Gynecol Infertil.* 8(2):33–40 (in Persian).
45. Bahadoran P, Rokni FK, Fahami F. (2011). Investigating the therapeutic effect of vaginal cream containing garlic and thyme compared to clotrimazole cream for the treatment of mycotic vaginitis. *Iran J Nurs Midwifery Res.* 15(Suppl. 1):343–349.
46. Brinker FJ. (1995). *Eclectic Dispensatory of Botanical Therapeutics*, vol. 2, sect. 1: *Native Healing Gifts*. Sandy: Eclectic Medical Publications, pp. 19–23.
47. Felter HW, Lloyd JU. (1898). *King's American Dispensatory*.
48. Ellingwood F. (1919). *The American Materia Medica, Therapeutics and Pharmacognosy*.
49. Cook W. (1869). *The Physio-medical Dispensatory*.
50. Bigelow J. (1817–1821). *American Medical Botany*.
51. Siegers C, Bodinet C, Ali SS, Siegers CP. (2003). Bacterial deconjugation of arbutin by *Escherichia coli*. *Phytomed.* 10(Suppl. 4):58–60.
52. Holopainen M, Jabodar L, Seppanen-Laakso T. et al. (1988). Antimicrobial activity of some Finnish ericaceous plants. *Acta Pharmacol Fenn.* 97(4):197–202.
53. Efstratiou E, Hussain AI, Nigam PS, Moore JE, Ayub MA, Rao JR. (2012). Antimicrobial activity of *Calendula officinalis* petal extracts against fungi, as well as Gram-negative and Gram-positive clinical pathogens. *Complement Ther Clin Pract.* 18(3):173–176.
54. Roopashree TS, Dang R, Shobha Rani RH, Narendra C. (2008). Antibacterial activity of antipsoriatic herbs: *Cassia tora, Momordica charantia* and *Calendula officinalis*. *Int J Appl Res Nat Prod.* 1:20–28.
55. Pazhohideh Z, Mohammadi S, Bahrami N, Mojab F, Abedi P, Maraghi, E. (2018). The effect of *Calendula officinalis* versus metronidazole on bacterial vaginosis in women: A double-blind randomized controlled trial. *J Adv Pharmacol Tech Res.* 9(1):15–19.
56. Saffari E, Mohammad-Alizadeh-Charandabi S, Adibpour M, Mirghafourvand M, Javadzadeh Y. (2017). Comparing the effects of

Calendula officinalis and clotrimazole on vaginal candidiasis: A randomized controlled trial. *Women & Health.* 57(10):1145–1160.
57. Naser B, Lund B, Henneicke-von Zepelin HH, Köhler G, Lehmacher W, Scaglione F. (2005). A randomized, double-blind, placebo-controlled, clinical dose-response trial of an extract of *Baptisia*, *Echinacea* and *Thuja* for the treatment of patients with common cold. *Phytomed.* 12(10):715–722.
58. Reitz HD, Hergarten H. (1990). Immunmodulatoren mit pflanzlichen Wirkstoffen–2. Teil: eine wissenschaftliche Studie am Beispiel Esberitox® N. *Notabene Medici.* 20:304–306, 362–366.
59. Zimmer M. (1985). Gezielte konservative Therapie der akuten Sinusitis in der HNO-Praxis. *Therapiewoche.* 35:4024–4028.
60. Felter HW, Lloyd JU. (1898). *King's American Dispensatory.*
61. Cech NB, Junio HA, Ackermann LW, Kavanaugh JS, Horswill AR. (2012). Quorum quenching and antimicrobial activity of goldenseal (*Hydrastis canadensis*) against methicillin-resistant Staphylococcus aureus (MRSA). *Planta Med.* 78(14):1556–1561.
62. Han Y, Lee JH. (2005). Berberine synergy with amphotericin B against disseminated candidiasis in mice. *Biol Pharmacol Bull.* 28(3):541–544.
63. Soffar SA, Metwali DM, Abdel-Aziz SS, el-Wakil HS, Saad GA. (2001). Evaluation of the effect of a plant alkaloid (berberine derived from *Berberis aristata*) on *Trichomonas vaginalis* in vitro. *J Egypt Soc Parasitol.* 31(3):893–904.
64. Han Y, Lee JH. (2005). Berberine synergy with amphotericin B against disseminated candidiasis in mice. *Biol Pharmacol Bull.* 28(3):541–544.
65. Masoudi M, Kopaei MR, Miraj S. (2016). Comparison between the efficacy of metronidazole vaginal gel and Berberis vulgaris (*Berberis vulgaris*) combined with metronidazole gel alone in the treatment of bacterial vaginosis. *Electronic Physician.* 8(8):2818–2827.
66. Di Vito M, Mattarelli P, Modesto M, Girolamo A. et al. (2015). In vitro activity of tea tree oil vaginal Suppositories against *Candida* spp. and probiotic vaginal microbiota. *Phytother Res.* 29(10):1628–1633.
67. Mertas A, Garbusińska A, Szliszka E, Jureczko A, Kowalska M, Król W. (2015). The influence of tea tree oil (*Melaleuca alternifolia*) on fluconazole activity against fluconazole-resistant *Candida albicans* strains. *BioMed Res Int.* 590470.
68. Di Vito M, Fracchiolla G, Mattarelli P, Modesto M, Tamburro A. et al. (2016). Probiotic and tea tree oil treatments improve therapy of vaginal candidiasis: A preliminary clinical study. *Med J Obstet Gynecol.* 4(4):1090.

69. Cook W. (1869). *The Physio-medical Dispensatory.*
70. Felter HW, Lloyd JU. (1890). *King's American Dispensatory.*
71. Viollon C, Chaumont JP. (1994). Antifungal properties of essential oils and their main components upon *Cryptococcus neoformans. Mycopathologia.* 128(3):151–153.
72. Didry N, Dubreuil L, Pinkas M. (1993). Activité antibactérienne du thymol, du carvacrol et de l'aldéhyde cinnamique seuls ou associés [Antibacterial activity of thymol, carvacrol and cinnamaldehyde alone or in combination]. *Pharmazie.* 48(4):301–304.
73. Tabak M, Armon R, Potasman I, Neeman I. (1996). In vitro inhibition of *Helicobacter pylori* by extracts of thyme. *J Appl Bacteriol.* 80(6):667–672.
74. Yassin MT, Abdel-Fattah Mostafa A, Al-Askar AA, Shaban RM, Sayed SRM. (2022). In vitro antimicrobial activity of *Thymus vulgaris* extracts against some nosocomial and food poisoning bacterial strains. *Process Biochem.* 115:152–159.
75. Khan K, Shah R, Gautam M, Patil S. (2007). Clue cells. *Indian J Sex Transm Dis.* 28(2):1085.
76. Braga PC, Dal Sasso M, Culici M, Spallino A. (2010). Inhibitory activity of thymol on native and mature *Gardnerella vaginalis* biofilms: In vitro study. *Arzneimittelforschung.* 60(11):675–681.
77. Jafri H, Ahmad I. (2020). *Thymus vulgaris* essential oil and thymol inhibit biofilms and interact synergistically with antifungal drugs against drug resistant strains of *Candida albicans* and *Candida tropicalis. Journal de Mycologie Médicale.* 30(1):100911.
78. Fouladi Z, Afshari P, Gharibi T, Dabbagh MA. (2009). The comparison of *Zataria multiflora* boiss (Avishan Shirazi) and clotrimazol vaginal cream in the treatment of candidiasis vaginitis. *Iran South Med J.* 12(3):214–224.
79. Bahadoran P, Rokni FK, Fahami F. (2011). Investigating the therapeutic effect of vaginal cream containing garlic and thyme compared to clotrimazole cream for the treatment of mycotic vaginitis. *Iran J Nurs Midwifery Res.* 15(Suppl. 1):343–349.
80. Murina F, Vicariotto F, Di Francesco S. (2018). Thymol, eugenol and lactobacilli in a medical device for the treatment of bacterial vaginosis and vulvovaginal candidiasis. *New Microbiol.* 41(3):220–224.
81. Kohlert C, Schindler G, März RW, Abel G. et al. (2002). Systemic availability and pharmacokinetics of thymol in humans. *J Clin Pharmacol.* 42(7):731–737.
82. Takada M, Agata I, Sakamoto M, Yagi N, Hayashi N. (1979). On the metabolic detoxication to thymol in rabbit and man. *J Toxicol Sci.* 4:341–350.

83. Zhou Y, Xu W, Hong K, Li H, Zhang J, Chen X. et al. (2019). Therapeutic effects of probiotic *Clostridium butyricum* WZ001 on bacterial vaginosis in mice. *J Appl Microbiol*. 127:565–575.
84. Sabbatini S, Monari C, Ballet N, Mosci P, Decherf AC, Pélerin F. et al. (2018). *Saccharomyces cerevisiae*-based probiotic as novel antimicrobial agent for therapy of bacterial vaginosis. *Virulence*. 9:954–966.
85. Jang SJ, Lee K, Kwon B, You HJ, Ko G. (2019). Vaginal lactobacilli inhibit growth and hyphae formation of *Candida albicans*. *Sci Rep*. 9(1):8121.
86. Neri A, Sabah G, Samra Z. (1993). Bacterial vaginosis in pregnancy treated with yoghurt. *Acta Obstet Gynecol Scand*. 72(1):17–19.
87. Chimura T, Funayama T, Murayama K, Numazaki M. (1995). Ecological treatment of bacterial vaginosis. *Jpn J Antibiot*. 48(3):432–436. In Japanese.
88. Vujic G, Jajac Knez A, Despot Stefanovic V, Kuzmic Vrbanovic V. (2013). Efficacy of orally applied probiotic capsules for bacterial vaginosis and other vaginal infections: A double-blind, randomized, placebo-controlled study. *Eur J Obstet Gynecol Reprod Biol*. 168(1):75–79.
89. Wang Z, He Y, Zheng Y. (2019). Probiotics for the treatment of bacterial vaginosis: A meta-analysis. *Int J Environ Res Public Health*. 16(20):3859.
90. Falagas ME, Betsi GI, Athanasiou S. (2006). Probiotics for prevention of recurrent vulvovaginal candidiasis: A review. *J Antimicrob Chemother*. 58(2):266–272.
91. Zakeri S, Esmaeilzadeh S, Gorji N, Memariani Z, Moeini R, Bijani A. (2020). The effect of *Achillea millefolium* L. on vulvovaginal candidiasis compared with clotrimazole: A randomized controlled trial. *Complement Ther Med*. 52:102483.
92. Saghafi N, Karjalian M, Ghazanfarpour M, Khorsand I. et al. (2018). The effect of a vaginal suppository formulation of dill (*Anethum graveolens*) in comparison to clotrimazole vaginal tablet on the treatment of vulvovaginal candidiasis. *J Obstet Gynaecol*. 38(7):985–988.
93. El-Sherbiny GM, El Sherbiny ET. (2011). The effect of *Commiphora molmol* (Myrrh) in treatment of *Trichomoniasis vaginalis* infection. *Iran Red Cresc Med J*. 13(7):480–486.
94. Abouali N, Moghimipour E, Mahmoudabadi AZ, Namjouyan F, Abbaspoor Z. (2019). The effect of curcumin-based and clotrimazole vaginal cream in the treatment of vulvovaginal candidiasis. *J Fam Med Prim Care*. 8(12):3920–3924.
95. Dovigo LN, Carmello JC, de Souza Costa CA, Vergani CE. et al. (2013). Curcumin-mediated photodynamic inactivation of *Candida albicans* in a murine model of oral candidiasis. *Med Mycol*. 51:243–251.

96. Mendling W, Brasch J. (2012). Guideline vulvovaginal candidiasis (2010) of the German Society for Gynecology and Obstetrics, the Working Group for Infections and Infectimmunology in Gynecology and Obstetrics, the German Society of Dermatology, the Board of German Dermatologists and the German Speaking Mycological Society. *Mycoses*. 55(Suppl. 3):1–13.
97. Lee W, Lee DG. (2014). An antifungal mechanism of curcumin lies in membrane-targeted action within *Candida albicans*. *Int Union Biochem Mole Bio Life*. 66:780–785.
98. Masoudi M, Miraj S, Rafieian-Kopaei M. (2016). Comparison of the effects of *Myrtus communis* L, *Berberis vulgaris* and metronidazole vaginal gel alone for the treatment of bacterial vaginosis. *J Clin Diagn Res*. 10(3):4–7.
99. Roozbahani F, Kariman N, Mojab F, Nasiri M. (2013). Effect of *Myrtus communis* capsule on vaginal candidiasis treatment. *Pejouhandeh J*. 18(5):242–249.
100. Janani F, Akbari S, Delfan B, Tolabi T, Ebrahimzadeh F, Motamedi M. (2010). A comparative study of effect of myrtus vaginal cream and clotrimazol vaginal cream in the treatment of vaginal candidiasis. *Yafteh*. 13(1):32–41.
101. Askari SF, Jahromi BN, Dehghanian A, Zarei A. et al. (2020). Effect of a novel herbal vaginal suppository containing myrtle and oak gall in the treatment of vaginitis: A randomized clinical trial. *Daru: J Fac Pharm, Tehran Univ Medical Sciences*. 28(2):603–614.
102. Al-Saimary IE, Bakr SS, Jaffar T, Al-Saimary AE, Salim H, Al-Muosawi R. (2002). Effects of some plant extracts and antibiotics on *Pseudomonas aeruginosa* isolated from various burn cases. *Saudi Med J*. 7:802–805.
103. Sobel JD. (2000). Bacterial vaginosis. *Ann Rev Med*. 1:349–356.
104. Hosseinzadeh H, Khoshdel M, Ghorbani M. (2011). Antinociceptive, anti-inflammatory effects and acute toxicity of aqueous and ethanolic extracts of *Myrtus communis* L aerial parts in mice. *J Acupunct Meridian Stud*. 4:242–247.
105. Rossi A, Di Paola R, Mazzon E, Genovese T. et al. (2009). Myrtucommulone from *Myrtus communis* exhibits potent anti-inflammatory effectiveness in vivo. *J Pharmacol Exp Ther*. 1:76–86.
106. Fard FA, Zahrani ST, Bagheban AA, Mojab F. (2015). Therapeutic effects of *Nigella sativa* linn (Black Cumin) on *Candida albicans* vaginitis. *Arch Clin Infect Dis*. 10(1):e22991.
107. Mehni S, Tork Zahrani S, Taheri Sarvtin M, Mojab F, Mirzaei M, Vazirnasab H. (2015). Therapeutic effects of *Bunium perscicum* boiss (Black Zira) on *Candida albicans* vaginitis. *Biom Pharmacol J*. 8(2):1103–1109.

108. Mousavi MS, Keshavarz T, Montaseri H, Pakshir K. et al. (2010). A comparative study on the therapeutic effect of the propolis vaginal cream and clotrimazol on candida vulvovaginitis in reproductive aged women. *J Isfahan Med Sch*. 28(117):1099–1107.
109. Baery N, Nejad AG, Amin M, Mahroozade S. et al. (2018). Effect of vaginal suppository on bacterial vaginitis based on Persian medicine (Iranian traditional medicine): A randomised double blind clinical study. *J Obstet Gynec*. 38(8):1110–1114.
110. Ahangari F, Farshbaf-Khalili A, Javadzadeh Y, Adibpour M, Sadeghzadeh Oskouei B. (2019). Comparing the effectiveness of *Salvia officinalis*, clotrimazole and their combination on vulvovaginal candidiasis: A randomized, controlled clinical trial. *J Obstet Gynaecol Res*. 45(4):897–907.
111. Shabanian S, Khalili S, Lorigooini Z, Malekpour A, Heidari-Soureshjani S. (2017). The effect of vaginal cream containing ginger in users of clotrimazole vaginal cream on vaginal candidiasis. *J Adv Pharmacol Technol Res*. 8:80–84.
112. Arbabi M, Delavari M, Fakhrieh Kashan Z, Taghizadeh M, Hooshyar H. (2016). Ginger (*Zingiber officinale*) induces apoptosis in *Trichomonas vaginalis* in vitro. *Int J Reprod Biomed*. 14(11):691–698.
113. Mallo N, Lamas J, Leiro JM. (2013). Hydrogenosome metabolism is the key target for antiparasitic activity of resveratrol against *Trichomonas vaginalis*. *Antimicrob Agents Chemother*. 57(6):2476–2484.
114. Kashan ZF, Arbabi M, Delavari M, Hooshyar H, Taghizadeh M, Joneydy Z. (2015). Effect of *Verbascum thapsus* ethanol extract on induction of apoptosis in *Trichomonas vaginalis* in vitro. *Infect Disord Drug Targets*. 15(2):125–130.
115. Antonio MA, Rabe LK, Hillier SL. (2005). Colonization of the rectum by *Lactobacillus* species and decreased risk of bacterial vaginosis. *J Infect Dis*. 192(3):394–398.
116. Tilg H. (2010). Obesity, metabolic syndrome, and microbiota: Multiple interactions. *J Clin Gastroenterol*. 44 (Suppl. 1):S16–18.
117. Parsapure R, Rahimiforushani A, Majlessi F, Montazeri A, Sadeghi R, Garmarudi G. (2016). Impact of health-promoting educational intervention on lifestyle (nutrition behaviors, physical activity and mental health) related to vaginal health among reproductive-aged women with vaginitis. *Iran Red Cresc Med J*. 18(10):e37698.
118. Neggers YH, Nansel TR, Andrews WW, Schwebke JR, Yu KF, Goldenberg RL, Klebanoff MA. (2007). Dietary intake of selected nutrients affects bacterial vaginosis in women. *J Nutr*. 137(9):2128–2133.

119. Neggers YH, Nansel TR, Andrews WW, Schwebke JR, Yu KF, Goldenberg RL, Klebanoff MA. (2007). Dietary intake of selected nutrients affects bacterial vaginosis in women. *J Nutr*. 137(9):2128–2133.
120. Dunlop AL, Taylor RN, Tangpricha V, Fortunato S, Menon R. (2011). Maternal vitamin D, folate, and polyunsaturated fatty acid status and bacterial vaginosis during pregnancy. *Infect Dis Obstet Gynec*. 216217.
121. Tohill BC, Heilig CM, Klein RS, Rompalo A, Cu-Uvin S, Piwoz EG. et al. (2007). Nutritional biomarkers associated with gynecological conditions among US women with or at risk of HIV infection. *Am J Clin Nutr*. 85(5):1327–1334.
122. Christian P, Labrique AB, Ali H, Richman MJ, Wu L, Rashid M, West KP Jr. (2011). Maternal vitamin A and β-carotene supplementation and risk of bacterial vaginosis: A randomized controlled trial in rural Bangladesh. *Am J Clin Nutr*. 94(6):1643–1649.
123. Westney OE, Westney LS, Johnson AA, Knight EM. et al. (1994). Nutrition, genital tract infection, hematologic values, and premature rupture of membranes among African American Women. *J Nutr*. 124(6 Suppl.):987S–993S.
124. Bodnar LM, Krohn MA, Simhan HN. (2009). Maternal vitamin D deficiency is associated with bacterial vaginosis in the first trimester of pregnancy. *J Nutr*. 139(6):1157–1161.
125. Thoma ME, Klebanoff MA, Rovner AJ, Nansel TR, Neggers Y, Andrews WW. et al. (2011). Bacterial vaginosis is associated with variation in dietary indices. *J Nutr*. 141(9):1698–1704.
126. Tuddenham S, Ghanem KG, Caulfield LE, Rovner AJ. et al. (2019). Associations between dietary micronutrient intake and molecular-bacterial vaginosis. *Reprod Health*. 16(1):151.
127. Wang H, Li S, Fang S, Yang X, Feng J. (2018). Betaine improves intestinal functions by enhancing digestive enzymes, ameliorating intestinal morphology, and enriching intestinal microbiota in high-salt stressed rats. *Nutrients*. 10(7):907.
128. Watson CJ, Calabretto H. (2007). Comprehensive review of conventional and non-conventional methods of management of recurrent vulvovaginal candidiasis. *Aust NZ J Obstet Gynaec*. 47(4):262–272.
129. Zeng X, Zhang Y, Zhang T, Xue Y, Xu H. (2018). Risk factors of vulvovaginal candidiasis among women of reproductive age in Xi'an: A cross-sectional study. *Biomed Res Int*. 9703754.
130. Ehrström SM, Kornfeld D, Thuresson J, Rylander E. (2005). Signs of chronic stress in women with recurrent candida vulvovaginitis. *Am J Obstet Gynecol*. 193(4):1376–1381.

131. Zeng X, Zhang Y, Zhang T, Xue Y, Xu H, An R. (2018). Risk factors of vulvovaginal candidiasis among women of reproductive age in Xi'an: A cross-sectional study. *Biomed Res Int*. 9703754.
132. Ogouyèmi-Hounto A, Adisso S, Djamal J. et al. (2014). Place of vulvovaginal candidiasis in the lower genital tract infections and associated risk factors among women in Benin. *Journal de Mycologie Médicale*. 24(2):100–105.
133. Chassot F, Negri MFN, Svidzinski AE. et al. (2008). Can intrauterine contraceptive devices be a *Candida albicans* reservoir? *Contraception*. 77(5):355–359.
134. Zeng X, Zhang Y, Zhang T, Xue Y, Xu H, An R. (2018). Risk factors of vulvovaginal candidiasis among women of reproductive age in Xi'an: A cross-sectional study. *Biomed Res Int*. 9703754.

Chapter 6: Ovarian cysts

1. Pavlik EJ, Ueland FR, Miller RW, Ubellacker JM. et al. (2013). Frequency and disposition of ovarian abnormalities followed with serial transvaginal ultrasonography. *Obstet Gynecol*. 122(2 Pt 1):210–217.
2. American College of Obstetricians and Gynecologists' Committee on Practice Bulletins—Gynecology. (2016). Practice Bulletin No. 174: Evaluation and Management of Adnexal Masses. *Obstet Gynecol*. 128(5):e210–e226.
3. Mobeen S, Apostol R. (2021). Ovarian cyst. In: *StatPearls*. [Internet]. Treasure Island, FL: StatPearls Publishing.
4. Stany MP, Hamilton CA. (2008). Benign disorders of the ovary. *Obstet Gynecol Clin North Am*. 35(2):271–284.
5. Holt VL, Cushing-Haugen KL, Daling JR. (2003). Oral contraceptives, tubal sterilization, and functional ovarian cyst risk. *Obstet Gynecol*. 102(2):252–258.
6. Jain KA. (2002). Sonographic spectrum of hemorrhagic ovarian cysts. *J Ultrasound Med*. 21(8):879–886.
7. Pradhan P, Thapa M. (2014). Dermoid cyst and its bizarre presentation. *J Nepal Med Assoc*. 52(194):837–844.
8. Grimes DA, Jones LB, Lopez LM, Schulz KF. (2009). Oral contraceptives for functional ovarian cysts. *Cochrane Database Syst Rev*. 2:CD006134.
9. Glanc P, Salem S, Farine D. (2008). Adnexal masses in the pregnant patient: A diagnostic and management challenge. *Ultrasound Q*. 24(4):225–240.

10. Sohrabvand F, Kamalinejad M, Tansaz M, Vazifekhah S. et al. (2016). Comparative study of the effects of treatment with herbal product Shilanum and high-dose contraceptive pills on functional ovarian cysts. *Int J Curr Res*. 8(9):39365–39368.

Chapter 7: Polycystic ovary syndrome

1. Rosenfield RL, Ehrmann DA. (2016). The pathogenesis of Polycystic Ovary Syndrome (PCOS): The hypothesis of PCOS as functional ovarian hyperandrogenism revisited. *Endocrine Rev*. 37(5):467–520.
2. Barthelmess EK, Naz RK. (2014). Polycystic ovary syndrome: Current status and future perspective. *Front Biosci*. (*Elite ed*.). 6:104–119.
3. Liu T, Cui Yq, Zhao H. et al. (2015). High levels of testosterone inhibit ovarian follicle development by repressing the FSH signaling pathway. *J Huazhong Univ Sci Technol. [Med. Sci.]*. 35:723–729.
4. Zhang Sw, Zhou J, Gober HJ, Leung WT, Wang L. (2021). Effect and mechanism of berberine against polycystic ovary syndrome. *Biomed Pharmacotherapy*. 138:111468.
5. Apter D, Bützow T, Laughlin GA, Yen SS. (1994). Accelerated 24-hour luteinizing hormone pulsatile activity in adolescent girls with ovarian hyperandrogenism: Relevance to the developmental phase of polycystic ovarian syndrome. *J Clin Endocrinol Metab*. 79(1):119–125.
6. Baptiste CG, Battista MC, Trottier A, Baillargeon JP. (2010). Insulin and hyperandrogenism in women with polycystic ovary syndrome. *J Steroid Biochem Mol Biol*. 122(1–3):42–52.
7. Rosenfield RL, Ehrmann DA. (2016). The pathogenesis of Polycystic Ovary Syndrome (PCOS): The hypothesis of PCOS as functional ovarian hyperandrogenism revisited. *Endocrine Rev*. 37(5):467–520.
8. Toprak S, Yönem A, Çakır B, Güler S, Azal Ö, Özata M, Çorakçı A. (2001). Insulin resistance in nonobese patients with polycystic ovary syndrome. *Horm Res*. 55:65–70.
9. Dunaif A. (1997). Insulin resistance and the polycystic ovary syndrome: Mechanism and implications for pathogenesis. *Endocr Rev*. 18:774–800.
10. Shaaban Z, Khoradmehr A, Jafarzadeh Shirazi MR, Tamadon A. (2019). Pathophysiological mechanisms of gonadotropins- and steroid hormones-related genes in etiology of polycystic ovary syndrome. *Iran J Basic Med Sci*. 22(1):3–16.
11. Yki-Jarvinen H, Makimattila S, Utriainen T, Rutanen EM. (1995). Portal insulin concentrations rather than insulin sensitivity regulate serum sex

hormone-binding globulin and insulin-like growth factor binding protein 1 in vivo. *J Clin Endocrinol Metab.* 80:3227–3232.
12. Farrell K, Antoni MH. (2010). Insulin resistance, obesity, inflammation, and depression in polycystic ovary syndrome: Biobehavioral mechanisms and interventions. *Fertil. Steril.* 94(5):1565–1574.
13. Zheng SH, Du DF, Li XL. (2017). Leptin levels in women with polycystic ovary syndrome: A systematic review and a meta-analysis. *Reprod Sci.* 24(5):656–670.
14. Chakrabarti J. (2013). Serum leptin level in women with polycystic ovary syndrome: Correlation with adiposity, insulin, and circulating testosterone. *Annals Med Health Sci Res.* 3(2):191–196.
15. Hardie L, Trayhurn P, Abramovich D, Fowler P. (1997). Circulating leptin in women: A longitudinal study in the menstrual cycle and during pregnancy. *Clin Endocrinol.* (Oxford). 47:101–106.
16. Sir-Petermann T, Maliqueo M, Palomino A, Vantman D, Recabarren SE, Wildt L. (1999). Episodic leptin release is independent of luteinizing hormone secretion. *Hum Reprod.* 14:2695–2699.
17. Chakrabarti J. (2013). Serum leptin level in women with polycystic ovary syndrome: Correlation with adiposity, insulin, and circulating testosterone. *Annals Med Health Sci Res.* 3(2):191–196.
18. Vidal H, Auboeuf D, De Vos P, Staels B, Riou JP, Auwerx J. et al. (1996). The expression of ob gene is not actually regulated by insulin and fasting in human abdominal subcutaneous adipose tissue. *J Clin Invest.* 98:251–255.
19. Majumdar A, Mangal NS. (2013). Hyperprolactinemia. *J Human Reprod Sci.* 6(3):168–175.
20. Liu T, Cui YQ, Zhao H. et al. (2015). High levels of testosterone inhibit ovarian follicle development by repressing the FSH signaling pathway. *J Huazhong Univ Sci Technol. [Med. Sci.].* 35:723–729.
21. Zhang Sw, Zhou J, Gober HJ, Leung WT, Wang L. (2021). Effect and mechanism of berberine against polycystic ovary syndrome. *Biomed Pharmacotherapy.* 138:111468.
22. Yildiz BO, Woods KS, Stanczyk F, Bartolucci A, Azziz R. (2004). Stability of adrenocortical steroidogenesis over time in healthy women and women with polycystic ovary syndrome. *J Clin Endocrinol Metab.* 89(11):5558–5562.
23. Blank SK, McCartney CR, Marshall JC. (2006). The origins and sequelae of abnormal neuroendocrine function in polycystic ovary syndrome. *Hum Reprod Update.* 12(4):351–361.

24. Singla R, Gupta Y, Khemani M, Aggarwal S. (2015). Thyroid disorders and polycystic ovary syndrome: An emerging relationship. *Indian J Endocrinol Metab.* 19(1):25–29.
25. Kim JY, Tfayli H, Michaliszyn SF, Lee S, Nasr A, Arslanian S. (2017). Anti-Müllerian hormone in obese adolescent girls with polycystic ovary syndrome. *J Adolesc Health.* 60(3):333–339.
26. Pigny P, Merlen E, Robert Y, Cortet-Rudelli C, Decanter C, Jonard S, Dewailly D. (2003). Elevated serum level of anti-Mullerian hormone in patients with polycystic ovary syndrome: Relationship to the ovarian follicle excess and to the follicular arrest. *J Clin Endocrinol Metab.* 88(12):5957–5962.
27. Xu J, Bishop CV, Lawson MS, Park BS, Xu F. (2016). Anti-Müllerian hormone promotes pre-antral follicle growth, but inhibits antral follicle maturation and dominant follicle selection in primates. *Hum Reprod.* 31(7):1522–1530.
28. Eyvazzadeh AD, Pennington KP, Pop-Busui R, Sowers MF, Zubieta JK, Smith YR. (2009). The role of the endogenous opioid system in polycystic ovary syndrome. *Fertil Steril.* 92(1):1–12.
29. Webster DE, Lu J, Chen SN, Farnsworth NR, Wang ZJ. (2006). Activation of the mu-opiate receptor by *Vitex agnus-castus* methanol extracts: Implication for its use in PMS. *J Ethnopharmacol.* 106(2):216–221.
30. Webster DE, He Y, Chen SN, Pauli GF, Farnsworth NR, Wang ZJ. (2011). Opioidergic mechanisms underlying the actions of *Vitex agnus-castus* L. *Biochem Pharmacol.* 81(1):170–177.
31. Rhyu MR, Lu J, Webster DE, Fabricant DS, Farnsworth NR, Wang ZJ. (2006). Black cohosh (*Actaea racemosa*, *Cimicifuga racemosa*) behaves as a mixed competitive ligand and partial agonist at the human mu opiate receptor. *J Agric Food Chem.* 54(26):9852–9857.
32. Torres PJ, Siakowska M, Banaszewska B, Pawelczyk L, Duleba AJ, Kelley ST, Thackray VG. (2018). Gut microbial diversity in women with polycystic ovary syndrome correlates with hyperandrogenism. *J Clin Endocrinol Metab.* 103(4):1502–1511.
33. Liu SM, Shen Y, Li J, Han FJ. (2019). Research progress of berberine on prevention and treatment of endometrial cancer related to polycystic ovary syndrome based on anti-inflammatory mechanism. *Chin Pharmacol.* 30(16):2294–2297.
34. Seidlova-Wuttke D, Eder N, Stahnke V, Kammann M, Stecher G, Haunschild J, Wessels JT, Wuttke W. (2012). *Cimicifuga racemosa* and its triterpene-saponins prevent the metabolic syndrome and deterioration

of cartilage in the knee joint of ovariectomized rats by similar mechanisms. *Phytomed.* 19(8–9):846–853.
35. El-Mehiry HF. (2017). Biological activities of *Vitex agnus-castus* (L.) leaves in diabetes control in high fat/high fructose fed female rats. *Res J Specific Education.* 5:529–553.
36. Wuttke W, Jarry H, Christoffel V, Spengler B, Seidlová-Wuttke D. (2003). Chaste tree (*Vitex agnus-castus*)—pharmacology and clinical indications. *Phytomed.* 10(4):348–357.
37. Haidari F, Banaei-Jahromi N, Zakerkish M, Ahmadi K. (2020). The effects of flaxseed supplementation on metabolic status in women with polycystic ovary syndrome: A randomized open-labeled controlled clinical trial. *Nutr J.* 19(1):8.
38. Pourjafari F, Haghpanah T, Sharififar F, Nematollahi-Mahani SN, Afgar A, Ezzatabadipour M. (2021). Evaluation of expression and serum concentration of anti-mullerian hormone as a follicle growth marker following consumption of fennel and flaxseed extract in first-generation mice pups. *BMC Complement Med Ther.* 21(1):90.
39. Wiweko B, Susanto CA. (2017). The effect of metformin and cinnamon on serum anti-mullerian hormone in women having PCOS: A double-blind, randomized, controlled trial. *J Hum Reprod Sci.* 10(1):31–36.
40. Shamasbi SG, Ghanbari-Homayi S, Mirghafourvand M. (2020). The effect of probiotics, prebiotics, and synbiotics on hormonal and inflammatory indices in women with polycystic ovary syndrome: A systematic review and meta-analysis. *Eur J Nutr.* 59(2):433–450.
41. Zhang Y, Liu W, Liu D, Zhao T, Tian, H. (2016). Efficacy of *Aloe vera* supplementation on prediabetes and early non-treated diabetic patients: A systematic review and meta-analysis of randomized controlled trials. *Nutrients.* 8(7):388.
42. Suksomboon N, Poolsup N, Punthanitisarn S. (2016). Effect of Aloe vera on glycaemic control in prediabetes and type 2 diabetes: A systematic review and meta-analysis. *J Clin Pharmacol Ther.* 41(2):180–188.
43. Huseini HF, Kianbakht S, Hajiaghaee R, Dabaghian FH. (2012). Anti-hyperglycemic and anti-hypercholesterolemic effects of *Aloe vera* leaf gel in hyperlipidemic type 2 diabetic patients: A randomized double-blind placebo-controlled clinical trial. *Planta Med.* 78:311–316.
44. Tehrani HG, Allahdadian M, Zarre F, Ranjbar H, Allahdadian F. (2017). Effect of green tea on metabolic and hormonal aspect of polycystic ovarian syndrome in overweight and obese women suffering from polycystic ovarian syndrome: A clinical trial. *J Educ Health Promotion.* 6:36.

45. Chan CC, Koo MW, Ng EH, Tang OS, Yeung WS, Ho PC. (2006). Effects of Chinese green tea on weight, and hormonal and biochemical profiles in obese patients with polycystic ovary syndrome—a randomized placebo-controlled trial. *J Soc Gynecol Investig*. 13(1):63–68.
46. Borzoei A, Rafraf M, Niromanesh S, Farzadi L, Narimani F, Doostan F. (2018). Effects of cinnamon supplementation on antioxidant status and serum lipids in women with polycystic ovary syndrome. *J Tradit Complement Med*. 8(1):128–133.
47. Lemay A, Dodin S, Kadri N. et al. (2002). Flaxseed dietary supplement versus hormone replacement therapy in hypercholesterolemic menopausal women. *Obstet Gynecol* 100:495–504.
48. Murray MT. (2020). *Glycyrrhiza glabra* (Licorice). In Pizzorno JE, Murray MT (eds). *Textbook of Natural Medicine*, 5th ed. St Louis, MO: Elsevier, pp. 641–647.
49. Armanini D, De Palo CB, Mattarello M.J. (2003). Effect of licorice on the reduction of body fat mass in healthy subjects. *J Endocrinol Invest*. 26:646–650.
50. Chen JT, Tominaga K, Sato Y, Anzai H, Matsuoka R. (2010). Maitake mushroom (*Grifola frondosa*) extract induces ovulation in patients with polycystic ovary syndrome: A possible monotherapy and a combination therapy after failure with first-line clomiphene citrate. *J Altern Complement Med*. 16(12):1295–1299.
51. Rafraf M, Zemestani M, Asghari-Jafarabadi M. (2015). Effectiveness of chamomile tea on glycemic control and serum lipid profile in patients with type 2 diabetes. *J Endocrinol Invest*. 38:163–170.
52. Zemestani M, Rafraf M, Asghari-Jafarabadi M. (2016). Chamomile tea improves glycemic indices and antioxidants status in patients with type 2 diabetes mellitus. *Nutrition*. 32(1):66–72.
53. Heidary M, Yazdanpanahi Z, Dabbaghmanesh MH, Parsanezhad ME, Emamghoreishi M, Akbarzadeh M. (2018). Effect of chamomile capsule on lipid- and hormonal-related parameters among women of reproductive age with polycystic ovary syndrome. *J Res Med Sci*. (Isfahan). 23:33.
54. Naeimi SA, Tansaz M, Sohrabvand F, Hajimehdipoor H. et al. (2018). Assessing the effect of processed *Nigella sativa* on oligomenorrhea and amenorrhea in patients with polycystic ovarian syndrome: A pilot study. *Int J Pharmacol Sci Res*. 9(11):4716–4722.
55. Vuksan V, Sung MK, Sievenpiper JL, Stavro PM. et al. (2008). Korean red ginseng (*Panax ginseng*) improves glucose and insulin regulation in well-controlled, type 2 diabetes: Results of a randomized, double-blind,

placebo-controlled study of efficacy and safety. *Nutr Metab Cardiovasc Dis.* 18:46–56.
56. Shishtar E, Sievenpiper JL, Djedovic V, Cozma AI. et al. (2014). The effect of ginseng (The Genus Panax) on glycemic control: A systematic review and meta-analysis of randomized controlled clinical trials. *PLoS One.* 9:e107391.
57. Jovanovski E, Lea-Duvnjak-Smircic, Komishon A, Au-Yeung F. et al. (2020). Vascular effects of combined enriched Korean Red ginseng (*Panax ginseng*) and American ginseng (*Panax quinquefolius*) administration in individuals with hypertension and type 2 diabetes: A randomized controlled trial. *Complement Ther Med.* 49:102338.
58. Haj-Husein I, Tukan S, Alkazaleh F. (2016). The effect of marjoram (*Origanum majorana*) tea on the hormonal profile of women with polycystic ovary syndrome: A randomised controlled pilot study. *J Hum Nutr Diet.* 29(1):105–111.
59. Jamilian M, Asemi Z. (2016). The effects of soy isoflavones on metabolic status of patients with polycystic ovary syndrome. *J Clin Endocrinol Metab.* 101(9):3386–3394.
60. Samani NB, Jokar A, Soveid M, Heydari M, Mosavat SH. (2016). Efficacy of the hydroalcoholic extract of *Tribulus terrestris* on the serum glucose and lipid profile of women with diabetes mellitus: A double-blind randomized placebo-controlled clinical trial. *J Evid Based Complement Altern Med.* 21:NP91–NP97.
61. Bashtian MH, Emami SA, Mousavifar N, Esmaily HA, Mahmoudi M, Poor AHM. (2013). Evaluation of fenugreek (*Trigonella foenum-graceum* L.), effects seeds extract on insulin resistance in women with polycystic ovarian syndrome. *Iran J Pharm Res.* 12(2):475.
62. Arablou T, Aryaeian N, Valizadeh M, Sharifi F, Hosseini A, Djalali M. (2014). The effect of ginger consumption on glycemic status, lipid profile and some inflammatory markers in patients with type 2 diabetes mellitus. *Int J Food Sci Nutr.* 65:515–520.
63. Arablou T, Aryaeian N, Valizadeh M, Sharifi F, Hosseini A, Djalali M. (2014). The effect of ginger consumption on glycemic status, lipid profile and some inflammatory markers in patients with type 2 diabetes mellitus. *Int J Food Sci Nutr.* 65:515–520.
64. Seidlova-Wuttke D, Eder N, Stahnke V, Kammann M. et al. (2012). *Cimicifuga racemosa* and its triterpene-saponins prevent the metabolic syndrome and deterioration of cartilage in the knee joint of ovariectomized rats by similar mechanisms. *Phytomed.* 19(8–9):846–853.

65. Seidlová-Wuttke D, Jarry H, Becker T, Christoffel V, Wuttke W. (2003). Pharmacology of *Cimicifuga racemosa* extract BNO 1055 in rats: Bone, fat and uterus. *Maturitas.* 44(Suppl. 1):S39–S50.
66. Moser C, Vickers SP, Brammer R, Cheetham SC, Drewe J. (2014). Antidiabetic effects of the *Cimicifuga racemosa* extract Ze 450 in vitro and in vivo in ob/ob mice. *Phytomed.* 21(11):1382–1389.
67. Shokoohi M, Abtahi-Eivary SH, Moghimian M, Hajizadeh H. (2018). The effect of *Galega officinalis* on hormonal and metabolic profile in a rat model of Polycystic Ovary Syndrome (PCOS). *Int J Women's Health Reprod Sci.* 6(3).
68. Nakamura Y, Tsumura Y, Tonogai Y, Shibata T. (1999). Fecal steroid excretion is increased in rats by oral administration of gymnemic acids contained in *Gymnema sylvestre* leaves. *J Nutr.* 129(6):1214–1222.
69. Preuss HG, Jarrell ST, Scheckenbach R, Lieberman S, Anderson RA. (1998). Comparative effects of chromium, vanadium and *Gymnema sylvestre* on sugar-induced blood pressure elevations in SHR. *J Am Coll Nutr.* 17(2):116–123.
70. Preuss HG, Garis RI, Bramble JD, Bagchi D. et al. (2005). Efficacy of a novel calcium/potassium salt of (-)-hydroxycitric acid in weight control. *Int J Clin Pharmacol Res.* 25(3):133–144.
71. Zhang Y, Liu W, Liu D, Zhao T, Tian, H. (2016). Efficacy of *Aloe vera* supplementation on prediabetes and early non-treated diabetic patients: A systematic review and meta-analysis of randomized controlled trials. *Nutrients.* 8(7):388.
72. Rhee Y, Brunt A. (2016). Flaxseed supplementation improved insulin resistance in obese glucose intolerant people: A randomized crossover design. *Nutr J.* 10:44.
73. Jamilian M, Asemi Z. (2016). The effects of soy isoflavones on metabolic status of patients with polycystic ovary syndrome. *J Clin Endocrinol Metab.* 101(9):3386–3394.
74. Fuhrman B, Volkova N, Kaplan M, Presser D, Attias J, Hayek T, Aviram M. (2002). Antiatherosclerotic effects of licorice extract supplementation on hypercholesterolemic patients: Increased resistance of LDL to atherogenic modifications, reduced plasma lipid levels, and decreased systolic blood pressure. *Nutrition.* 18(3):268–273.
75. Bnouham M, Ziyyat A, Mekhfi H, Tahri A, Legssyer A. (2006). Medicinal plants with potential antidiabetic activity—a review of ten years of herbal medicine research (1990–2000). *Int J Diabetes Metab.* 14:1–25.

76. Rafraf M, Zemestani M, Asghari-Jafarabadi M. (2015). Effectiveness of chamomile tea on glycemic control and serum lipid profile in patients with type 2 diabetes. *J Endocrinol Invest*. 38:163–170.
77. Zemestani M, Rafraf M, Asghari-Jafarabadi M. (2016). Chamomile tea improves glycemic indices and antioxidants status in patients with type 2 diabetes mellitus. *Nutrition*. 32(1):66–72.
78. Heidary M, Yazdanpanahi Z, Dabbaghmanesh MH, Parsanezhad ME, Emamghoreishi M, Akbarzadeh M. (2018). Effect of chamomile capsule on lipid- and hormonal-related parameters among women of reproductive age with polycystic ovary syndrome. *J Res Med Sci*. (Isfahan). 23:33.
79. Naeimi SA, Tansaz M, Sohrabvand F, Hajimehdipoor H. et al. (2018). Assessing the effect of processed *Nigella sativa* on oligomenorrhea and amenorrhea in patients with polycystic ovarian syndrome: A pilot study. *Int J Pharmacol Sci Res*. 9(11):4716–4722.
80. Shishtar E, Sievenpiper JL, Djedovic V, Cozma AI. et al. (2014). The effect of ginseng (The Genus Panax) on glycemic control: A systematic review and meta-analysis of randomized controlled clinical trials. *PLoS One*. 9:e107391.
81. Jovanovski E, Lea-Duvnjak-Smircic, Komishon A, Au-Yeung F. et al. (2020). Vascular effects of combined enriched Korean Red ginseng (*Panax ginseng*) and American ginseng (*Panax quinquefolius*) administration in individuals with hypertension and type 2 diabetes: A randomized controlled trial. *Complement Ther Med*. 49:102338.
82. Seidlová-Wuttke D, Eder N, Stahnke V, Kammann M, Stecher G, Haunschild J, Wessels JT, Wuttke W. (2012). *Cimicifuga racemosa* and its triterpene-saponins prevent the metabolic syndrome and deterioration of cartilage in the knee joint of ovariectomized rats by similar mechanisms. *Phytomed*. 19(8–9):846–853.
83. Seidlová-Wuttke D, Jarry H, Becker T, Christoffel V, Wuttke W. (2003). Pharmacology of *Cimicifuga racemosa* extract BNO 1055 in rats: Bone, fat and uterus. *Maturitas*. 44(Suppl. 1):S39–S50.
84. Moser C, Vickers SP, Brammer R, Cheetham SC, Drewe J. (2014). Antidiabetic effects of the *Cimicifuga racemosa* extract Ze 450 in vitro and in vivo in ob/ob mice. *Phytomed*. 21(11):1382–1389.
85. Ştefănescu R, Tero-Vescan A, Negroiu A, Aurică E, Vari CE. (2020). A comprehensive review of the phytochemical, pharmacological, and toxicological properties of *Tribulus terrestris* L. *Biomolecules*. 10(5):752.

86. Fuhrman B, Volkova N, Kaplan M, Presser D, Attias J, Hayek T, Aviram M. (2002). Antiatherosclerotic effects of licorice extract supplementation on hypercholesterolemic patients: Increased resistance of LDL to atherogenic modifications, reduced plasma lipid levels, and decreased systolic blood pressure. *Nutrition.* 18(3):268–273.
87. Devaraj S, Jialal R, Jialal I, Rockwood R. (2008). A pilot randomized placebo controlled trial of 2 *Aloe vera* supplements in patients with prediabetes/metabolic syndrome. *Planta Med.* 74:SL77.
88. Choi HC, Kim SJ, Son KY, Oh BJ, Cho BL. (2013). Metabolic effects of *Aloe vera* gel complex in obese prediabetes and early non-treated diabetic patients: Randomized controlled trial. *Nutrition.* 29:1110–1114.
89. Borzoei A, Rafraf M, Niromanesh S, Farzadi L, Narimani F, Doostan F. (2018). Effects of cinnamon supplementation on antioxidant status and serum lipids in women with polycystic ovary syndrome. *J Tradit Complement Med.* 8(1):128–133.
90. Tehrani HG, Allahdadian M, Zarre F, Ranjbar H, Allahdadian F. (2017). Effect of green tea on metabolic and hormonal aspect of polycystic ovarian syndrome in overweight and obese women suffering from polycystic ovarian syndrome: A clinical trial. *J Educ Health Promotion.* 6:36.
91. Chan CC, Koo MW, Ng EH, Tang OS, Yeung WS, Ho PC. (2006). Effects of Chinese green tea on weight, and hormonal and biochemical profiles in obese patients with polycystic ovary syndrome—a randomized placebo-controlled trial. *J Soc Gynecol Investig.* 13(1):63–68.
92. Rhee Y, Brunt. (2011). A Flaxseed supplementation improved insulin resistance in obese glucose intolerant people: A randomized crossover design. *Nutr J.* 10:44.
93. Murray MT. (2020). *Glycyrrhiza glabra* (Licorice). In Pizzorno JE, Murray MT (eds). *Textbook of Natural Medicine*, 5th ed. St Louis, MO: Elsevier, pp. 641–647.
94. Armanini D, De Palo CB, Mattarello MJ. (2003). Effect of licorice on the reduction of body fat mass in healthy subjects. *J Endocrinol Invest.* 26:646–650.
95. Woodgate DE, Conquer JA. (2003). Effects of a stimulant-free dietary supplement on body weight and fat loss in obese adults: A six-week exploratory study. *Curr Ther Res.* 64(4):248–262.
96. Moser C, Vickers SP, Brammer R, Cheetham SC, Drewe J. (2014). Antidiabetic effects of the *Cimicifuga racemosa* extract Ze 450 in vitro and in vivo in ob/ob mice. *Phytomed.* 21(11):1382–1389.

97. Jazani AM, Nazemiyeh H, Tansaz M, Bazargani HS. et al. (2018). Celery plus anise versus metformin for the treatment of oligomenorrhea in polycystic ovary syndrome: A triple-blind randomized clinical trial. *Iran Red Cresc Med J*. 20(5):e67181.
98. Tehrani HG, Allahdadian M, Zarre F, Ranjbar H, Allahdadian F. (2017). Effect of green tea on metabolic and hormonal aspect of polycystic ovarian syndrome in overweight and obese women suffering from polycystic ovarian syndrome: A clinical trial. *J Educ Health Promotion*. 6:36.
99. Chan CC, Koo MW, Ng EH, Tang OS, Yeung WS, Ho PC. (2006). Effects of Chinese green tea on weight, and hormonal and biochemical profiles in obese patients with polycystic ovary syndrome—a randomized placebo-controlled trial. *J Soc Gynecol Investig*. 13(1):63–68.
100. Nowak DA, Snyder DC, Brown AJ, Demark-Wahnefried W. (2007). The effect of flaxseed supplementation on hormonal levels associated with polycystic ovarian syndrome: A case study. *Curr Top Nutraceutical Res*. 5:177–181.
101. Sturgeon SR, Heersink JL, Volpe SL, Bertone-Johnson ER. et al. (2008). Effect of dietary flaxseed on serum levels of estrogens and androgens in postmenopausal women. *Nutr Cancer*. 60:612–618.
102. Nowak DA, Snyder DC, Brown AJ, Demark-Wahnefried WP. (2007). The effect of flaxseed supplementation on hormonal levels associated with polycystic ovarian syndrome: A case study. *Curr Top Nutraceutical Res*. 5:177–181.
103. Armanini D, Mattarello MJ, Fiore C, Bonanni G, Scaroni C, Sartorato P, Palermo M. (2004). Licorice reduces serum testosterone in healthy women. *Steroids*. 69(11–12):763–736.
104. Grant P. (2010). Spearmint herbal tea has significant anti-androgen effects in polycystic ovarian syndrome. A randomized controlled trial. *Phytother Res*. 24(2):186–188.
105. Akdoğan M, Tamer MN, Cüre E, Cüre MC, Köroğlu BK, Delibaş N. (2007). Effect of spearmint (*Mentha spicata* Labiatae) teas on androgen levels in women with hirsutism. *Phytother Res*. 21(5):444–447.
106. Haj-Husein I, Tukan S, Alkazaleh F. (2016). The effect of marjoram (*Origanum majorana*) tea on the hormonal profile of women with polycystic ovary syndrome: A randomised controlled pilot study. *J Hum Nutr Diet*. 29(1):105–111.
107. Yaginuma T, Isumi R, Yasui H, Arai T, Kawabata M. (1982). Effect of traditional herbal medicine on serum testosterone levels and its

induction of regular ovulation in hyperandrogenic and oligomenorrheic women. *Nihon Sanka Fujinka Gakkai Zasshi*. 34(7):939–944.
108. Takahashi K, Yoshino K, Shirai T, Nishigaki A, Araki Y, Kitao M. (1988). Effect of a traditional herbal medicine (*shakuyaku-kanzo-to*) on testosterone secretion in patients with polycystic ovary syndrome detected by ultrasound. *Nihon Sanka Fujinka Gakkai Zasshi*. 40(6):789–792.
109. Yaginuma T, Isumi R, Yasui H, Arai T, Kawabata M. (1982). Effect of traditional herbal medicine on serum testosterone levels and its induction of regular ovulation in hyperandrogenic and oligomenorrheic women. *Nihon Sanka Fujinka Gakkai Zasshi*. 34(7):939–944.
110. Takahashi K, Kitao M. (1994). Effect of TJ-68 (*shakuyaku-kanzo-to*) on polycystic ovarian disease. *Int J Fertil Menopausal Stud*. 39(2):69–76.
111. Aizawa H, Niimura M. (1996). Serum androgen levels in woman with *Acne vulgaris*: The effect of *shakuyaku-knazo-to* (SM). *Skin Research*. 38:37–41.
112. Jamilian M, Asemi Z. (2016). The effects of soy isoflavones on metabolic status of patients with polycystic ovary syndrome. *J Clin Endocrinol Metab*. 101(9):3386–3394.
113. Azouz AA, Ali SE, Abd-Elsalam RM, Emam SR. et al. (2021). Modulation of steroidogenesis by *Actaea racemosa* and vitamin C combination, in letrozole induced polycystic ovarian syndrome rat model: Promising activity without the risk of hepatic adverse effect. *Chin Med*. 16(1):36.
114. Jelodar G, Askari K. (2012). Effect of *Vitex agnus-castus* fruits hydroalcoholic extract on sex hormones in rat with induced Polycystic Ovary Syndrome (PCOS). *Physiol. Pharmacol*. 16:62–69.
115. Amann W. (1975). *Acne vulgaris* and *Agnus castus* (Agnolyt). *Z Allgemeinmed*. 51(35):1645–1648.
116. Sultan C, Terraza A, Devillier C, Carilla E, Briley M, Loire C, Descomps B. (1984). Inhibition of androgen metabolism and binding by a liposterolic extract of "Serenoa repens B" in human foreskin fibroblasts. *J Steroid Biochem*. 20(1):515–519.
117. Fan CW, Cieri-Hutcherson NE, Hutcherson TC. (2021). Systematic review of black cohosh (*Cimicifuga racemosa*) for management of polycystic ovary syndrome-related infertility. *J Pharmacol Pract*. 8971900211012244.
118. Kumarapeli M, Karunagoda K, Perera PK. (2018). A randomized clinical trial to evaluate the efficacy of *Satapushpashatavari* powered drug

with *Satapushpa-shatavari grita* for the management of Polycystic Ovary Syndrome (PCOS). *Int J Pharmacol Sci Res.* 9(6):2494–2499.
119. Jazani AM, Nazemiyeh H, Tansaz M, Bazargani HS. et al. (2018). Celery plus anise versus metformin for the treatment of oligomenorrhea in polycystic ovary syndrome: A triple-blind randomized clinical trial. *Iran Red Cresc Med J.* 20(5):e67181.
120. Kort DH, Lobo RA. (2014). Preliminary evidence that cinnamon improves menstrual cyclicity in women with polycystic ovary syndrome: A randomized controlled trial. *Am J Obstet Gynecol.* 211(5):487e1–487e6.
121. Wiweko B, Susanto CA. (2017). The effect of metformin and cinnamon on serum anti-mullerian hormone in women having PCOS: A double-blind, randomized, controlled trial. *J Hum Reprod Sci.* 10(1):31–36.
122. Hajimonfarednejad M, Nimrouzi M, Heydari M, Zarshenas MM, Raee MJ, Jahromi BN. (2018). Insulin resistance improvement by cinnamon powder in polycystic ovary syndrome: A randomized double-blind placebo controlled clinical trial. *Phytother Res.* 32(2):276–283.
123. Wang JG, Anderson RA, Graham GM III, Chu MC, Sauer MV, Guarnaccia MM. et al. (2007). The effect of cinnamon extract on insulin resistance parameters in polycystic ovary syndrome: A pilot study. *Fertil Steril.* 88(1):240–243.
124. Chen JT, Tominaga K, Sato Y, Anzai H, Matsuoka R. (2010). Maitake mushroom (*Grifola frondosa*) extract induces ovulation in patients with polycystic ovary syndrome: A possible monotherapy and a combination therapy after failure with first-line clomiphene citrate. *J Altern Complement Med.* 16(12):1295–1299.
125. Naeimi SA, Tansaz M, Sohrabvand F, Hajimehdipoor H, Nabimeybodi R, Saber S. et al. (2018). Assessing the effect of processed *Nigella sativa* on oligomenorrhea and amenorrhea in patients with polycystic ovarian syndrome: A pilot study. *Int J Pharmacol Sci Res.* 9(11):4716–4722.
126. Ushiroyama T, Ikeda A, Sakai M, Hosotani T, Suzuki Y, Tsubokura S, Ueki M. (2001). Effects of *unkei-to*, an herbal medicine, on endocrine function and ovulation in women with high basal levels of luteinizing hormone secretion. *J Reprod Med.* 46(5):451–456.
127. Ushiroyama T, Ikeda A, Higashio S, Hosotani T, Yamashita H, Yamashita Y, Suzuki Y, Ueki M. (2003). *Unkei-to* for correcting luteal phase defects. *J Reprod Med.* 48(9):729–734.
128. Yaginuma TI, Izumi R, Yasui H, Arai T, Kawabata M. (1982). Effect of traditional herbal medicine on serum testosterone levels and its

induction of regular ovulation in hyperandrogenic and oligomenorrheic women. *Nihon Sanka Fujinka Gakkai Zasshi.* 34(7):939–944.

129. Takahashi K, Yoshino K, Shirai T, Nishigaki A, Araki Y, Kitao M. (1988). Effect of a traditional herbal medicine (*shakuyaku-kanzo-to*) on testosterone secretion in patients with polycystic ovary syndrome detected by ultrasound. *Nihon Sanka Fujinka Gakkai Zasshi.* 40(6):789–792.

130. Swaroop A, Jaipuriar AS, Gupta SK, Bagchi M, Kumar P, Preuss HG, Bagchi D. (2015). Efficacy of a novel fenugreek seed extract (*Trigonella foenum-graecum*, FurocystTM) in Polycystic Ovary Syndrome (PCOS). *Int J Med Sci.* 12(10):825–831.

131. Ghahremaninasab P, Shahnazi M, Khalili AF, Hamdi K. (in press). The effects of combined low-dose oral contraceptives and *Vitex agnus* on the improvement of clinical and paraclinical parameters of polycystic ovarian syndrome: A triple-blind, randomized, controlled clinical trial. *Iran Red Cresc Med J.* e37510. Published online 2016.

132. Shayan A, Masoumi SZ, Shobeiri F, Tohidi S, Khalili A. (2016). Comparing the effects of agnugol and metformin on oligomenorrhea in patients with polycystic ovary syndrome: A randomized clinical trial. *J Clin Diag Res.* 10(12):QC13–QC16.

133. Milewicz A, Gejdel E, Sworen H, Sienkiewicz K, Jedrzejak J, Teucher T, Schmitz H. (1993). *Vitex agnus castus* extract in the treatment of luteal phase defects due to latent hyperprolactinemia. Results of a randomized placebo-controlled double-blind study. *Arzneimittelforschung.* 43(7):752–756.

134. Gerhard II, Patek A, Monga B, Blank A, Gorkow C. (1998). Mastodynon(R) bei weiblicher Sterilität. *Forsch Komplementarmed.* 5(6):272–278.

135. Eltbogen R, Litschgi M, Gasser UE, Flueeli A, Nebel S, Zahner C. (2014). *Vitex agnus-castus* extract (ZE440) improves symptoms in women with menstrual cycle irregularities. *Reprod Endocrin.* 28:86–91.

136. Bergmann J, Luft B, Boehmann S, Runnebaum B, Gerhard I. (2000). Die wirksamkeit des komplexmittels Phyto-Hypophyson L bei weiblicher, hormonell bedingter sterilität [The efficacy of the complex medication Phyto-Hypophyson L in female, hormone-related sterility. A randomized, placebo-controlled clinical double-blind study]. *Forsch Komplementarmed Klass Naturheilkd.* 7(4):190–199.

137. Farzana F, Sulaiman A, Ruckmani A, Vijayalakshmi K, Karunya Lakshmi G, Shri RS. (2015). Effects of flax seeds supplementation in polycystic ovarian syndrome. *J Res Med Sci.* 31(1):113–119.

138. Lee JC, Pak SC, Lee SH, Lim SC, Bai YH, Jin CS, Kim JS, Na CS, Bae CS, Oh KS. (2003). The effect of herbal medicine on nerve growth factor in estradiol valerate-induced polycystic ovaries in rats. *Am J Chin Med.* 31(06):885–895.
139. Yaginuma T, Isumi R, Yasui H, Arai T, Kawabata M. (1982). Effect of traditional herbal medicine on serum testosterone levels and its induction of regular ovulation in hyperandrogenic and oligomenorrheic women. *Nihon Sanka Fujinka Gakkai Zasshi.* 34(7):939–944.
140. Takahashi K, Kitao M. (1994). Effect of TJ-68 (*shakuyaku-kanzo-to*) on polycystic ovarian disease. *Int J Fertil Menopausal Stud.* 139(2):69–76.
141. Abbasian Z, Jafari Barmak M, Barazesh F, Ghavamizadeh M, Mirzaei A. (2020). Therapeutic efficacy of *Trifolium pratense* L. on letrozole induced polycystic ovary syndrome in rats. *Plant Sci Today.* 7(3):501–507.
142. Tabakova P, Dimitrov M, Tashkov B. (1984). *Clinical Studies on the Preparation Tribestan in Women with Endocrine Infertility or Menopausal Syndrome.* Sofia, Bulgaria: 1st Obstetrical and Gynecological Hospital.
143. Shahin AY, Mohammed SA. (2014). Adding the phytoestrogen *Cimicifugae racemosae* to clomiphene induction cycles with timed intercourse in polycystic ovary syndrome improves cycle outcomes and pregnancy rates—a randomized trial. *Gynecol Endocrinol.* 30(7):505–510.
144. Kamel HH. (2013). Role of phyto-oestrogens in ovulation induction in women with polycystic ovarian syndrome. *Eur J Obstet Gynecol Reprod Biol.* 168(1):60–63.
145. Yang P, Li L, Yang D, Wang C, Peng H, Huang H. et al. (2017). Effect of peony-glycyrrhiza decoction on amisulpride-induced hyperprolactinemia in women with schizophrenia: A preliminary study. *Evid Based Complement Alternat Med.* 7901670.
146. Jelodar G, Masoomi S, Rahmanifar F. (2018). Hydroalcoholic extract of flaxseed improves polycystic ovary syndrome in a rat model. *Iran J Basic Med Sci.* 21(6):645–650.
147. Sadeghpour N, Khaki AA, Najafpour A, Dolatkhah H, Montaseri A. (2015). Study of *Foeniculum vulgare* (fennel) seed extract effects on serum level of estrogen, progesterone and prolactin in mouse. *Crescent J Med Biol Sci.* 2:59–63.
148. Atashpour S, Jahromi HK, Jahromi ZK, Maleknasab M. (2017). Comparison of the effects of ginger extract with clomiphene citrate on sex hormones in rats with polycystic ovarian syndrome. *Int J Reprod Biomed.* 15(9):561.

149. Yuan HN, Wang CY, Sze CW, Tong Y, Tan QR, Feng XJ. et al. (2008). A randomized, crossover comparison of herbal medicine and bromocriptine against risperidone-induced hyperprolactinemia in patients with schizophrenia. *J Clin Psychopharmacol.* 28(3):264–370.
150. Milewicz A, Gejdel E, Sworen H, Sienkiewicz K, Jedrzejak J, Teucher T, Schmitz H. (1993). *Vitex agnus castus* extract in the treatment of luteal phase defects due to latent hyperprolactinemia. Results of a randomized placebo-controlled double-blind study. *Arzneimittelforschung.* 43(7):752–756.
151. Gerhard II, Patek A, Monga B, Blank A, Gorkow C. (1998). Mastodynon(R) bei weiblicher Sterilität. *Forsch Komplementarmed.* 5(6):272–278.
152. Eltbogen R, Litschgi M, Gasser UE, Flueeli A, Nebel S, Zahner C. (2014). *Vitex agnus-castus* extract (ZE440) improves symptoms in women with menstrual cycle irregularities. *Reprod Endocrin.* 28:86–91.
153. Bergmann J, Luft B, Boehmann S, Runnebaum B, Gerhard I. (2000). Die wirksamkeit des komplexmittels Phyto-Hypophyson L bei weiblicher, hormonell bedingter sterilität [The efficacy of the complex medication Phyto-Hypophyson L in female, hormone-related sterility. A randomized, placebo-controlled clinical double-blind study]. *Forsch Komplementarmed Klass Naturheilkd.* 7(4):190–199.
154. Geavlete P, Multescu R, Geavlete B. (2011). *Serenoa repens* extract in the treatment of benign prostatic hyperplasia. *Therap Advances Urol.* 3(4):193–198.
155. Van Coppenolle F, Le Bourhis X, Carpentier F, Delaby G. et al. (2000). Pharmacological effects of the lipidosterolic extract of *Serenoa repens* (Permixon) on rat prostate hyperplasia induced by hyperprolactinemia: Comparison with finasteride. *Prostate.* 43(1):49–58.
156. Seidlova-Wuttke D, Eder N, Stahnke V, Kammann M, Stecher G, Haunschild J, Wessels JT, Wuttke W. (2012). *Cimicifuga racemosa* and its triterpene-saponins prevent the metabolic syndrome and deterioration of cartilage in the knee joint of ovariectomized rats by similar mechanisms. *Phytomed.* 19(8–9):846–853.
157. Luo J, Qi J, Wang W, Luo Z, Liu L, Zhang G, Zhou Q, Liu J, Peng X. (2019). Antiobesity effect of flaxseed polysaccharide via inducing satiety due to leptin resistance removal and promoting lipid metabolism through the AMP-Activated Protein Kinase (AMPK) signaling pathway. *J Agric Food Chem.* 67(25):7040–7049.

158. Wuttke W, Jarry H, Christoffel V, Spengler B, Seidlová-Wuttke D. (2003). Chaste tree (*Vitex agnus castus*)—pharmacology and clinical indications. *Phytomed.* 10(4):348–357.
159. Fan CW, Cieri-Hutcherson NE, Hutcherson TC. (2021). Systematic review of black cohosh (*Cimicifuga racemosa*) for management of polycystic ovary syndrome-related infertility. *J Pharmacol Pract.* 8971900211012244.
160. Ushiroyama T, Ikeda A, Sakai M, Hosotani T, Suzuki Y, Tsubokura S, Ueki M. (2001). Effects of *unkei-to*, an herbal medicine, on endocrine function and ovulation in women with high basal levels of luteinizing hormone secretion. *J Reprod Med.* 46(5):451–456.
161. Nasri S, Oryan S, Rohani AH, Amin GR. (2007). The effects of *Vitex agnus castus* extract and its interaction with dopaminergic system on LH and testosterone in male mice. *Pak J Biol Sci.* 10(14):2300–2307.
162. Kamel HH. (2013). Role of phyto-oestrogens in ovulation induction in women with polycystic ovarian syndrome. *Eur J Obstet Gynecol Reprod Biol.* 168(1):60–63.
163. Jazani AM, Nazemiyeh H, Tansaz M, Bazargani HS. et al. (2018). Celery plus anise versus metformin for the treatment of oligomenorrhea in polycystic ovary syndrome: A triple-blind randomized clinical trial. *Iran Red Cresc Med J.* 20(5):e67181.
164. Ghavi F, Shakeri F. (2015). Effects of fennel on serum hormone levels in students with polycystic ovary syndrome. *Avicenna J Phytomed.* 5:42–43.
165. Heidary M, Yazdanpanahi Z, Dabbaghmanesh MH, Parsanezhad ME, Emamghoreishi M, Akbarzadeh M. (2018). Effect of chamomile capsule on lipid- and hormonal-related parameters among women of reproductive age with polycystic ovary syndrome. *J Res Med Sci.* (Isfahan). 23:33.
166. Takahashi K, Kitao M. (1994). Effect of TJ-68 (*shakuyaku-kanzo-to*) on polycystic ovarian disease. *Int J Fertil Menopausal Stud.* 39(2):69–76.
167. Wiweko B, Susanto CA. (2017). The effect of metformin and cinnamon on serum anti-mullerian hormone in women having PCOS: A double-blind, randomized, controlled trial. *J Hum Reprod Sci.* 10(1):31–36.
168. Kumarapeli M, Karunagoda K, Perera PK. (2018). A randomized clinical trial to evaluate the efficacy of *Satapushpashatavari* powered drug with *Satapushpa-shatavari grita* for the management of Polycystic Ovary Syndrome (PCOS). *Int J Pharmacol Sci Res.* 9(6):2494–2499.

169. Kumarapeli M, Karunagoda K, Perera PK. (2018). A randomized clinical trial to evaluate the efficacy of *Satapushpashatavari* powered drug with *Satapushpa-shatavari grita* for the management of Polycystic Ovary Syndrome (PCOS). *Int J Pharmacol Sci Res.* 9(6):2494–2499.
170. Farzana F, Sulaiman A, Ruckmani A, Vijayalakshmi K, Karunya Lakshmi G, Shri RS. (2015). Effects of flax seeds supplementation in polycystic ovarian syndrome. *J Res Med Sci.* 31(1):113–119.
171. Jalilian N, Modarresi M, Rezaie M, Ghaderi L, Bozorgmanesh M. (2013). Phytotherapeutic management of polycystic ovary syndrome: Role of aerial parts of wood betony (*Stachys lavandulifolia*). *Phytother* 27(11):1708–1713.
172. Swaroop A, Jaipuriar AS, Gupta SK, Bagchi M, Kumar P, Preuss HG, Bagchi D. (2015). Efficacy of a novel fenugreek seed extract (*Trigonella foenum-graecum*, FurocystTM) in Polycystic Ovary Syndrome (PCOS). *Int J Med Sci.* 12(10):825–831.
173. Bashtian MH, Emami SA, Mousavifar N, Esmaily HA, Mahmoudi M, Poor AHM. (2013). Evaluation of fenugreek (*Trigonella foenum-graceum* L.), effects seeds extract on insulin resistance in women with polycystic ovarian syndrome. *Iran J Pharm Res.* 12(2):475–481.
174. Lee JC, Pak SC, Lee SH, Lim SC, Bai YH, Jin CS, Kim JS, Na CS, Bae CS, Oh KS. (2003). The effect of herbal medicine on nerve growth factor in estradiol valerate-induced polycystic ovaries in rats. *Am J Chin Med.* 31(06):885–895.
175. Mehraban M, Jelodar G, Rahmanifar F. (2020). A combination of spearmint and flaxseed extract improved endocrine and histomorphology of ovary in experimental PCOS. *J Ovarian Res.* 13(1):32.
176. Abbasian Z, Jafari Barmak M, Barazesh F, Ghavamizadeh M, Mirzaei A. (2020). Therapeutic efficacy of *Trifolium pratense* L. on letrozole induced polycystic ovary syndrome in rats. *Plant Sci Today.* 7(3):501–507.
177. Dehghan A, Esfandiari A, Bigdeli SM. (2012). Alternative treatment of ovarian cysts with *Tribulus terrestris* extract: A rat model. *Reprod Domest Anim.* 47(1):e12–e15.
178. Kumarapeli M, Karunagoda K, Perera PK. (2018). A randomized clinical trial to evaluate the efficacy of *Satapushpashatavari* powered drug with *Satapushpa-shatavari grita* for the management of Polycystic Ovary Syndrome (PCOS). *Int J Pharmacol Sci Res.* 9(6):2494–2499.
179. Grant P. (2010). Spearmint herbal tea has significant anti-androgen effects in polycystic ovarian syndrome. A randomized controlled trial. *Phytother Res.* 24(2):186–188.

180. Akdoğan M, Tamer MN, Cüre E, Cüre MC, Köroğlu BK, Delibaş N. (2007). Effect of spearmint (*Mentha spicata* Labiatae) teas on androgen levels in women with hirsutism. *Phytother Res.* 21(5):444–447.
181. Nowak DA, Snyder DC, Brown AJ, Demark-Wahnefried W. (2007). The effect of flaxseed supplementation on hormonal levels associated with polycystic ovarian syndrome: A case study. *Curr Top Nutraceutical Res.* 5:177–181.
182. Sturgeon SR, Heersink JL, Volpe SL, Bertone-Johnson ER, Puleo E, Stanczyk FZ. et al. (2008). Effect of dietary flaxseed on serum levels of estrogens and androgens in postmenopausal women. *Nutr Cancer.* 60:612–618.
183. Nowak DA, Snyder DC, Brown AJ, Demark-Wahnefried W. (2007). The effect of flaxseed supplementation on hormonal levels associated with polycystic ovarian syndrome: A case study. *Curr Top Nutraceutical Res.* 5:177–181.
184. Javidnia K, Dastgheib L, Mohammadi Samani S, Nasiri A. (2003). Antihirsutism activity of Fennel (fruits of *Foeniculum vulgare*) extract. A double-blind placebo controlled study. *Phytomed.* 10(6–7):455–458.
185. Javidnia K, Dastgheib L, Mohammadi Samani S, Nasiri A. (2003). Antihirsutism activity of Fennel (fruits of *Foeniculum vulgare*) extract. A double-blind placebo controlled study. *Phytomed.* 10(6–7):455–458.
186. Akha O, Rabiei K, Kashi Z, Bahar A, Zaeif-Khorasani E, Kosaryan M. et al. (2014). The effect of fennel (*Foeniculum vulgare*) gel 3% in decreasing hair thickness in idiopathic mild to moderate hirsutism, a randomized placebo controlled clinical trial. *Caspian J Intern Med.* 5:26–29.
187. Faghihi G, Iraji F, Abtahi-Naeini B, Saffar B, Saffaei A. et al. (2015). Complementary therapies for idiopathic hirsutism: Topical licorice as promising option. *Evid Based Complement Alt. Med.* 659041.
188. Azouz AA, Ali SE, Abd-Elsalam RM, Emam SR, Galal MK. et al. (2021). Modulation of steroidogenesis by *Actaea racemosa* and vitamin C combination, in letrozole induced polycystic ovarian syndrome rat model: Promising activity without the risk of hepatic adverse effect. *Chin Med.* 16(1):36.
189. Seidlová-Wuttke D, Hesse O, Jarry H, Christoffel V, Spengler B, Becker T, Wuttke W. (2003). Evidence for selective estrogen receptor modulator activity in a black cohosh (*Cimicifuga racemosa*) extract: Comparison with estradiol-17beta. *Eur J Endocrinol.* 149(4):351–362.
190. Seidlová-Wuttke D, Hesse O, Jarry H, Christoffel V, Spengler B, Becker T, Wuttke W. (2003). Evidence for selective estrogen receptor

modulator activity in a black cohosh (*Cimicifuga racemosa*) extract: Comparison with estradiol-17beta. *Eur J Endocrinol.* 149(4):351–362.
191. Seidlová-Wuttke D, Eder N, Stahnke V, Kammann M, Stecher G, Haunschild J, Wessels JT, Wuttke W. (2012). *Cimicifuga racemosa* and its triterpene-saponins prevent the metabolic syndrome and deterioration of cartilage in the knee joint of ovariectomized rats by similar mechanisms. *Phytomed.* 19(8–9):846–853.
192. Seidlová-Wuttke D, Jarry H, Becker T, Christoffel V, Wuttke W. (2003). Pharmacology of *Cimicifuga racemosa* extract BNO 1055 in rats: Bone, fat and uterus. *Maturitas.* 44(Suppl. 1):S39–S50.
193. Moser C, Vickers SP, Brammer R, Cheetham SC, Drewe J. (2014). Antidiabetic effects of the *Cimicifuga racemosa* extract Ze 450 in vitro and in vivo in ob/ob mice. *Phytomed.* 21(11):1382–1389.
194. Rachoń D, Vortherms T, Seidlová-Wuttke D, Wuttke W. (2008). Effects of black cohosh extract on body weight gain, intra-abdominal fat accumulation, plasma lipids and glucose tolerance in ovariectomized Sprague-Dawley rats. *Maturitas.* 60(3–4):209–215.
195. Shahin AY, Mohammed SA. (2014). Adding the phytoestrogen *Cimicifugae racemosae* to clomiphene induction cycles with timed intercourse in polycystic ovary syndrome improves cycle outcomes and pregnancy rates—a randomized trial. *Gynecol Endocrinol.* 30(7):505–510.
196. Kamel HH. (2013). Role of phyto-oestrogens in ovulation induction in women with polycystic ovarian syndrome. *Eur J Obstet Gynecol Reprod Biol.* 168(1):60–63.
197. Akilen R, Tsiami A, Devendra D, Robinson N. (2012). Cinnamon in glycaemic control: Systematic review and meta analysis. *Clin Nutr.* 31(5):609–615.
198. Leach MJ, Kumar S. (2012). Cinnamon for diabetes mellitus. *Cochrane Database Syst Rev.* 9:CD007170.2.
199. Heibashy M, Mazen G, Shahin M. (2013). Metabolic changes and hormonal disturbances in polycystic ovarian syndrome rats and the amelioration effects of metformin and/or cinnamon extraction. *J Am Sci.* 9(12):54–62.
200. Hajimonfarednejad M, Nimrouzi M, Heydari M, Zarshenas MM, Raee MJ, Jahromi BN. (2018). Insulin resistance improvement by cinnamon powder in polycystic ovary syndrome: A randomized double-blind placebo controlled clinical trial. *Phytother Res.* 32(2):276–283.
201. Wang JG, Anderson RA, Graham GM III, Chu MC, Sauer MV, Guarnaccia MM, Lobo RA. (2007). The effect of cinnamon extract on

insulin resistance parameters in polycystic ovary syndrome: A pilot study. *Fertil Steril.* 88(1):240–243.
202. Borzoei A, Rafraf M, Asghari-Jafarabadi M. (2018). Cinnamon improves metabolic factors without detectable effects on adiponectin in women with polycystic ovary syndrome. *Asia Pac J Clin Nutr.* 27(3):556–563.
203. Heydarpour F, Hemati N, Hadi A, Moradi S, Mohammadi E, Farzaei MH. (2020). Effects of cinnamon on controlling metabolic parameters of polycystic ovary syndrome: A systematic review and meta-analysis. *J Ethnopharmacol.* 254:112741.
204. Kort DH, Lobo RA. (2014). Preliminary evidence that cinnamon improves menstrual cyclicity in women with polycystic ovary syndrome: A randomized controlled trial. *Am J Obstet Gynecol.* 211(5):487e1–487e6.
205. Allen RW, Schwartzman E, Baker WL, Coleman CI, Phung OJ. (2013). Cinnamon use in type 2 diabetes: An updated systematic review and meta-analysis. *Ann Fam Med.* 11(5):452–459.
206. Wiweko B, Susanto CA. (2017). The effect of metformin and cinnamon on serum anti-mullerian hormone in women having PCOS: A double-blind, randomized, controlled trial. *J Hum Reprod Sci.* 10(1):31–36.
207. Medagama AB. (2015). The glycaemic outcomes of cinnamon, a review of the experimental evidence and clinical trials. *Nutr J.* 14:108.
208. Armanini D, Castello R, Scaroni C, Bonanni G, Faccini G. et al. (2007). Treatment of polycystic ovary syndrome with spironolactone and licorice. *Eur J Obstet Gynecol Reprod.* 131:61–67.
209. Armanini D, Mattarello MJ, Fiore C, Bonanni G, Scaroni C. et al. (2004). Licorice reduces serum testosterone in healthy women. *Steroids.* 69:763–766.
210. Tamura Y, Nishikawa T, Yamada K, Yamamoto M, Kumagai A. (1979). Effects of glycyrrhetinic acid and its derivatives on Δ 4-5α- and 5β-reductase in rat liver. *Arzneimittel-Forschung.* 29(4):647–649.
211. Ko BS, Jang JS, Hong SM, Sung SR, Lee JE, Lee MY, Jeon WK, Park S. (2007). Changes in components, glycyrrhizin and glycyrrhetinic acid, in raw *Glycyrrhiza uralensis* Fisch, modify insulin sensitizing and insulinotropic actions. *Biosci Biotechnol Biochem.* 71(6):1452–1461.
212. Josephs RA, Guinn JS, Harper ML, Askari F. (2001). Liquorice consumption and salivary testosterone concentrations. *Lancet.* 358(9293):1613–1614.
213. Lee JC, Pak SC, Lee SH, Lim SC, Bai YH, Jin CS, Kim JS, Na CS, Bae CS, Oh KS. (2003). The effect of herbal medicine on nerve growth factor in

estradiol valerate-induced polycystic ovaries in rats. *Am J Chin Med.* 31(6):885–895.
214. Armanini D, De Palo CB, Mattarello MJ, Spinella P, Zaccaria M, Ermolao A. et al. (2003). Effect of licorice on the reduction of body fat mass in healthy subjects. *J Endocrinol Invest.* 26(7):646–650.
215. Fuhrman B, Volkova N, Kaplan M, Presser D, Attias J, Hayek T, Aviram M. (2002). Antiatherosclerotic effects of licorice extract supplementation on hypercholesterolemic patients: Increased resistance of LDL to atherogenic modifications, reduced plasma lipid levels, and decreased systolic blood pressure. *Nutrition.* 18(3):268–273.
216. Armanini D, Mattarello MJ, Fiore C, Bonanni G, Scaroni C, Sartorato P. et al. (2004). Licorice reduces serum testosterone in healthy women. *Steroids.* 69(11–12):763–766.
217. Mattarello MJ, Benedini S, Fiore C, Camozzi V, Sartorato P, Luisetto G, Armanini D. (2006). Effect of licorice on PTH levels in healthy women. *Steroids.* 71(5):403–408.
218. Armanini D, Castello R, Scaroni C, Bonanni G, Faccini G, Pellati D. et al. (2007). Treatment of polycystic ovary syndrome with spironolactone plus licorice. *Eur J Obstet Gynecol Reprod Biol.* 131(1):61–67.
219. Faghihi G, Iraji F, Abtahi-Naeini B, Saffar B, Saffaei A. et al. (2015). Complementary therapies for idiopathic hirsutism: Topical licorice as promising option. *Evid Based Complement Alt. Med.* 659041.
220. Ota A, Ulrih NP. (2017). An overview of herbal products and secondary metabolites used for management of type two diabetes. *Front Pharmacol.* 8:436.
221. Tiwari P, Mishra BN, Sangwan NS. (2014). Phytochemical and pharmacological properties of *Gymnema sylvestre*: An important medicinal plant. *Biomed Res Int.* 830285.
222. Shimizu K, Ozeki M, Lino A, Nakajyo S, Urakawa N, Atsuchi M. (2001). Structure-activity relationships of triterpenoid derivatives extracted from *Gymnema inodorum* leaves on glucose absorption. *Jpn J Pharmacol* 86(2):223–229.
223. Yoshioka S. (1986). Inhibitory effects of gymnemic acid and an extract from the leaves of *Zizyphus jujuba* on glucose absorption in the rat small intestine. *J Yonago Med Assoc.* 37:142–154.
224. Fushiki T, Kojima A, Imoto T, Inoue K, Sugimoto E. (1992). An extract of *Gymnema sylvestre* leaves and purified gymnemic acid inhibits glucose-stimulated gastric inhibitory peptide secretion in rats. *J Nutr.* 122(12):2367–2373.

225. Sugihara Y, Nojima H, Matsuda H, Murakami T, Yoshikawa M, Kimura I. (2000). Antihyperglycemic effects of gymnemic acid IV, a compound derived from *Gymnema sylvestre* leaves in streptozotocin-diabetic mice. *J Asian Natural Prod Res.* 2(4):321–327.
226. Shanmugasundaram ER, Gopinath KL, Shanmugasundaram KR, Rajendran VM. (1990). Possible regeneration of the islets of Langerhans in streptozotocin-diabetic rats given *Gymnema sylvestre* leaf extracts. *J Ethnopharmacol.* 30(3):265–279.
227. Nakamura Y, Tsumura Y, Tonogai Y, Shibata T. (1999). Fecal steroid excretion is increased in rats by oral administration of gymnemic acids contained in *Gymnema sylvestre* leaves. *J Nutr.* 129(6):1214–1222.
228. Preuss HG, Jarrell ST, Scheckenbach R, Lieberman S, Anderson RA. (1998). Comparative effects of chromium, vanadium and *Gymnema sylvestre* on sugar-induced blood pressure elevations in SHR. *J Am Coll Nutr.* 17(2):116–123.
229. Preuss HG, Garis RI, Bramble JD, Bagchi D. et al. (2005). Efficacy of a novel calcium/potassium salt of (-)-hydroxycitric acid in weight control. *Int J Clin Pharmacol Res.* 25(3):133–144.
230. Brala PM, Hagen RL. (1983). Effects of sweetness perception and calorie value of a preload on short term intake. *Physiol Behav.* 30(1):1–9.
231. Woodgate DE, Conquer JA. (2003). Effects of a stimulant-free dietary supplement on body weight and fat loss in obese adults: A six- week exploratory study. *Curr Ther Res.* 64(4):248–262.
232. ClinicalTrials.gov. (2016). Effect of *Gymnema sylvestre* on metabolic syndrome and insulin. Available at: https://clinicaltrials.gov/ct2/show/NCT02370121.
233. Bnouham M, Ziyyat A, Mekhfi H, Tahri A, Legssyer A. (2006). Medicinal plants with potential antidiabetic activity—a review of ten years of herbal medicine research (1990–2000). *Int J Diabetes Metab.* 14:1–25.
234. Baskaran K, Ahamath BK, Shanmugasundaram KR, Shanmugasundaram ER. (1990). Antidiabetic effect of leaf extract from *Gymnema sylvestre* in non-insulin-dependent diabetes mellitus patients. *J Ethnopharmacol.* 30(3):295–300.
235. Stracquadanio M, Ciotta L, Palumbo MA. (2018). Effects of myo-inositol, gymnemic acid, and L-methylfolate in polycystic ovary syndrome patients. *Gynecol Endocrinol.* 34(6):495–501.
236. Akdogan M, Ozguner M, Kocak A, Oncu M, Cicek E. (2004). Effects of peppermint teas on plasma testosterone, follicle-stimulating hormone,

and luteinizing hormone levels and testicular tissue in rats. *Urology.* 64(2):394–398.
237. Grant P. (2010). Spearmint herbal tea has significant anti-androgen effects in polycystic ovarian syndrome. A randomized controlled trial. *Phytother Res.* 24(2):186–188.
238. Akdoğan M, Tamer MN, Cüre E, Cüre MC, Köroğlu BK, Delibaş N. (2007). Effect of spearmint (*Mentha spicata* Labiatae) teas on androgen levels in women with hirsutism. *Phytother Res.* 21(5):444–447.
239. Yuan HN, Wang CY, Sze CW, Tong Y, Tan QR, Feng XJ. et al. (2008). A randomized, crossover comparison of herbal medicine and bromocriptine against risperidone-induced hyperprolactinemia in patients with schizophrenia. *J Clin Psychopharmacol.* 28(3):264–370.
240. Yamada K, Kanba S, Yagi G, Asai M. (1999). Herbal medicine (*skakuyaku-kanzo-to*) in the treatment of risperidone-induced amenorrhea. *J Clin Psychopharmacol.* 19:380–381.
241. Man SC, Li XB, Wang HH, Yuan HN, Wang HN, Zhang RG. et al. (2016). Peony-glycyrrhiza decoction for antipsychotic-related hyperprolactinemia in women with schizophrenia: A randomized controlled trial. *J Clin Psychopharmacol.* 36(6):572–579.
242. Aboraya A, Fullen JE, Ponieman BL, Makela EH, Latocha M. (2004). Hyperprolactinemia associated with risperidone. A case report and review of literature. *Psychiatry* (Edgmont). (3):29–31.
243. Yang P, Li L, Yang D, Wang C, Peng H, Huang H. et al. (2017). Effect of peony-glycyrrhiza decoction on amisulpride-induced hyperprolactinemia in women with schizophrenia: A preliminary study. *Evid Based Complement Alternat Med.* 7901670.
244. Aizawa H, Niimura M. (1996). Serum androgen levels in woman with *Acne vulgaris*: The effect of *shakuyaku-knazo-to* (SM). *Skin Research.* 38:37–41.
245. Takeuchi T, Nishii O, Okamura T, Yaginuma T. (1989). Effect of traditional herbal medicine, *shakuyaku-kanzo-to* on total and free serum testosterone levels. *Am J Chin Med.* 17(1–2):35–44.
246. Takahashi K, Kitao M. (1994). Effect of TJ-68 (*shakuyaku-kanzo-to*) on polycystic ovarian disease. *Int J Fertil Menopausal Stud.* 39(2):69.
247. Yaginuma T, Izumi R, Yasui H, Arai T, Kawabata M. (1982). Effect of traditional herbal medicine on serum testosterone levels and its induction of regular ovulation in hyperandrogenic and oligomenorrheic women. *Nihon Sanka Fujinka Gakkai Zasshi.* 34(7):939–944.

248. Takahashi K, Yoshino K, Shirai T, Nishigaki A, Araki Y, Kitao M. (1988). Effects of traditional medicine (*Shakuyaku-kanzo-to*) on testosterone secretion in patients with polycystic ovarian syndrome detected by ultrasound. *Nihon Sanka Fujinka Gakkai Zasshi.* 40(6):789–792.
249. Buck AC. (2004). Is there a scientific basis for the therapeutic effects of *Serenoa repens* in benign prostatic hyperplasia? Mechanisms of action. *J Urol.* 172(5 Pt 1):1792–1799.
250. Geavlete P, Multescu R, Geavlete B. (2011). *Serenoa repens* extract in the treatment of benign prostatic hyperplasia. *Ther Adv Urol.* 3(4):193–198.
251. Tacklind J, MacDonald R, Rutks I, Wilt TJ. (2009). *Serenoa repens* for benign prostatic hyperplasia. *Cochrane Database Syst Rev.* (2):CD001423.
252. Sinescu I, Geavlete P, Multescu R, Gangu C, Miclea F. et al. (2011). Long-term efficacy of *Serenoa repens* treatment in patients with mild and moderate symptomatic benign prostatic hyperplasia. *Urol Int.* 86(3):284–289.
253. Vinarov AZ, Spivak LG, Platonova DV, Rapoport LM, Korolev DO. (2019). 15 years' survey of safety and efficacy of *Serenoa repens* extract in benign prostatic hyperplasia patients with risk of progression. *Urologia.* 86(1):17–22.
254. Sultan C, Terraza A, Devillier C, Carilla E, Briley M, Loire C, Descomps B. (1984). Inhibition of androgen metabolism and binding by a liposterolic extract of "Serenoa repens B" in human foreskin fibroblasts. *J Steroid Biochem.* 20(1):515–519.
255. Sultan C, Terraza A, Devillier C, Carilla E, Briley M, Loire C, Descomps B. (1984). Inhibition of androgen metabolism and binding by a liposterolic extract of "Serenoa repens B" in human foreskin fibroblasts. *J Steroid Biochem.* 20(1):515–519.
256. Düker EM, Kopanski L, Schweikert HU. Inhibition of 5-reductase activity by extracts from *Sabal serrulata. Planta Med.* 55:587.
257. Scaglione F, Lucini V, Pannacci M, Caronno A, Leone C. (2008). Comparison of the potency of different brands of *Serenoa repens* extract on 5alpha-reductase types I and II in prostatic co-cultured epithelial and fibroblast cells. *Pharmacol.* 82:270–275.
258. Di Silverio F, D'Eramo G, Lubrano C, Flammia G, P, Sciarra A, Palma E, Caponera M, Sciarra F. (1992). Evidence that *Serenoa repens* extract displays an antiestrogenic activity in prostatic tissue of benign prostatic hypertrophy patients. *Eur Urol.* 21:309–314.

259. Geavlete P, Multescu R, Geavlete B. (2011). *Serenoa repens* extract in the treatment of benign prostatic hyperplasia. *Therap Adv Urol.* 3(4):193–198.
260. Van Coppenolle F, Le Bourhis X, Carpentier F, Delaby G, Cousse H, Raynaud JP, Dupouy JP, Prevarskaya N. (2000). Pharmacological effects of the lipidosterolic extract of *Serenoa repens* (Permixon) on rat prostate hyperplasia induced by hyperprolactinemia: comparison with finasteride. *Prostate.* 43(1):49–58.
261. Prager N. (2002). A randomized double-blind placebo controlled trial to determine the effectiveness of botanically derived inhibitors of 5 alpha reductase in the treatment of androgenetic alopecia. *J Altern Complent Med.* 8:413–452.
262. Fasculo C. (2004). Effectiveness of *Serenoa repens* in androgenetic alopecia. *JDDG, 6.2004 (Band 2). 552 Abstracts, 4th Intercontinental Meeting of Hair Research Societies.*
263. Tosti A. (2008). Ketoil® shampoo (ketaconazole 0.5%, *Serenoa repens*, taurine) Vs ketaconazole 1% shampoo (Triatop®) in patients with dandruff and seborrheic dermatitis. *Abstract Book, 13th Annual Meeting of European Hair Research Society.* Genoa, Italy. pp. 3–5.
264. Yousefi M, Barikbin B, Givrad S, Moravvej H, Khoshnoudi R. (2009). The effectiveness of the extract of *Serenoa repens* (saw palmetto) in idiopathic facial hirsutism. *Iran J Dermatol.* 12(4).
265. Gerhard II, Patek A, Monga B, Blank A, Gorkow C. (1985). Mastodynon(R) bei weiblicher Sterilität. *Forsch Komplementarmed.* 5(6):272–278.
266. Eltbogen R, Litschgi M, Gasser UE, Flueeli A, Nebel S, Zahner C. (2014). *Vitex agnus-castus* extract (ZE440) improves symptoms in women with menstrual cycle irregularities. *Reprod Endocrin.* 28:86–91.
267. Bergmann J, Luft B, Boehmann S, Runnebaum B, Gerhard I. (2000). Die wirksamkeit des komplexmittels Phyto-Hypophyson L bei weiblicher, hormonell bedingter sterilität [The efficacy of the complex medication Phyto-Hypophyson L in female, hormone-related sterility. A randomized, placebo-controlled clinical double-blind study]. *Forsch Komplementarmed Klass Naturheilkd.* 7(4):190–199.
268. Milewicz A, Gejdel E, Sworen H, Sienkiewicz K, Jedrzejak J, Teucher T, Schmitz H. (1993). *Vitex agnus castus* extract in the treatment of luteal phase defects due to latent hyperprolactinemia. Results of a randomized placebo-controlled double-blind study. *Arzneimittelforschung* 43(7):752–756.

269. Soleymanzadeh F, Mahmoodi M, Shahidi S. (2020). Effect of *Vitex agnus-castus* ethanolic extract on sex hormones in streptozotocin-induced diabetic rats. *J Fam Reprod Health*. 14(2):102–105.
270. Wuttke W, Jarry H, Christoffel V, Spengler B, Seidlová-Wuttke D. (2003). Chaste tree (*Vitex agnus-castus*)—pharmacology and clinical indications. *Phytomed*. 10(4):348–357.
271. Jelodar G, Askari K. (2012). Effect of *Vitex agnus-castus* fruits hydroalcoholic extract on sex hormones in rat with induced polycystic ovary syndrome (PCOS). *Physiol Pharmacol*. 16:62–69.
272. Ghahremaninasab P, Shahnazi M, Khalili AF, Hamdi K. (in press). The effects of combined low-dose oral contraceptives and *Vitex agnus* on the improvement of clinical and paraclinical parameters of polycystic ovarian syndrome: A triple-blind, randomized, controlled clinical trial. *Iran Red Cresc Med J*. e37510. Published online 2016.
273. Shayan, A., Masoumi, S. Z., Shobeiri, F., Tohidi, S., & Khalili, A. (2016). Comparing the effects of agnugol and metformin on oligomenorrhea in patients with polycystic ovary syndrome: A randomized clinical trial. *J Clin Diag Res*. 10(12):QC13–QC16.
274. Jazani AM, Nazemiyeh H, Tansaz M, Bazargani HS. et al. (2018). Celery plus anise versus metformin for the treatment of oligomenorrhea in polycystic ovary syndrome: A triple-blind randomized clinical trial. *Iran Red Cresc Med J*. 20(5):e67181.
275. Kumarapeli M, Karunagoda K, Perera PK. (2018). A randomized clinical trial to evaluate the efficacy of *Satapushpashatavari* powered drug with *Satapushpa-shatavari grita* for the management of Polycystic Ovary Syndrome (PCOS). *Int J Pharmacol Sci Res*. 9(6):2494–2499.
276. Wang Y, Fu X, Xu J, Wang Q, Kuang H. (2016). Systems pharmacology to investigate the interaction of berberine and other drugs in treating polycystic ovary syndrome. *Sci Rep*. 6:28089.
277. Bone K, Mills S. (2013). *Principles and Practice of Phytotherapy*. 2nd ed. London: Elsevier.
278. Liu CS, Zheng YR, Zhang YF, Long XY. (2016). Research progress on berberine with a special focus on its oral bioavailability. *Fitoterapia*. 109:274–282.
279. Ko BS, Choi SB, Park SK, Jang JS, Kim YE, Park S. (2005). Insulin sensitizing and insulinotropic action of berberine from *Cortidis rhizoma*. *Biol Pharmacol Bull*. 28(8):1431–1437.
280. Imenshahidi M, Hosseinzadeh H. (2019). Berberine and barberry (*Berberis vulgaris*): A clinical review. *Phytother Res*. 33(3):504–523.

281. Wei W, Zhao H, Wang A, Sui M. et al. (2012). A clinical study on the short-term effect of berberine in comparison to metformin on the metabolic characteristics of women with polycystic ovary syndrome. *Eur J Endocrinol.* 166(1):99–105.
282. An Y, Zhang Y, Lu H, Li L, Sun Z. (2016). Effect of berberine on clinical, metabolic and endocrine indexes and pregnancy outcome in women with polycystic ovary syndrome undergoing IVF treatment. *Modern J Integ Trad Chin West Med.* 25(5):459–462, 466.
283. Li MF, Zhou XM, Li XL. (2018). The effect of berberine on Polycystic Ovary Syndrome patients with Insulin Resistance (PCOS-IR): A meta-analysis and systematic review. *Evidence-Based Complement Alt Med.* 2532935.
284. Wei W, Zhao H, Wang A, Sui M. et al. (2012). A clinical study on the short-term effect of berberine in comparison to metformin on the metabolic characteristics of women with polycystic ovary syndrome. *Eur J Endocrinol.* 166(1):99–105.
285. Li L, Li C, Pan P, Chen X, Wu X, Ng EH, Yang, D. (2015). A single arm pilot study of effects of berberine on the menstrual pattern, ovulation rate, hormonal and metabolic profiles in anovulatory Chinese women with polycystic ovary syndrome. *PloS One.* 10(12):e0144072.
286. Kuang H. (2014). *Clinical Study on Berberine in the Treatment of Insulin Resistance in Women with Polycystic Ovary Syndrome.* Guangzhou University of Chinese Medicine.
287. Li X, Kuang H, Luo Y. (2017). Clinical observation of berberine in intervening insulin resistance of polycystic ovary syndrome. *J Guangzhou Univ Trad Chin Med.* 2:172–177.
288. Wang L, Kong Y, Ren Y, Shen M. (2011). Therapeutic effect of berberine combined with diformin for women with Polycystic Ovary Syndrome and Insulin Resistance. *J Zhejiang University Trad Chin Med.* 35(5):713–715.
289. Tehrani HG, Allahdadian M, Zarre F, Ranjbar H, Allahdadian F. (2017). Effect of green tea on metabolic and hormonal aspect of polycystic ovarian syndrome in overweight and obese women suffering from polycystic ovarian syndrome: A clinical trial. *J Educ Health Promotion.* 6:36.
290. Wu CH, Lu FH, Chang CS, Chang TC, Wang RH, Chang CJ. (2003). Relationship among habitual tea consumption, percent body fat, and body fat distribution. *Obes Res.* 11:1088–1095.
291. Iso H, Date C, Wakai K, Fukui M, Tamakoshi A. (2006). JACC Study Group. The relationship between green tea and total caffeine intake

and risk for self-reported type 2 diabetes among Japanese adults. *Ann Intern Med.* 144:554–562.
292. Heshmati J, Golab F, Morvaridzadeh M, Potter E, Akbari-Fakhrabadi M, Farsi F, Tanbakooei S, Shidfar F. (2020). The effects of curcumin supplementation on oxidative stress, Sirtuin-1 and peroxisome proliferator activated receptor γ coactivator 1α gene expression in polycystic ovarian syndrome (PCOS) patients: A randomized placebo-controlled clinical trial. *Diabetes Metab Syndr.* 14(2):77–82.
293. Heshmati J, Moini A, Sepidarkish M. et al. (2021). Effects of curcumin supplementation on blood glucose, insulin resistance, and androgens in patients with polycystic ovary syndrome: A randomized double-blind placebo-controlled clinical trial. *Phytomed.* 80:153395.
294. Jamilian M, Foroozanfard F, Kavossian E, Aghadavod E, Shafabakhsh R, Hoseini A, Asemi Z. (2020). Effects of curcumin on body weight, glycemic control and serum lipids in women with polycystic ovary syndrome: A randomized, double-blind, placebo-controlled trial. *Clin Nutr ESPEN.* 36:128–133.
295. Azhdari M, Karandish M, Mansoori A. (2019). Metabolic benefits of curcumin supplementation in patients with metabolic syndrome: A systematic review and meta-analysis of randomized controlled trials. *Phytother Res.* 33:1289–1301.
296. Na LX, Yan BL, Jiang S, Cui HL, Li Y, Sun CH. (2014). Curcuminoids target decreasing serum adipocyte-fatty acid binding protein levels in their glucose-lowering effect in patients with type 2 diabetes. *Biomed Environ Sci.* 27(11):902–906.
297. Na LX, Li Y, Pan HZ. et al. (2013). Curcuminoids exert glucose-lowering effect in type 2 diabetes by decreasing serum free fatty acids: A double-blind, placebo-controlled trial. *Molec Nutr Food Res.* 57(9):1569–1577.
298. Nistico S, Tamburi F, Bennardo L, Dastoli S, Schipani G, Caro G, Fortuna MC, Rossi A. (2019). Treatment of telogen effluvium using a dietary supplement containing *Boswellia serrata, Curcuma longa,* and *Vitis vinifera*: Results of an observational study. *Dermatol Ther.* 32:e12842.
299. Jelodar G, Masoomi S, Rahmanifar F. (2018). Hydroalcoholic extract of flaxseed improves polycystic ovary syndrome in a rat model. *Iran J Basic Med Sci.* 21(6):645–650.
300. Mokaberinejad R, Rampisheh Z, Aliasl J, Akhtari E. (2019). The comparison of fennel infusion plus dry cupping versus metformin in

management of oligomenorrhoea in patients with polycystic ovary syndrome: A randomised clinical trial. *J Obstet Gynaecol.* 39(5):652–658.
301. Mohebbi-Kian E, Mohammad-Alizadeh-Charandabi S, Bekhradi R. (2014). Efficacy of fennel and combined oral contraceptive on depot medroxyprogesterone acetate-induced amenorrhea: A randomized placebo-controlled trial. *Contraception.* 90:440–446.
302. Ghavi F, Shakeri F. (2015). Effects of fennel on serum hormone levels in students with polycystic ovary syndrome. *Avicenna J Phytomed.* 5:42–43.
303. Javidnia K, Dastgheib L, Mohammadi Samani S, Nasiri A. (2003). Antihirsutism activity of fennel (fruits of *Foeniculum vulgare*) extract. A double-blind placebo controlled study. *Phytomed.* 10(6–7):455–458.
304. Akha O, Rabiei K, Kashi Z, Bahar A, Zaeif-Khorasani E, Kosaryan M. et al. (2014). The effect of fennel (*Foeniculum vulgare*) gel 3% in decreasing hair thickness in idiopathic mild to moderate hirsutism, a randomized placebo controlled clinical trial. *Caspian J Intern Med.* 5(1):26–29.
305. Zangeneh FZ, Minaee B, Amirzargar A, Ahangarpour A, Mousavizadeh K. (2010). Effects of chamomile extract on biochemical and clinical parameters in a rat model of polycystic ovary syndrome. *J Reprod Infertil.* 11(3):169–174.
306. Farideh ZZ, Bagher M, Ashraf A, Akram A, Kazem M. (2010). Effects of chamomile extract on biochemical and clinical parameters in a rat model of polycystic ovary syndrome. *J Reprod Infertil* 11(3):169–174.
307. Heidary M, Yazdanpanahi Z, Dabbaghmanesh MH, Parsanezhad ME, Emamghoreishi M, Akbarzadeh M. (2018). Effect of chamomile capsule on lipid- and hormonal-related parameters among women of reproductive age with polycystic ovary syndrome. *J Res Med Sci.* (Isfahan). 23:33.
308. Rafraf M, Zemestani M, Asghari-Jafarabadi M. (2015). Effectiveness of chamomile tea on glycemic control and serum lipid profile in patients with type 2 diabetes. *J Endocrinol Invest.* 38:163–170.
309. Zemestani M, Rafraf M, Asghari-Jafarabadi M. (2016). Chamomile tea improves glycemic indices and antioxidants status in patients with type 2 diabetes mellitus. *Nutrition.* 32(1):66–72.
310. Taghvaee Javanshir S, Yaghmaei P, Hajebrahimi Z. (2018). Thymoquinone ameliorates some endocrine parameters and histological alteration in a rat model of polycystic ovary syndrome. *Internat J Reprod Biomed.* 16(4):275–284.

311. Fararh KM, Atoji Y, Shimizu Y, Takewaki T. (2002). Isulinotropic properties of *Nigella sativa* oil in streptozotocin plus nicotinamide diabetic hamster. *Res Vet Sci.* 73(3):279–282.
312. Alimohammadi S, Hobbenaghi R, Javanbakht J, Kheradmand D. et al. (2013). Protective and antidiabetic effects of extract from *Nigella sativa* on blood glucose concentrations against streptozotocin (STZ)-induced diabetic in rats: An experimental study with histopathological evaluation. *Diagnost Path.* 8:137.
313. Naeimi SA, Tansaz M, Sohrabvand F, Hajimehdipoor H. et al. (2018). Assessing the effect of processed *Nigella sativa* on oligomenorrhea and amenorrhea in patients with polycystic ovarian syndrome: A pilot study. *Int J Pharmacol Sci Res.* 9(11):4716–4722.
314. Perez Gutierrez RM. (2012). Inhibition of advanced glycation end-product formation by *Origanum majorana* L. in vitro and in streptozotocin-induced diabetic rats. *Evidence-Based Complement Alt Med.* 598638.
315. Haj-Husein I, Tukan S, Alkazaleh F. (2016). The effect of marjoram (*Origanum majorana*) tea on the hormonal profile of women with polycystic ovary syndrome: A randomised controlled pilot study. *J Hum Nutr Diet.* 29(1):105–111.
316. Ushiroyama T, Ikeda A, Sakai M, Hosotani T, Suzuki Y, Tsubokura S, Ueki M. (2001). Effects of *unkei-to,* an herbal medicine, on endocrine function and ovulation in women with high basal levels of luteinizing hormone secretion. *J Reprod Med.* 46(5):451–456.
317. Moosavifar N, Mohammadpour AH, Jallali M, Karimiz G, Saberi H. (2010). Evaluation of effect of silymarin on granulosa cell apoptosis and follicular development in patients undergoing *in vitro* fertilization. *East Mediterr Health J.* 16:642–645.
318. Taher MA, Atia YA, Amin MK. (2012). Improving an ovulation rate in women with polycystic ovary syndrome by using silymarin. *J Res Med Sci.* 12:1–8.
319. Voroneanu L, Nistor I, Dumea R, Apetrii M, Covic A. (2016). Silymarin in type 2 diabetes mellitus: A systematic review and meta-analysis of randomized controlled trials. *J Diabetes Res.* 5147468.
320. Srichamroen A, Thomson ABR, Field CJ, Basu TK. (2009). In vitro intestinal glucose uptake is inhibited by galactomannan from Canadian fenugreek seed (*Trigonella foenumgraecum* L.) in genetically lean and obese rats. *Nutr Res.* 29(1):49–54.
321. Al-Habori M, Raman A, Lawrence MJ, Skett P. (2021). In vitro effect of fenugreek extracts on intestinal sodium dependent glucose

uptake and hepatic glycogen phosphorylase A. *Int J Exp Diabetes Res.* 2(2):91–99.
322. Swaroop A, Jaipuriar AS, Gupta SK, Bagchi M, Kumar P, Preuss HG, Bagchi D. (2015). Efficacy of a novel fenugreek seed extract (*Trigonella foenum-graecum*, FurocystTM) in Polycystic Ovary Syndrome (PCOS). *Int J Med Sci.* 12(10):825–831.
323. Bashtian MH, Emami SA, Mousavifar N, Esmaily HA, Mahmoudi M, Poor AHM. (2013). Evaluation of fenugreek (*Trigonella foenum-graecum* L.), effects seeds extract on insulin resistance in women with polycystic ovarian syndrome. *Iran J Pharm Res.* 12(2):475–481.
324. Sharma RD, Sarkar A, Hazara DK, Mishra B. et al. (1996). Use of fenugreek seed powder in the management of non-insulin dependent diabetes mellitus. *Nutr Res.* 16(8):1331–1339.
325. Sharma RD, Raghuram TC, Rao NS. (1990). Effect of fenugreek seeds on blood glucose and serum lipids in type I diabetes. *Eur J Clin Nutr.* 44(4):301–306.
326. Gupta A, Gupta R, Lal B. (2001). Effect of *Trigonella foenumgraecum* (fenugreek) seeds on glycaemic control and insulin resistance in type 2 diabetes mellitus: A double blind placebo controlled study. *J Assoc Physicians India.* 49:1057–1061.
327. Gaddam A, Galla C, Thummisetti S, Marikanty RK, Palanisamy UD, Rao PV. (2015). Role of fenugreek in the prevention of type 2 diabetes mellitus in prediabetes. *J Diabetes Metab Disord.* 14:1–10.
328. Puri D, Prabhu KM, Murthy PS. (2002). Mechanism of action of a hypoglycemic principle isolated from fenugreek seeds. *Indian J Physiol Pharmacol.* 46(4):457–462.
329. Bordia A, Verma SK, Srivastava KC. (1997). Effect of ginger (*Zingiber officinale* Rosc.) and fenugreek (*Trigonella foenumgraecum* L.) on blood lipids, blood sugar and platelet aggregation in patients with coronary artery disease. *Prostaglandins Leukot Essent Fatty Acids.* 56(5):379–384.
330. Lu FR, Shen L, Qin Y, Gao L, Li H, Dai Y. (2008). Clinical observation on *Trigonella foenumgraecum* L. total saponins in combination with sulfonylureas in the treatment of type 2 diabetes mellitus. *Chin J Integr Med.* 14(1):56–60.
331. Ştefănescu R, Tero-Vescan A, Negroiu A, Aurică E, Vari CE. (2020). A comprehensive review of the phytochemical, pharmacological, and toxicological properties of *Tribulus terrestris* L. *Biomolecules.* 10(5):752.
332. Dehghan A, Esfandiari A, Bigdeli SM. (2012). Alternative treatment of ovarian cysts with *Tribulus terrestris* extract: A rat model. *Reprod Domest Anim.* 47(1):e12–e15.

333. Samani NB, Jokar A, Soveid M, Heydari M, Mosavat SH. (2016). Efficacy of the hydroalcoholic extract of Tribulus terrestris on the serum glucose and lipid profile of women with diabetes mellitus: A double-blind randomized placebo-controlled clinical trial. *J Evidence-Based Complement Altern Med.* 21:NP91–NP97.
334. Tabakova P, Dimitrov M, Tashkov B. (1984). *Clinical Studies on the Preparation Tribestan in Women with Endocrine Infertility or Menopausal Syndrome.* Sofia, Bulgaria: 1st Obstetrical and Gynecological Hospital.
335. Arentz S, Smith CA, Abbott J, Fahey P, Cheema BS, Bensoussan A. (2017). Combined lifestyle and herbal medicine in overweight women with Polycystic Ovary Syndrome (PCOS): A randomized controlled trial. *Phytotherapy Res.* 31(9):1330–1340.
336. Maharjan R, Nagar PS, Nampoothiri L. (2010). Effect of *Aloe barbadensis* Mill. formulation on letrozole induced polycystic ovarian syndrome rat model. *J Ayurveda Integr Med.* 1(4):273–279.
337. Desai BN, Maharjan RH, Nampoothiri LP. (2012). *Aloe barbadensis* Mill. formulation restores lipid profile to normal in a letrozole-induced polycystic ovarian syndrome rat model. *Pharmacog Res.* 4(2):109–115.
338. Devaraj S, Jialal R, Jialal I, Rockwood R. (2008). A pilot randomized placebo controlled trial of 2 *Aloe vera* supplements in patients with pre-diabetes/metabolic syndrome. *Planta Med.* 74:SL77.
339. Choi HC, Kim SJ, Son KY, Oh BJ, Cho BL. (2013). Metabolic effects of *Aloe vera* gel complex in obese prediabetes and early non-treated diabetic patients: Randomized controlled trial. *Nutrition.* 29:1110–1114.
340. Suksomboon N, Poolsup N, Punthanitisarn S. (2016). Effect of *Aloe vera* on glycaemic control in prediabetes and type 2 diabetes: A systematic review and meta-analysis. *J Clin Pharmacol Ther.* 41(2):180–188.
341. Huseini HF, Kianbakht S, Hajiaghaee R, Dabaghian FH. (2012). Antihyperglycemic and anti-hypercholesterolemic effects of *Aloe vera* leaf gel in hyperlipidemic type 2 diabetic patients: A randomized double-blind placebo-controlled clinical trial. *Planta Med.* 78:311–316.
342. Zhang Y, Liu W, Liu D, Zhao T, Tian H. (2016). Efficacy of *Aloe vera* supplementation on prediabetes and early non-treated diabetic patients: A systematic review and meta-analysis of randomized controlled trials. *Nutrients.* 8(7):388.
343. Shokoohi M, Abtahi-Eivary SH, Moghimian M, Hajizadeh H. (2018). The effect of *Galega officinalis* on hormonal and metabolic profile in a rat model of Polycystic Ovary Syndrome (PCOS). *Intern J Women's Health Reprod Sci.* 6(3).

344. Bailey CJ. (2017). Metformin: Historical overview. *Diabetologia.* 60(9):1566–1576.
345. Mehraban M, Jelodar G, Rahmanifar F. (2020). A combination of spearmint and flaxseed extract improved endocrine and histomorphology of ovary in experimental PCOS. *J Ovarian Res.* 13(1):32.
346. Choi JH, Jang M, Kim EJ, Lee MJ. et al. (2020). Korean red ginseng alleviates dehydroepiandrosterone-induced polycystic ovarian syndrome in rats via its antiinflammatory and antioxidant activities. *J Ginseng Res.* 44(6):790–798.
347. Jung JH, Park HT, Kim T, Jeong MJ, Lim SC. et al. (2011). Therapeutic effect of Korean red ginseng extract on infertility caused by polycystic ovaries. *J Ginseng Res.* 35(2):250–255.
348. Pak SC, Kim SE, Oh DM, Shim KM, Jeong MJ. et al. (2009). Effect of Korean red ginseng extract in a steroid-induced polycystic ovary murine model. *Arch Pharmacol Res.* 32(3):347–352.
349. Pak SC, Lim SC, Nah SY, Lee J, Hill JA, Bae CS. (2005). Role of Korean red ginseng total saponins in rat infertility induced by polycystic ovaries. *Fertil Steril.* 84(Suppl. 2):1139–1143.
350. Vuksan V, Sung MK, Sievenpiper JL, Stavro PM, Jenkins AL. et al. (2008). Korean red ginseng (*Panax ginseng*) improves glucose and insulin regulation in well-controlled, type 2 diabetes: Results of a randomized, double-blind, placebo-controlled study of efficacy and safety. *Nutr Metab Cardiovasc Dis.* 18:46–56.
351. Shishtar E, Sievenpiper JL, Djedovic V, Cozma AI. et al. (2014). The effect of ginseng (The Genus Panax) on glycemic control: A systematic review and meta-analysis of randomized controlled clinical trials. *PLoS One.* 9:e107391.
352. Jovanovski E, Lea-Duvnjak-Smircic, Komishon A, Au-Yeung F. et al. (2020). Vascular effects of combined enriched Korean red ginseng (*Panax ginseng*) and American ginseng (*Panax quinquefolius*) administration in individuals with hypertension and type 2 diabetes: A randomized controlled trial. *Complement Ther Med.* 49:102338.
353. Abbasian Z, Jafari Barmak M, Barazesh F, Ghavamizadeh M, Mirzaei A. (2020). Therapeutic efficacy of *Trifolium pratense* L. on letrozole induced polycystic ovary syndrome in rats. *Plant Sci Today.* 7(3):501–507.
354. Ghorbanibirgani A, Khalili A, Zamani L. (2013). The efficacy of stinging nettle (*Urtica dioica*) in patients with benign prostatic hyperplasia: A randomized double-blind study in 100 patients. *Iran Red Cresc Med J.* 15(1):9–10.

355. Bandariyan E, Mogheiseh A, Ahmadi A. (2021). The effect of lutein and *Urtica dioica* extract on in vitro production of embryo and oxidative status in polycystic ovary syndrome in a model of mice. *BMC Complement Med Ther.* 21(1):55.
356. Atashpour S, Jahromi HK, Jahromi ZK, Maleknasab M. (2017). Comparison of the effects of ginger extract with clomiphene citrate on sex hormones in rats with polycystic ovarian syndrome. *Int J Reprod Biomed.* 15(9):561.
357. Arablou T, Aryaeian N, Valizadeh M, Sharifi F, Hosseini A, Djalali M. (2014). The effect of ginger consumption on glycemic status, lipid profile and some inflammatory markers in patients with type 2 diabetes mellitus. *Int J Food Sci Nutr.* 65:515–520.
358. Palomba S, Falbo A, Giallauria F. et al. (2010). Six weeks of structured exercise training and hypocaloric diet increases the probability of ovulation after clomiphene citrate in overweight and obese patients with polycystic ovary syndrome: A randomized controlled trial. *Hum Reprod.* 25(11):2783–2791.
359. Moran LJ, Ko H, Misso M, Marsh K, Noakes M. et al. (2013). Dietary composition in the treatment of polycystic ovary syndrome: A systematic review to inform evidence-based guidelines. *J Acad Nutr Diet.* 113(4):520–545.
360. Soares NP, Santos AC, Costa EC. et al. (2016). Diet-induced weight loss reduces DNA damage and cardiometabolic risk factors in overweight/obese women with polycystic ovary syndrome. *Ann Nutr Metab.* 68(3):220–227.
361. Rondanelli M, Perna S, Faliva M, Monteferrario F, Repaci E, Allieri F. (2014). Focus on metabolic and nutritional correlates of polycystic ovary syndrome and update on nutritional management of these critical phenomena. *Arch Gynecol Obstet.* 290(6):1079–1092.
362. Papakonstantinou E, Kechribari I, Mitrou P. et al. (2016). Effect of meal frequency on glucose and insulin levels in women with polycystic ovary syndrome: A randomised trial. *Eur J Clin Nutr.* 70(5):588–594.
363. Pearce KL, Noakes M, Keogh J, Clifton PM. (2008). Effect of carbohydrate distribution on postprandial glucose peaks with the use of continuous glucose monitoring in type 2 diabetes. *Am J Clin Nutr.* 87:638–644.
364. Kang X, Wang C, Lifang L. et al. (2013). Effects of different proportion of carbohydrate in breakfast on postprandial glucose excursion in normal glucose tolerance and impaired glucose regulation subjects. *Diabetes Technol Ther.* 15(7):569–574.

365. Papavasiliou K, Papakonstantinou E. (2017). Nutritional support and dietary interventions for women with polycystic ovary syndrome. *Nutr Diet Suppl.* 9:63–85.
366. Nestler JE, Powers LP, Matt DW, Steingold KA. et al. (1991). A direct effect of hyperinsulinemia on serum sex hormone-binding globulin levels in obese women with polycystic ovary syndrome. *J Clin Endocrinol Metab.* 72(1):83–91.
367. Cutillas-Tolín A, Arense-Gonzalo JJ, Mendiola J, Adoamnei E. et al. (2021). Are dietary indices associated with polycystic ovary syndrome and Its phenotypes? A preliminary study. *Nutrients.* 13(2):313.
368. Xiong YL, Liang XY, Yang X, Li Y, Wei LN. (2011). Low-grade chronic inflammation in the peripheral blood and ovaries of women with polycystic ovarian syndrome. *Eur J Obstet Gynecol Reprod Biol.* 159(1):148–150.
369. Gonzalez F. (2012). Inflammation in polycystic ovary syndrome: Underpinning of insulin resistance and ovarian dysfunction. *Steroids.* 77(4):300–305.
370. Asemi Z, Samimi M, Tabassi Z, Shakeri H, Sabihi SS, Esmaillzadeh A. (2014). Effects of DASH diet on lipid profiles and biomarkers of oxidative stress in overweight and obese women with polycystic ovary syndrome: A randomized clinical trial. *Nutrition.* 30:1287–1293.
371. Asemi Z, Esmaillzadeh A. (2015). DASH diet, insulin resistance, and serum hs-CRP in polycystic ovary syndrome: A randomized controlled clinical trial. *Horm Metab Res.* 47(3):232–238.
372. Azadi-Yazdi M, Karimi-Zarchi M, Salehi-Abargouei A, Fallahzadeh H, Nadjarzadeh A. (2017). Effects of Dietary Approach to Stop Hypertension diet on androgens, antioxidant status and body composition in overweight and obese women with polycystic ovary syndrome: A randomised controlled trial. *J Hum Nutr Diet.* 30(3):275–283.
373. Foroozanfard F, Rafiei H, Samimi M, Gilasi HR, Gorjizadeh R, Heidar Z, Asemi Z. (2017). The effects of Dietary Approaches to Stop Hypertension diet on weight loss, anti-Müllerian hormone and metabolic profiles in women with polycystic ovary syndrome: A randomized clinical trial. *Clin Endocrinol.* (Oxford). 87(1):51–58.
374. Azadi-Yazdi M, Karimi-Zarchi M, Salehi-Abargouei A, Fallahzadeh H, Nadjarzadeh A. (2017). Effects of Dietary Approach to Stop Hypertension diet on androgens, antioxidant status and body composition in overweight and obese women with polycystic ovary syndrome: A randomised controlled trial. *J Hum Nutr Diet.* 30:275–283.

375. Asemi Z, Esmaillzadeh A. (2015). DASH diet, insulin resistance, and serum hs-CRP in polycystic ovary syndrome: A randomized controlled clinical trial. *Horm Metab Res.* 47(3):232–238.
376. Asemi Z Samimi M, Tabassi Z, Shakeri H, Sabihi SS, Esmaillzadeh A. (2014). Effects of DASH diet on lipid profiles and biomarkers of oxidative stress in overweight and obese women with polycystic ovary syndrome: A randomized clinical trial. *Nutrition.* 30(11–12):1287–1293.
377. Barrea L, Arnone A, Annunziata G, Muscogiuri G, Laudisio D. et al. (2019). Adherence to the Mediterranean diet, dietary patterns and body composition in women with Polycystic Ovary Syndrome (PCOS). *Nutrients.* 11(10):2278.
378. Papavasiliou K, Papakonstantinou E. (2017). Nutritional support and dietary interventions for women with polycystic ovary syndrome. *Nutr Diet Suppl.* 9:63–85.
379. Sharman MJ, Kraemer WJ, Love DM, Avery NG, Gomez AL, Scheett TP. et al. (2002). A ketogenic diet favorably affects serum biomarkers for cardiovascular disease in normal-weight men. *J Nutr.* 132(7):1879–1885.
380. Sharman MJ, Kraemer WJ, Love DM, Avery NG, Gomez AL, Scheett TP. et al. (2002). A ketogenic diet favorably affects serum biomarkers for cardiovascular disease in normal-weight men. *J Nutr.* 132(7):1879–1885.
381. Graff SK, Mário FM, Alves BC, Spritzer PM. (2013). Dietary glycemic index is associated with less favorable anthropometric and metabolic profiles in polycystic ovary syndrome women with different phenotypes. *Fertil Steril.* 100(4):1081–1088.
382. Barr S, Reeves S, Sharp K, Jeanes YM. (2013). An isocaloric low glycemic index diet improves insulin sensitivity in women with polycystic ovary syndrome. *J Acad Nutr Diet.* 113(11):1523–1531.
383. Kasim-Karakas SE, Almario RU, Cunningham W. (2009). Effects of protein versus simple sugar intake on weight loss in polycystic ovary syndrome (according to the National Institutes of Health criteria). *Fertil Steril.* 92(1):262–270.
384. Kasim-Karakas SE, Cunningham WM, Tsodikov A. (2007). Relation of nutrients and hormones in polycystic ovary syndrome. *Am J Clin Nutr.* 85(3):688–694.
385. Hajishafiee M, Askari G, Iranj B. et al. (2016). The effect of n-3 polyunsaturated fatty acid supplementation on androgen status in patients with polycystic ovary syndrome: A systematic review and meta-analysis of clinical trials. *Horm Metab Res.* 48(5):281–289.
386. Nadjarzadeh A, Firouzabadi RD, Daneshbodi NV, Lotfi MH, Mozaffari-Khosravi H. (2013). The effect of omega-3 supplementation on

androgen profile and menstrual status in women with polycystic ovary syndrome: A randomized clinical trial. *Iran J Reprod Med.* 11(8):665–672.
387. Sadeghi A, Djafarian K, Mohammadi H, Shab-Bidar S. (2016). Effect of omega-3 fatty acids supplementation on insulin resistance in women with polycystic ovary syndrome: Meta-analysis of randomized controlled trials. *Diabetes Metab Syndr.* 11(2):157–162.
388. Phelan N, O'Connor A, Kyaw Tun T. et al. (2011). Hormonal and metabolic effects of polyunsaturated fatty acids in young women with polycystic ovary syndrome: Results from a cross-sectional analysis and a randomized, placebo-controlled, crossover trial. *Am J Clin Nutr.* 93(3):652–662.
389. Sadeghi A, Djafarian K, Mohammadi H, Shab-Bidar S. (2016). Effect of omega-3 fatty acids supplementation on insulin resistance in women with polycystic ovary syndrome: Meta-analysis of randomized controlled trials. *Diabetes Metab Syndr.* 11(2):157–162.
390. Khani B, Mardanian F, Fesharaki SJ. (2017). Omega-3 supplementation effects on polycystic ovary syndrome symptoms and metabolic syndrome. *J Res Med Sci.* 22:64.
391. Azadi-Yazdi M, Nadjarzadeh A, Khosravi-Boroujeni H, Salehi-Abargouei A. (2017). The effect of vitamin D supplementation on the androgenic profile in patients with polycystic ovary syndrome: A systematic review and meta-analysis of clinical trials. *Horm Metab Res.* 49(3):174–179.
392. Krul-Poel YH, Snackey C, Louwers Y. et al. (2013). The role of vitamin D in metabolic disturbances in polycystic ovary syndrome: A systematic review. *Eur J Endocrinol.* 169(6):853–865.
393. Jamilian M, Razavi M, Fakhrie Kashan Z, Ghandi Y, Bagherian T, Asemi Z. (2015). Metabolic response to selenium supplementation in women with polycystic ovary syndrome: A randomized, double-blind, placebo-controlled trial. *Clin Endocrinol.* 82(6):885–891.
394. Foroozanfard F, Jamilian M, Jafari Z. et al. (2015). Effects of zinc supplementation on markers of insulin resistance and lipid profiles in women with polycystic ovary syndrome: A randomized, double-blind, placebo-controlled trial. *Exp Clin Endocrinol Diabetes.* 123(4):215–220.
395. Bahmani F, Karamali M, Shakeri H, Asemi Z. (2014). The effects of folate supplementation on inflammatory factors and biomarkers of oxidative stress in overweight and obese women with polycystic ovary syndrome: A randomized, double-blind, placebo-controlled clinical trial. *Clin Endocrinol.* 81(4):582–587.

396. Costello RB, Dwyer JT, Merkel JM. (2019). Chromium supplements in health and disease. In: Vincent JB, ed. *The Nutritional Biochemistry of Chromium*, 3rd edn. Cambridge, MA: Elsevier, pp. 219–259.
397. Jamilian M, Asemi Z. (2015). Chromium supplementation and the effects on metabolic status in women with polycystic ovary syndrome: A randomized, double-blind, placebo-controlled trial. *Ann Nutr Metab.* 67(1):42–48.
398. Thakker D, Raval A, Patel I, Walia R. (2015). N-acetylcysteine for polycystic ovary syndrome: A systematic review and meta-analysis of randomized controlled clinical trials. *Obstet Gynecol Internat.* 817849.
399. Mostajeran F, Tehrani HG, Rahbary B. (2018). N-acetylcysteine as an adjuvant to letrozole for induction of ovulation in infertile patients with polycystic ovary syndrome. *Adv Biomed Res.* 7:100.
400. Salehpour S, Sene AA, Saharkhiz N, Sohrabi MR, Moghimian F. (2012). N-acetylcysteine as an adjuvant to clomiphene citrate for successful induction of ovulation in infertile patients with polycystic ovary syndrome. *J Obstet Gynaecol Res.* 38(9):1182–1186.
401. Maged AM, Elsawah H, Abdelhafez A, Bakry A, Mostafa WA. (2015). The adjuvant effect of metformin and N-acetylcysteine to clomiphene citrate in induction of ovulation in patients with polycystic ovary syndrome. *Gynecol Endocrinol.* 31(8):635–638.
402. Tovar J, Nilsson A, Johansson M, Björk I. (2014). Combining functional features of whole-grain barley and legumes for dietary reduction of cardiometabolic risk: A randomised cross-over intervention in mature women. *Br J Nutr.* 111(4):706–714.
403. He FF, Li YM. (2020). Role of gut microbiota in the development of insulin resistance and the mechanism underlying polycystic ovary syndrome: A review. *J Ovarian Res.* 13:1–13.
404. Liu R, Zhang C, Shi Y, Zhang F, Li L. et al. (2017). Dysbiosis of gut microbiota associated with clinical parameters in polycystic ovary syndrome. *Front Microbiol.* 8:324.
405. Torres PJ, Siakowska M, Banaszewska B, Pawelczyk L. et al. (2018). Gut microbial diversity in women with polycystic ovary syndrome correlates with hyperandrogenism. *J Clin Endocrinol Metab.* 103:1502–1511.
406. Sanchez HN, Moroney JB, Gan H, Shen T. et al. (2020). B cell-intrinsic epigenetic modulation of antibody responses by dietary fiber-derived short-chain fatty acids. *Nat Commun.* 11:1–19.
407. Bhathena SJ, Velasquez MT. (2002). Beneficial role of dietary phytoestrogens in obesity and diabetes. *Am J Clin Nutr.* 76(6):1191–1201.

408. Fang K, Dong H, Wang D, Gong J, Huang W, Lu F. (2016). Soy isoflavones and glucose metabolism in menopausal women: A systematic review and meta-analysis of randomized controlled trials. *Mol Nutr Food Res.* 60(7):1602–1614.
409. Zhang YB, Chen WH, Guo JJ, Fu ZH, Yi C, Zhang M, Na XL. (2013). Soy isoflavone supplementation could reduce body weight and improve glucose metabolism in non-Asian postmenopausal women—a meta-analysis. *Nutrition.* 29(1):8–14.
410. Jamilian M, Asemi Z. (2016). The effects of soy isoflavones on metabolic status of patients with polycystic ovary syndrome. *J Clin Endocrinol Metab.* 101(9):3386–3394.
411. Forouhari S, Heidari Z, Tavana Z, Salehi M, Sayadi M. (2013). The effect of soya on some hormone levels in women with polycystic ovary syndrome (balance diet): A cross over randomized clinical trial. *Bull Env Pharmacol Life Sci.* 3(1):246–250.
412. Luo J, Qi J, Wang W, Luo Z, Liu L, Zhang G, Zhou Q, Liu J, Peng X. (2019). Antiobesity effect of flaxseed polysaccharide via inducing satiety due to leptin resistance removal and promoting lipid metabolism through the AMP-activated Protein Kinase (AMPK) signaling pathway. *J Agric Food Chem.* 67(25):7040–7049.
413. Jelodar G, Masoomi S, Rahmanifar F. (2018). Hydroalcoholic extract of flaxseed improves polycystic ovary syndrome in a rat model. *Iran J Basic Med Sci.* 21(6):645–650.
414. Farzana F, Sulaiman A, Ruckmani A, Vijayalakshmi K, Karunya Lakshmi G, Shri RS. (2015). Effects of flax seeds supplementation in polycystic ovarian syndrome. *J Res Med Sci.* 31(1):113–119.
415. Adlercreutz H, Höckerstedt K, Bannwart C, Bloigu S, Hämäläinen E, Fotsis T, Ollus A. (1987). Effect of dietary components, including lignans and phytoestrogens, on enterohepatic circulation and liver metabolism of estrogens and on sex hormone binding globulin (SHBG). *J Ster Biochem.* 27(4–6):1135–1144.
416. Martin ME, Haourigui M, Pelissero C, Benassayag C, Nunez EA. (1996). Interactions between phytoestrogens and human sex steroid binding protein. *Life Sci.* 58(5):429–436.
417. Sturgeon SR, Heersink JL, Volpe SL, Bertone-Johnson ER. et al. (2008). Effect of dietary flaxseed on serum levels of estrogens and androgens in postmenopausal women. *Nutr Cancer.* 60(5):612–618.
418. Wang C, Mäkelä T, Hase T, Adlercreutz H, Kurzer MS. (1994). Lignans and flavonoids inhibit aromatase enzyme in human preadipocytes. *Steroid Biochem Mol Biol.* 50(3–4):205–212.

419. Hutchins AM, Martini MC, Olson BA, Thomas W, Slavin JL. (2001). Flaxseed consumption influences endogenous hormone concentrations in postmenopausal women. *Nutr Cancer.* 39(1):58–65.
420. Cristoni A, Di Pierro F, Bombardelli E. (2000). Botanical derivatives for the prostate. *Fitoterapia.* 71(1):S21–S28.
421. Mani UV, Mani I, Biswas M, Kumar SN. (2011). An open-label study on the effect of flax seed powder (*Linum usitatissimum*) supplementation in the management of diabetes mellitus. *J Diet Suppl.* 8:257–265.
422. Lemay A, Dodin S, Kadri N, Jacques H, Forest JC. (2002). Flaxseed dietary supplement versus hormone replacement therapy in hypercholesterolemic menopausal women. *Obstet Gynecol.* 100(3):495–504.
423. Edel AL, Rodriguez-Leyva D, Maddaford TG, Caligiuri SP. et al. (2015). Dietary flaxseed independently lowers circulating cholesterol and lowers it beyond the effects of cholesterol-lowering medications alone in patients with peripheral artery disease. *J Nutr.* 145(4): 749–757.
424. Ibrügger S, Kristensen M, Mikkelsen MS, Astrup A. (2012). Flaxseed dietary fiber supplements for suppression of appetite and food intake. *Appetite.* 58:490–495.
425. Tehrani HG, Allahdadian M, Zarre F, Ranjbar H, Allahdadian F. (2017). Effect of green tea on metabolic and hormonal aspect of polycystic ovarian syndrome in overweight and obese women suffering from polycystic ovarian syndrome: A clinical trial. *J Educ Health Promotion.* 6:36.
426. Wu CH, Lu FH, Chang CS, Chang TC, Wang RH, Chang CJ. (2003). Relationship among habitual tea consumption, percent body fat, and body fat distribution. *Obes Res.* 11:1088–1095.
427. Iso H, Date C, Wakai K, Fukui M, Tamakoshi A, JACC Study Group. (2006). The relationship between green tea and total caffeine intake and risk for self-reported type 2 diabetes among Japanese adults. *Ann Intern Med.* 144:554–562.
428. Tsitsimpikou C, Tsarouhas K, Kioukia-Fougia N. et al. (2014). Diet & lifestyle dietary supplementation with tomato-juice in patients with metabolic syndrome: A suggestion to alleviate detrimental clinical factors. *Food Chem Toxicol.* 74:9–13.

Chapter 8: Endometriosis

1. Kitawaki J. (2002). Endometriosis: The pathophysiology as an estrogen-dependent disease. *J Steroid Biochem Mol Biol.* 83:149–155.

2. Whitehill K, Yong PJ, Williams C. (2012). Clinical predictors of endometriosis in the infertility population: Is there a better way to determine who needs a laparoscopy? *J Obstet Gynaecol Can.* 34(6):552–557.
3. Stefansson H, Geirsson RT, Steinthorsdottir V. et al. (2002). Genetic factors contribute to the risk of developing endometriosis. *Hum Reprod.* 17(3):555–559.
4. Mounsey A, Wilgus A. (2006). Diagnosis and management of endometriosis. *Am Fam Phys.* 74:594–600.
5. Meresman GF, Auge L. (2002). Oral contraceptives suppress cell proliferation and enhance apoptosis of eutopic endometrial tissue from patients with endometriosis. *Fertil Steril.* 77:1141–1147.
6. Vercellini P. (2003). Progestogens for endometriosis: Forward to the past. *Hum Reprod Update.* 9:387–396.
7. Burney RO, Giudice L. (2012). Pathogenesis and pathophysiology of endometriosis. *Fertil Steril.* 98:511–519.
8. Kitawaki J. (2002). Endometriosis: The pathophysiology as an estrogen-dependent disease. *J Steroid Biochem Mol Biol.* 83:149–155.
9. Ilhan M, Gürağaç Dereli FT, Akkol EK. (2019). Novel drug targets with traditional herbal medicines for overcoming endometriosis. *Current Drug Delivery.* 16(5):386–399.
10. Halme J, Hammond MG, Hulka JF, Raj SG, Talbert LM. (1984). Retrograde menstruation in healthy women and in patients with endometriosis. *Obstet Gynecol.* 64(2):151–154.
11. Giudice LC, Kao LC. (2004). Endometriosis. *Lancet.* 364:1789–1799.
12. Wu MY, Ho HN. (2003). The role of cytokines in endometriosis. *Am J Reprod Immunol.* 49:285–296.
13. Szyllo K. (2003). The involvement of T lymphocytes in the pathogenesis of endometriotic tissues overgrowth in women with endometriosis. *Mediators Inflamm.* 12:131–138.
14. Augoulea A, Mastorakos G, Lambrinoudaki I, Christodoulakos G, Creatsas G. (2009). The role of the oxidative-stress in the endometriosis-related infertility. *Gynecol Endocrinol.* 25:75–81.
15. Scutiero G, Iannone P, Bernardi G, Bonaccorsi G, Spadaro S. et al. (2017). Oxidative stress and endometriosis: A systematic review of the literature. *Oxid Med Cell Longev.* 7265238.
16. Santulli P, Marcellin L, Noël JC, Borghese B, Fayt I. et al. (2012). Sphingosine pathway deregulation in endometriotic tissues. *Fertil Steril.* 97:904–911.
17. Burney RO, Giudice LC. (2012). Pathogenesis and pathophysiology of endometriosis. *Fertil Steril.* 98:511–519.

18. Iarmolinskaia MI, Molotkov AS, Bezhenar' VF, Shved NI, Ivashchenko TE, Baranov VS. (2014). Association of matrix metalloproteinases' polymorphisms of MMP3 and MMP9 with development of genital endometriosis. *Genetika*. 50(2):230–235.
19. Yang H, Liu J, Fan Y. (2016). Associations between various possible promoter polymorphisms of MMPs genes and endometriosis risk: A meta-analysis. *Europ J Obstet Gynecol Reprod Biol*. 205:174–188.
20. Borghese B, Mondon F, Noël JC, Fayt I, Mignot TM, Vaiman D, Chapron C. (2008). Gene expression profile for ectopic versus eutopic endometrium provides new insights into endometriosis oncogenic potential. *Mol Endocrinol*. 22:2557–2562.
21. Kerbel RS. (2008). Tumor angiogenesis. *N Engl J Med*. 358:2039–2049.
22. Zhang H, Zhao X, Liu S, Li J, Wen Z, Li M. (2010). 17betaE2 promotes cell proliferation in endometriosis by decreasing PTEN via NFkappaB-dependent pathway. *Mol Cell Endocrinol*. 317:31–43.
23. Hardee ME, Zagzag D. (2012). Mechanisms of glioma-associated neovascularization. *Am J Pathol*. 181:1126–1141.
24. Kokawa K, Shikone T, Nakano R. (1996). Apoptosis in the human uterine endometrium during the menstrual cycle. *J Clin Endocrinol Metab*. 81:4144–4147.
25. Vaskivuo TE, Stenbäck F, Karhumaa P, Risteli J, Dunkel L, Tapanainen JS. (2000). Apoptosis and apoptosis-related proteins in human endometrium. *Mol Cell Endocrinol*. 165:75–83.
26. Sinaii N, Cleary SD, Ballweg ML. et al. (2002). High rates of autoimmune and endocrine disorders, fibromyalgia, chronic fatigue syndrome and atopic diseases among women with endometriosis: A survey analysis. *Hum Reprod*. 17(10):2715–2724.
27. Murphy AJ, Guyre PM, Wira CR, Pioli PA. (2009). Estradiol regulates expression of estrogen receptor ERalpha46 in human macrophages. *PLoS One*. 4:e5539.
28. Olivares C, Ricci A, Bilotas M, Barañao RI, Meresman G. (2011). The inhibitory effect of celecoxib and rosiglitazone on experimental endometriosis. *Fertil Steril*. 96(2):438–433.
29. Jana S, Chatterjee K, Ray AK, DasMahapatra P, Swarnakar S, Ramchandran R. (2016). Regulation of matrix metalloproteinase-2 activity by COX-2-PGE2-pAKT axis promotes angiogenesis in endometriosis. *PLoS One*. 11(10):e0163540.
30. Vallée A, Lecarpentier Y. (2020). Curcumin and endometriosis. *Int J Mol Sci*. 21(7):2440.

31. Hulboy DL, Rudolph LA, Matrisian LM. (1997). Matrix metalloproteinases as mediators of reproductive function. *Mol Hum Reprod.* 3:27–45.
32. Yang H, Liu J, Fan Y. (2016). Associations between various possible promoter polymorphisms of MMPs genes and endometriosis risk: A meta-analysis. *Europ J Obstet Gynecol Reprod Biol.* 205:174–188.
33. Iarmolinskaia MI, Molotkov AS, Bezhenar' VF, Shved NI, Ivashchenko TE, Baranov VS. (2014). Association of matrix metalloproteinases' polymorphisms of MMP3 and MMP9 with development of genital endometriosis. *Genetika.* 50(2):230–235.
34. Bulun SE, Cheng YH, Pavone ME, Yin P, Imir G. et al. (2010). 17beta-hydroxysteroid dehydrogenase-2 deficiency and progesterone resistance in endometriosis. *Seminars Reprod Med.* 28(1):44–50.
35. Vázquez-Martínez ER, Bello-Alvarez C, Hermenegildo-Molina AL, Solís-Paredes M, Parra-Hernández S. et al. (2020). Expression of membrane progesterone receptors in eutopic and ectopic endometrium of women with endometriosis. *Biomed Res Int.* 2196024.
36. Poorasamy J, Patil JSSA. (2022). Progesterone resistance in endometriosis. *EMJ Repro Health.* 8(1):51–63.
37. Yang JZ, Agarwal SK. (2000). Subchronic exposure to 2,3,7, 8-tetrachlorodibenzo-p-dioxin modulates the pathophysiology of endometriosis in the cynomolgus monkey. *Toxicol Sci.* 56:374–381.
38. Yrjanheikki E. (1989). *Levels of PCBs, PCDDs, and PCDFs in Breast Milk: Results of Coordinated Inter-Laboratory Quality Control Studies and Analytical Field Studies.* Copenhagen: World Health Organization.
39. Guo SW. (2004). The link between exposure to dioxin and endometriosis: A critical reappraisal of primate data. *Gynecol Obstet Invest.* 57:157–173.
40. Porpora MG. (2006). Increased levels of polychlorobiphenyls in Italian women with endometriosis. *Chemosphere.* 63:1361–1367.
41. Fraga MF, Ballestar E. (2005). Epigenetic differences arise during the lifetime of monozygotic twins. *Proc Natl Acad Sci USA.* 102:10604–10609.
42. Bischoff F, Simpson JL. (2004). Genetics of endometriosis: Heritability and candidate genes. *Best Pract Res Clin Obstet Gynaecol.* 18:219–232.
43. Guo SW. (2009). Epigenetics of endometriosis. *Mol Hum Reprod.* 15:587–607.
44. Olive DL, Stohs GF, Metzger DA, Franklin RR. (1985). Expectant management and hydrotubations in the treatment of endometriosis-associated infertility. *Fertil Steril.* 44:35–41.
45. Della Corte L, Noventa M, Ciebiera M, Magliarditi M. et al. (2020). Phytotherapy in endometriosis: An up-to-date review. *J Complement Integr Med.* 17(3).

46. Meresman GF, Götte M, Laschke MW. (2021). Plants as source of new therapies for endometriosis: A review of preclinical and clinical studies. *Hum Reprod Update.* 27(2):367–392.
47. Bina F, Soleymani S, Toliat T, Hajimahmoodi M, Tabarrai M, Abdollahi M, Rahimi R. (2019). Plant-derived medicines for treatment of endometriosis: A comprehensive review of molecular mechanisms. *Pharmacol Res.* 139:76–90.
48. Celik O, Ersahin A, Acet M, Celik N, Baykus Y, Deniz R, Ozerol E, Ozerol I. (2016). Disulfiram, as a candidate NF-κB and proteasome inhibitor, prevents endometriotic implant growing in a rat model of endometriosis. *Eur Rev Med Pharmacol Sci.* 20:4380–4389.
49. Soares SR, Martínez-Varea A, Hidalgo-Mora JJ, Pellicer A. (2012). Pharmacologic therapies in endometriosis: A systematic review. *Fertil Steril.* 98:529–555.
50. Reis FM, Petraglia F, Taylor RN. (2013). Endometriosis: Hormone regulation and clinical consequences of chemotaxis and apoptosis. *Hum Reprod Update.* 19:406–418.
51. Schmid D, Woehs F, Svoboda M, Thalhammer T, Chiba P, Moeslinger T. (2009). Aqueous extracts of *Cimicifuga racemosa* and phenolcarboxylic constituents inhibit production of proinflammatory cytokines in LPS-stimulated human whole blood. *Can J Physiol Pharmacol.* 87(11):963–972.
52. Wuttke W, Jarry H, Seidlová-Wuttke D. (2006). *Cimicifuga* extract for the treatment of climacteric complaints. *J Endocrinol Reprod.* 10(2):106–110.
53. Park SY, Kim HJ, Lee SR, Choi YH, Jeong K, Chung H. (2016). Black cohosh inhibits 17β-estradiol-induced cell proliferation of endometrial adenocarcinoma cells. *Gynecol Endocrinol.* 32(10):840–843.
54. Ruhlen RL, Sun GY, Sauter ER. (2008). Black cohosh: Insights into its mechanism(s) of action. *Integr Med Insights.* 3:21–32.
55. Yang CL, Chik SC, Li JC, Cheung BK, Lau AS. (2009). Identification of the bioactive constituent and its mechanisms of action in mediating the anti-inflammatory effects of black cohosh and related *Cimicifuga* species on human primary blood macrophages. *J Med Chem.* 52(21):6707–6715.
56. Düker EM, Kopanski L, Jarry H, Wuttke W. (1991). Effects of extracts from *Cimicifuga racemosa* on gonadotropin release in menopausal women and ovariectomized rats. *Planta Med.* 57(5):420–424.
57. Kamel HH. (2013). Role of phyto-oestrogens in ovulation induction in women with polycystic ovarian syndrome. *Eur J Obstet Gynecol Reprod Biol.* 168(1):60–63.

58. Shahin AY, Mohammed SA. (2014). Adding the phytoestrogen *Cimicifugae racemosae* to clomiphene induction cycles with timed intercourse in polycystic ovary syndrome improves cycle outcomes and pregnancy rates—a randomized trial. *Gynecol Endocrinol.* 30(7):505–510.
59. Küpeli Akkol E, Demirel MA, Bahadır Acıkara O, Süntar I, Ergene B, Ilhan M, Ozbilgin S, Saltan G, Keleş H, Tekin M. (2015). Phytochemical analyses and effects of *Alchemilla mollis* (Buser) Rothm. and *Alchemilla persica* Rothm. in rat endometriosis model. *Arch Gynecol Obstet.* 292(3):619–628.
60. Sun YX, Liu JC, Liu DY. (2011). Phytochemicals and bioactivities of *Anemone raddeana* Regel: A review. *Pharmazie.* 66:813–821.
61. Sun Y, Li M, Liu J. (2008). Haemolytic activities and adjuvant effect of *Anemone raddeana* saponins (ARS) on the immune responses to ovalbumin in mice. *Int Immunopharmacol.* 8:1095–1102.
62. Hao DC, Gu X, Xiao P. (2017). *Anemone* medicinal plants: Ethnopharmacology, phytochemistry and biology. *Acta Pharmacol Sin B.* 7(2):146–158.
63. Hao DC, Xiao PG, Ma H, Peng Y, He CN. (2015). Mining chemodiversity from biodiversity: Pharmacophylogeny of medicinal plants of the Ranunculaceae. *Chin J Nat Med.* 13:507–520.
64. Lee TH, Huang NK, Lai TC, Yang AT, Wang GJ. (2008). Anemonin, from *Clematis crassifolia*, potent and selective inducible nitric oxide synthase inhibitor. *J Ethnopharmacol.* 116:518–527.
65. Xiao K, Cao ST, Jiao le F, Lin FH, Wang L, Hu CH. (2016). Anemonin improves intestinal barrier restoration and influences TGF-β1 and EGFR signaling pathways in LPS-challenged piglets. *Innate Immun.* 22(5):344–352.
66. Duan H. (2006). Effect of anemonin on NO, ET-1 and ICAM-1 production in rat intestinal microvascular endothelial cells. *J Ethnopharmacol.* 104(3):362–366.
67. Jia D, Han B, Yang S, Zhao J. (2014). Anemonin alleviates nerve injury after cerebral ischemia and reperfusion (i/r) in rats by improving antioxidant activities and inhibiting apoptosis pathway. *J Mol Neurosci.* 53(2):271–279.
68. Tan C, Zhu W, Lu Y. (2002). Aloin, cinnamic acid and sophorcarpidine are potent inhibitors of tyrosinase. *Chin Med J.* (Engl). 115(12):1859–1862.
69. Martin ML, Ortíz de Urbina AV, Montero MJ, Carrón R, San Román L. (1988). Pharmacologic effects of lactones isolated from *Pulsatilla alpina* subsp. *Apiifolia*. *J Ethnopharmacol.* 24(2–3):185–191.

70. Preethi KC, Kuttan G, Kuttan R. (2009). Anti-inflammatory activity of flower extract of *Calendula officinalis* Linn. and its possible mechanism of action. *Indian J Exp Biol.* 47(2):113–120.
71. Popovic M, Kourinovic B, Mimica-Dukic N, Vojinovic-Miloradav M, Djordjevic A. (2000). Combined effects of plant extracts and xenobiotics on liposomal lipid peroxidation. Part II. Marigold extract-CCl_4/fullerenol. *Oxid Commun.* 23:178–186.
72. Yasukawa K, Akihisa T, Oinuma H, Kaminaga T, Kanno H. et al. (1996). Inhibitory effect of taraxastane-type triterpenes on tumor promotion by 12-O-tetradecanoylphorbol-13-acetate in two-stage carcinogenesis in mouse skin. *Oncology.* 53:341–344.
73. Poordast T, Najib FS, Tanide N, Kanani A, Mokhtari M, Chaman-Ara K. (2019). Comparing the effects of triptorelin and *Calendula officinalis* on size and pathology of induced endometriosis in rats. *J Endometr Pelvic Pain Disord.* 11(3):132–136.
74. Zhai Z, Liu Y, Wu L, Senchina DS, Wurtele ES, Murphy PA, Kohut ML, Cunnick JE. (2007). Enhancement of innate and adaptive immune functions by multiple *Echinacea* species. *J Med Food.* 10(3):423–434.
75. Zhai Z, Liu Y, Wu L, Senchina DS, Wurtele ES, Murphy PA, Kohut ML, Cunnick JE. (2007). Enhancement of innate and adaptive immune functions by multiple *Echinacea* species. *J Med Food.* 10(3):423–434.
76. Matthias A, Banbury L, Stevenson LM, Bone KM, Leach DN, Lehmann RP. (2007). Alkylamides from *Echinacea* modulate induced immune responses in macrophages. *Immunol Invest.* 36(2):117–130.
77. Guiotto P, Woelkart K, Grabnar I, Voinovich D, Perissutti B, Invernizzi S. et al. (2008). Pharmacokinetics and immunomodulatory effects of phytotherapeutic lozenges (bonbons) with *Echinacea purpurea* extract. *Phytomed.* 15:547–554.
78. Percival SS. (2000). Use of *Echinacea* in medicine. *Biochem Pharmacol.* 60(2):155–158.
79. Raduner S, Majewska A, Chen JZ, Xie XQ, Hamon J, Faller B. et al. (2006). Alkylamides from *Echinacea* are a new class of cannabinomimetics. Cannabinoid type 2 receptor-dependent and -independent immunomodulatory effects. *J Biol Chem.* 281:14192–14206.
80. Woelkart K, Bauer R. (2007). The role of alkamides as an active principle of *Echinacea*. *Planta Med.* 73:615–623.
81. Chicca A, Raduner S, Pellati F, Strompen T, Altmann KH, Schoop R. et al. Synergistic immunomopharmacological effects of N-alkylamides in *Echinacea purpurea* herbal extracts. *Int Immunopharmacol.* 9:850–858.

82. Woelkart K, Xu W, Pei Y, Makriyannis A, Picone RP, Bauer R. (2005). The endocannabinoid system as a target for alkamides from *Echinacea angustifolia* roots. *Planta Med.* 71:701–705.
Pacher P, Bátkai S, Kunos G. (2006). The endocannabinoid system as an emerging target of pharmacotherapy. *Pharmacol Rev.* 58:389–462.
83. Barnes J, Anderson LA, Gibbons S, Phillipson JD. (2005). *Echinacea* species (*Echinacea angustifolia* (DC.). Hell, *Echinacea pallida* (Nutt.), Nutt *Echinacea purpurea* (L.) Moench): A review of their chemistry, pharmacology and clinical properties. *J Pharm Pharmacol.* 57:929–954.
84. Liang Y, Zhou Y, Shen P. (2004). NF-kappaB and its regulation on the immune system. *Cell Mol Immunol.* 1:343–350.
85. Matthias A, Banbury L, Bone KM, Leach DN, Lehmann RP. (2008). *Echinacea* alkylamides modulate induced immune responses in T-cells. *Fitoterapia.* 79:53–58.
86. Sharma M, Schoop R. Hudson JB. (2009). *Echinacea* as an antiinflammatory agent: The influence of physiologically relevant parameters. *Phytother Res.* 23:863–867.
87. Yang R, Yuan BC, Ma YS, Zhou S, Liu Y. (2017). The anti-inflammatory activity of licorice, a widely used Chinese herb. *Pharm Biol.* 55(1):5–18.
88. Park SY, Kwon SJ, Lim SS, Kim JK, Lee KW, Park JH. (2016). Licoricidin, an active compound in the hexane/ethanol extract of *Glycyrrhiza uralensis*, inhibits lung metastasis of 4t1 murine mammary carcinoma cells. *Int J Mol Sci.* 17(6):934.
89. Yang R, Yuan BC, Ma YS, Zhou S, Liu Y. (2017). The anti-inflammatory activity of licorice, a widely used Chinese herb. *Pharm Biol.* 55(1):5–18.
90. La VD, Tanabe S, Bergeron C, Gafner S, Grenier D. (2011). Modulation of matrix metalloproteinase and cytokine production by licorice isolates licoricidin and licorisoflavan A: Potential therapeutic approach for periodontitis. *J Periodontol.* 82(1):122–128.
91. Okimasu E, Moromizato Y, Watanabe S, Sasaki J, Shiraishi N, Morimoto YM. et al. (1983). Inhibition of phospholipase A2 and platelet aggregation by glycyrrhizin, an antiinflammation drug. *Acta Med Okayama.* 37(5):385–391.
92. Trombetta D, Giofrè SV, Tomaino A, Raciti R, Saija A, Cristani M. et al. (2014). Selective COX-2 inhibitory properties of dihydrostilbenes from liquorice leaves—in vitro assays and structure/activity relationship study. *Nat Prod Commun.* 9(12):1761–1764.
93. La VD, Tanabe S, Bergeron C, Gafner S, Grenier D. (2011). Modulation of matrix metalloproteinase and cytokine production by licorice isolates licoricidin and licorisoflavan A: Potential therapeutic approach for periodontitis. *J Periodontol.* 82(1):122–128.

94. Namavar Jahromi B, Farrokhnia F, Tanideh N, Vijayananda Kumar P, Parsanezhad ME, Alaee S. (2019). Comparing the effects of *Glycyrrhiza glabra* root extract, a cyclooxygenase-2 inhibitor (Celecoxib) and a gonadotropin-releasing hormone analog (Diphereline) in a rat model of endometriosis. *Int J Fert Steril.* 13(1):45–50.
95. Wang XR, Hao HG, Chu L. (2017). Glycyrrhizin inhibits LPS-induced inflammatory mediator production in endometrial epithelial cells. *Microb Pathog.* 109:110–113.
96. Bina F, Soleymani S, Toliat T, Hajimahmoodi M, Tabarrai M, Abdollahi M. et al. (2019). Plant-derived medicines for treatment of endometriosis: A comprehensive review of molecular mechanisms. *Pharmacol Res.* 139:76–90.
97. Qi JJ, Li XX, Diao YF, Liu PL, Wang DL, Bai CY. et al. (2020). Asiatic acid supplementation during the in vitro culture period improves early embryonic development of porcine embryos produced by parthenogenetic activation, somatic cell nuclear transfer and in vitro fertilization. *Theriogenol.* 142:26–33.
98. Cao S, Wang W, Nan F, Liu Y, Wei S, Li F. et al. (2018). Asiatic acid inhibits LPS-induced inflammatory response in endometrial epithelial cells. *Microbia Pathogen.* 116:195–199.
99. Kong D, Fu P, Zhang Q, Ma X, Jiang P. (2019). Protective effects of Asiatic acid against pelvic inflammatory disease in rats. *Exp Ther Med.* 17(6):4687–4692.
100. Liu M, Dai Y, Li Y. et al. (2008). Madecassoside isolated from *Centella asiatica* herbs facilitates burn wound healing in mice. *Planta Med.* 74(8):809–815.
101. Cook W. (1869). *The Physio-medical Dispensatory.*
102. Felter HW. (1922). *The Eclectic Materia Medica, Pharmacology and Therapeutics.*
103. Ellingwood F. (1908). *Ellingwood's Therapeutist*, vol. 2.
104. Jarboe CH, Schmidt CM, Nicholson JA, Zirvi KA. (1966). Uterine relaxant properties of *Viburnum. Nature.* 212:837.
105. Cometa MF, Parisi L, Palmery M, Meneguz A, Tomassini L. (2009). In vitro relaxant and spasmolytic effects of constituents from *Viburnum prunifolium* and HPLC quantification of the bioactive isolated iridoids. *J Ethnopharmacol.* 123:201–207.
106. Munch JC, Pratt HJ. (1941). Studies on *Viburnum* XI: Bioassay methods. *Pharm Arch.* 12:88–91.
107. Grote IW, Woods M. (1947). Studies on *Viburnum* III: The uterine sedative action of various fractions. *J Am Pharm Assoc.* 36:191–192.

108. Cometa MF, Parisi L, Palmery M, Meneguz A, Tomassini L. (2009). In vitro relaxant and spasmolytic effects of constituents from *Viburnum prunifolium* and HPLC quantification of the bioactive isolated iridoids. *J Ethnopharmacol.* 123:201–207.
109. Evans WE, Harne WG, Krantz JC. (1942). A uterine principle from *Viburnum prunifolium*. *J Pharmacol.* 75:174–177.
Hörhammer L, Wagner H, Reinhardt H. (1967). On new constituents from the barks of *Viburnum prunifolium* L. *J Am Pharm Ass.* 34:205–207.
110. Saltan G, Suntar I, Ozbilgin S, Ilhan M, Demirel MA, Oz BE, Keles H, Akkol EK. (2016). *Viburnum opulus* L.: A remedy for the treatment of endometriosis demonstrated by rat model of surgically-induced endometriosis. *J Ethnopharmacol.* 193:450–455.
111. Balansard G, Chausse D, Boukef K. et al. (1983). Selection criteria for a Viburnum extract, *Viburnum prunifolium* L., as a function of its veinotonic and spasmolytic action. *Plantes Med Phytother.* 17(3):123–132.
112. Choudhary MI, Azizuddin, Jalil S, Nawaz SA, Khan KM, Tareen RB. et al. (2009). Antiinflammatory and lipoxygenase inhibitory compounds from *Vitex agnus-castus*. *Phytother Res.* 23:1336–1339.
113. Chan EWC, Wong SK, Chan HT. (2018). Casticin from *Vitex* species: A short review on its anticancer and anti-inflammatory properties. *J Integr Med.* 16(3):147–152.
114. Jarry H, Leonhardt S, Gorkow C, Wuttke W. (1994). In vitro prolactin but not LH and FSH release is inhibited by compounds in extracts of *Agnus castus*: Direct evidence for a dopaminergic principle by the dopamine receptor assay. *Exp Clin Endocrinol.* 102(6):448–454.
115. Novella-Maestre E, Carda C, Noguera I, Ruiz-Saurí A, García-Velasco JA, Simón C, Pellicer A. (2009). Dopamine agonist administration causes a reduction in endometrial implants through modulation of angiogenesis in experimentally induced endometriosis. *Hum Reprod.* 24(5):1025–1035.
116. Dericks-Tan JS, Schwinn P, Hildt C. (2003). Dose-dependent stimulation of melatonin secretion after administration of *Agnus castus*. *Exp Clin Endocrinol Diabetes.* 111(1):44–46.
Diaz BL, Llaneza PC. (2008). Endocrine regulation of the course of menopause by oral melatonin: First case report. *Menopause.* 15(2):388–392.
117. Marino JL, Holt VL, Chen C, Davis S. (2008). Shift work, *hCLOCK* T3111C polymorphism, and endometriosis risk. *Epidemiol.* 19(3):477–484.
118. Guney M, Oral B, Karahan N, Mungan T. (2008). Regression of endometrial explants in a rat model of endometriosis treated melatonin. *Fertil Steril.* 89(4):934–942.

119. Chuffa LGA, Seiva FRF, Fávaro WJ, Teixeira GR, Amorim JPA. et al. (2011). Melatonin reduces LH, 17 beta-estradiol and induces differential regulation of sex steroid receptors in reproductive tissues during rat ovulation. *Reprod Biol Endocrinol.* 9:108.
120. Yilmaz B, Kilic S, Aksakal O, Ertas IE, Tanrisever GG. et al. (2015). Melatonin causes regression of endometriotic implants in rats by modulating angiogenesis, tissue levels of antioxidants and matrix metalloproteinases. *Arch Gynecol Obstet.* 292:209–216.
121. Paul S, Bhattacharya P, Das Mahapatra P, Swarnakar S. (2010). Melatonin protects against endometriosis via regulation of matrix metalloproteinase-3 and an apoptotic pathway. *J Pineal Res.* 49:156–168.
122. Shrestha S, Zhu J, Wang Q, Du X, Liu F. et al. (2017). Melatonin potentiates the antitumor effect of curcumin by inhibiting IKKβ/NF-κB/COX-2 signaling pathway. *Int J Oncol.* 51:1249–1260.
123. Eltbogen R, Litschgi M, Gasser UE, Flueeli A, Nebel S, Zahner C. (2014). *Vitex agnus-castus* extract (ZE440) improves symptoms in women with menstrual cycle irregularities. *Reprod Endocrinol.* 28:86–91.
124. Gerhard I, Patek A, Monga B, Blank A, Gorkow C. (1998). Mastodynon® for Female Infertility. Randomized placebo controlled, clinical double-blind study. *Forschende Komplementärmedizin/Res Compl Med.* 5(6):272–278.
125. Milewicz A, Gejdel E, Sworen H, Sienkiewicz K, Jedrzejak J, Teucher T, Schmitz H. (1993). *Vitex agnus castus* extract in the treatment of luteal phase defects due to latent hyperprolactinemia. Results of a randomized placebo-controlled double-blind study. *Arzneimittelforschung.* 43(7):752–756.
126. Zamani M, Mansour Ghanaei M, Farimany M, Nasrollahie SH. (2007). Efficacy of mefenamic acid and *Vitex* in reduction of menstrual blood loss and Hb changes in patients with a complaint of menorrhagia. *Iran J Obstet Gynecol Infertil.* 10(1):79–86.
127. El-Sharaky AS, Newairy AA, Kamel MA, Eweda SM. (2009). Protective effect of ginger extract against bromobenzene-induced hepatotoxicity in male rats. *Food Chem Toxicol.* 47:1584–1590.
128. Ahmed RS, Suke SG, Seth V, Chakraborti A, Tripathi AK, Banerjee BD. (2008). Protective effects of dietary ginger (*Zingiber officinale* Rosc.) on lindane-induced oxidative stress in rats. *Phytother Res.* 22:902–906.
129. Lantz RC, Chen GJ, Sarihan M, Sólyom AM, Jolad SD, Timmermann BN. (2007). The effect of extracts from ginger rhizome on inflammatory mediator production. *Phytomed.* 14:123–128.

130. Tjendraputra E, Tran VH, Liu-Brennan D, Roufogalis BD, Duke CC. (2001). Effect of ginger constituents and synthetic analogues on cyclo-oxygenase-2 enzyme in intact cells. *Bioorganic Chem*. 29:156–163.
131. Mallikarjuna K, Sahitya Chetan P, Sathyavelu Reddy K, Rajendra W. (2008). Ethanol toxicity: Rehabilitation of hepatic antioxidant defense system with dietary ginger. *Fitoterapia*. 79:174–178.
132. Pan MH, Hsieh MC, Kuo JM, Lai CS, Wu H, Sang S. et al. (2008). [6]-Shogaol induces apoptosis in human colorectal carcinoma cells via ROS production, caspase activation, and GADD 153 expression. *Mol Nutr Food Res*. 52:527–537.
133. Habib SH, Makpol S, Abdul Hamid NA, Das S, Ngah WZ, Yusof YA. (2008). Ginger extract (*Zingiber officinale*) has anti-cancer and anti-inflammatory effects on ethionine-induced hepatoma rats. *Clinics* (Sao Paulo). 63:807–813.
134. Rhode J, Fogoros S, Zick S, Wahl H, Griffith KA, Huang J. et al. (2007). Ginger inhibits cell growth and modulates angiogenic factors in ovarian cancer cells. *BMC Complement Altern Med*. 7:44.
135. Dugasani S, Pichika MR, Nadarajah VD, Balijepalli MK, Tandra S, Korlakunta JN. (2010). Comparative antioxidant and anti-inflammatory effects of [6]-gingerol, [8]-gingerol, [10]-gingerol and [6]-shogaol. *J Ethnopharmacol*. 127:515–520.
136. Lee HS, Seo EY, Kang NE, Kim WK. (2008). [6]-Gingerol inhibits metastasis of MDA-MB-231 human breast cancer cells. *J Nutr Biochem*. 19:313–319.
137. Nigam N, Bhui K, Prasad S, George J, Shukla Y. (2009). [6]-Gingerol induces reactive oxygen species regulated mitochondrial cell death pathway in human epidermoid carcinoma A431 cells. *Chem Biol Interact*. 181:77–84.
138. Shukla Y, Prasad S, Tripathi C, Singh M, George J, Kalra N. (2007). *In vitro* and *in vivo* modulation of testosterone mediated alterations in apoptosis related proteins by [6]-gingerol. *Mol Nutr Food Res*. 51:1492–1502.
139. Chen CX, Barrett B, Kwekkeboom KL. (2016). Efficacy of oral ginger (*Zingiber officinale*) for dysmenorrhea: A systematic review and meta-analysis. *Evid Based Comp Alt Med*. 6295737.
140. Daily JW, Zhang X, Kim DS, Park S. (2015). Efficacy of ginger for alleviating the symptoms of primary dysmenorrhea: A systematic review and meta-analysis of randomized clinical trials. *Pain Med*. 16(12):2243–2255.

141. Kohama T, Herai K, Inoue M. (2007). Effect of French maritime pine bark extract on endometriosis as compared with leuprorelin acetate. *J Reprod Med.* 52(8):703–708.
142. Ergenoglu AM, Yeniel AO, Erbas O, Aktug H, Yildirim N, Ulukus M, Taskiran D. (2013). Regression of endometrial implants by resveratrol in an experimentally induced endometriosis model in rats. *Reprod Sci.* 20:1230–1236.
143. Kolahdouz Mohammadi R, Arablou T. (2017). Resveratrol and endometriosis: In vitro and animal studies and underlying mechanisms (Review). *Biomed Pharmacotherapy.* 19:220–228.
144. Rudzitis-Auth J, Menger MD, Laschke MW. (2013). Resveratrol is a potent inhibitor of vascularization and cell proliferation in experimental endometriosis. *Hum Reprod.* 28:1339–1347.
145. Bruner-Tran KL, Osteen KG, Taylor HS, Sokalska A, Haines K, Duleba A.J. (2011). Resveratrol inhibits development of experimental endometriosis *in vivo* and reduces endometrial stromal cell invasiveness *in vitro*. *Biol Reprod.* 84:106–112.
146. Herington JL, Crispens MA, Carvalho-Macedo AC, Camargos AF, Lebovic DI, Bruner-Tran KL, Osteen KG. (2011). Development and prevention of postsurgical adhesions in a chimeric mouse model of experimental endometriosis. *Fertil Steril.* 95(4):1295–1301.e1.
147. Taylor HS, Osteen KG, Bruner-Tran KL, Lockwood CJ, Krikun G, Sokalska A, Duleba AJ. (2011). Novel therapies targeting endometriosis. *Reprod Sci.* 18:814–823.
148. Cenksoy PO, Oktem M, Erdem O. et al. (2015). A potential novel treatment strategy: Inhibition of angiogenesis and inflammation by resveratrol for regression of endometriosis in an experimental rat model. *Gynecol Endocrinol.* 31(3):219–224.
149. Taguchi A, Wada-Hiraike, Kawana K. et al. (2014). Resveratrol suppresses inflammatory responses in endometrial stromal cells derived from endometriosis: A possible role of the sirtuin 1 pathway. *J Obstet Gynaecol Res.* 40(3):770–778.
150. Amaya SC, Savaris RF, Filipovic CJ. et al. (2014). Resveratrol and endometrium: A closer look at an active ingredient of red wine using in vivo and in vitro models. *Reprod Sci.* 21(11):1362–1369.
151. Maia H Jr, Haddad C, Pinheiro N, Casoy J. (2012). Advantages of the association of resveratrol with oral contraceptives for management of endometriosis-related pain. *Int J Women's Health.* 4:543–549.

152. Mendes da Silva D, Gross LA, Neto E de, Lessey BA, Savaris RF. (2017). The use of resveratrol as an adjuvant treatment of pain in endometriosis: A randomized clinical trial. *J Endoc Soc.* 1(4):359–369.
153. Wong AS, Che CM, Leung KW. (2015). Recent advances in ginseng as cancer therapeutics: A functional and mechanistic overview. *Nat Prod Rep.* 32:256–272.
154. Wong AS, Che CM, Leung KW. (2015). Recent advances in ginseng as cancer therapeutics: A functional and mechanistic overview. *Nat Prod Rep.* 32:256–272.
    Wang C, Cai Y, Anderson S, Yuan C. (2015). Ginseng metabolites on cancer chemoprevention: An angiogenesis link? *Diseases.* 3(3):193–204.
155. Yue PYK, Wong DYL, Wu PK. et al. (2006). The angiosuppressive effects of 20(R)- ginsenoside Rg3. *Biochem Pharmacol.* 72(4):437–445.
156. Cao Y, Ye Q, Zhuang M. et al. (2017). Ginsenoside Rg3 inhibits angiogenesis in a rat model of endometriosis through the VEGFR-2-mediated PI3K/Akt/mTOR signaling pathway. *PLoS One.* 12(11): e0186520.
157. Li Z, Zhi MC, Li XL. (2007). Control study of ginsenosides and gestrinone on the treatment of endometriosis rats. *Chin J Obstet Gynecol.* 42:417–418.
158. Song ZY, Li Z, Zhi MC, Jiang YH. (2006). The observation of inhibition effect of ginsenoside Rg3 on endometriosis rats model. *Chin Remed Clin.* 6:255–256.
159. Kim, MK, Lee SK, Park JH. et al. (2017). Ginsenoside Rg3 decreases fibrotic and invasive nature of endometriosis by modulating miRNA-27b: In vitro and In vivo studies. *Sci Rep.* 7(1).
160. Long JR, Li Z. (2012). Ginsenoside Rg3 in combination with surgery in patients with stage III-IV endometriosis: A clinical control trial. *Chin Remed Clin.* 12:720–724.
161. González-Ramos R, Van Langendonckt A, Defrère S. Lousse JC. et al. (2010). Involvement of the nuclear factor-kappaB pathway in the pathogenesis of endometriosis. *Fertil Steril.* 94(6):1985–1994.
162. González-Ramos R, Donnez J, Defrère S, Leclercq I. et al. (2007). Nuclear factor-kappa B is constitutively activated in peritoneal endometriosis. *Mol Hum Reprod.* 13(7):503–509.
163. Lousse JC, Van Langendonckt A, González-Ramos R, Defrère S, Renkin E, Donnez J. (2008). Increased activation of nuclear factor-kappa B (NF-kappaB) in isolated peritoneal macrophages of patients with endometriosis. *Fertil Steril.* 90:217–220.

164. Lin FL, Wu SJ, Lee SC, Ng LT. (2009). Antioxidant, antioedema and analgesic activities of *Andrographis paniculata* extracts and their active constituent andrographolide. *Phytother Res*. 23:958–964.
165. Sulaiman MR, Zakaria ZA, Abdul Rahman A. et al. (2009). Antinociceptive and antiedematogenic activities of andrographolide isolated from *Andrographis paniculata* in animal models. *Biol Res Nurs*. 11(3):293–301.
166. Zheng Y, Liu X, Guo SW. (2012). Therapeutic potential of andrographolide for treating endometriosis. *Hum Reprod*. 27:1300–1313.
167. Xia YF, Ye BQ, Li YD. (2004). Andrographolide attenuates inflammation by inhibition of NF-kappa B activation through covalent modification of reduced cysteine 62 of p50. *J Immunol*. 173:4207–4217.
168. Abu-Ghefreh AA, Canatan H, Ezeamuzie, CI. (2009). In vitro and in vivo anti-inflammatory effects of andrographolide. *Int Immunopharmacol*. 9:313–318.
169. Hidalgo MA, Romero A, Figueroa J. et al. (2005). Andrographolide interferes with binding of nuclear factor-kappaB to DNA in HL-60-derived neutrophilic cells. *Br J Pharmacol*. 144:680–686.
170. Hsieh CY, Hsu MJ, Hsiao G. et al. (2011). Andrographolide enhances nuclear factor-kappaB subunit p65 Ser536 dephosphorylation through activation of protein phosphatase 2A in vascular smooth muscle cells. *J Biol Chem*. 286:5942–5955.
171. Mao X, Wang Y, Carter AV, Zhen X, Guo SX. (2011). The retardation of myometrial infiltration, reduction of uterine contractility, and alleviation of generalized hyperalgesia in mice with induced adenomyosis by levo-tetrahydropalmatine (l-THP) and andrographolide. *Reprod Sci*. 18:1025–1037.
172. Li B, Chen M, Liu X, Guo SW. (2013). Constitutive and tumor necrosis factor-alpha-induced activation of nuclear factor-kappaB in adenomyosis and its inhibition by andrographolide. *Fertil Steril*. 100:568–577.
173. Li B, Chen M, Liu X, Guo SW. (2013). Constitutive and tumor necrosis factor-alpha-induced activation of nuclear factor-kappaB in adenomyosis and its inhibition by andrographolide. *Fertil Steril*. 100:568–577.
174. Zheng W, Cao L, Xu Z, Ma Y, Liang X. (2018). Anti-angiogenic alternative and complementary medicines for the treatment of endometriosis: A review of potential molecular mechanisms. *Complement Alternat Med*. 4128984.
175. Burgos RA, Hancke JL, Bertoglio JC. et al. (2009). Efficacy of an *Andrographis paniculata* composition for the relief of rheumatoid arthritis

symptoms: A prospective randomized placebo-controlled trial. *Clin Rheumatol.* 28:931–946.
176. Liu X, Yu S, Guo SW. (2014). A pilot study on the use of andrographolide to treat symptomatic adenomyosis. *Gynecol Min Invasive Ther.* 3:119–126.
177. Henning SM, Niu Y, Lee NH, Thames GD, Minutti RR, Wang H, Go VL, Heber D. (2004). Bioavailability and antioxidant activity of tea flavanols after consumption of green tea, black tea, or a green tea extract supplement. *Am J Clin Nutr.* 80:1558–1564.
178. Xu H, Lui WT, Chu CY, Ng PS, Wang CC, Rogers MS. (2009). Anti-angiogenic effects of green tea catechin on an experimental endometriosis mouse model. *Hum Reprod.* 24:608–618.
179. Laschke MW, Schwender C, Scheuer C, Vollmar B, Menger MD. (2008). Epigallocatechin-3-gallate inhibits estrogen-induced activation of endometrial cells *in vitro* and causes regression of endometriotic lesions *in vivo. Hum Reprod.* 23:2308–2318.
180. Laschke MW, Schwender C, Scheuer C, Vollmar B, Menger MD. (2008). Epigallocatechin-3-gallate inhibits estrogen-induced activation of endometrial cells *in vitro* and causes regression of endometriotic lesions *in vivo. Hum Reprod.* 23:2308–2318.
181. Xu H, Becker CM, Lui WT, Chu CY, Davis TN, et al. (2011). Green tea epigallocatechin-3-gallate inhibits angiogenesis and suppresses vascular endothelial growth factor C/vascular endothelial growth factor receptor 2 expression and signaling in experimental endometriosis in vivo. *Fertil Steril.* 96(4):1021–1028.
182. Wang CC, Xu H, Man GC, Zhang T, Chu KO. et al. (2013). Prodrug of green tea epigallocatechin-3-gallate (Pro-EGCG) as a potent anti-angiogenesis agent for endometriosis in mice. *Angiogenesis.* 16:59–69.
183. Xu H, Lui WT, Chu CY, Ng PS, Wang CC. et al. (2009). Anti-angiogenic effects of green tea catechin on an experimental endometriosis mouse model. *Hum Reprod.* 24:608–618.
184. Ricci AG, Olivares CN, Bilotas MA, Baston JI, Singla JJ, Meresman GF, Baranao RI. (2013). Natural therapies assessment for the treatment of endometriosis. *Hum Reprod.* 28:178–188.
185. Rao SD, Pagidas K. (2010). Epigallocatechin-3-gallate, a natural polyphenol, inhibits cell proliferation and induces apoptosis in human ovarian cancer cells. *Anticancer Res.* 30:2519–2523.
186. Zaveri NT. (2006). Green tea and its polyphenolic catechins: Medicinal uses in cancer and noncancer applications. *Life Sci.* 78:2073–2080.

187. Zhang D, Al-Hendy M, Richard-Davis G, Montgomery-Rice V, Rajaratnam V, Al-Hendy A. (2010). Antiproliferative and proapoptotic effects of epigallocatechin gallate on human leiomyoma cells. *Fertil Steril.* 94:1887–1893.
188. Zhang D, Al-Hendy M, Richard-Davis G, Montgomery-Rice V, Sharan C, Rajaratnam V, Khurana A, Al-Hendy A. (2010). Green tea extract inhibits proliferation of uterine leiomyoma cells in vitro and in nude mice. *Am J Obstet Gynecol.* 202:289e1–289e9.
189. Matsuzaki S, Darcha C. (2014). Antifibrotic properties of epigallocatechin-3-gallate in endometriosis. *Hum Reprod.* 29(8):1677–1687.
190. Xu H, Becker CM, Lui WT, Chu CY, Davis TN. et al. (2011). Green tea epigallocatechin-3-gallate inhibits angiogenesis and suppresses vascular endothelial growth factor C/vascular endothelial growth factor receptor 2 expression and signaling in experimental endometriosis in vivo. *Fertil Steril.* 96(4):1021–1028.
191. Ricci AG, Olivares CN, Bilotas NA. et al. (2013). Natural therapies assessment for the treatment of endometriosis. *Hum Reprod.* 28(1):178–188.
192. Park S, Lim W, Bazer FW, Song G. (2017). Naringenin induces mitochondriamediated apoptosis and endoplasmic reticulum stress by regulating MAPK and AKT signal transduction pathways in endometriosis cells. *Mole Hum Reprod.* 23(12):842–854.
193. Li Q, Wang Y, Zhang L. et al. (2016). Naringenin exerts anti-angiogenic effects in human endothelial cells: Involvement of ERRα/VEGF/KDR signaling pathway. *Fitoterapia.* 111:78–86.
194. Arablou T, Kolahdouz-Mohammadi R. (2018). Curcumin and endometriosis: Review on potential roles and molecular mechanisms. *Biomed Pharmacother.* 97:91–97.
195. Soetikno V, Sari FR, Lakshmanan AP, Arumugam S, Harima M, Suzuki K, Kawachi H, Watanabe K. (2013). Curcumin alleviates oxidative stress, inflammation, and renal fibrosis in remnant kidney through the Nrf2-keap1 pathway. *Mol Nutr Food Res.* 57:1649–1659.
196. Vallée A, Lecarpentier Y. (2020). Curcumin and endometriosis. *Int J Mol Sci.* 21(7):2440.
197. Chowdhury I, Banerjee S, Driss A, Xu W, Mehrabi S, Nezhat C, Sidell N, Taylor RN, Thompson WE. (2019). Curcumin attenuates proangiogenic and proinflammatory factors in human eutopic endometrial stromal cells through the NF-κB signaling pathway. *J Cell Physiol.* 234:6298–6312.

198. Jana S, Rudra DS, Paul S, Snehasikta S. (2012). Curcumin delays endometriosis development by inhibiting MMP-2 activity. *Indian J Biochem Biophys.* 49:342–348.
199. Jana S, Paul S, Swarnakar S. (2012). Curcumin as anti-endometriotic agent: Implication of MMP-3 and intrinsic apoptotic pathway. *Biochem Pharmacol.* 83(6):797–804.
200. Swarnakar S, Paul S. (2009). Curcumin arrests endometriosis by down-regulation of matrix metalloproteinase-9 activity. *Indian J Biochem Biophys.* 46:59–65.
201. Zhang Y, Cao H, Yu Z, Peng HY, Zhang CJ. (2013). Curcumin inhibits endometriosis endometrial cells by reducing estradiol production. *Iran J Reprod Med.* 11(5):415–422.
202. Kim KH, Lee EN, Park JK. Lee JR, Kim JH. et al. (2012). Curcumin attenuates TNF-α-induced expression of intercellular adhesion molecule-1, vascular cell adhesion molecule-1 and proinflammatory cytokines in human endometriotic stromal cells. *Phytother Res.* 26(7):1037–1047.
203. Jana SK, Chakravarty B, Chaudhury K. (2014). Letrozole and curcumin loaded-PLGA nanoparticles: A therapeutic strategy for endometriosis. *J Nanomedine Biother Discov.* 4:123.
204. Kim KH, Lee EN, Park JK. et al. (2012). Curcumin attenuates TNF-α-induced expression of intercellular adhesion molecule-1, vascular cell adhesion molecule-1 and proinflammatory cytokines in human endometriotic stromal cells. *Phytother Res.* 26(7):1037–1047.
205. Kim KH, Lee EN, Park JK. et al. (2012). Curcumin attenuates TNF-α-induced expression of intercellular adhesion molecule-1, vascular cell adhesion molecule-1 and proinflammatory cytokines in human endometriotic stromal cells. *Phytother Res.* 26(7):1037–1047.
206. Zhang Y, Cao H, Hu YY, Wang H, Zhang CJ. (2011). Inhibitory effect of curcumin on angiogenesis in ectopic endometrium of rats with experimental endometriosis. *Int J Mol Med.* 27(1):87–94.
207. Jana S, Paul S, Swarnakar S. (2012). Curcumin as anti-endometriotic agent: Implication of MMP-3 and intrinsic apoptotic pathway. *Biochem Pharmacol.* 83(6):797–804.
208. Kizilay G, Uz YH, Seren G. et al. (2017). In vivo effects of curcumin and deferoxamine in experimental endometriosis. *Adv Clinic Experimental Med.* 26(2):207–213.
209. Vallée A, Lecarpentier Y. (2020). Curcumin and endometriosis. *Int J Mol Sci.* 21(7):2440.

210. Williams CS, Mann M, DuBois RN. (1999). The role of cyclooxygenases in inflammation, cancer, and development. *Oncogene.* 18:7908–7916.
211. Arablou T, Kolahdouz-Mohammadi R. (2018). Curcumin and endometriosis: Review on potential roles and molecular mechanisms. *Biomed Pharmacother.* 97:91–97.
212. Kim KH, Lee EN, Park JK. Lee JR, Kim JH. et al. (2012). Curcumin attenuates TNF-α-induced expression of intercellular adhesion molecule-1, vascular cell adhesion molecule-1 and proinflammatory cytokines in human endometriotic stromal cells. *Phytother Res.* 26(7):1037–1047.
213. Zhang Y, Cao H, Hu YY, Wang H, Zhang CJ. (2011). Inhibitory effect of curcumin on angiogenesis in ectopic endometrium of rats with experimental endometriosis. *Int J Mol Med.* 27(1):87–94.
214. Cao H, Wei YX, Zhou Q, Zhang Y, Guo XP, Zhang J. (2017). Inhibitory effect of curcumin in human endometriosis endometrial cells via downregulation of vascular endothelial growth factor. *Mol Med Reports.* 16(4):5611–5617.
215. Zhang Y, Cao H, Yu Z, Peng HY, Zhang CJ. (2013). Curcumin inhibits endometriosis endometrial cells by reducing estradiol production. *Iran J Reprod Med.* 11(5):415–422.
216. Fadus MC, Lau C, Bikhchandani J, Lynch HT. (2017). Curcumin: An age-old anti-inflammatory and anti-neoplastic agent. *J Trad Complement Med.* 7(3):339–346.
217. Rudzitis-Auth J, Krbel C, Scheuer C, Menger MD, Laschke MW. (2012). Xanthohumol inhibits growth and vascularization of developing endometriotic lesions. *Hum Reprod.* 27(6):1735–1744.
218. Ilhan M, Suntar I, Demirel MA, Yesilada E, Keles H, Kupeli Akkol E. (2016). A mixture of St. John's wort and sea buckthorn oils regresses endometriotic implants and affects the levels of inflammatory mediators in peritoneal fluid of the rat: A surgically induced endometriosis model. *Taiwan J Obstet Gynecol.* 55:786–790.
219. Wu H, Wei W, Song L, Zhang L, Chen Y, Hu X. (2007). Paeoniflorin induced immune tolerance of mesenteric lymph node lymphocytes via enhancing beta 2-adrenergic receptor desensitization in rats with adjuvant arthritis. *Int Immunopharmacol.* 7:662–673.
220. He DY, Dai SM. (2011). Anti-inflammatory and immunomodulatory effects of *Paeonia lactiflora* pall., a traditional Chinese herbal medicine. *Front Pharmacol.* 2:10.
221. Zhou Q, Li ZG. (2003). Pharmacology and therapeutic usages of total glucosides of paeony in autoimmune diseases. *Zhongguo Xin Yao Yu Lin Chuang Za Zhi.* 22:687–691.

222. Shuai ZW, Xu JH, Liu S, Wei W, Xu SQ, Xu SY. (2003). Clinical observation of total glucosides of paeony in the treatment of systemic lupus erythematosus. *Zhongguo Zhong Xi Yi Jie He Za Zhi.* 23:188–191 (in Chinese).
223. He DY, Dai SM. (2011). Anti-inflammatory and immunomodulatory effects of *Paeonia lactiflora* pall., a traditional Chinese herbal medicine. *Front Pharmacol.* 2:10.
224. Jin Z, Huang J, Zhu Z. (2017). Baicalein reduces endometriosis by suppressing the viability of human endometrial stromal cells through the nuclear factor-kappaB pathway *in vitro*. *Exp Ther Med.* 14:2992–2998.
225. Zhou ZH, Weng Q, Zhou JH, Zhou J. (2012). Extracts of *Salvia miltiorrhiza* Bunge on the cytokines of rat endometriosis models. *Afric J Trad Complement Altern Med.* 9(3):303–314.
226. Lu ML, Li Y, Zeng RL. et al. (2016). Effect of *Salviae miltiorrhizae* on stromal cells MMP-9 mRNA and protein expression of endometriosis. *J New Chin Med.* 48(4):278–280.
227. Lin LG, Liu QY, Ye Y. (2014). Naturally occurring homoiso-flavonoids and their pharmacological activities. *Planta Med.* 80:1053–1066.
228. Cosar E, Mamillapalli R, Moridi I, Duleba A, Taylor HS. (2018). Serum microRNA biomarkers regulated by simvastatin in a primate model of endometriosis. *Reprod Sci.* 1933719118765971.
229. Chavez M, Chavez P. (1999). Feverfew. *Hosp Pharm.* 34:436–461.
Heptinstall S, Groenewegen WA, Spangenberg P, Loesche W. (1987). Extracts of feverfew may inhibit platelet behavior via neutralization of sulphydryl groups. *J Pharm Pharmacol.* 39:459–465.
230. Heptinstall S, Groenewegen S, Spangenberg P, Losche W. (1988). Inhibition of platelet behaviour by feverfew: A mechanism of action involving sulphydryl groups. *Folia Haematol Int Mag Klin Morphol Blutforsch.* 115:447–449.
231. Pugh WJ, Sambo K. (1988). Prostaglandin synthetase inhibitors in feverfew. *J Pharm Pharmacol.* 40:743–745.
232. Makheja AN, Bailey JM. (1982). A platelet phospholipase inhibitor from the medicinal herb feverfew (*Tanacetum parthenium*). *Prostaglandins Leukot Med.* 8:653–660.
233. Collier HO, Butt NM, McDonald WJ, Saeed SA. (1980). Extract of feverfew inhibits prostaglandin biosynthesis. *Lancet.* 2:922–923.
234. Brown AM, Edwards CM, Davey MR, Power JB, Lowe KC. (1997). Pharmacological activity of feverfew (*Tanacetum parthenium* [L.] Schultz-Bip.): Assessment by inhibition of human polymorphonuclear leukocyte chemiluminescence *in vitro*. *J Pharm Pharmacol.* 49:558–561.

235. Sumner H, Salan U, Knight DW, Hoult JR. (1992). Inhibition of 5-lipoxygenase and cyclo-oxygenase in leukocytes by feverfew. Involvement of sesquiterpene lactones and other components. *Biochem Pharmacol.* 43:2313–2320.
236. Pattrick M, Heptinstall S, Doherty M. (1989). Feverfew in rheumatoid arthritis: A double blind, placebo controlled study. *Ann Rheum Dis.* 48:547–549.
237. Smith TH, Liu X. (2001). Feverfew extracts and the sesquiterpene lactone parthenolide inhibit intercellular adhesion molecule-1 expression in human synovial fibroblasts. *Cell Immunol.* 209:89–96.
238. Setty AR, Sigal AH. (2005). Herbal medications commonly used in the practice of rheumatology: Mechanisms of action, efficacy, and side effects. *Semin Arthritis Rheum.* 34:773–784.
239. Pareek A, Suthar M, Rathore GS, Bansal V. (2011). Feverfew (*Tanacetum parthenium* L.): A systematic review. *Pharmacog Rev.* 5:103–110.
240. Sur R, Martin K, Liebel F, Lyte P, Shapiro S, Southall M. (2009). Anti-inflammatory activity of parthenolide-depleted feverfew (*Tanacetum parthenium*). *Inflammopharmacol.* 17(1):42–49.
241. Pareek A, Suthar M, Rathore GS, Bansal V. (2011). Feverfew (*Tanacetum parthenium* L.): A systematic review. *Pharmacog Rev.* 5:103–110.
242. Kwok BH, Koh B, Ndubuisi MI, Elofsson M, Crews CM. (2001). The anti-inflammatory natural product parthenolide from the medicinal herb feverfew directly binds to and inhibits IkappaB kinase. *Chem Biol.* 8(8):759–766.
243. Collier HO, Butt NM, McDonald WJ, Saeed SA. (1980). Extract of feverfew inhibits prostaglandin biosynthesis. *Lancet.* 2:922–923.
244. Brown AM, Edwards CM, Davey MR, Power JB, Lowe KC. (1997). Pharmacological activity of feverfew (*Tanacetum parthenium* [L.] Schultz-Bip.): Assessment by inhibition of human polymorphonuclear leukocyte chemiluminescence *in vitro. J Pharm Pharmacol.* 49:558–561.
245. Neill LA, Barrett ML, Lewis GP. (1987). Extracts of feverfew inhibit mitogen-induced human peripheral blood mononuclear cell proliferation and cytokine mediated responses: A cytotoxic effect. *Br J Clin Pharmacol.* 23:81–83.
246. Barsby RW, Salan U, Knight DW, Hoult JR. (1992). Feverfew extracts and parthenolide irreversibly inhibit vascular responses of the rabbit aorta. *J Pharm Pharmacol.* 44(9):737–740.
    Barsby RW, Salan U, Knight DW, Hoult JR. (1993). Feverfew and vascular smooth muscle: Extracts from fresh and dried plants show

opposing pharmacological profiles, dependent upon sesquiterpene lactone content. *Planta Med.* 59:20–25.

Barsby RW, Knight DW, McFadzean I. (1993). A chloroform extract of the herb feverfew blocks voltage-dependent potassium currents recorded from single smooth muscle cells. *J Pharm Pharmacol.* 45(7):641–645.

247. Hardin SR. (2007). Cat's claw: An Amazonian vine decreases inflammantion in osteoarthritis. *Complement Ther Clin Pract.* 13(1):25–28.
248. Nogueira Neto J, Coelho TM, Aguiar GC, Carvalho LR, de Araújo AG, Girão MJ, Schor E. (2011). Experimental endometriosis reduction in rats treated with *Uncaria tomentosa* (cat's claw) extract. *Eur J Obstet Gynecol Reprod Biol.* 154(2):205–208.
249. Nogueira Neto J, Coelho TM, Aguiar GC, Carvalho LR, de Araújo AG, Girão MJ, Schor E. (2011). Experimental endometriosis reduction in rats treated with *Uncaria tomentosa* (cat's claw) extract. *Eur J Obstet Gynecol Reprod Biol.* 154(2):205–208.
250. Nogueira Neto J, Cavalcante FL, Carvalho RA, Rodrigues TG, Xavier MS, Furtado PG, Schor E. (2011). Contraceptive effect of *Uncaria tomentosa* (cat's claw) in rats with experimental endometriosis. *Acta Cir Bras.* 26(Suppl. 2):15–19.
251. Armour M, Middleton A, Lim S, Sinclair J, Varjabedian D, Smith CA. (2021). Dietary practices of women with endometriosis: A cross-sectional survey. *J Altern Complement Med.* 27(9):771–777.
252. Krabbenborg I, de Roos N, van der Grinten P, Nap A. (2021). Diet quality and perceived effects of dietary changes in Dutch endometriosis patients: An observational study. *Reprod Biomed Online.* 43(5):952–961.
253. Vennberg Karlsson J, Patel H, Premberg A. (2020). Experiences of health after dietary changes in endometriosis: A qualitative interview study. *BMJ Open.* 10(2):e032321.
254. Nirgianakis K, Egger K, Kalaitzopoulos DR, Lanz S, Bally L, Mueller MD. (2021). Effectiveness of dietary interventions in the treatment of endometriosis: A systematic review. *Reprod Sci.* 29(1):26–42.
255. Ott J, Nouri K, Hrebacka D, Gutschelhofer S, Huber J, Wenzl R. (2012). Endometriosis and nutrition—recommending a Mediterranean diet decreases endometriosis-associated pain: An experimental observational study. *J Aging Res Clin Practice.* 1:162–166.
256. Jurkiewicz-Przondziono J, Lemm M, Kwiatkowska-Pamuła A, Ziółko E, Wójtowicz MK. (2017). Influence of diet on the risk of developing endometriosis. *Ginekol Pol.* 88(2):96–102.

257. Heilier JF, Donnez J, Nackers F. et al. (2007). Environmental and host-associated risk factors in endometriosis and deep endometriotic nodules: A matched case-control study. *Environ Res.* 103(1):121–129.
258. Parazzini F, Chiaffarino F, Surace M. et al. (2004). Selected food intake and risk of endometriosis. *Hum Reprod.* 19(8):1755–1759.
259. Mier-Cabrera J, Aburto-Soto T, Burrola-Méndez S. et al. (2009). Women with endometriosis improved their peripheral antioxidant markers after the application of a high antioxidant diet. *Reprod Biol Endocrinol.* 7:54.
260. Sesti F, Pietropolli A, Capozzolo T, Broccoli P, Pierangeli S, Bollea MR, Piccione E. (2007). Hormonal suppression treatment or dietary therapy versus placebo in the control of painful symptoms after conservative surgery for endometriosis stage III-IV. A randomized comparative trial. *Fertil Steril.* 88(6):1541–1547.
261. Huijs E, Nap A. (2020). The effects of nutrients on symptoms in women with endometriosis: A systematic review. *Reprod Biomed Online.* 41(2):317–328.
262. Darling AM, Chavarro JE, Malspeis S. et al. (2013). A prospective cohort study of vitamins B, C, E, and multivitamin intake and endometriosis. *J Endometr.* 5(1):17–26.
263. Parazzini F, Viganò P, Candiani M, Fedele L. (2013). Diet and endometriosis risk: A literature review. *Reprod Biomed Online.* 26(4):323–336.
264. Nodler JL, Harris HR, Chavarro JE, Frazier AL, Missmer SA. (2020). Dairy consumption during adolescence and endometriosis risk. *Am J Obstet Gynecol.* 222(3):257.e1–257.e16.
265. Harris HR, Chavarro JE, Malspeis S, Willett WC, Missmer SA. (2013). Dairy-food, calcium, magnesium, and vitamin D intake and endometriosis: A prospective cohort study. *Am J Epidemiol.* 177(5):420–430.
266. Parazzini F, Chiaffarino F, Surace M. et al. (2004). Selected food intake and risk of endometriosis. *Hum Reprod.* 19(8):1755–1759.
267. Tsuchiya M, Miura T, Hanaoka T, Iwasaki M, Sasaki H, Tanaka T. et al. (2007). Effect of soy isoflavones on endometriosis: Interaction with estrogen receptor 2 gene polymorphism. *Epidemiol.* 18(3):402–408.
268. Lin LG, Liu QY, Ye Y. (2014). Naturally occurring homoisoflavonoids and their pharmacological activities. *Planta Med.* 80(13):1053–1066.
269. Sutrisno S, Aprina H, Simanungkalit HM. et al. (2018). Genistein modulates the estrogen receptor and suppresses angiogenesis and inflammation in the murine model of peritoneal endometriosis. *J Trad Complement Med.* 8(2):278–281.

270. Noel JC, Anaf V, Fayt I, Wespes E. (2006). Ureteral mullerian carcinosarcoma (mixed mullerian tumor) associated with endometriosis occurring in a patient with a concentrated soy isoflavones supplementation. *Arch Gynecol Obstet.* 274(6):389–392.
271. Harris HR, Chavarro JE, Malspeis S, Willett WC, Missmer SA. (2013). Dairy-food, calcium, magnesium, and vitamin D intake and endometriosis: A prospective cohort study. *Am J Epidemiol.* 177(5):420–430.
272. Tian SS, Jiang FS, Zhang K. et al. (2013). Flavonoids from the leaves of *Carya cathayensis* Sarg. inhibit vascular endothelial growth factor-induced angiogenesis. *Fitoterapia.* 92(1):34–40.
273. Zhang M, Liu C, Zhang Z. et al. (2014). A new flavonoid regulates angiogenesis and reactive oxygen species production. *Adv Exper Med Biol.* 812:149–155.
274. Li Q, Wang Y, Zhang L. et al. (2016). Naringenin exerts anti-angiogenic effects in human endothelial cells: Involvement of ERRα/VEGF/KDR signaling pathway. *Fitoterapia.* 111:78–86.
275. Park S, Lim W, Bazer FW, Song G. (2017). Naringenin induces mitochondriamediated apoptosis and endoplasmic reticulum stress by regulating MAPK and AKT signal transduction pathways in endometriosis cells. *Mol Hum Reprod.* 23(12):842–854.
276. Missmer SA, Chavarro JE, Malspeis S. et al. (2010). A prospective study of dietary fat consumption and endometriosis risk. *Hum Reprod.* 25(6):1528–1535.
277. Parazzini F, Chiaffarino F, Surace M. et al. (2004). Selected food intake and risk of endometriosis. *Hum Reprod.* 19(8):1755–1759.
278. Chiaffarino F, Bravi F, Cipriani S. et al. (2014). Coffee and caffeine intake and risk of endometriosis: A meta-analysis. *Eur J Nutr.* 53(7):1573–1579.
279. Lucero J, Harlow BL, Barbieri RL. et al. (2001). Early follicular phase hormone levels in relation to patterns of alcohol, tobacco, and coffee use. *Fertil Steril.* 76(4):723–729.
280. De Giorgio R, Volta U, Gibson PR. (2016). Sensitivity to wheat, gluten and FODMAPs in IBS: Facts or fiction? *Gut.* 65(1):169–178.
281. Black CJ, Staudauer HM, Ford AC. (2021). Efficacy of a low FODMAP diet in irritable bowel syndrome: Systematic review and network meta-analysis. *Gut.* 71(6):1117–1126.
282. Ek M, Roth B, Ekström P, Valentin L, Bengtsson M, Ohlsson B. (2015). Gastrointestinal symptoms among endometriosis patients—a case-cohort study. *BMC Women's Health.* 15(1):59.

283. Jess T, Frisch M, Jørgensen KT, Pedersen BV, Nielsen NM. (2012). Increased risk of inflammatory bowel disease in women with endometriosis: A nationwide Danish cohort study. *Gut.* 61(9):1279–1283.
284. Moore JS, Gibson PR, Perry RE, Burgell RE. (2017). Endometriosis in patients with irritable bowel syndrome: Specific symptomatic and demographic profile, and response to the low FODMAP diet. *Aust N Z J Obstet Gynaecol.* 57(2):201–205.
285. Matalliotakis IM, Cakmak H, Fragouli YG. et al. (2008). Epidemiological characteristics in women with and without endometriosis in the Yale series. *Arch Gynecol Obstet.* 277(5):389–393.
286. Trabert B, Peters U, De Roos AJ. et al. (2011). Diet and risk of endometriosis in a population-based case-control study. *Br J Nutr.* 105(3):459–467.
287. Heilier JF, Donnez J, Nackers F. et al. (2007). Environmental and host-associated risk factors in endometriosis and deep endometriotic nodules: A matched case-control study. *Environ Res.* 103(1):121–129.
288. Britton JA, Westhoff C, Howe GR. et al. (2000). Diet and benign ovarian tumors (United States). *Cancer Causes Control.* 11(5):389–401.
289. Parazzini F, Chiaffarino F, Surace M. et al. (2004). Selected food intake and risk of endometriosis. *Hum Reprod.* 19(8):1755–1759.
290. Savaris AL, do Amaral VF. (2011). Nutrient intake, anthropometric data and correlations with the systemic antioxidant capacity of women with pelvic endometriosis. *Eur J Obstet Gynecol Reprod Biol.* 158(2):314–318.

Chapter 9: Uterine fibroids (uterine leiomyomas)

1. Baird DD, Dunson DB, Hill MC. et al. (2003). High cumulative incidence of uterine leiomyoma in black and white women: Ultrasound evidence. *Am J Obstet Gynecol.* 188(1):100–107.
2. Cook H, Ezzati M, Segars JH, McCarthy K. (2010). The impact of uterine leiomyomas on reproductive outcomes. *Minerva Ginecol.* 62(3):225–236.
3. Catherino WH, Parrott E, Segars J. (2011). Proceedings from the National Institute of Child Health and Human Development conference on the Uterine Fibroid Research Update Workshop. *Fertil Steril.* 95(1):9–12.
4. Sozen I, Arici A. (2002). Interactions of cytokines, growth factors, and the extracellular matrix in the cellular biology of uterine leiomyomata. *Fertil Steril.* 78(1):1–12.
5. Barker NM, Carrino DA, Caplan AI. et al. (2016). Proteoglycans in leiomyoma and normal myometrium: Abundance, steroid hormone control, and implications for pathophysiology. *Reprod Sci.* 23(3):302–309.

Fujisawa C, Castellot JJ. Jr. (2014). Matrix production and remodeling as therapeutic targets for uterine leiomyoma. *J Cell Commun Signal.* 8(3):179–194.
6. Wallach EE, Vlahos NF. (2004). Uterine myomas: An overview of development, clinical features, and management. *Obstet Gynecol.* 104(2):393–406.
7. Flake GP, Moore AB, Sutton D, Kissling GE, Horton J. et al. (2013). The natural history of uterine leiomyomas: Light and electron microscopic studies of fibroid phases, interstitial ischemia, inanosis, and reclamation. *Obstet Gynecol Int.* 528376.
8. Bulun SE. (2013). Uterine fibroids. *N Engl J Med.* 369(14):1344–1355.
9. Richards PA, Tiltman AJ. (1996). Anatomical variation of the oestrogen receptor in the non-neoplastic myometrium of fibromyomatous uteri. *Virchows Archiv.* 428(6):347–351.
10. Bulun SE, Imir G, Utsunomiya H. et al. (2005). Aromatase in endometriosis and uterine leiomyomata. *J Steroid Biochem Mol Biol.* 95(1–5):57–62.
11. Olmos Grings A, Lora V, Dias Ferreira G, Simoni Brum I, Von Eye Corleta H, Capp E. (2012). Protein expression of estrogen receptors α and β and aromatase in myometrium and uterine leiomyoma. *Gynecol Obstet Invest.* 73(2):113–117.
12. Park S, Ramachandran S, Kwon S. et al. (2008). Upregulation of ATP-sensitive potassium channels for estrogen-mediated cell proliferation in human uterine leiomyoma cells. *Gynecol Endocrinol.* 24(5):250–256.
13. Ishikawa H, Ishi K, Ann Serna V, Kakazu R, Bulun SE, Kurita T. (2010). Progesterone is essential for maintenance and growth of uterine leiomyoma. *Endocrinol.* 151(6):2433–2442.
14. Ying Z, Weiyuan Z. (2009). Dual actions of progesterone on uterine leiomyoma correlate with the ratio of progesterone receptor A:B. *Gynecol Endocrinol.* 25(8):520–523.
15. Kurachi O, Matsuo H, Samoto T, Maruo T. (2001). Tumor necrosis factor-α expression in human uterine leiomyoma and its down-regulation by progesterone. *J Clin Endocrinol Metab.* 86(5):2275–2280.
16. Payson M, Leppert P, Segars J. (2006). Epidemiology of myomas. *Obstet Gynecol Clin N Am.* 33(1):1–11.
17. Faerstein E, Szklo M, Rosenshein NB. (2001). Risk factors for uterine leiomyoma: A practice-based case-control study. II. Atherogenic risk factors and potential sources of uterine irritation. *Am J Epidemiol.* 153(1):11–19.
18. Boynton-Jarrett R, Rich-Edwards J, Malspeis S, Missmer SA, Wright R. (2005). A prospective study of hypertension and risk of uterine leiomyomata. *Am J Epidemiol.* 161:628–638.

19. Hocutt JE. (1979). Uterine fibroids and hypertension. *Del Med J.* 51:697–699.
20. He Y, Zeng Q, Li X, Liu B, Wang P. (2013). The association between subclinical atherosclerosis and uterine fibroids. *PLoS One.* 8(2):e57089.
21. Matsumoto T, Sagawa N, Mukoyama M, Tanaka I, Itoh H, Goto M. et al. (1996). Type 2 angiotensin II receptor is expressed in human myometrium and uterine leiomyoma and is down-regulated during pregnancy. *J Clin Endocrinol Metab.* 81(12):4366–4372.
22. Rüster C, Wolf G. (2013). The role of the renin-angiotensin-aldosterone system in obesity-related renal diseases. *Semin Nephrol.* 33(1):44–53.
23. Kalupahana NS, Moustaid-Moussa N. (2012). The renin-angiotensin system: A link between obesity, inflammation and insulin resistance. *Obes Rev.* 13(2):136–149.
24. Dixon D, Flake GP, Moore AB. et al. (2002). Cell proliferation and apoptosis in human uterine leiomyomas and myometria. *Virchows Archiv.* 441(1):53–62.
25. Protic O, Toti P, Islam MS. et al. (2016). Possible involvement of inflammatory/reparative processes in the development of uterine fibroids. *Cell Tissue Res.* 364(2):415–427.
26. Stewart EA, Nowak RA. (1996). Leiomyoma-related bleeding: A classic hypothesis updated for the molecular era. *Hum Reprod Update.* 2(4):295–306.
27. Norian JM, Malik M, Parker CY. et al. (2009). Transforming Growth Factor β3 regulates the versican variants in the extracellular matrix-rich uterine leiomyomas. *Reprod Sci.* 16(12):1153–1164.
28. Ciavattini A, Di Giuseppe J, Stortoni P, Montik N. et al. (2013). Uterine fibroids: Pathogenesis and interactions with endometrium and endomyometrial junction. 173184.
29. Sozen I, Arici A. (2002). Interactions of cytokines, growth factors, and the extracellular matrix in the cellular biology of uterine leiomyomata. *Fertil Steril.* 78(1):1–12.
30. Austin DJ, Nowak RA, Stewart EA. (1999). Onapristone suppresses prolactin production in explant cultures of leiomyoma. *Gynecol Obstet Invest.* 47(4):268–271.
31. Navarro A, Yin P, Monsivais D. et al. (2012). Genome-wide DNA methylation indicates silencing of tumor suppressor genes in uterine leiomyoma. *PLoS One.* 7(3):e33284.
32. Maekawa R, Sato S, Yamagata Y. et al. (2013). Genome-wide DNA methylation analysis reveals a potential mechanism for the pathogenesis and development of uterine leiomyomas. *PLoS One.* 8(6):e66632.

33. Huyck KL, Panhuysen CI, Cuenco KT. et al. (2008). The impact of race as a risk factor for symptom severity and age at diagnosis of uterine leiomyomata among affected sisters. *Am J Obstet Gynecol*. 198(2):168.e1–168.e9.
34. Williams A. (2017). Uterine fibroids—what's new?. *F1000Research*. 6:2109.
35. Marshall LM, Spiegelman D, Goldman MB. et al. (1998). A prospective study of reproductive factors and oral contraceptive use in relation to the risk of uterine leiomyomata. *Fertil Steril*. 70:432–439.
36. Donnez J, Dolmans M. (2016). Uterine fibroid management: From the present to the future. *Hum Reprod Update*. 22(6):665–686.
37. Vines AI, Nguyen TTX, Ta M, Esserman D, Baird DD. (2011). Self-reported daily stress, squelching of anger and the management of daily stress and the prevalence of uterine leiomyomata: The ultrasound screening study. *Stress Health*. 27:e188–194.
38. Vines AI, Ta M, Esserman DA. (2010). The association between self-reported major life events and the presence of uterine fibroids. *Women's Health Issues*. 20(4):294–298.
39. Summers WE, Watson RL, Wooldridge WH. et al. (1971). Hypertension, obesity and fibromyomata uteri, as a syndrome. *Arch Intern Med*. 128:750–754.
40. Shikora SA, Niloff JM, Bistrian BR, Forse RA, Blackburn GL. (1991). Relationship between obesity and uterine leiomyomata. *Nutrition*. 7(4):251–255.
41. Takeda T, Sakata M, Isobe A, Miyake A, Nishimoto F, Ota Y. et al. (2008). Relationship between metabolic syndrome and uterine leiomyomas: A case-control study. *Gynecol Obstet Invest*. 66:14–17.
42. Ross RK, Pike MC, Vessey MP. et al. (1986). Risk factors for uterine fibroids: Reduced risk associated with oral contraceptives. *BMJ (Clin Res Ed.)*. 293:359–362.
43. Marshall LM, Spiegelman D, Manson JE. et al. (1998). Risk of uterine leiomyomata among premenopausal women in relation to body size and cigarette smoking. *Epidemiol*. 9:511–517.
44. Shozu M, Murakami K, Inoue M. (2004). Aromatase and leiomyoma of the uterus. *Semin Reprod Med*. 22(1):51–60.
45. Nepomnaschy PA, Welch K, McConnell D, Strassmann BI, England BG. (2004). Stress and female reproductive function: A study of daily variations in cortisol, gonadotrophins, and gonadal steroids in a rural Mayan population. *Am J Hum Biol*. 16(5):523–532.
46. Vines AI, Ta M, Esserman DA. (2010). The association between self-reported major life events and the presence of uterine fibroids. *Women's Health Issues*. 20(4):294–298.

47. Kim JJ, Sefton EC. (2012). The role of progesterone signaling in the pathogenesis of uterine leiomyoma. *Mol Cell Endocrinol.* 358(2):223–231.
48. Trivedi P, Abreo M. (2009). Predisposing factors for fibroids and outcome of laparoscopic myomectomy in infertility. *J Gynecol Endosc Surg.* 1(1):47–56.
49. Sachdev S, Reyes MC, Snyder, PJ. (2020). Ectopic prolactin secretion from a uterine leiomyoma. *J Endocr Soc.* 4(4):bvaa035.
50. Catherino WH, Leppert PC, Stenmark MH. et al. (2004). Reduced dermatopontin expression is a molecular link between uterine leiomyomas and keloids. *Genes Chromosomes Cancer.* 40(3):204–217.
51. Csupor-Löffler B, Hajdú A, Zupkó I. et al. (2009). Antiproliferative effect of flavonoids and sesquiterpenoids from *Achillea millefolium* s.l. on cultured human tumour cell lines. *Phytother Res.* 23(5):672–676.
52. Khan Au, Gilani AH. (2011). Blood pressure lowering, cardiovascular inhibitory and bronchodilatory actions of *Achillea millefolium*. *Phytother Res.* 25(4):577–583.
53. Dall'Acqua S, Bolego C, Cignarella A, Gaion RM, Innocenti G. (2011). Vasoprotective activity of standardized *Achillea millefolium* extract. *Phytomed.* 18(12):1031–1036.
54. Jenabi E, Fereidoony B. (2015). Effect of *Achillea millefolium* on relief of primary dysmenorrhea: A doubleblind randomized clinical trial. *J Pediatr Adolesc Gynecol.* 28:402–404.
55. Sachdev S, Reyes MC, Snyder, PJ. (2020). Ectopic prolactin secretion from a uterine leiomyoma. *J Endocr Soc.* 4(4):bvaa035.
56. Novella-Maestre E, Carda C, Noguera I. et al. (2009). Dopamine agonist administration causes a reduction in endometrial implants through modulation of angiogenesis in experimentally induced endometriosis. *Hum Reprod.* 24(5):1025–1035.
57. Wuttke W, Seidlová-Wuttke D. (2015). Black cohosh (*Cimicifuga racemosa*) is a non-estrogenic alternative to hormone replacement therapy. *Clin Phytosci.* 1:12.
58. Park SY, Kim HJ, Lee SR, Choi YH, Jeong K, Chung H. (2016). Black cohosh inhibits 17β-estradiol-induced cell proliferation of endometrial adenocarcinoma cells. *Gynecol Endocrinol.* 32(10):840–843.
59. Schmid D, Gruber M, Woehs F, Prinz S. et al. (2009). Inhibition of inducible nitric oxide synthesis by *Cimicifuga racemosa* (*Actaea racemosa*, black cohosh) extracts in LPS-stimulated RAW 264.7 macrophages. *J Pharm Pharmacol.* 61(8):1089–1096.

60. Ruhlen RL, Sun GY, Sauter ER. (2008). Black cohosh: Insights into its mechanism(s) of action. *Integr Med Insights*. 3:21–32.
61. Xi S, Liske E, Wang S, Liu J, Zhang Z, Geng L. et al. (2014). Effect of isopropanolic *Cimicifuga racemosa* extract on uterine fibroids in comparison with tibolone among patients of a recent randomized, double blind, parallel-controlled study in Chinese women with menopausal symptoms. *Evid Based Complement Alternat Med*. 2717686.
62. Vlaisavljević S, Jelača S, Zengin G, Mimica-Dukić N, Berežni S, Miljić M, Stevanović ZD. (2019). *Alchemilla vulgaris* agg. (Lady's mantle) from central Balkan: Antioxidant, anticancer and enzyme inhibition properties. *RSC Advances*. 9(64):37474–37483.
63. Ibrahim OHM, Abo-Elyousr KAM, Asiry KA, Alhakamy NA, Mousa MAA. (2022). Phytochemical characterization, antimicrobial activity and in vitro antiproliferative potential of *Alchemilla vulgaris* auct root extract against prostate (PC-3), breast (MCF-7) and colorectal adenocarcinoma (Caco-2) cancer cell lines. *Plants* (Basel). 11(16):2140.
64. Jelača S, Dajić-Stevanović Z, Vuković N, Kolašinac S. et al. (2022). Beyond traditional use of *Alchemilla vulgaris*: Genoprotective and antitumor activity in vitro. *Molecules* (Basel). 27(23):8113.
65. Petcu P, Androronescu E. (1979). Treatment of juvenile menometrorrhagia with *Alchemilla vulgaris* fluid extract. *Clujul Med*. 52(3):266–270.
66. Boericke W. (1901). *Boericke's Materia Medica: The Tinctures*.
67. Schumann E. (1939). Newer concepts of blood coagulation and control of haemorrhage. *Am J Obstet Gynecol*. 38:1002–1007.
68. Steinberg A. Segal HI, Parris HM. (1940). Role of oxalic acid and certain related dicarboxylic acids in the control of haemorrhage. *Ann Otol Rhinol Laryngol*. 49:1008–1021.
69. Kuroda K, Takagi K. (1968). Physiologically active substance in *Capsella bursa-pastoris*. *Nature*. 220(168):707–708.
70. Kuroda K, Akao M. (1981). Antitumor and anti-intoxication activities of fumaric acid in cultured cells. *Gann*. 72(5):777–782.
71. Shipochliev T. (1981). Uterotonic action of extracts from a group of medicinal plants. *Vet Med Nauki*. 18(4):94–98.
72. Shipochliev T. (1981). Uterotonic action of extracts from a group of medicinal plants. *Vet Med Nauki*. 18(4):94–98.
73. Alqasoumi SI, Al-Rehaily AJ, AlSheikh AM, Abdel-Kader MS. (2008). Evaluation of the hepatoprotective effect of *Ephedra foliate, Alhagi maurorum, Capsella bursa-pastoris* and *Hibiscus sabdariffa* against experimentally induced liver injury in rats. *Nat Prod Sci*. 14(2):95–99.

74. Alqasoumi SI. (2007). Isolation and chemical structure elucidation of hepatoprotective constituents from plants used in traditional medicine in Saudi Arabia. PhD thesis, College of Pharmacy, King Saud University.
75. Grosso C, Vinholes J, Silva LR, de Pinho BG. et al. (2011). Chemical composition and biological screening of *Capsella bursa-pastoris*. *Brazil J Pharmacog*. 21(4):635–644.
76. Takada Y, Andreeff M, Aggarwal BB. (2005). Indole-3-carbinol suppresses NF-κB and κBα kinase activation, causing inhibition of expression of NF-κB-regulated antiapoptotic and metastatic gene products and enhancement of apoptosis in myeloid and leukemia cells. *Blood*. 106:641–649.
77. Benson JM, Shepherd DM. (2013). Dietary ligands of the aryl hydrocarbon receptor induce anti-inflammatory and immunoregulatory effects on murine dendritic cells. *Toxicol Sci*. 124:327–338.
78. Chen YH, Dai HJ, Chang HP. (2003). Suppression of inducible nitric oxide production by indole and isothiocyanate derivatives from Brassica plants in stimulated macrophages. *Planta Med*. 69:696–700.
79. Tsai JT, Liu HC, Chen YH. (2010). Suppression of inflammatory mediators by cruciferous vegetable-derived indole-3-carbinol and phenylethyl isothiocyanate in lipopolysaccharide-activated macrophages. *Mediators Inflamm*. 293642.
80. Jiang J, Kang TB, Shim DW, Oh NH. et al. (2013). Indole-3-carbinol inhibits LPS-induced inflammatory response by blocking TRIF-dependent signaling pathway in macrophages. *Food Chem Toxicol*. 57:256–261.
81. Ping J, Li JT, Liao ZX, Shang L, Wang H. (2011). Indole-3-carbinol inhibits hepatic stellate cells proliferation by blocking NADPH oxidase/reactive oxygen species/p38 MAPK pathway. *Eur J Pharmacol*. 650:656–662.
82. Guan H, Chen C, Zhu L, Cui C. et al. (2012). Indole-3-carbinol blocks platelet-derived growth factor-stimulated vascular smooth muscle cell function and reduces neointima formation in vivo. *J Nutr Biochem*. 24:62–69.
83. Kunimasa K, Kobayashi T, Kaji K, Ohta T. (2010). Antiangiogenic effects of indole-3-carbinol and 3,3'-diindolylmethane are associated with their differential regulation of ERK1/2 and Akt in tube-forming HUVEC. *J Nutr*. 140:1–6.
84. Naafe M, Kariman N, Keshavarz Z, Khademi N, Mojab F, Mohammadbeigi A. (2018). Effect of hydroalcoholic extracts of *Capsella bursa-pastoris* on heavy menstrual bleeding: A randomized clinical trial. *J Altern Complement Med*. 24(7):694–700.

85. Ghalandari S, Kariman N, Sheikhan Z, Mojab F, Mirzaei M, Shahrahmani H. (2017). Effect of hydroalcoholic extract of *Capsella bursa pastoris* on early postpartum hemorrhage: A clinical trial study. *J Altern Complement Med*. 23(10):794–799.
86. Zhang D, Al-Hendy M, Richard-Davis G, Montgomery-Rice V. et al. (2010). Antiproliferative and proapoptotic effects of epigallocatechin gallate on human leiomyoma cells. *Fertil Steril*. 94:1887–1893.
87. Zhu BT, Shim JY, Nagai M, Bai HW. (2008). Molecular modelling study of the mechanism of high-potency inhibition of human catechol-O-methyltransferase by (-)-epigallocatechin-3-o-gallate. *Xenobiotica*. 38:130–146.
88. Jung YD, Kim MS, Shin BA, Chay KO. et al. (2001). EGCG, a major component of green tea, inhibits tumour growth by inhibiting VEGF induction in human colon carcinoma cells. *Br J Cancer*. 84:844–850.
89. Zhang D, Al-Hendy M, Richard-Davis G, Montgomery-Rice V. et al. (2010). Green tea extract inhibits proliferation of uterine leiomyoma cells in vitro and in nude mice. *Am J Obstet Gynecol*. 202:289.e.281–e.289.
90. Ozercan IH, Sahin N, Akdemir F, Onderci M. et al. (2008). Chemoprevention of fibroid tumors by [-]-epigallocatechin-3-gallate in quail. *Nutr Res*. 228:92–97.
91. Roshdy E, Rajaratnam V, Maitra S, Sabry M. et al. (2013). Treatment of symptomatic uterine fibroids with green tea extract: A pilot randomized controlled clinical study. *Int J Women's Health*. 5:477–486.
92. Porcaro G, Santamaria A, Giordano D, Angelozzi P. (2020). Vitamin D plus epigallocatechin gallate: A novel promising approach for uterine myomas. *Eur Rev Med Pharmacol Sci*. 24(6):3344–3351.
93. Kim D, Ramachandran S, Baek S, Kwon SH. et al. (2008). Induction of growth inhibition and apoptosis in human uterine leiomyoma cells by isoliquiritigenin. *Reprod Sci*. 15:552–558.
94. Feldman M. Santos J, Grenier D. (2011). Comparative evaluation of two structurally related flavonoids, isoliquiritigenin and liquiritigenin, for their oral infection therapeutic potential. *J Nat Prod*. 74:1862–1867.
95. Watanabe Y, Nagai Y, Honda H, Okamoto N. et al. (2016). Isoliquiritigenin attenuates adipose tissue inflammation in vitro and adipose tissue fibrosis through inhibition of innate immune responses in mice. *Sci Rep*. 6:23097.
96. Li J, Kang SW, Kim JL, Sung HY, Kwun IS, Kang YH. (2010). Isoliquiritigenin entails blockade of tgf-beta1-Smad signaling for retarding high glucose-induced mesangial matrix accumulation. *J Agric Food Chem*. 58:3205–3212.

97. Yang R, Yuan BC, Ma YS, Zhou S, Liu Y. (2017). The anti-inflammatory activity of licorice, a widely used Chinese herb. *Pharm Biol.* 55(1):5–18.
98. Yang R, Yuan BC, Ma YS, Zhou S, Liu Y. (2017). The anti-inflammatory activity of licorice, a widely used Chinese herb. *Pharm Biol.* 55(1):5–18.
99. Park SY, Kwon SJ, Lim SS, Kim JK, Lee KW, Park JH. (2016). Licoricidin, an active compound in the hexane/ethanol extract of *Glycyrrhiza uralensis*, inhibits lung metastasis of 4T1 murine mammary carcinoma cells. *Int J Mol Sci.* 17(6):934.
100. La VD, Tanabe S, Bergeron C, Gafner S, Grenier D. (2011). Modulation of matrix metalloproteinase and cytokine production by licorice isolates licoricidin and licorisoflavan A: Potential therapeutic approach for periodontitis. *J Periodontol.* 82(1):122–128.
101. Lloyd JU, Lloyd CG. (1884–1887). *Drugs and Medicines of North America.*
102. Ellingwood F. (1919). *The American Materia Medica, Therapeutics and Pharmacognosy.*
103. Wu HL, Chuang TY, Al-Hendy A, Diamond MP, Azziz R, Chen YH. (2015). Berberine inhibits the proliferation of human uterine leiomyoma cells. *Fertil Steril.* 103:1098–1106.
104. Chuang TY, Min J, Wu HL, McCrary C, Layman LC. et al. (2017). Berberine inhibits uterine leiomyoma cell proliferation via downregulation of cyclooxygenase 2 and pituitary tumor-transforming gene 1. *Reprod Sci.* 24(7):1005–1013.
105. Sun Y, Xun K, Wang Y, Chen X. (2009). A systematic review of the anticancer properties of berberine, a natural product from Chinese herbs. *Anticancer Drugs.* 20:757–769.
106. Fu L, Chen W, Guo W, Wang J, Tian Y. et al. (2013). Berberine targets AP-2/hTERT, NF-kappaB/COX-2, HIF-1alpha/VEGF and cytochrome-C/caspase signaling to suppress human cancer cell growth. *PLoS One.* 8:e69240.
107. Lee TK, Kim DI, Han JY, Kim CH. (2004). Inhibitory effects of *Scutellaria barbata* D. Don. and *Euonymus alatus* Sieb. on aromatase activity of human leiomyomal cells. *Immunopharmacol Immunotoxicol.* 26:315–327.
108. Wang D, Wang W, Zhou Y, Wang J, Jia D, Wong HK, Zhang ZJ. (2015). Studies on the regulatory effect of peony-glycyrrhiza decoction on prolactin hyperactivity and underlying mechanism in hyperprolactinemia rat model. *Neurosci Lett.* 606:60–65.
109. Sakamoto S, Mitamura T, Iwasawa M, Kitsunai H, Shindou K. et al. (1998). Conservative management for perimenopausal women with

uterine leiomyomas using Chinese herbal medicines and synthetic analogs of gonadotropin-releasing hormone. *In Vivo.* 12:333–337.
110. Yuan HN, Wang CY, Sze CW, Tong Y, Tan QR, Feng XJ. et al. (2008). A randomized, crossover comparison of herbal medicine and bromocriptine against risperidone-induced hyperprolactinemia in patients with schizophrenia. *J Clin Psychopharmacol.* 28(3):264–370.
111. Yamada K, Kanba S, Yagi G, Asai M. (1997). Effectiveness of herbal medicine (*Shakuyaku-kanzo-to*) for neuroleptic-induced hyperprolactinemia. *J Clin Psychopharmacol.* 17(3):234–235.
112. Yamada K, Kanba S, Murata T, Fukuzawa M, Terashi B, Yagi G. et al. (1996). Effectiveness of *shakuyaku-kanzo-to* in neuroleptic-induced hyperprolactinemia: A preliminary report. *Psychiatry Clin Neurosci.* 50(6):341–342.
113. Man SC, Li XB, Wang HH, Yuan HN, Wang HN, Zhang RG. et al. (2016). Peony-glycyrrhiza decoction for antipsychotic-related hyperprolactinemia in women with schizophrenia: A randomized controlled trial. *J Clin Psychopharmacol.* 36(6):572–579.
114. Takeuchi T, Nishii O, Okamura T, Yaginuma T. (1991). Effect of paeoniflorin, glycyrrhizin and glycyrrhetic acid on ovarian androgen production. *Am J Chin Med.* 19(1):73–78.
115. Bulun SE, Imir G, Utsunomiya H. et al. (2005). Aromatase in endometriosis and uterine leiomyomata. *J Steroid Biochem Mol Biol.* 95(1–5): 57–62.
116. Ellingwood F. (1919). *The American Materia Medica, Therapeutics and Pharmacognosy.*
117. Ellingwood F. (1908). *Ellingwood's Therapeutics,* vol. 2.
118. Ellingwood F. (1908). *Ellingwood's Therapeutics,* vol. 2.
119. Sunila ES, Hamsa TP, Kuttan G. (2011). Effect of *Thuja occidentalis* and its polysaccharide on cell-mediated immune responses and cytokine levels of metastatic tumor-bearing animals. *Pharma Biol.* 49(10):1065–1073.
120. Torres A, Vargas Y, Uribe D, Carrasco C, Torres C. et al. (2016). Proapoptotic and anti-angiogenic properties of the α/β-thujone fraction from *Thuja occidentalis* on glioblastoma cells. *J Neurooncol.* 128:9–19.
121. Siveen KS, Kuttan G. (2011). Augmentation of humoral and cell mediated immune responses by thujone. *Int Immunopharmacol.* 11:1967–1975.
122. Caruntu S, Ciceu A, Olah NK, Don I, Hermenean A, Cotoraci C. (2020). *Thuja occidentalis* L. (Cupressaceae): Ethnobotany, phytochemistry and biological activity. *Molecules* (Basel). 25(22):5416.

123. Sachdev S, Reyes MC, Snyder PJ. (2020). Ectopic prolactin secretion from a uterine leiomyoma. *J Endoc Soc.* 4(4):bvaa035.
124. Novella-Maestren E, Carda C, Noguera I. et al. (2009). Dopamine agonist administration causes a reduction in endometrial implants through modulation of angiogenesis in experimentally induced endometriosis. *Hum Reprod.* 24(5):1025–1035.
125. Wuttke W, Seidlová-Wuttke D. (2015). Black cohosh (*Cimicifuga racemosa*) is a non-estrogenic alternative to hormone replacement therapy. *Clin Phytosci.* 1:12.
126. Jarry H, Leonhardt S, Gorkow C, Wuttke W. (1994). In vitro prolactin but not LH and FSH release is inhibited by compounds in extracts of *Agnus castus*: Direct evidence for a dopaminergic principle by the dopamine receptor assay. *Exp Clin Endocrinol.* 102(6):448–454.
127. Dericks-Tan JS, Schwinn P, Hildt C. (2003). Dose-dependent stimulation of melatonin secretion after administration of *Agnus castus*. *Exp Clin Endocrinol Diabetes.* 111(1):44–46.
128. Dericks-Tan JS, Schwinn P, Hildt C. (2003). Dose-dependent stimulation of melatonin secretion after administration of *Agnus castus*. *Exp Clin Endocrinol Diabetes.* 111(1):44–46.
Diaz BL, Llaneza PC. (2008). Endocrine regulation of the course of menopause by oral melatonin: First case report. *Menopause.* 15(2):388–392.
129. Lin PH, Tung YT, Chen HY, Chiang YF, Hong HC. et al. (2020). Melatonin activates cell death programs for the suppression of uterine leiomyoma cell proliferation. *J Pineal Res.* 68(1):e12620.
130. Gaginella TS, Phillips SF. (1975). Ricinoleic acid: Current view of an ancient oil. *Am J Dig Dis.* 20:1171–1177.
131. Vieira C, Evangelista S, Cirillo R, Terracciano R, Lippi A, Maggi CA, Manzini S. (2000). Antinociceptive activity of ricinoleic acid, a capsaicin-like compound devoid of pungent properties. *Eur J Pharmacol.* 407(1–2):109–116.
132. Maier M, Staupendahl D, Duerr HR, Refior HJ. (1999). Castor oil decreases pain during extracorporeal shock wave application. *Arch Orthop Trauma Surg.* 119(7–8):423–427.
133. Keaton D, Myatt D. (1992). Effects of castor oil on lymphocytes subsets. Presented at: AANP Conference, 2–6 September 1992. The Buttes, Tempe, Arizona.
134. Arslan GG, Eser I. (2011). An examination of the effect of castor oil packs on constipation in the elderly. *Complement Ther Clin Pract.* 17:58–62.

135. Grady H. (1998). Immunomodulation through castor oil packs. *J Naturopath Med*. 7:84–89.
136. He DY, Dai SM. (2011). Anti-inflammatory and immunomodulatory effects of *Paeonia lactiflora* pall., a traditional Chinese herbal medicine. *Front Pharmacol*. 2:10.
137. Wu H, Wei W, Song L, Zhang L, Chen Y, Hu X. (2007). Paeoniflorin induced immune tolerance of mesenteric lymph node lymphocytes via enhancing beta2-adrenergic receptor desensitization in rats with adjuvant arthritis. *Int Immunopharmacol*. 7:662–673.
138. Malik M, Mendoza M, Payson M, Catherino WH. (2009). Curcumin, a nutritional supplement with antineoplastic activity, enhances leiomyoma cell apoptosis and decreases fibronectin expression. *Fertil Steril*. 91:2177–2184.
139. Chen X, Chen X, Shi X, Gao Z, Guo Z. (2020). Curcumin attenuates endothelial cell fibrosis through inhibiting endothelial-interstitial transformation. *Clin Exp Pharmacol Physiol*. 47(7):1182–1192.
140. Tsuiji K, Takeda T, Li B, Wakabayashi A, Kondo A, Kimura T, Yaegashi N. (2011). Inhibitory effect of curcumin on uterine leiomyoma cell proliferation. *Gynecol Endocrinol*. 27:512–517.
141. Biswas S, Chen S, Liang G, Feng B, Cai L, Khan ZA, Chakrabarti S. (2019). Curcumin analogs reduce stress and inflammation indices in experimental models of diabetes. *Front Endocrinol*. (Lausanne). 10:887.
142. Jana S, Paul S, Swarnakar S. (2012). Curcumin as anti-endometriotic agent: Implication of MMP-3 and intrinsic apoptotic pathway. *Biochem Pharmacol*. 83(6):797–804.
143. Kim KH, Lee EN, Park JK, Lee JR, Kim JH. et al. (2012). Curcumin attenuates TNF-alpha-induced expression of intercellular adhesion molecule-1, vascular cell adhesion molecule-1 and proinflammatory cytokines in human endometriotic stromal cells. *Phytother Res*. 26:1037–1047.
144. Zhang Y, Cao H, Yu Z, Peng HY, Zhang CJ. (2013). Curcumin inhibits endometriosis endometrial cells by reducing estradiol production. *Iran J Reprod Med*. 11(5):415–422.
145. He Y, Zeng Q, Li X, Liu B, Wang P. (2013). The association between subclinical atherosclerosis and uterine fibroids. *PLoS One*. 8(2):e57089.
146. Catherino WH, Parrott E, Segars J. (2011). Proceedings from the National Institute of Child Health and Human Development Conference on the Uterine Fibroid Research Update Workshop. *Fertil Steril*. 95:9–12.

147. Maia Jr H, Haddad C, Pinheiro N. et al. (2012). Advantages of the association of resveratrol with oral contraceptives for management of endometriosis-related pain. *Int J Women's Health.* 4:543–549.
148. Wise LA, Radin RG, Palmer JR, Kumanyika SK, Rosenberg L. (2010). A prospective study of dairy intake and risk of uterine leiomyomata. *Am J Epidemiol.* 171(2):221–232.
149. Chiaffarino F, Parazzini F, La Vecchia C, Chatenoud L. et al. (1999). Diet and uterine myomas. *Obstet Gynecol.* 94:395–398.
150. Wise LA, Radin RG, Palmer JR, Kumanyika SK, Boggs DA, Rosenberg L. (2011). Intake of fruit, vegetables, and carotenoids in relation to risk of uterine leiomyomata. *Am J Clin Nutr.* 94:1620–1631.
151. Atkinson C, Lampe JW, Scholes D. et al. (2006). Lignan and isoflavone excretion in relation to uterine fibroids: A case-control study of young to middle-aged women in the United States. *Am J Clin Nutr.* 84(3):587–593.
152. Heber D. (2007). Plant foods and phytochemicals in human health. In Berdanier CD, Dwyer J, Feldman EB. (eds). *Handbook of Nutrition and Food*, 2nd ed. Boca Raton: CRC Press, pp. 1175–1181.
153. Vines AI, Ta M, Esserman DA. (2010). The association between self-reported major life events and the presence of uterine fibroids. *Women's Health Issues.* 20:294–298.
Vines AI, Nguyen TTX, Ta M, Esserman D, Baird DD. (2011). Self-reported daily stress, squelching of anger and the management of daily stress and the prevalence of uterine leiomyomata: The ultrasound screening study. *Stress Health.* 27:e188–e194.
154. Dallman MF, Pecoraro N, Akana SF, la Fleur SE, Gomez F. et al. (2003). Chronic stress and obesity: A new view of "comfort food". *Proc Natl Acad Sci USA.* 100(11):696–701.
DeFronzo R, Ferrannini E. (1991). Insulin resistance: A multifaceted syndrome responsible for NIDDM, obesity, hypertension, dyslipidemia, and atherosclerotic cardiovascular disease. *Diabetes Care.* 14(3):173–194.
155. Wise LA, Palmer JR, Harlow BL. et al. (2004). Risk of uterine leiomyomata in relation to tobacco, alcohol and caffeine consumption in the Black Women's Health Study. *Hum Reprod.* 19:1746–1754.
156. Islam MS, Giampieri F, Janjusevic M, Gasparrini M, Forbes-Hernandez TY. et al. (2017). An anthocyanin rich strawberry extract induces apoptosis and ROS while decreases glycolysis and fibrosis in human uterine leiomyoma cells. *Oncotarget.* 8:23575–23587.

157. Giampieri F, Islam MS, Greco S, Gasparrini M, Forbes Hernandez TY. et al. (2019). Romina: A powerful strawberry with in vitro efficacy against uterine leiomyoma cells. *J Cell Physiol*. 234:7622–7633.
158. Roshdy E, Rajaratnam V, Maitra S, Sabry M, Allah ASA, Al-Hendy A. (2013). Treatment of symptomatic uterine fibroids with green tea extract: A pilot randomized controlled clinical study. *Int J Women's Health*. 5:477–486.
159. Al-Hendy A, Salama SA. (2008). Catechol-O-methyltransferase polymorphism is associated with increased uterine leiomyoma risk in different ethnic groups. *J Soc Gynecol Investig*. 13(2):136–144.
160. Dalton-Brewer N. (2016). The role of complementary and alternative medicine for the management of fibroids and associated symptomatology. *Curr Obste Gynec Rports*. 5:110–118.
161. Shushan A, Ben-Bassat H, Mishani E. et al. (2007). Inhibition of leiomyoma cell proliferation in vitro by genistein and the protein tyrosine kinase inhibitor TKS050. *Fertil Steril*. 87(1):127–135.
Moore AB, Castro L, Yu L. et al. (2007). Stimulatory and inhibitory effects of genistein on human uterine leiomyoma cell proliferation are influenced by the concentration. *Hum Reprod*. 22(10):2623–2631.
162. Di X, Yu L, Moore AB, Castro L. et al. (2008). A low concentration of genistein induces estrogen receptor-alpha and insulin-like growth factor-I receptor interactions and proliferation in uterine leiomyoma cells. *Hum Reprod*. 23:1873–1883.
163. Moore AB, Castro L, Yu L. et al. (2007). Stimulatory and inhibitory effects of genistein on human uterine leiomyoma cell proliferation are influenced by the concentration. *Hum Reprod*. 22(10):2623–2631.
164. Di X, Andrews DMK, Tucker CJ, Yu L. et al. (2012). A high concentration of genistein down-regulates activin A, Smad3 and other TGF-β pathway genes in human uterine leiomyoma cells. *Exp Mol Med*. 44:281–292.
165. Sahin K, Akdemir F, Tuzcu M, Sahin N. et al. (2009). Genistein suppresses spontaneous oviduct tumorigenesis in quail. *Nutr Cancer*. 61:799–806.
166. Sahin K, Ozercan R, Onderci M, Sahin N, Gursu MF. et al. (2004). Lycopene supplementation prevents the development of spontaneous smooth muscle tumors of the oviduct in Japanese quail. *Nutr Cancer*. 50(2):181–189.
167. Sahin K, Ozercan R, Onderci M, Sahin N, Khachik F, Seren S, Kucuk O. (2007). Dietary tomato powder supplementation in the prevention of leiomyoma of the oviduct in the . quail. *Nutr Cancer*. 59(1):70–75.

168. Hwang ES, Bowen PE. (2002). Can the consumption of tomatoes or lycopene reduce cancer risk? *Integr Cancer Ther.* 1(2):121–132.
169. Li K, Huang T, Zheng J, Wu K, Li D. (2014). Effect of marine-derived n-3 polyunsaturated fatty acids on C-reactive protein, interleukin 6 and tumor necrosis factor α: A meta-analysis. *PLoS One.* 9(2):e88103.
170. Islam MS, Castellucci C, Fiorini R, Greco S, Gagliardi R. et al. (2018). Omega-3 fatty acids modulate the lipid profile, membrane architecture, and gene expression of leiomyoma cells. *J Cell Physiol.* 233(9):7143–7156.
171. Greco S, Islam MS, Zannotti A, Delli Carpini G, Giannubilo SR. et al. (2020). Quercetin and indole-3-carbinol inhibit extracellular matrix expression in human primary uterine leiomyoma cells. *Reprod Biomed Online.* 40(4):593–602.
172. Islam MS, Afrin S, Brennan J, Segars J. (2020). The active phytochemical of cruciferous vegetables, sulforaphane, reduces proliferation and inflammation of uterine fibroid cells. Meeting: The Basic Science of Uterine Fibroids. National Institute of Environmental Health Sciences. Research Triangle Park, California.
173. Thompson ME, Racine EF. (2011). Serum micronutrient concentrations and risk for uterine fibroids. *J Women's Health* (Larchmt). 20(6):915–922.
174. Ciebiera M, Ali M, Zgliczyńska M, Skrzypczak M, Al-Hendy A. (2020). Vitamins and uterine fibroids: Current data on pathophysiology and possible clinical relevance. *Int J Mol Sci.* 21(15):5528.
175. Boettger-Tong H, Shipley G, Hsu CJ, Stancel GM. (1997). Cultured human uterine smooth muscle cells are retinoid responsive. *Proc Soc Exp Biol Med.* 215(1):59–65.
176. Ben-Sasson H, Ben-Meir A, Shushan A, Karra L, Rojansky N, Klein BY, Levitzki R, Ben-Bassat H. (2011). All-trans-retinoic acid mediates changes in PI3K and retinoic acid signaling proteins of leiomyomas. *Fertil Steril.* 95(6):2080–2086.
177. Gamage SD, Bischoff ED, Burroughs KD, Lamph WW, Gottardis MM, Walker CL, Fuchs-Young R. (2000). Efficacy of LGD1069 (Targretin), a retinoid X receptor-selective ligand, for treatment of uterine leiomyoma. *J Pharmacol Exp Ther.* 295:677–681.
178. Sabry M, Halder SK, Allah ASA, Roshdy E, Rajaratnam V, Al-Hendy A. (2013). Serum vitamin D_3 level inversely correlates with uterine fibroid volume in different ethnic groups: A cross-sectional observational study. *Int J Women's Health.* 5:93–100.
179. Bulun SE. (2013). Uterine fibroids. *N Engl J Med.* 369:1344–1355.

180. Sabry M, Halder SK, Allah ASA, Roshdy E, Rajaratnam V, Al-Hendy A. (2013). Serum vitamin D_3 level inversely correlates with uterine fibroid volume in different ethnic groups: A cross-sectional observational study. *Int J Women's Health.* 5:93–100.
181. Wetmore JB, Kimber C, Mahnken JD, Stubbs JR. (2016). Cholecalciferol v. Ergocalciferol for 25-hydroxyvitamin D (25(OH)D) repletion in chronic kidney disease: A randomised clinical trial. *Br J Nutr.* 116:2074–2081.
182. Halder S, Sharan C, Hendy A. (2012). 1,25-dihydroxyvitamin D3 treatment shrinks uterine leiomyoma tumors in the Eker rat model. *Biol Reprod.* 86(4)(Article 116):1–10.
183. Ciavattini A, Delli Carpini G, Serri M, Vignini A, Sabbatinelli J, Tozzi A, Aggiusti A, Clemente N. (2016). Hypovitaminosis D and "small burden" uterine fibroids: Opportunity for a vitamin D supplementation. *Medicine* (Baltimore). 95:e5698.
184. Arjeh S, Darsareh F, Asl ZA, Kutenaei MA. (2020). Effect of oral consumption of Vitamin D on uterine fibroids: A randomized clinical trial. *Complement Ther Clin Pract.* 39:101159.
185. Porcaro G, Santamaria A, Giordano D, Angelozzi P. (2020). Vitamin D plus epigallocatechin gallate: A novel promising approach for uterine myomas. *Eur Rev Med Pharmacol Sci.* 24:3344–3351.

Chapter 10: Cervical dysplasia

1. Trimble CL, Piantadosi S, Gravitt P. et al. (2005). Spontaneous regression of high-grade cervical dysplasia: Effects of human papillomavirus type and HLA phenotype. *Clin Cancer Res.* 11:4717–1423.
2. Munoz N, Bosch FX, de Sanjose S. et al. (2003). Epidemiologic classification of human papillomavirus types associated with cervical cancer. *N Engl J Med.* 348:518–527.
3. Skyldberg B, Fujioka K, Hellstrom AC. et al. (2001). Human papillomavirus infection, centrosome aberration, and genetic stability in cervical lesions. *Mod Pathol.* 14:279–284.
4. Smith JS, Muñoz N, Herrero R. et al. (2002). Evidence for *Chlamydia trachomatis* as a human papillomavirus cofactor in the etiology of invasive cervical cancer in Brazil and the Philippines. *J Infect Dis.* 185:324–331.
5. Heley S. (2003). Human papillomavirus: Beware the infection you can't see. *Aust Fam Phys.* 32:311–315.

6. Fischer N. (2002). *Chlamydia trachomatis* infection in cervical intraepithelial neoplasia and invasive carcinoma. *Eur J Gynaecol Oncol.* 23:247–250.
7. Koshiyama M. (2019). The effects of the dietary and nutrient intake on gynecologic cancers. *Healthcare* (Basel). 7(3):88.
8. Chen X, Jiang J, Shen H, Hu Z. (2011). Genetic susceptibility of cervical cancer. *J Biomed Res.* 25(3):155–164.
9. Hogewoning CJ, Bleeker MC, van den Brule AJ. et al. (2003). Condom use promotes regression of cervical intraepithelial neoplasia and clearance of human papillomavirus: A randomized clinical trial. *Int J Cancer.* 107(5):811–816.
10. Maruthur NM, Bolen SD, Brancati FL, Clark JM. (2009). The association of obesity and cervical cancer screening: A systematic review and meta-analysis. *Obesity* (Silver Spring, Md). 17(2):375–381.
11. Louie KS, de Sanjose S, Diaz M, Castellsagué X, Herrero R, Meijer CJ, Shah K, Franceschi S, Muñoz N, Bosch FX. & International Agency for Research on Cancer Multicenter Cervical Cancer Study Group. (2009). Early age at first sexual intercourse and early pregnancy are risk factors for cervical cancer in developing countries. *Brit J Cancer.* 100(7):1191–1197.
12. Castellsagué X, Muñoz N. (2003). Cofactors in human papillomavirus carcinogenesis—role of parity, oral contraceptives, and tobacco smoking. *J Natl Cancer Inst Monogr.* 31:20–28.
13. Kuebler U, Fischer S, Mernone L. et al. (2021). Is stress related to the presence and persistence of oncogenic human papillomavirus infection in young women? *BMC Cancer* 21:419.
14. Trimble CL, Piantadosi S, Gravitt P. et al. (2005). Spontaneous regression of high-grade cervical dysplasia: Effects of human papillomavirus type and HLA phenotype. *Clin Cancer Res.* 11:4717–1423.
15. Zhai L, Tumban E. (2016). Gardasil-9: A global survey of projected efficacy. *Antiviral Res.* 130:101–109.
16. Yang DY, Bracken K. (2016). Update on the new 9-valent vaccine for human papillomavirus prevention. *Canad Fam Phys./Medecin de famille canadien.* 62(5):399–402.
17. Freeman LW. (2009). *Complementary and Alternative Medicine: A Research-Based Approach.* London: Elsevier.
18. Shen L, Gwak SR, Cui ZY, Joo JC, Park SJ. (2021). Astragalus-containing Chinese herbal medicine combined with chemotherapy for cervical cancer: A systematic review and meta-analysis. *Front Pharmacol.* 12:587021.

19. Issa AY, Volate SR, Muga SJ, Nitcheva D, Smith T, Wargovich MJ. (2007). Green tea selectively targets initial stages of intestinal carcinogenesis in the AOM-ApcMin mouse model. *Carcinogenesis.* 28(9):1978–1984.
20. Li WG, Li QH, Tan Z. (2005). Epigallocatechin gallate induces telomere fragmentation in HeLa and 293 but not in MRC-5 cells. *Life Sci.* 76(15):1735–1746.
21. Yokoyama M, Noguchi M, Nakao Y, Pater A, Iwasaka T. (2004). The tea polyphenol, (-)-epigallocatechin gallate effects on growth, apoptosis, and telomerase activity in cervical cell lines. *Gynecol Oncol.* 92(1):197–204.
22. Zou C, Liu H, Feugang JM, Hao Z, Chow HH, Garcia F. (2010). Green tea compound in chemoprevention of cervical cancer. *Int J Gynec Cancer.* 20(4):617–624.
23. Ahn WS, Yoo J, Huh SW. et al. (2003). Protective effects of green tea extracts (polyphenon E and EGCG) on human cervical lesions. *Eur J Cancer Prev.* 12:383–390.
24. Jia Y, Hu T, Hang CY, Yang R, Li X. et al. (2012). Case-control study of diet in patients with cervical cancer or precancerosis in Wufeng, a high incidence region in China. *Asian Pac J Cancer Prev.* 13(10):5299–5302.
25. Tomeh MA, Hadianamrei R, Zhao X. (2019). A review of curcumin and its derivatives as anticancer agents. *Int J Mol Sci.* 20(5):1033.
26. Giordano A, Tommonaro G. (2019). Curcumin and cancer. *Nutrients.* 11(10):2376.
27. Cheng AL, Hsu CH, Lin JK, Hsu MM, Ho YF. et al. (2001). Phase I clinical trial of curcumin, a chemopreventive agent, in patients with high-risk or pre-malignant lesions. *Anticancer Res.* 21:2895–2900.
28. Tayyem RF, Heath DD, Al-Delaimy WK, Rock CL. (2006). Curcumin content of turmeric and curry powders. *Nutr Cancer.* 55(2):126–131.
29. Aguilar-Velázquez G, Espinosa D, Ordaz-Pichardo C. (2018). Effects of homeopathic dilutions of *Echinacea angustifolia* and *Thuja occidentalis* on cervical cancer cells. *Homeopathy.* 107(S 01):55–78.
30. De Rosa N, Giampaolino P, Lavitola G, Morra I, Formisano C, Nappi C, Bifulco G. (2019). Effect of immunomodulatory supplements based on *Echinacea angustifolia* and *Echinacea purpurea* on the posttreatment relapse incidence of genital condylomatosis: A prospective randomized study. *Biomed Res Int.* 3548396.
31. Jin H, Song C, Zhao Z, Zhou G. (2020). *Ganoderma lucidum* polysaccharide, an extract from *Ganoderma lucidum*, exerts suppressive effect on

cervical cancer cell malignancy through mitigating epithelial-mesenchymal and JAK/STAT5 signaling pathway. *Pharmacol.* 105(7–8):461–470.
32. Barbieri A, Quagliariello V, Del Vecchio V, Falco M, Luciano A. et al. (2017). Anticancer and anti-inflammatory properties of *Ganoderma lucidum* extract effects on melanoma and triple-negative breast cancer treatment. *Nutrients.* 9(3):210.
33. Kong M, Yao Y, Zhang H. (2019). Antitumor activity of enzymatically hydrolyzed *Ganoderma lucidum* polysaccharide on U14 cervical carcinoma-bearing mice. *Int J Immunopathol Pharmacol.* 33:2058738419869489.
34. Ali NAKM, Saeed HA, Othman RT. (2018). Immunostimulatory and anti-inflammatory effect of *Gannoderma lucidum* on breast cancer patients. *Asian Pacific J Cancer Biol.* 3(2):51–57.
35. Liang LD, He T, Du TW, Fan YG, Chen DS, Wang Y. (2015). Ginsenoside-Rg5 induces apoptosis and DNA damage in human cervical cancer cells. *Mol Med Rep.* 11(2):940–946.
36. Huynh DTN, Jin Y, Myung CS, Heo KS. (2021). Ginsenoside Rh1 induces MCF-7 cell apoptosis and autophagic cell death through ROS-mediated Akt signaling. *Cancers* (Basel). 213(8):1892.
37. Aguilar-Velázquez G, Espinosa D, Ordaz-Pichardo C. (2018). Effects of homeopathic dilutions of *Echinacea angustifolia* and *Thuja occidentalis* on cervical cancer cells. *Homeopathy.* 107(S 01):55–78.
38. Pal A, Das S, Basu S, Kundu R. (2022). Apoptotic and autophagic death union by *Thuja occidentalis* homeopathic drug in cervical cancer cells with thujone as the bioactive principle. *J Integr Med.* 20(5):463–472.
39. Matić IZ, Juranić Z, Savikin K, Zdunić G, Nađvinski N, Godevac D. (2013). Chamomile and marigold tea: Chemical characterization and evaluation of anticancer activity. *Phytother Res.* 27(6):852–858.
40. Barnaulov OD, Denisenko PP. (1980). Antiulcerogenic action of the decoction from flowers of *Filipendula ulmaria*. *Pharmacol Toxicol.* 43:700–705.
41. Barnaulov OD, Kumkov AV, Khalikova NA, Kozhina IS, Shukhobodskii BA. (1977). Chemical compostition and primary evaluation of the properties from *Filipendula ulmaria* and *Maxim* flowers. *Rastit Resur.* 13(4):661–669.
42. Beukelman CJ, Halkes SBA, Kroes BH, Labadie RP, Van den Berg AJJ, Van Dijk H. (1977). In vitro immunomodulatory activity of *Filipendula ulmaria*. *Phytother Res.* 11:518–520.
43. Kruglova MJ, Olennikov DN, Kruglov DS. (2013). New flavonoid glycoside and other components taken from *Filpendula* genus plants. *Planta Med.* 79-PJ27.

44. Peresun'ko AP, Bespalov VG, Limarenko AI, Aleksandrov VA. (1993). Clinico-experimental study of using plant preparations from the flowers of *Filipendula ulmaria* (L.) Maxim for the treatment of precancerous changes and prevention of uterine cervical cancer. *Vopr Onkol*. 39(7–12):291–295. In Russian.
45. Peresun'ko AP, Bespalov VG, Limarenko AI, Aleksandrov VA. (1993). Clinico-experimental study of using plant preparations from the flowers of *Filipendula ulmaria* (L.) Maxim for the treatment of precancerous changes and prevention of uterine cervical cancer. *Vopr Onkol*. 39(7–12):291–295. In Russian.
46. Nikakhtar Z, Hasanzadeh M, Hamedi SS. et al. (2018). The efficacy of vaginal suppository based on myrtle in patients with cervicovaginal human papillomavirus infection: A randomized, double-blind, placebo trial. *Phytother Res*. 32:2002–2008.
47. Abou Baker DH. (2020). *Achillea millefolium* L. ethyl acetate fraction induces apoptosis and cell cycle arrest in human cervical cancer (HeLa) cells. *Annals Agric Sci*. 65(1):42–48.
48. Mahata S, Bharti AC, Shukla S. et al. (2011). Berberine modulates AP-1 activity to suppress HPV transcription and downstream signaling to induce growth arrest and apoptosis in cervical cancer cells. *Mol Cancer*. 10:39.
49. Đilas S, Knez Ž, Ćetković-Simin D, Tumbas V. et al. (2012). In vitro antioxidant and antiproliferative activity of three rosemary (*Rosmarinus officinalis* L.) extract formulations. *Int J Food Sci Technol*. 47:2052–2062.
50. Greenlee H, Abascal K, Yarnell E, Ladas E. (2007). Clinical applications of *Silybum marianum* in oncology. *Integr Cancer Ther*. 6(2):158–165.
51. Venezuela RF, Mosmann JP, Mugas ML, Kiguen AX, Nuñez Montoya SC, Konigheim BS, Cuffini CG. (2021). Dandelion root extract affects the proliferation, survival and migration of cervical cancer cell lines. *Res Square*. Preprint and under revision *BMC Complementary Med Ther*.
52. Ansari JA, Ahmad MK, Khan AR, Fatima N, Khan HJ, Rastogi N. et al. (2016). Anticancer and antioxidant activity of *Zingiber officinale* Roscoe rhizome. *Indian J Exp Biol*. 54:767–773.
53. Rastogi N, Duggal S, Singh SK, Porwal K, Srivastava VK. et al. (2015). Proteasome inhibition mediates p53 reactivation and anti-cancer activity of 6-gingerol in cervical cancer cells. *Oncotarget*. 6(41):43310–43325.
54. Liu Q, Peng YB, Qi LW, Cheng XL, Xu XJ. et al. (2012). The cytotoxicity mechanism of 6-shogaol-treated HeLa human cervical cancer cells revealed by label-free shotgun proteomics and bioinformatics analysis. *Evid Based Complement Alternat Med*. 278652.

55. Nikakhtar Z, Hasanzadeh M, Hamedi SS. et al. (2018). The efficacy of vaginal suppository based on myrtle in patients with cervicovaginal human papillomavirus infection: A randomized, double-blind, placebo trial. *Phytother Res.* 32:2002–2008.
56. Hung YC, Pan TL, Hu WL. (2016). Roles of reactive oxygen species in anticancer therapy with *Salvia miltiorrhiza* Bunge. *Oxid Med Cell Longev.* 5293284.
57. Wu X, Yang Z, Dang H, Peng H, Dai Z. (2017). Baicalein inhibits the proliferation of cervical cancer cells through the GSK3ß-dependent pathway. *Oncol Res.* 26(4):645–653.
58. Shrimali D, Shanmugam MK, Kumar AP. et al. (2013). Targeted abrogation of diverse signal transduction cascades by emodin for the treatment of inflammatory disorders and cancer. *Cancer Letters.* 341(2):139–149.
59. Wang Y, Yu HZ, Zhang Y, Liu Y, Ge X, Wu X. (2013). Emodin induces apoptosis of human cervical cancer HeLa cells via intrinsic mitochondrial and extrinsic death receptor pathway. *Cancer Cell Int.* 13(1, article 71).
60. Yang J, Li J, Sun M, Chen K. (2014). Studies of traditional Chinese medicine monomer on HeLa cell of cervical cancer. *Pak J Pharm Sci.* 27(4 Suppl.):1063–1068.
61. Hosono S, Matsuo K, Kajiyama H, Hirose K, Suzuki T, Kawase T, Kidokoro K, Nakanishi T, Hamajima N, Kikkawa F, Tajima K, Tanaka H. (2010). Association between dietary calcium and vitamin D intake and cervical carcinogenesis among Japanese women. *Eur J Clin Nutr.* 64(4):400–409.
62. Awad KS. *Ph.D. Thesis.* Kent State University; Kent, OH, USA: 2007. Inhibition of Human Papilloma Virus E6 Oncogene Function by Mammalian Lignans Activates p53 Tumor Supressor Protein and Induces Apoptosis in Cervical Cancer Cells.
63. Barchitta M, Maugeri A, Quattrocchi A, Agrifoglio O, Scalisi A, Agodi A. (2018). The association of dietary patterns with high-risk human papillomavirus infection and cervical cancer: A cross-sectional study in Italy. *Nutrients.* 10:469.
64. Siegel EM, Salemi JL, Villa LL, Ferenczy A, Franco EL, Giuliano AR. (2010). Dietary consumption of antioxidant nutrients and risk of incident cervical intraepithelial neoplasia. *Gynecol. Oncol.* 118:289–294.
65. Borgdorff H, Gautam R, Armstrong SD, et al. (2016). Cervicovaginal microbiome dysbiosis is associated with proteome changes related to alterations of the cervicovaginal mucosal barrier. *Mucosal Immunol.* 9:621–633.

66. Verhoeven Veronique,[a] Renard Nathalie,[a] Makar Amin,[d] Royen Paul Van,[a] Bogers John-Paul,[a,b] Lardon Filip,[c] Peeters Marc,[c] Baay Marc[c]. (2013). Probiotics enhance the clearance of human papillomavirus-related cervical lesions, *European Journal of Cancer Prevention.* 22(1):46–51.
67. Xiong Y, Cui L, Bian C, Zhao X, Wang X. (2020). Clearance of human papillomavirus infection in patients with cervical intraepithelial neoplasia: A systemic review and meta-analysis. *Medicine (Baltimore).* 99(46):e23155.
68. Xiong Y, Cui L, Bian C, Zhao X, Wang X. (2020). Clearance of human papillomavirus infection in patients with cervical intraepithelial neoplasia: A systemic review and meta-analysis. *Medicine (Baltimore).* 99(46):e23155.
69. Sedjo RL, Roe DJ, Abrahamsen M, Harris RB, Craft N, Baldwin S, Giuliano AR. (2002). Vitamin A, carotenoids, and risk of persistent oncogenic human papillomavirus infection. *Cancer Epidemiol. Biomarkers Prev.* 11:876–884.
70. Feng CY, Lin M, Lakhaney D, Sun HK, Dai XB, Zhao FH, Qiao YL. (2011). The association between dietary intake and cervical intraepithelial neoplasia grade 2 or higher among women in a high-risk rural area of China. *Arch. Gynecol. Obstet.* 284:973–980.
71. Hwang JH, Lee JK, Kim TJ, Kim MK. (2010). The association between fruit and vegetable consumption and HPV viral load in high-risk HPV-positive women with cervical intraepithelial neoplasia. *Cancer Causes Control.* 21:51–59.
72. Chih HJ, Lee AH, Colville L, Binns CW, Xu DA. (2013). A review of dietary prevention of human papillomavirus-related infection of the cervix and cervical intraepithelial neoplasia. *Nutr. Cancer.* 65:317–328. doi: 10.1080/01635581.2013.757630.
73. Atalah E, Urteaga C, Rebolledo A, Villegas RA, Medina E, Csendes A. (2001). Diet, smoking and reproductive history as risk for cervical cancer. *Rev. Med. Chil.* 129:597–603.
74. Tomita LY, Roteli-Martins CM, Villa LL, Franco EL, Cardoso MA. (2011). BRINCA Study Team Associations of dietary dark-green and deep-yellow vegetables and fruits with cervical intraepithelial neoplasia: Modification by smoking. *Br. J. Nutr.* 105:928–937.
75. Barchitta M, Maugeri A, Quattrocchi A, Agrifoglio O, Scalisi A, Agodi A. (2018). The association of dietary patterns with high-risk human papillomavirus infection and cervical cancer: A cross-sectional study in Italy. *Nutrients.* 10:469.

76. Schiff MA, Patterson RE, Baumgartner RN, Masuk M, van Asselt-King L, Wheeler CM, Becker TM. (2001). Serum carotenoids and risk of cervical intraepithelial neoplasia in Southwestern American Indian women. *Cancer Epidemiol Biomarkers Prev.* 10(11):1219–1222.
77. Nagata C, Shimizu H, Yoshikawa H. et al. (1999). Serum carotenoids and vitamins and risk of cervical dysplasia from a case–control study in Japan. *Br J Cancer.* 81:1234–1237.
78. Sedjo RL, Papenfuss MR, Craft NE, Giuliano AR. (2003). "Effect of plasma micronutrients on clearance of oncogenic human papillomavirus (HPV) infection (United States)." *Cancer Causes Control.* 14(4):319–326.
79. Ono A, Koshiyama M, Nakagawa M, Watanabe Y, Ikuta E, Seki K, Oowaki M. (2020). The Preventive Effect of Dietary Antioxidants on Cervical Cancer Development. *Medicina.* 56:604.
   Giuliano AR, Siegel EM, Roe DJ, Ferreira S, Baggio ML, Galan L, Duarte-Franco E, Villa LL, Rohan TE, Marshall JR, et al. (2003). HPV Natural History Study. Dietary intake and risk of persistent human papillomavirus (HPV) infection: The Ludwig-McGill HPV Natural History Study. *J. Infect Dis.* 188:1508–1516.
   Vahedpoor Z, Jamilian M, Bahmani F, Aghadavod E, Karamali M, Kashanian M, Asemi Z. Effects of long-term vitamin D supplementation on regression and metabolic status of cervical intraepithelial neoplasia: A randomized, double-blind, placebo-controlled trial. *Horm. Cancer.* 2017:58–67.
80. Siegel EM, Salemi JL, Villa LL, Ferenczy A, Franco EL, Giuliano AR. (2010). Dietary consumption of antioxidant nutrients and risk of incident cervical intraepithelial neoplasia. *Gynecol. Oncol.* 118:289–294.
81. Palan PR, Mikhail MS, Shaban DW, Romney SL. (2003). Plasma concentrations of coenzyme Q10 and tocopherols in cervical intraepithelial neoplasia and cervical cancer. *Eur J Cancer Prev.* 12(4):321–326.
82. Sepkovic DW, Stein J, Carlisle AD, Ksieski HB, Auborn K, Bradlow HL. (2009). Diindolylmethane inhibits cervical dysplasia, alters estrogen metabolism, and enhances immune response in the K14-HPV16 transgenic mouse model. *Cancer Epidemiol Biomarkers Prev.* 18(11):2957–2964.
83. Naik R. et al. (2006). A randomized phase II trial of indole-3-carbinol in the treatment of vulvar intraepithelial neoplasia, *Int J Gynecol Cancer.* 16:786–790.
84. Ono A, Koshiyama M, Nakagawa M, Watanabe Y, Ikuta E, Seki K, Oowaki M. (2020). The Preventive Effect of Dietary Antioxidants on Cervical Cancer Development. *Medicina.* 56:604.

85. Giuliano AR, Siegel EM, Roe DJ, Ferreira S, Baggio ML, Galan L, Duarte-Franco E, Villa LL, Rohan TE, Marshall JR, et al. (2003). HPV Natural History Study. Dietary intake and risk of persistent human papillomavirus (HPV) infection: The Ludwig-McGill HPV Natural History Study. *J. Infect Dis.* 188:1508–1516.
86. Hwang JH, Kim MK, Lee JK. (2010). Dietary supplements reduce the risk of cervical intraepithelial neoplasia. *Int. J. Gynecol. Cancer.* 20:398–403.
87. Yeo AS, Schiff MA, Montoya G, Masuk M, van Asselt-King L, Becker TM. (2000). Serum micronutrients and cervical dysplasia in Southwestern American Indian women. *Nutr. Cancer.* 38:141–150.
88. Chih HJ, Lee AH, Colville L, Binns CW, Xu DA. (2013). A review of dietary prevention of human papillomavirus-related infection of the cervix and cervical intraepithelial neoplasia. *Nutr. Cancer.* 65:317–328.
89. DaZhi Chen, Karen Auborn. (1999). Fish oil constituent docosahexaenoic acid selectively inhibits growth of human papillomavirus immortalized keratinocytes, *Carcinogenesis.* 20(2):249–254.
90. Di Domenico F, Foppoli C, Coccia R, Perluigi M. (2012). Antioxidants in cervical cancer: chemopreventive and chemotherapeutic effects of polyphenols. *Biochim Biophys Acta.* 1822(5):737–747.
91. Moga MA, Dimienescu OG, Arvatescu CA, Mironescu A, Dracea L, Ples L. (2016). The Role of Natural Polyphenols in the Prevention and Treatment of Cervical Cancer-An Overview. *Molecules.* 21(8):1055.
92. Jakubowicz-Gil J, Paduch R, Piersiak T, Głowniak K, Gawron A, Kandefer-Szerszeń M. (2005). The effect of quercetin of pro-apoptotic activity of cisplatin in HeLa cells. *Biochem. Pharmacol.* 69:1343–1350. doi: 10.1016/j.bcp.2005.01.022.
93. Lin C, Yu Y, Zhao HG, Yang A, Yan H, Cui Y. (2012). Combination of quercetin with radiotherapy enhances tumor radiosensitivity in vitro and in vivo. *Radiother. Oncol.* 104:395–400.
94. Xu Y, Xin Y, Diao Y, Lu C, Fu J, Luo L, Yin Z. (2011). Synergistic effects of apigenin and paclitaxel on apoptosis of cancer cells. *PLoS ONE.* 6:29169. doi: 10.1371/journal.pone.0029169.
95. Lo YL, Wang W. (2013). Formononetin potentiates epirubicininduced apoptosis via ROS production in HeLa cells in vitro. *Chem. Biol. Interact.* 205:188–197.

    Lo YL, Wang W, Ho CT. (2012). 7,3′,4′-Trihydroxyisoflavone modulates multidrug resistance transporters and induces apoptosis via production of reactive oxygen species. *Toxicology.* 302:221–232.

96. Shin JI, Shim JH, Kim KH, Choi HS, Kim JW, Lee HG, Kim BY, Park SN, Park OJ, Yoon DY. (2008). Sensitization of the apoptotic effect of gamma-irradiation in genistein-pretreated CaSki cervical cancer cells. *J. Microbiol. Biotechnol.* 18:523–531.
97. Singh M, Bhui K, Singh R, Shukla Y. (2013). Tea polyphenols enhance cisplatin chemosensitivity in cervical cancer cells via induction of apoptosis. *Life Sci.* 93:7–16.
98. Ahn WS, Yoo J, Huh SW, Kim CK, Lee JM, Namkoong SE, Bae S-M, Lee IP. (2003). Protective effects of green tea extracts (polyphenon E and EGCG) on human cervical lesions. *Eur. J. Cancer Prev.* 12:383–390.
99. Cheng AL, Hsu CH, Lin JK, Hsu MM, Ho YF, Shen TS, Ko JY, Lin J-T, Lin B-R, Wu MS, et al. (2001). Phase I clinical trial of curcumin, a chemopreventive agent, in patients with high-risk or pre-malignant lesions. *Anticancer Res.* 21:2895–2900.
100. Obhielo E, Ezeanochie M, Olokor OO, Okonkwo A, Gharoro E. (2019). The Relationship between the Serum Level of Selenium and Cervical Intraepithelial Neoplasia: A Comparative Study in a Population of Nigerian Women. *Asian Pacific journal of cancer prevention: APJCP.* 20(5):1433–1436.
101. Xie Y, Wang J, Zhao X, Zhou X, Nie X, Li C, Huang F, Yuan H. (2018). Higher serum zinc levels may reduce the risk of cervical cancer in Asian women: A meta-analysis. *The Journal of international medical research.* 46(12):4898–4906.
102. Cheng YM, Tsai CC, Hsu YC. (2016). Sulforaphane, a dietary isothiocyanate, induces G2/M arrest in cervical cancer cells through cyclinB1 downregulation and GADD45β/CDC2 association. *Int. J. Mol. Sci.* 17:1530.
103. Chih HJ, Lee AH, Colville L, Binns CW, Xu DA. (2013). A review of dietary prevention of human papillomavirus-related infection of the cervix and cervical intraepithelial neoplasia. *Nutr. Cancer.* 65:317–328.
104. Zhang X, Dai B, Zhang B, Wang Z. (2012). Vitamin A and risk of cervical cancer: a meta-analysis. *Gynecol Oncol.* 124(2):366–373.
105. Ono A, Koshiyama M, Nakagawa M, Watanabe Y, Ikuta E, Seki K, Oowaki M. (2020). The Preventive Effect of Dietary Antioxidants on Cervical Cancer Development. *Medicina.* 56:604.
106. Kwanbunjan K, Saengkar P, Cheeramakara C, Thanomsak W, Benjachai W, Laisupasin P, Buchachart K, Songmuaeng K, Boontaveeyuwat N. (2005). Low folate status as a risk factor for cervical dysplasia in Thai women. *Nutr. Res.* 25:641–654.

107. Weinstein SJ, Ziegler RG, Frongillo EA Jr, Colman N, Sauberlich HE, Brinton LA, Hamman RF, Levine RS, Mallin K, Stolley PD, Bisogni CA. (2001). Low serum and red blood cell folate are moderately, but non-significantly associated with increased risk of invasive cervical cancer in U.S. women. *J Nutr.* 131(7):2040–2048.
108. Kwanbunjan K, Saengkar P, Cheeramakara C, Tangjitgamol S, Chitcharoenrung K. (2006). Vitamin B12 status of Thai women with neoplasia of the cervix uteri. *Southeast Asian J Trop Med Public Health.* 37(Suppl. 3):178–183.
109. Alberg AJ, Selhub J, Shah KV, Viscidi RP, Comstock GW, Helzlsouer KJ. (2000). The risk of cervical cancer in relation to serum concentrations of folate, vitamin B12, and homocysteine. *Cancer Epidemiol Biomarkers Prev.* 9(7):761–764.
110. Flatley JE, McNeir K, Balasubramani L, Tidy J, Stuart EL, Young TA, Powers HJ. (2009). Folate status and aberrant DNA methylation are associated with HPV infection and cervical pathogenesis. *Cancer Epidemiol Biomarkers Prev.* 18(10):2782–2789.
111. Pathak S, Bhatla N, Singh N. (2012). Cervical cancer pathogenesis is associated with one-carbon metabolism. *Mol Cell Biochem.* 369(1–2):1–7.
112. Tong, Seo-yun, Mi Kyung Kim, Jae Kwan Lee, Jong Min Lee, Sang Woon Choi, Simonetta Friso, Eun-Seop Song, Kwang Beom Lee, and Jung Pil Lee. (2011). "Common Polymorphisms in Methylenetetrahydrofolate Reductase Gene Are Associated with Risks of Cervical Intraepithelial Neoplasia and Cervical Cancer in Women with Low Serum Folate and Vitamin B12." *Cancer Causes & Control.* 22(1):63–72.
113. Wassertheil-Smoller S, Romney SL, Wylie-Rosett J, Slagle S, Miller G, Lucido D, Duttagupta C, Palan PR. (1981). Dietary vitamin C and uterine cervical dysplasia. *Am J Epidemiol.* 114(5):714–724.
114. Vahedpoor Z, Jamilian M, Bahmani F, Aghadavod E, Karamali M, Kashanian M, Asemi Z. (2017). Effects of Long-Term Vitamin D Supplementation on Regression and Metabolic Status of Cervical Intraepithelial Neoplasia: A Randomized, Double-Blind, Placebo-Controlled Trial. *Horm Cancer.* 8(1):58–67.
115. Siegel EM, Craft NE, Duarte-Franco E, Villa LL, Franco EL, Giuliano AR. (2007). Associations between serum carotenoids and tocopherols and type-specific HPV persistence: The Ludwig-McGill cohort study. *Int. J. Cancer.* 120:672–680.
116. Palan PR, Mikhai MS, Shaban DW, Romney SL. (2003). Plasma concentrations of coenzyme Q10 and tocopherols on cervical intraepithelial neoplasia and cervical cancer. *Eur. J. Cancer Prev.* 12:321–326.

117. Beck MA. (2001). Antioxidants and viral infections: Host immune response and viral pathogenicity. *J. Am. Coll. Nutr.* 20:384S–388S; discussion 96S–97S.

Chapter 11: Benign breast disorders

1. Watt-Boolsen S, Emus HC, Junge J. (1982). Fibrocystic disease and mastalgia. A histological and enzyme-histochemical study. *Dan Med Bull.* 29(5):252–254.
2. Jørgensen J, Watt-Boolsen S. (1985). Cyclical mastalgia and breast pathology. *Acta Chir Scand.* 151(4):319–321.
3. Lumachi F, Ermani M, Brandes AA, Boccagni P, Polistina F. et al. (2002). Breast complaints and risk of breast cancer. Population-based study of 2,879 self-selected women and long-term follow-up. *Biomed Pharmacother.* 56(2):88–92.
4. Ader DN, Browne MW. (1987). Prevalence and impact of cyclic mastalgia in a United States clinic-based sample. *Am J Obstet Gynecol.* 177(1):126–132.
5. Ader DN, Shriver CD, Browne MW. (1999). Cyclical mastalgia: Premenstrual syndrome or recurrent pain disorder? *J Psychosom Obstet Gynaecol.* 20(4):198–202.
6. Jenkins PL, Jamil N, Gateley C, Mansel RE. (1993). Psychiatric illness in patients with severe treatment-resistant mastalgia. *Gen Hosp Psychiatry.* 15(1):55–57.
7. Colegrave S, Holcombe C, Salmon P. (2001). Psychological characteristics of women presenting with breast pain. *J Psychosom Res.* 50(6):303–307.
8. Fox H, Walker LG, Heys SD, Ah-See AK, Eremin O. (1997). Are patients with mastalgia anxious, and does relaxation therapy help? *Breast.* 6:138–142.
9. Ramirez AJ, Jarrett SR, Hamed H, Smith P, Fentiman IS. (1995). Psychosocial adjustment of women with mastalgia. *Breast.* 4:48–51.
10. Davies EL, Gateley CA, Miers M, Mansel RE. (1998). The long-term course of mastalgia. *J R Soc Med.* 91(9):462–464.
11. Mansel RE. (1994). ABC of breast diseases. Breast pain. *BMJ.* 309(6958):866–868.
12. McNicholas MM, Heneghan JP, Milner MH, Tunney T, Hourihane JB, MacErlaine DP. (1994). Pain and increased mammographic density in women receiving hormone replacement therapy: A prospective study. *AJR Am J Roentgenol.* 163(2):311–315.

13. Davies EL, Gateley CA, Miers M, Mansel RE. (1998). The long-term course of mastalgia. *J R Soc Med*. 91(9):462–464.
14. Preece PE, Mansel RE, Bolton PM, Hughes LM, Baum M, Gravelle IH. (1976). Clinical syndromes of mastalgia. *Lancet*. 2(7987):670–673.
15. Malherbe K, Khan M, Fatima S. (2021). Fibrocystic breast disease. In: *StatPearls* [Internet]. Treasure Island, FL: StatPearls Publishing [2022].
16. Li TT, Kang CS, Li HZ, Xue JP, Yang QM, Lyu J. (2019). Value of shear wave elastrography image classification in the diagnosis of breast masses. *Zhonghua Zhong Liu Za Zhi*. 41(7):540–545.
17. Cloete DJ, Minne C, Schoub PK, Becker JHR. (2018). Magnetic resonance imaging of fibroadenoma-like lesions and correlation with Breast Imaging-Reporting and Data System and Kaiser scoring system. *SA J Radiol*. 22(2):1532.
18. Eskandari A, Alipour S. (2019). Hormone replacement therapy and breast diseases: A matter of concern for the gynecologist. *Arch Breast Cancer*. 63:113–119.
19. Macias H, Hinck L. (2012). Mammary gland development. *Wiley Interdiscip Rev Dev Biol*. 1(4):533–557.
20. Malherbe K, Khan M, Fatima S. (2021). Fibrocystic breast disease. In: *StatPearls* [Internet]. Treasure Island, FL: StatPearls Publishing [2022].
21. Olsson HL, Olsson ML. (2020). The menstrual cycle and risk of breast cancer: A review. *Front Oncol*. 10:21.
22. Kour A, Sharma S, Sambyal V, Guleria K, Singh NR. et al. (2019). Risk factor analysis for breast cancer in premenopausal and postmenopausal women of Punjab, India. *Asian Pac J Cancer Prev*. 20(11):3299–3304.
23. Cole EN, Sellwood RA, England PC, Griffiths K. (1977). Serum prolactin concentrations in benign breast disease throughout the menstrual cycle. *Eur J Cancer*. [1965]. 13(6):597–603.
24. Milligan D, Drife JO, Short RV. (1975). Changes in breast volume during normal menstrual cycle and after oral contraceptives. *BMJ*. 14(5995):494–496.
25. Boyd NF, McGuire V, Shannon P. (1988). Effect of a low-fat high-carbohydrate diet on symptoms of cyclical mastopathy. *Lancet*. 2:128–132.
26. Goodwin PJ, Miller A, Del Giudice ME, Singer W, Connelly P, Ritchie JW. (1998). Elevated high-density lipoprotein cholesterol and dietary fat intake in women with cyclic mastopathy. *Am J Obstet Gynecol*. 179(2):430–437.

27. Goodwin PJ, Rose DP, Boyar A, Haley N, Cohen C, Lahti H, Strong LE. (1985). Low fat diet in fibrocystic disease of the breast with cyclical mastalgia: a feasibility study. *Am J Clin Nutr.* 41:856.
28. Rose DP, Boyar AP, Cohen C, Strong LE. (1987). Effect of a low-fat diet on hormone levels in women with cystic breast disease. I. Serum steroids and gonadotropins. *J Natl Cancer Inst.* 78(4):623–626.
29. Ader DN, South-Paul J, Adera T. et al. (2001). Cyclycal mastalgia: Prevalence and associated health and behavioral factors. *J Psychosom Obstet Gynecol.* 22:71–76.
30. Felter HW, Lloyd JU. (1898). *King's American Dispensatory.*
31. Felter HW, Lloyd JU. (1898). *King's American Dispensatory.*
32. Sekhavat L, Zare Tarzejani T, Kholase Zadeh P. (2009). The effect of *Vitex agnus-castus* on mastalgia in women. *Iran South Med J.* 11(2):147–152.
33. Halaska M, Beles P, Gorkow C, Sieder C. (1998). Treatment of cyclical mastalgia with a solution containing a *Vitex agnus castus* extract: Results of a placebo-controlled double-blind study. *Breast.* 8(4):175–181.
34. Moridani AS. (2015). Effect of *Nigella sativa* and *Vitex agnus* on severity mastalgia during pregnancy. *School of Nursing and Midwifery J, Tehran University of Medical Sciences.*
35. Loch EG, Selle H, Boblitz N. (2000). Treatment of premenstrual syndrome with a phytopharmaceutical formulation containing *Vitex agnus castus. J Women's Health Gend Based Med.* 9(3):315–320.
36. Ooi SL, Watts S, McClean R, Pak SC. (2020). *Vitex agnus-castus* for the treatment of cyclic mastalgia: A systematic review and meta-analysis. *J Women's Health* (Larchmt). 29(2):262–278.
37. Mirghafourvand M, Mohammad-Alizadeh, Charandabi S, Ahmadpour P, Javadzadeh Y. (2016). Effects of *Vitex agnus* and flaxseed on cyclic mastalgia: A randomized controlled trial. *Comp Ther Med.* 24:90–95.
38. Mirmolaei S, Olfatbakhsh A, Fallahhosseini H, Kazemnejad E, Sotodeh A. (2016). The effect of Vitagnus on cyclic breast pain in women of reproductive age. *J Babol University of Medical Sciences.* 18(9):7–13.
39. Sheidaei S, Irani M, Ghazanfarpour M. (2019). The effect of herbal medicines and supplements on mastalgia: A systematic review and meta-analysis of clinical trials in Iran. *Iran J Obstet Gynec Infertil.* 22(3):87–98.
40. Rajaby Gharaiy N, Shahnazi M, Yavari Kia P, Javadzadeh Y. (2017). The effect of cinnamon on cyclical breast pain. *Iran Red Cres Med J.* 19(6):e26442.

41. Khayat S, Fanael H, Pourmohsen M. (2016). The effect of curcumin on premenstrual syndrome symptoms: A double-blind randomized clinical trial. *J Nursing Midwifery, Urmia University of Medical Sciences*. 13(11):935–944.
42. Gouhar M, Mehran A, Ahmadi M, Surmaghi MS, Akhoundzadeh S. (2005). Effect of *Hypericum perforatum* L. for treatment of premenstrual syndrome. *J Med Plants*. 3(15):33–42.
43. Ingram D, Hickling C, West L, Mahe LJ, Dunbar PM. (2002). A double-blind randomized controlled trial of isoflavones in the treatment of cyclical mastalgia. *Breast*. 11(2):170–174.
44. Vaziri F, Lari MZ, Dehaghani AS, Salehi M, Sadeghpour H. et al. (2014). Comparing the effects of dietary flaxseed and omega-3 fatty acids supplement on cyclical mastalgia in Iranian women: A randomized clinical trial. *Int J Family Med*. 174532.
45. Goss P, Li T, Theriault M, Pinto S, Thompson L. (2000). Effects of dietary flaxseed in women with cyclical mastalgia. *Breast Cancer Res Treat*. 64(1):49.
46. Mirghafourvand M, Mohammad-Alizadeh, Charandabi S, Ahmadpour P, Javadzadeh Y. (2016). Effects of *Vitex agnus* and flaxseed on cyclic mastalgia: A randomized controlled trial. *Comp Ther Med*. 24:90–95.
47. Saghafi N, Rhkhshandeh H, Pourmoghadam N, Pourali L, Ghazanfarpour M. et al. (2018). Effectiveness of *Matricaria chamomilla* (chamomile) extract on pain control of cyclic mastalgia: A doubleblind randomised controlled trial. *J Obstet Gynecol*. 38(1):81–84.
48. Al-Ghamdi MS. (2001). The anti-inflammatory, analgesic and antipyretic activity of *Nigella sativa*. *J Ethnopharmacol*. 76(1):45–48.
49. Moridani AS. (2015). Effect of *Nigella sativa* and *Vitex agnus* on severity mastalgia during pregnancy. *School of Nursing and Midwifery J Tehran University of Medical Sciences*.
50. Mirmolaei ST, Olfatbakhsh A, Falah Huseini H, Kazemnezhad Leyli E, Sotoodeh Moridiani A. (2017). The effect of *Nigella sativa* syrup on the relief of cyclic mastalgia: A triple-blind randomized clinical trial. *J Hayat*. 23(1):33–43.
51. Taheri P, Ghazanfarpour M, Faridi H, Movahedinia S, Fazli B. (2022). Effectiveness of herbal medicines containing phytoestrogens to treat of cyclic mastalgia: A systematic review and meta-analysis. *Health Providers*. 1(2):55–65.

52. Zand RS, Jenkins DJ, Diamandis EP. (2000). Steroid hormone activity of flavonoids and related compounds. *Breast Cancer Res Treat.* 62(1):35–49.
53. McMichael-Phillips DF, Harding C. (1998). Effects of soy-protein supplementation on epithelial proliferation in the histologically normal human breast. *Am J Clin Nutr.* 68(6 Suppl.):1431S–1435S.
54. Lampe JW, Nishino Y, Ray RM, Wu C, Li W. et al. (2007). Plasma isoflavones and fibrocystic breast conditions and breast cancer among women in Shanghai, China. *Cancer Epidemiol Biomarkers Prev.* 16(12):2579–2586.
55. Wu C, Ray RM, Lin MG, Gao DL, Horner NK. et al. (2004). A case-control study of risk factors for fibrocystic breast conditions: Shanghai Nutrition and Breast Disease Study, China, 1995–2000. *Am J Epidemiol.* 160(10):945–960.
56. Berkey CS, Tamimi RM, Willett WC, Rosner B, Hickey M. et al. (2020). Adolescent alcohol, nuts, and fiber: Combined effects on benign breast disease risk in young women. *NPJ Breast Cancer.* 6(1):61.
57. Shannon J, King IB, Lampe JW, Gao DL, Ray RM, Lin MG, Stalsberg H, Thomas DB. (2009). Erythrocyte fatty acids and risk of proliferative and nonproliferative fibrocystic disease in women in Shanghai, China. *Am J Clin Nutr.* 89(1):265–276.
58. Vaziri F, Lari MZ, Dehaghani AS, Salehi M, Sadeghpour H. et al. (2014). Comparing the effects of dietary flaxseed and omega-3 fatty acids supplement on cyclical mastalgia in Iranian women: A randomized clinical trial. *Int J Family Med.* 174532.
59. Blommers J, de Lange-De Klerk ES, Kuik DJ, Bezemer PD, Meijer S. (2002). Evening primrose oil and fish oil for severe chronic mastalgia: A randomized, double-blind, controlled trial. *Am J Oolecol.* 187(5):1389–1394.
60. Salehi A, Momeni H, Seraji A. (2013). [The effect of evening primrose and *Vitex* on cyclic mastalgia in comparison with vitamin E: A randomized clinical trial]. *Sci Mag Yafte.* 15(2):95–109. In Persian.
61. Fathizadeh N, Takfallah L, Ehsanpour S, Namnabati M, Askari S. (2009). Effects of evening primrose oil and vitamin E on the severity of periodical breast pain. *Iran J Nurs Midwifery Res.* 13(3).
62. Blommers J, de Lange-De Klerk ES, Kuik DJ, Bezemer PD, Meijer S. (2002). Evening primrose oil and fish oil for severe chronic mastalgia: A randomized, double-blind, controlled trial. *Am J Obstet Gynecol.* 187(5):1389–1394.
63. Gateley CA, Maddox PR, Pritchard GA, Sheridan W, Harrison BJ. et al. (1992). Plasma fatty acid profiles in benign breast disorders. *Br J Surg.* 79(5):407–409.

64. Alvandipour M, Tayebi P, Alizadeh Navaie R, Khodabakhshi H. (2011). Comparison between effect of evening primrose oil and vitamin E in treatment of cyclic mastalgia. *J Babol Univ Med Sci*. 13(2):7–11. In Persian.
65. Murshid KR. (2011). A review of mastalgia in patients with fibrocystic breast changes and the non-surgical treatment options. *J Taibah University Medical Sciences*. 6(1):1–18.
66. Stonemetz D. (2008). A review of the clinical efficacy of evening primrose. *Holist Nurs Pract*. 22(3):171–174.
67. Samkari AA, Alsulami M, Bataweel L, Altaifi R, Altaifi A. et al. (2022). Body microbiota and its relationship with benign and malignant breast tumors: A systematic review. *Cureus*. 14(5):e25473.
68. Patrick L. (2008). Iodine: Deficiency and therapeutic considerations. *Altern Med Rev*. 13(2):116–127.
69. Estes NC. (1981). Mastodynia due to fibrocystic disease of the breast controlled with thyroid hormone. *Am J Surg*. 142:6.
70. Iodine Global Network. (2019). Global Scorecard of Iodine Nutrition.
71. Pearce EN. (2015). Is iodine deficiency reemerging in the United States? *AACE Clinical Case Reports*. 1:e81–e82.
72. Hess SY. (2010). The impact of common micronutrient deficiencies on iodine and thyroid metabolism: The evidence from human studies. *Best Pract Res Clin Endocrinol Metab*. 24(1):117–132.
73. Aceves C, Mendieta I, Anguiano B, Delgado-González E. (2021). Molecular iodine has extrathyroidal effects as an antioxidant, differentiator, and immunomodulator. *Int J Mol Sci*. 22(3):1228.
74. Southern AP, Jwayyed S. (2022). Iodine toxicity. In: *StatPearls* [Internet]. Treasure Island, FL: StatPearls Publishing.
75. Zhang J, Riby JE, Conde L, Grizzle WE, Cui X, Skibola CF. (2016). A *Fucus vesiculosus* extract inhibits estrogen receptor activation and induces cell death in female cancer cell lines. *BMC Complement Altern Med*. 16:151.
76. Zand RS, Jenkins DJ, Diamandis EP. (2000). Steroid hormone activity of flavonoids and related compounds. *Breast Cancer Res Treat*. 62(1):35–49.
77. McMichael-Phillips DF, Harding C. (1998). Effects of soy-protein supplementation on epithelial proliferation in the histologically normal human breast. *Am J Clin Nutr*. 68(6 Suppl.):1431S–1435S.
78. Lampe JW, Nishino Y, Ray RM, Wu C, Li W. et al. (2007). Plasma isoflavones and fibrocystic breast conditions and breast cancer among women in Shanghai, China. *Cancer Epidemiol Biomarkers Prev*. 16(12):2579–2586.

79. Vaziri F, Lari MZ, Dehaghani AS, Salehi M, Sadeghpour H. et al. (2014). Comparing the effects of dietary flaxseed and omega-3 fatty acids supplement on cyclical mastalgia in Iranian women: A randomized clinical trial. *Int J Family Med*. 174532.
80. Goss P, Li T, Theriault M, Pinto S, Thompson L. (2000). Effects of dietary flaxseed in women with cyclical mastalgia. *Breast Cancer Res Treat*. 64(1):49.
81. Mirghafourvand M, Mohammad-Alizadeh-Charandabi S, Ahmadpour P, Javadzadeh Y. (2016). Effects of *Vitex agnus* and flaxseed on cyclic mastalgia: A randomized controlled trial. *Complement Ther Med*. 24:90–95.
82. Rose DP, Boyar AP, Cohen C, Strong LE. (1987). Effect of a low-fat diet on hormone levels in women with cystic breast disease. I. Serum steroids and gonadotropins. *J Natl Cancer Inst*. 78(4):623–626.
83. Rose DP, Cohen LA, Berke B, Boyar AP. (1987). Effect of a low-fat diet on hormone levels in women with cystic breast disease. II. Serum radioimmunoassayable prolactin and growth hormone and bioactive lactogenic hormones. *J Natl Cancer Inst*. 78(4):627–631.
84. Boyd NF, McGuire V, Shannon P. (1988). Effect of a low-fat high-carbohydrate diet on symptoms of cyclical mastopathy. *Lancet*. 2:128–132.
85. Goodwin PJ, Miller A, Del Giudice ME, Singer W, Connelly P, Ritchie JW. (1988). Elevated high-density lipoprotein cholesterol and dietary fat intake in women with cyclic mastopathy. *Am J Obstet Gynecol*. 179(2):430–437.
86. Rohan TE, Negassa A, Caan B, Chlebowski RT, Curb JD. et al. (2008). Low-fat dietary pattern and risk of benign proliferative breast disease: A randomized, controlled dietary modification trial. *Cancer Prev Res.* (Phila.). 1(4):275–284.
87. Fentiman IS. (2000). Management of breast pain. In JR Harris, ME Lippman, M Morrow, CK Osborne (eds). *Diseases of the Breast*, 2nd ed. Philadelphia: Lippincott Williams & Wilkins, pp. 57–62.
88. Boyle CA, Berkowitz GS, LiVolsi VA, Ort S, Merino MJ, White C, Kelsey JL. (1984). Caffeine consumption and fibrocystic breast disease: A case-control epidemiologic study. *J Natl Cancer Inst*. 72(5):1015–1019.
89. Minton JP, Abou-Issa H. (1989). Nonendocrine theories of the etiology of benign breast disease. *World J Surg*. 13(6):680–684.
90. Bespalov VG, Barash NIu, Ivanova OA, Krzhivitskiĭ PI, Semiglazov VF. et al. (2004). Study of an antioxidant dietary supplement "Karinat" in patients with benign breast disease. *Vopr Onkol*. 50(4):467–472. In Russian.

91. Ding H, Yang Y, Wei S, Spicer LJ, Kenéz Á. et al. (2021). Influence of N-acetylcysteine on steroidogenesis and gene expression in porcine placental trophoblast cells. *Theriogenol*. 161:49–56.
92. Kashi EA, Salmani AA, Shafagh S, Mousavi GA, Mousavi N, Heydari M, Hajian A. (2022). Effects of oral N-acetyl cysteine on pain and plasma biochemical parameters in fibrocystic breast disorder: A randomized controlled trial. *Surg Open Sci*. 10:69–73.
93. Ghent WR, Eskin BA, Low DA, Hill LP. (1993). Iodine replacement in fibrocystic disease of the breast. *Can J Surg*. 36:453–460.
94. Kessler JH. (2004). The effect of supraphysiologic levels of iodine on patients with cyclic mastalgia. *Breast J*. 10(4):328–336.
95. Cann SA, van Netten JP, van Netten C. (2000). Hypothesis: Iodine, selenium and the development of breast cancer. *Cancer Causes Control*. 11:121–127.
96. Mansel RE, Das T, Baggs GE, Noss MJ, Jennings WP. et al. (2018). A randomized controlled multicenter trial of an investigational liquid nutritional formula in women with cyclic breast pain associated with fibrocystic breast changes. *J Women's Health* (Larchmt.). 27(3):333–340.
97. Bezpalov VG, Barash NIu, Ivanova OA, Semënov II, Aleksandrov VA, Semiglazov VF. (2005). Investigation of the drug "Mamoclam" for the treatment of patients with fibroadenomatosis of the breast. *Vopr Onkol*. 51(2):236–241. In Russian.
98. Band PR, Deschamps M, Falardeau M, Ladouceur J, Cote J. (1984). Treatment of benign breast disease with vitamin A. *Prev Med*. 13(5):549–554.
99. Soltany S, Alavy Toussy J. (2014). The effect of vitamin B6 on cyclic and non-cyclic mastalgia. *Adv Environ Biol*. 2014:2936–2939.
100. Goyal A. (2011). Breast pain. BMJ Clin Evid. 0812.
101. Shobeiri F, Oshvandi K, Nazari M. (2015). Clinical effectiveness of vitamin E and vitamin B6 for improving pain severity in cyclic mastalgia. *Iran J Nurs Midwifery Res*. 20(6):723–727.
102. Meyer EC, Sommers DK, Reitz CJ, Mentis H. (1990). Vitamin E and benign breast disease. *Surgery*. 107(5):549–551.
103. Parsay S, Olfati F, Nahidi S. (2009). Therapeutic effects of vitamin E on cyclic mastalgia. *Breast J*. 15(5):510–514.
104. Pruthi S, Wahner-Roedler DL, Torkelson CJ, Cha SS, Thicke LS, Hazelton JH, Bauer BA. (2010). Vitamin E and evening primrose oil for management of cyclical mastalgia: A randomized pilot study. *Altern Med Rev*. 15(1):59–67.

105. Chamras H, Barsky SH, Ardashian A, Navasartian D, Heber D, Glaspy JA. (2005). Novel interactions of vitamin E and estrogen in breast cancer. *Nutr Cancer.* 52(1):43–48.
106. Ataollahi M, Akbari SA, Mojab F, Alavi Majd H. (2015). The effect of wheat germ extract on premenstrual syndrome symptoms. *Iran J Pharm Res.* 14(1):159–166.
107. Mason BR, Page KA, Fallon K. (1999). An analysis of movement and discomfort of the female breast during exercise and the effects of breast support in three cases. *J Sci Med Sport.* 2(2):134–144.
108. Ader DN, South-Paul J, Adera T. et al. (2001). Cyclycal mastalgia: Prevalence and associated health and behavioral factors. *J Psychosom Obstet Gynecol.* 22:71–76.
109. Fox H, Walker LG, Heys SD, Ah-See AK, Eremin O. (1997). Are patients with mastalgia anxious, and does relaxation therapy help? *Breast.* 6:138–142.
110. Bhatti DS, Bokhari MHT, Khan MAA. (2022). Smoking and fibrocystic changes in the breast: A case report of a lifelong smoker and changes in breast parenchyma. *Cureus.* 14(6):e26384.

Chapter 12: Lichen sclerosus

1. Regauer S, Liegl B, Reich O. (2005). Early vulvar lichen sclerosus: A histopathological challenge. *Histopathol.* 47:340–347.
2. Bleeker MC, Visser PJ, Overbeek LI, Beurden Mv, Berkhof J. (2016). Lichen sclerosus: Incidence and risk of vulvar squamous cell carcinoma. *Cancer Epidemiol Biomarkers Prev.* 25:1224–1230.
3. Singh N, Ghatage P. (2020). Etiology, clinical features, and diagnosis of vulvar lichen sclerosus: A scoping review. *Obstet Gynecol Int.* 7480754.
4. Tran DA, Tan X, Macri CJ, Goldstein AT, Fu SW. (2019). Lichen sclerosus: An autoimmunopathogenic and genomic enigma with emerging genetic and immune targets. *Int J Biol Sci.* 15(7):1429–1439.
5. Sheinis M, Selk A. (2018). Development of the Adult Vulvar Lichen Sclerosus Severity Scale—A Delphi consensus exercise for item generation. *J Low Genit Tract Dis.* 22(1):66–73.
6. Fistarol SK, Itin PH. (2013). Diagnosis and treatment of lichen sclerosus: An update. *Am J Clin Dermatol.* 14(1):27–47.
7. Günthert AR, Faber M, Knappe G, Hellriegel S, Emons G. (2008). Early onset vulvar lichen sclerosus in premenopausal women and oral contraceptives. *Eur J Obstet Gynecol Reprod Biol.* 137(1):56–60.

8. Tran DA, Tan X, Macri CJ, Goldstein AT, Fu SW. (2019). Lichen sclerosus: An autoimmunopathogenic and genomic enigma with emerging genetic and immune targets. *Int J Biol Sci.* 15(7):1429–1439.
9. Higgins CA, Cruickshank ME. (2012). A population-based case-control study of aetiological factors associated with vulval lichen sclerosus. *J Obstet Gynaec.* 32:271–275.
10. Cooper SM, Ali I, Baldo M, Wojnarowska F. (2008). The association of lichen sclerosus and erosive lichen planus of the vulva with autoimmune disease: A case-control study. *Arch Dermatol.* 144:1432–1435.
11. Aidé S, Lattario FR, Almeida G, do Val IC, da Costa M. (2010). Epstein-Barr virus and human papillomavirus infection in vulvar lichen sclerosus. *J Low Genit Tract Dis.* 14(4):319–322.
12. Virgili A, Minghetti S, Borghi A, Corazza M. (2013). Long-term maintenance therapy for vulvar lichen sclerosus: The results of a randomized study comparing topical vitamin E with an emollient. *Eur J Dermatol.* 23(2):189–194.
13. Kapadia GJ, Azuine MA, Tokuda H, Takasaki M, Mukainaka T, Konoshima T, Nishino H. (2002). Chemopreventive effect of resveratrol, sesamol, sesame oil and sunflower oil in the Epstein-Barr virus early antigen activation assay and the mouse skin two-stage carcinogenesis. *Pharmacol. Res.* 45:499–505.
14. Bailey E. (1945). Treatment of leprosy. *Nature.* 155:601.
15. Brinkhaus B, Lindner M, Schuppan D, Hahn EG. (2000). Chemical, pharmacological and clinical profile of the East Asian medical plant *Centella asiatica*. *Phytomed.* 7:427–448.
16. Hashim P. (2014). The effect *of Centella asiatica*, vitamins, glycolic acid and their mixtures preparations in stimulating collagen and fibronectin synthesis in cultured human skin fibroblast. *Pak J Pharm Sci.* 27:233–237.
17. Bonté F, Dumas M, Chaudagne C, Meybeck A, Bonte F, Dumas M, Chaudagne C, Meybeck A. (1994). Influence of Asiatic acid, madecassic acid, and asiaticoside on human collagen I synthesis. *Planta Med.* 60:133–135.
18. Darnis F, Orcel L, de Saint-Maur PP, Mamou P. (1979). Note sur l'utilisation de l'extrait titre de *Centella asiatica* au cours des hepatopathies chroniques. *Sem Des Hop.* 55:1749–1750.
19. Ilegra C. (1981). Comparative capillaroscopic study of certain bioflavonoids and total triterpenic fractions of *Centella asiatica* in venous insufficiency. *Clin Ther.* 99:507–513.

20. Rosen H, Blumenthal A, McCallum J. (1967). Effect of asiaticoside on wound healing in the rat. *Proc Soc Exp Biol Med.* 125:279–280.
21. Incandela L, Cesarone MR, Cacchio M, De Sanctis MT, Santavenere C. et al. (2001). Total triterpenic fraction of *Centella asiatica* in chronic venous insufficiency and in high-perfusion microangiopathy. *Angiology.* 52:S9–13.
22. Widgerow AD, Chait LA, Stals R, Stals PJ. (2000). New innovations in scar management. *Aesthetic Plast Surg.* 24:227–234.
23. Shukla A, Rasik AM, Dhawan BN. (1999). Asiaticoside-induced elevation of antioxidant levels in healing wounds. *Phytother Res.* 13:50–54.
24. Shukla A, Rasik AM, Jain GK, Shankar R, Kulshrestha, Dhawan BN. (1999). In vitro and in vivo wound healing activity of asiaticoside isolated from *Centella asiatica*. *J Ethnopharmacol.* 65(1):1–11.
25. Lee J, Jung E, Kim Y, Park J, Park J. et al. (2006). Asiaticoside induces human collagen I synthesis through TGF-beta receptor I kinase (TbetaRI kinase)—independent Smad signaling. *Planta Med.* 72(4):324–328.
26. Widgerow AD, Chait LA, Stals R, Stals PJ. (2000). New innovations in scar management. *Aesth Plast Surg.* 24:227–234.
27. Kimura Y, Sumiyoshi M, Samukawa KI, Satake N, Sakanaka M. (2008). Facilitating action of asiaticoside at low doses on burn wound repair and its mechanism. *Eur J Pharmacol.* 584(2–3):415–423.
28. Guseva G, Stravoitova MN, Mach ES. (1998). Madecassol treatment of systematic and localized scleroderma. *Ter Arkh.* 70:58–61.
29. Zalewski J, Mączyńska J, Bieżuńska-Kusiak K, Kulbacka J, Choromańska A. et al. (2019). *Calophyllum inophyllum* in vaginitis treatment: Stimulated by electroporation with an in vitro approach. *Adv Clin Exp Med.* 28(2):223–228.
30. Hagedorn M. (1989). Genitaler vulvärer Lichen sclerosus bei Geschwistern [Genital vulvar lichen sclerosis in 2 siblings]. *Z Hautkr.* 64(9):810, 813–814.
31. Ding H, Han C, Guo D, Chin YW, Ding Y, Kinghorn AD, D'Ambrisio SM. (2009). Selective induction of apoptosis of human oral cancer cell lines by avocado extracts via a ROS-mediated mechanism. *Nutr Cancer.* 61(3):348–356.
32. Borghi A, Corazza M, Minghetti S, Toni G, Virgili A. (2015). Avocado and soybean extracts as active principles in the treatment of mild-to-moderate vulvar lichen sclerosus: Results of efficacy and tolerability. *J Eur Acad Dermatol Venereol.* 29(6):1225–1230.

33. Lin TK, Zhong L, Santiago JL. (2017). Anti-inflammatory and skin barrier repair effects of topical application of some plant oils. *Int J Mol Sci.* 19(1):70.
34. Virgili A, Minghetti S, Borghi A, Corazza M. (2013). Long-term maintenance therapy for vulvar lichen sclerosus: The results of a randomized study comparing topical vitamin E with an emollient. *Eur J Dermatol.* 23(2):189–194.
35. Intahphuak S, Khonsung P, Panthong A. (2010). Anti-inflammatory, analgesic, and antipyretic activities of virgin coconut oil. *Pharm Biol.* 48(2):151–157.
36. Mori HM, Kawanami H, Kawahata H, Aoki M. (2016). Wound healing potential of lavender oil by acceleration of granulation and wound contraction through induction of TGF-β in a rat model. *BMC Complement Altern Med.* 16:144.
37. Zuzarte M, Gonçalves MJ, Cavaleiro, Canhoto J, Vale-Silva L, Silva MJ, Pinto E, Salgueiro L. (2011). Chemical composition and antifungal activity of the essential oils of *Lavandula viridis* L'Hér. *J Med Microbiol.* 60(5):612–618.
38. Ud-Din S, McGeorge D, Bayat A. (2016). Topical management of striae distensae (stretch marks): Prevention and therapy of striae rubrae and albae. *J Eur Acad Dermatol Venereol.* 30(2):211–222.
39. Katiyar SK. (2016). Dietary proanthocyanidins inhibit UV radiation-induced skin tumor development through functional activation of the immune system. *Mol Nutr Food Res.* 60(6):1374–1382.
40. Sahin K, Cross B, Sahin N, Ciccone K, Suleiman S. et al. (2015). Lycopene in the prevention of renal cell cancer in the TSC2 mutant Eker rat model. *Arch Biochem Biophys.* 572:36–39.
41. Lin Y, Yngve A, Lagergren J, Lu Y. (2014). A dietary pattern rich in lignans, quercetin and resveratrol decreases the risk of oesophageal cancer. *Br J Nutr.* 112(12):2002–2009.
42. Aoki H, Takada Y, Kondo S, Sawaya R, Aggarwal BB, Kondo Y. (2007). Evidence that curcumin suppresses the growth of malignant gliomas in vitro and in vivo through induction of autophagy: Role of Akt and extracellular signal-regulated kinase signaling pathways. *Mol Pharmacol.* 72(1):29–39.
43. Sideri M, Parazzini F, Rognoni MT, La Vecchia C, Negri E, Garsia S, Arnoletti E, Cecchetti G. (1989). Risk factors for vulvar lichen sclerosus. *Am J Obstet Gynecol.* 161(1):38–42.

44. Vieira-Baptista P, Lima-Silva J, Cavaco-Gomes J, Beires J, Martinez-de-Oliveira J. (2015). What differentiates symptomatic from asymptomatic women with lichen sclerosus? *Gynecol Obstet Invest*. 79(4):263–268.
45. Calista D, Cappelli MC, Foglietta F, Gambi A. (1994). Vitamins A and E in the treatment of atrophic lichen sclerosus of the vulva. *Specializzati Oggi—Dermatologia*. 3:12–14. In Italian.
46. Ronger S, Viallard AM, Meunier-Mure F, Chouvet B, Balme B, Thomas L. (2003). Oral calcitriol: A new therapeutic agent in cutaneous lichen sclerosus. *J Drugs Dermatol*. 2(1):23–28.
47. Vieira-Baptista P, Lima-Silva J, Cavaco-Gomes J, Beires J, Martinez-de-Oliveira J. (2015). What differentiates symptomatic from asymptomatic women with lichen sclerosus? *Gynecol Obstet Invest*. 79(4):263–268.
48. D'Antuono A, Bellavista S, Negosanti F, Zauli S, Baldi E, Patrizi A. (2011). Dermasilk briefs in vulvar lichen sclerosus: An adjuvant tool. *J Low Genit Tract Dis*. 15(4):287–291.

Chapter 13: Premenstrual syndrome (PMS)

1. Brice-Ytsma H, McDermott A. (2020). *Herbal Medicine in Treating Gynaecological Conditions: Herbs, Hormones, Pre-Menstrual Syndrome and Menopause*. London: Aeon.
2. Panossian A, Wikman G. (2010). Effects of adaptogens on the central nervous system and the molecular mechanisms associated with their stress–protective activity. *Pharmaceuticals* (Basel). 3(1):188–224.
3. Yarnell E, Abascal K. (2006). Botanical medicine for thyroid regulation. *Altern Comp Ther*. 12(3).
4. İşik H, Ergöl Ş, Aynioğlu Ö, Şahbaz A, Kuzu A, Uzun M. (2016). Premenstrual syndrome and life quality in Turkish health science students. *Turk J Med Sci*. 46(3):695–701.
   Bianco V, Cestari AM, Casati D, Cipriani S, Radici G, Valente I. (2014). Premenstrual syndrome and beyond: Lifestyle, nutrition, and personal facts. *Minerva Ginecol*. 66(4):365–375.
5. Fernández MM, Saulyte J, Inskip HM, Takkouche B. (2018). Premenstrual syndrome and alcohol consumption: A systematic review and meta-analysis. *BMJ Open*. 8(3):e019490.
6. Steiner JL, Crowell KT, Lang CH. (2015). Impact of alcohol on glycemic control and insulin action. *Biomol*. 5(4):2223–2246.

Chapter 14: Menopause

1. Brice-Ytsma H, McDermott A. (2020). *Herbal Medicine in Treating Gynaecological Conditions: Herbs, Hormones, Pre-Menstrual Syndrome and Menopause.* London: Aeon.

Section Two: Monographs of Herbs Frequently Used in Women's Health, Without a Hormonal Reputation
Achillea millefolium

1. Jones WHS. (1956). [Pliny, the Elder] *Naturalis Historia. English and Latin.* Cambridge, MA: Harvard University Press.
2. Solecki RS. (1975). Shanidar IV, a Neanderthal flower burial in northern Iraq. *Science.* 190:880–881.
3. Leroi-Gourhan A. (1975). The flowers found with Shanidar IV, a Neanderthal burial in Iraq. *Science.* 190:562–564.
   Leroi-Gourhan A. (1998). Shanidar et ses fleurs. *Paléorient.* 24(2):79–88.
4. Lietava J. (1992). Medicinal plants in a Middle Paleolithic grave Shanidar IV? *J Ethnopharmacol.* 35(3):263–266.
5. Jones WHS. (1956). [Pliny, the Elder] *Naturalis Historia. English and Latin.* Cambridge, MA: Harvard University Press.
6. Osbaldeston TA, Wood RPA (eds). (2000). *Dioscorides: De materia medica.* Johannesburg: Ibidis Press.
7. Felter HW, Lloyd JU. (1898). *King's American Dispensatory.*
8. Scudder JM. (1870). *Specific Medication and Specific Medicines.*
9. Felter HW, Lloyd JU. (1898). *King's American Dispensatory.*
10. Lloyd JU, Ellingwood F. (1919). *American Materia Medica.*
11. Kielczynski W. (1995). Phytotherapy for hypertension. *Mod Phytother.* 2(1).
12. Nemeth EI, Bernath J. (2008). Biological activities of yarrow species (*Achillea* spp.). *Curr Pharm Des.* 14(29):3151–3167.
13. Ali SI, Gopalakrishnan B, Venkatesalu V. (2017). Pharmacognosy, phytochemistry and pharmacological properties of *Achillea millefolium* L.: A review. *Phytother Res.* 31(8):1140–1161.
14. Ayoobi F, Shamsizadeh A, Fatemi I, Vakilian A, Allahtavakoli M, Hassanshahi G, Moghadam-Ahmadi A. (2017). Bio-effectiveness of the main flavonoids of *Achillea millefolium* in the pathophysiology of neurodegenerative disorders—a review. *Iran J Basic Med Sci.* 20(6):604–612.

15. Vitalini S, Beretta G, Iriti M, Orsenigo S, Basilico N. et al. (2011). Phenolic compounds from *Achillea millefolium* L. and their bioactivity. *Acta Biochim Pol.* 58(2):203–209.
16. Veryser L, Taevernier L, Wynendaele E, Verheust Y, Dumoulin A, De Spiegeleer B. (2017). N-alkylamide profiling of *Achillea ptarmica* and *Achillea millefolium* extracts by liquid and gas chromatography-mass spectrometry. *J Pharm Anal.* 7(1):34–47.
17. Nemeth EI, Bernath J. (2008). Biological activities of yarrow species (*Achillea* spp.). *Curr Pharm Des.* 14(29):3151–3167.
18. Hosseini MS, Hosseini F, Ahmadi A, Mozafari M, Amjadi I. (2019). Antiproliferative activity of *Hypericum perforatum*, *Achillea millefolium*, and *Aloe vera* in Interaction with the prostatic activity of CD82. *Rep Biochem Mol Biol.* 8(3):260–268.
19. Csupor-Löffler B, Hajdú Z, Zupkó I, Réthy B, Falkay G. et al. (2009). Antiproliferative effect of flavonoids and sesquiterpenoids from *Achillea millefolium* s.l. on cultured human tumour cell lines. *Phytother Res.* 23(5):672–676.
20. Lin LT, Liu LT, Chang LC, Lin CC. (2002). In vitro anti-hepatoma activity of fifteen natural medicines from Canada. *Phytother Res.* 16:440–444.
21. Tozyo T, Yoshimura Y, Sakurai K, Uchida N, Takeda Y, Nakai, Ishii H. (1994). Novel antitumor sesquiterpenoids in *Achillea millefolium*. *Chem Pharm Bull.* (Tokyo). 42:1096–1100.
22. Goldberg AS, Mueller EC, Eigen E, Desalva SJ. (1969). Isolation of the anti-inflammatory principles from *Achillea millefolium* (Compositae). *J Pharm Sci.* 58(8):938–941.
23. Choudhary MI, Jalil S, Todorova M, Trendafilova A, Mikhova B, Duddeck H, Rahman Au. (2007). Inhibitory effect of lactone fractions and individual components from three species of the *Achillea millefolium* complex of Bulgarian origin on the human neutrophils respiratory burst activity. *Nat Prod Res.* 21(11):1032–1036.
24. Maswadeh HM, Semreen MH, Naddaf AR. (2006). Anti-inflammatory activity of *Achillea* and *Ruscus* topical gel on carrageenan-induced paw edema in rats. *Acta Poloniae Pharmaceutica.* 63:277–280.
25. Benedek BI, Kopp B, Melzig MF. (2007). *Achillea millefolium* L. s.l.—is the anti-inflammatory activity mediated by protease inhibition? *J Ethnopharmacol.* 113(2):312–317.
26. Ramadan M, Goeters S, Watzer B, Krause E, Lohmann K, Bauer R, Hempel B, Imming P. (2006). Chamazulene carboxylic acid and matricin: A natural profen and its natura prodrug, identified through similarity to synthetic drug substances. *J Nat Prod.* 69:1041–1045.

27. Mahady GB, Pendland SL, Stoia A, Hamill FA, Fabricant D, Dietz BM, Chadwick LR. (2005). In vitro susceptibility of *Helicobacter pylori* to botanical extracts used traditionally for the treatment of gastrointestinal disorders. *Phytother Res*. 19:988–991.
28. Cáceres A. (1999). *Plantas de uso medicinal en Guatemala*. Universidad de San Carlos de Guatemala: Editorial Universitaria, pp. 268–270.
29. Frey FM, Meyers R. (2010). Antibacterial activity of traditional medicinal plants used by Haudenosaunee peoples of New York State. *BMC Complement Altern Med*. 10:64.
30. Candan F, Unlu M, Tepe B, Daferera D, Polissiou M, Sökmen A, Akpulat HA. (2003). Antioxidant and antimicrobial activity of the essential oil and methanol extracts of *Achillea millefolium* subsp. *millefolium Afan*. (Asteraceae). *J Ethnopharmacol*. 87(2–3):215–220.
31. Murnigsih T, Subeki, Matsuura H, Takahashi K, Yamasaki M. et al. (2005). Evaluation of the inhibitory activities of the extracts of Indonesian traditional medicinal plants against *Plasmodium falciparum* and *Babesia gibsoni*. *J Vet Med Sci*. 67(8):829–831.
32. Konyalioglu S, Karamenderes C. (2005). The protective effects of *Achillea* L. species native in Turkey against H(2)O(2)-induced oxidative damage in human erythrocytes and leucocytes. *J Ethnopharmacol*. 102(2):221–227.
33. Yaeesh S, Jamal Q, Khan AU, Gilani AH. (2006). Studies on hepatoprotective, antispasmodic and calcium antagonist activities of the aqueous-methanol extract of *Achillea millefolium*. *Phytother Res*. 20:546–551.
34. Lemmens-Gruber R, Marchart E, Rawnduzi P, Engel N, Benedek B, Kopp B. (2006). Investigation of the spasmolytic activity of the flavonoid fraction of *Achillea millefolium* s.l. on isolated guinea-pig ilea. *Arzneimittelforschung*. 56:582–588.
35. Molina-Hernandez M, Tellez-Alcantara NP, Diaz MA, Perez Garcia J, Olivera Lopez JI, Jaramillo MT. (2004). Anticonflict actions of aqueous extracts of flowers of *Achillea millefolium* L. vary according to the estrous cycle phases in Wistar rats. *Phytother Res*. 18:915–920.
36. Vazirinejad R, Ayoobi F, Arababadi MK, Eftekharian MM, Darekordi A. et al. (2014). Effect of aqueous extract of *Achillea millefolium* on the development of experimental autoimmune encephalomyelitis in C57BL/6 mice. *Ind J Pharmacol*. 46(3):303–308.
37. Benedek B, Geisz N, Jäger W, Thalhammer T, Kopp B. (2006). Choleretic effects of yarrow (*Achillea millefolium* s.l.) in the isolated perfused rat liver. *Phytomed*. 13:702–706.
38. Borrelli F, Romano B, Fasolino I, Tagliatatela-Scafati O, Aprea G. et al. (2012). Prokinetic effect of a standardized yarrow (*Achillea millefolium*)

extract and its constituent choline: Studies in the mouse and human stomach. *Neurogastroenterol Motil.* 24(2):164–171.
39. Cavalcanti AM, Hatsuko Baggio C, Freitas CS, Rieck L, de Sousa RS. et al. (2006). Safety and antiulcer efficacy studies of *Achillea millefolium* L. after chronic treatment in Wistar rats. *J Ethnopharmacol.* 107(2):277–284.
40. Hatsuko Baggio C, De Martini Otofuji G, Setim Freitas C, Brandão Torres, LM, Andrade Marques MC, Mesia-Vela S. (2008). Brazilian medicinal plants in gastrointestinal therapy. In RR Watson, VR Preedy (eds). *Botanical Medicine in Clinical Practice.* Wallingford, UK: CABI, pp. 46–51.
41. Potrich FB, Allemand A, da Silva LM, Do Santos AC, Hatsuko Baggio H. et al. (2010). Antiulcerogenic activity of hydroalcoholic extract of *Achillea millefolium* L.: Involvement of the antioxidant system. *J Ethnopharmacol.* 130(1):85–92.
42. Sellerberg U, Glasl H. (2000). Pharmacognostical examination concerning the hemostyptic effect of *Achillea millefolium* Aggregat. *Sci Pharm.* 68(2):201–206.
43. Yaeesh S, Jamal Q, Khan AU, Gilani AH. (2006). Studies on hepatoprotective, antispasmodic and calcium antagonist activities of the aqueous-methanol extract of *Achillea millefolium. Phytother Res.* 20:546–551.
44. Khan AU, Gilani AH. (2011). Blood pressure lowering, cardiovascular inhibitory and bronchodilatory actions of *Achillea millefolium. Phytother Res.* 25(4):577–583.
45. Jaenson TG, Pålsson K, BorgKarlson AK. (2006). Evaluation of extracts and oils of mosquito (Diptera: Culicidae) repellent plants from Sweden and Guinea-Bissau. *J Med Entomol.* 43:113–119.
46. Innocenti G, Vegeto E, S. Dall'Acqua S, Ciana P, Giorgetti M, Agradi E, Sozzi A, Fico G, Tomè F. (2007). In vitro estrogenic activity of *Achillea millefolium* L. *Phytomed.* 14:147–152.
47. Breinholt V, Larsen JC. (1998). Detection of weak estrogenic flavonoids using a recombinant years strain and a modified MCF7 cell proliferation assay. *Chem Res Toxicol.* 11:622–629.
48. Pain S, Altobelli C, Boher A, Cittadini L, Favre-Mercuret M. et al. (2011). Surface rejuvenating effect of *Achillea millefolium* extract. *Int J Cosmet Sci.* 33(6):535–542.
49. Dall'Acqua S, Bolego C, Cignarella A, Gaion RM, Innocenti G. (2011). Vasoprotective activity of standardized *Achillea millefolium* extract. *Phytomed.* 18(12):1031–1036.
50. Hajhashemi M, Ghanbari Z, Movahedi M, Rafieian M, Keivani A, Haghollahi F. (2018). The effect of *Achillea millefolium* and *Hypericum*

perforatum ointments on episiotomy wound healing in primiparous women. *J Matern Fetal Neonatal Med.* 31(1):63–69.
51. Vahid S, Dashti-Khavidaki S, Ahmadi F, Amini M, Salehi Surmaghi MH. (2012). Effect of herbal medicine *Achillea millefolium* on plasma nitrite and nitrate levels in patients with chronic kidney disease: A preliminary study. *Iran J Kidney Dis.* 6(5):350–354.
52. Mahler P. (1926). On the effect of bitterness on gastric juice secretion. *Z Ges Exp Med.* 51:267–277.
53. Ayoobi F, Moghadam-Ahmadi A, Amiri H, Vakilian A, Heidari M. et al. (2019). *Achillea millefolium* is beneficial as an add-on therapy in patients with multiple sclerosis: A randomized placebo-controlled clinical trial. *Phytomed.* 52:89–97.
54. Miranzadeh S, Adib-Hajbaghery M, Soleymanpoor L, Ehsani M. (2015). Effect of adding the herb *Achillea millefolium* on mouthwash on chemotherapy induced oral mucositis in cancer patients: A double-blind randomized controlled trial. *Eur J Oncol Nurs.* 19(3):207–213.
55. Jenabi E, Fereidoony B. (2015). Effect of *Achillea millefolium* on relief of primary dysmenorrhea: A doubleblind randomized clinical trial. *J Pediatr Adolesc Gynecol.* 28:402–404.
56. Kazemian A, Toghiani A, Shafiei K, Afshar H, Rafiei R, Memari M, Adibi P. (2017). Evaluating the efficacy of mixture of *Boswellia carterii*, *Zingiber officinale*, and *Achillea millefolium* on severity of symptoms, anxiety, and depression in irritable bowel syndrome patients. *J Res Med Sci.* 22(1):120.
57. Ryttig K, Schlamowitz PV, Warnoe O, Wilstrup F. (1991). Gitadyl versus ibuprofen in patients with osteoarthrosis. The result of a double-blind, randomized crossover study. *Ugeskr Laeg.* 153:2298–2299.
58. Binić I, Janković A, Janković D, Janković I, Vručinić Z. (2010). Evaluation of healing and antimicrobiological effects of herbal therapy on venous leg ulcer: Pilot study. *Phytother Res.* 24:277–282.

Alchemilla vulgaris

1. Savikin K, Zdunić G, Menković N, Zivković J, Cujić N, Tereščenko M, Bigović D. (2013). Ethnobotanical study on traditional use of medicinal plants in South-Western Serbia, Zlatibor district. *J Ethnopharmacol.* 146(3):803–810.
2. Matthiolus PA. (1626). *New-Kreuterbuch.*
3. Blackwell E. (1737). *A Curious Herbal, Containing Five Hundred Cuts of the Most Useful Plants, Which Are Now Used in the Practice of Physic.*

4. Künzle J. (1928). *Monatshefte für giftfreie Kräuterheilkunde des Krauterpfarrers*.
5. Madaus G. (1938). *Lehrbuch der Biologischen Heilmittel*.
6. Tasić-Kostov M, Arsić I, Pavlović D, Stojanović S, Najman S, Naumović S, Tadić V. (2019). Towards a modern approach to traditional use: *In vitro* and *in vivo* evaluation of *Alchemilla vulgaris* L. gel wound healing potential. *J Ethnopharmacol*. 238:111789.
7. Vlaisavljević S, Jelača S, Zengin G, Mimica-Dukić N, Berežni S, Miljić M, Stevanović ZD. (2019). *Alchemilla vulgaris* agg. (Lady's mantle) from central Balkan: Antioxidant, anticancer and enzyme inhibition properties. *RSC Adv*. 9(64):37474–37483.
8. Hedayat KM, Lapraz JC. (2019). *The Theory of Endobiogeny*, 4 vols. London: Academic Press.
9. Zava DT, Dollbaum CM, Blen M. (1998). Estrogen and progestin bioactivity of foods, herbs, and spices. *Proc Soc Exp Biol Med*. 217(3):369–378.
10. Bone K. (1997). Progesteronic herbs? *Modern Phytotherapist*. 3(2):14–16.
11. Yang P, Li L, Yang D, Wang C, Peng H, Huang H. et al. (2017). Effect of peony-glycyrrhiza decoction on amisulpride-induced hyperprolactinemia in women with schizophrenia: A preliminary study. *Evid Based Complement Alternat Med*. 7901670.
12. Shahin AY, Mohammed SA. (2014). Adding the phytoestrogen *Cimicifugae racemosae* to clomiphene induction cycles with timed intercourse in polycystic ovary syndrome improves cycle outcomes and pregnancy rates—a randomized trial. *Gynecol Endocrinol*. 30(7):505–510.
13. Kamel HH. (2013). Role of phyto-oestrogens in ovulation induction in women with polycystic ovarian syndrome. *Eur J Obstet Gynecol Reprod Biol*. 168(1):60–63.
14. Mohammed SK. (2020). Effect of *Alchemilla vulgaris* powder on the reproductive system and liver, spleen functions of female rats exposed to high dose of zinc sulfate in drinking water. Thesis, University of Kerbala.
15. Jonadet M, Meunier MT, Villie F, Bastide JP, Lamaison JL. (1986). Flavonoids extracted from *Ribes nigrum* L. and *Alchemilla vulgaris* L.: 1. In vitro inhibitory activities on elastase, trypsin and chymotrypsin. 2. Angioprotective activities compared in vivo. *J Pharmacol*. 17(1):21–27.
16. Boroja T, Mihailović V, Katanić J, Pan SP, Nikles S. et al. (2018). The biological activities of roots and aerial parts of *Alchemilla vulgaris* L. *S Afr J Bot*. 116:175–184.
17. Pawlaczyk I, Czerchawski L, Pilecki W, Lamer-Zarawska E, Gancarz R. (2009). Polyphenolic-polysaccharide compounds from selected medicinal plants of Asteraceae and Rosaceae families: Chemical

characterization and blood anticoagulant activity. *Carbohydrate Polymers.* 77(3):568–575.
18. Boroja T, Mihailović V, Katanić, J, Pan SP, Nikles S. et al. (2018). The biological activities of roots and aerial parts of *Alchemilla vulgaris* L. *S Afr J Bot.* 116:175–184.
19. Hamad I, Erol-Dayi O, Pekmez M, Onay-Ucar E, Arda N. (2007). Free radical scavenging activity and protective effects of *Alchemilla vulgaris* (L.). *J Biotechnol.* 131:S40–S41.
20. Filippova EI. (2017). Antiviral activity of lady's mantle (*Alchemilla vulgaris* L.) extracts against orthopoxviruses. *Bull Exp Biol Med.* 163(3):374–377.
21. Sufka KJ, Roach JT, Chambliss WG Jr, Broom SL, Feltenstein MW, Wyandt CM, Zeng L. (2001). Anxiolytic properties of botanical extracts in the chick social separation-stress procedure. *Psychopharmacol.* (Berlin). 153(2):219–224.
22. Shilova IV, Suslov NI, Samylina IA, Baeva VM, Lazareva NB, Mazin EV. (2020). Neuroprotective properties of common lady's mantle infusion. *Pharma Chem J.* 5311:1059–1062.
23. Kupeli Akkol E, Demirel MA, Bahadir Acikara O, Suntar I, Ergene B. et al. (2015). Phytochemical analyses and effects of *Alchemilla mollis* (Buser) Rothm. and *Alchemilla persica* Rothm. in rat endometriosis model. *Arch Gynecol Obstet.* 292:619–628.
24. Krivokuća M, Niketić M, Milenković M, Golić N, Masia C. et al. (2015). Anti-*Helicobacter pylori* activity of four *Alchemilla* species (Rosaceae). *Nat Prod Commun.* 10(8):1369–1371.
25. Ozbek H, Acikara OB, Keskin I, Kirmizi NI, Ozbilgin S. et al. (2017). Evaluation of hepatoprotective and antidiabetic activity of *Alchemilla mollis*. *Biomed Pharmacother.* 86:172–176.
26. Eshak M, Refat OG, Halaby MS, Elmetwaly EM, Omar AA. (2018). Effect of lion's foot (*Alchemilla vulgaris*) on liver and renal functions in rats induced by CCl4. *Food Nutr.* 9:46–62.
27. Jurić T, Katanić Stanković JS, Rosić G, Selaković D, Joksimović J. et al. (2020). Protective effects of *Alchemilla vulgaris* L. extracts against cisplatin-induced toxicological alterations in rats. *S Afr J Bot.* 128: 141–151.
28. Takır S, Altun IH, Sezgi B, Süzgeç-Selçuk S, Mat A, Uydeş-Doğan BS. (2015). Vasorelaxant and blood pressure lowering effects of *Alchemilla vulgaris*: A comparative study of methanol and aqueous extracts. *Pharmacogn Mag.* 11(41):163–169.
29. Slanc P, Doljak B, Kreft S, Lunder M, Janeš D, Štrukelj B. (2009). Screening of selected food and medicinal plant extracts for pancreatic lipase

inhibition: Inhibition of pancreatic lipase by plant extracts. *Phytother Res.* 23(6):874–877.
30. Nayal R, Abdullah K, Samah S. (2018). Phytochemical screening of *Alchemilla vulgaris, Sophora japonica, Crataegus azarolus,* and their inhibitory activity on lipase and α-amylase. *Int J Acad Sci Res.* 6(2):1–21.
31. Neagu E, Paun G, Albu C, Radu GL. (2015). Assessment of acetylcholinesterase and tyrosinase inhibitory and antioxidant activity of *Alchemilla vulgaris* and *Filipendula ulmaria* extracts. *J Taiwan Instit Chem Engineers.* 52:1–6.
32. Hwang E, Ngo HTT, Seo SA, Park B, Zhang M, Yi TH. (2018). Protective effect of dietary *Alchemilla mollis* on UVB-irradiated premature skin aging through regulation of transcription factor NFATc1 and Nrf2/ARE pathways. *Phytomed.* 39:125–136.
33. Shilova IV, Suslov NI, Samylina IA, Baeva VM, Lazareva NB, Mazin EV. (2020). Neuroprotective properties of common lady's mantle infusion. *Pharma Chem J.* 5311:1059–1062.
34. Vlaisavljević S, Jelača S, Zengin G, Mimica-Dukić N, Berežni S, Miljić M, Stevanović ZD. (2019). *Alchemilla vulgaris* agg. (Lady's mantle) from central Balkan: Antioxidant, anticancer and enzyme inhibition properties. *RSC Adv.* 9(64):37474–37483.
35. Ibrahim OHM, Abo-Elyousr KAM, Asiry KA, Alhakamy NA, Mousa MAA. (2022). Phytochemical characterization, antimicrobial activity and in vitro antiproliferative potential of *Alchemilla vulgaris* auct root extract against prostate (PC-3), breast (MCF-7) and colorectal adenocarcinoma (Caco-2) cancer cell lines. *Plants.* 11:2140.
36. Jelača S, Dajić-Stevanović Z, Vuković N, Kolašinac S, Trendafilova A. et al. (2022). Beyond traditional use of *Alchemilla vulgaris*: Genoprotective and antitumor activity in vitro. *Molecules* (Basel). 27(23):8113.
37. Shrivastava R, Cucuat N, John GW. (2007). Effects of *Alchemilla vulgaris* and glycerine on epithelial and myofibroblast cell growth and cutaneous lesion healing in rats. *Phytother Res.* 21(4):369–373.
38. Shrivastava RI, John GW. (2006). Treatment of aphthous stomatitis with topical *Alchemilla vulgaris* in glycerine. *Clin Drug Investig.* 26(10):567–573.
39. Petcu P, Andronescu E, Gheorgheci V. et al. (1979). Treatment of juvenile meno-metrorrhagia with *Alchemilla vulgaris* fluid extract. *Clucjul Med.* 52(3):266–270.
40. Said O, Saad B, Fulder S, Khalil K, Kassis E. (2011). Weight loss in animals and humans treated with "weighlevel", a combination of four

medicinal plants used in traditional Arabic and Islamic medicine. *Evid Based Complement Alternat Med.* 874538.

Anemone pulsatilla

1. Culpeper N. (1653). *The Complete Herbal.* Ware: Wordsworth Edition 1995.
2. Osbaldeston TA, Wood RPA (eds). (2000). *Dioscorides: De materia medica.* Johannesburg: Ibidis Press.
3. Gerard J. (1633). *The Herball or General History of Plants.* New York: Dover Publication Inc. 1975.
4. Culpeper N. (1653). *The Complete Herbal.* Ware: Wordsworth Edition 1995.
5. v. Störck A. (1771). *Abhandlung von dem heilsamen Gebrauch der Schwarzlichen Kuchenschelle (Pulsatilla nigricante).* Frankfurt.
6. Turner NJ. (1984). Counter-irritant and other medicinal uses of plants in Ranuculaceae by native peoples in British Columbia and neighbouring areas. *J Ethnopharmacol.* 11(2):181–201.
7. Felter HW, Lloyd JU. (1898). *King's American Dispensatory.*
8. Scudder JM. (1898). *The American Eclectic Materia Medica and Therapeutics.*
9. Felter HW. (1922). *The Eclectic Materia Medica, Pharmacology and Therapeutics.*
10. Palmer CD. (1919). *The Clinical Use of a Selection of Vegetable Remedies.*
11. Weiss RF. (1988). *Herbal Medicine.* Beaconsfield: Beaconsfield Publishers.
12. Mills S, Bone K. (2005). *The Essential Guide to Herbal Safety.* St Louis, MI: Elsevier-Churchill Livingstone.
13. Cao P, Wu FE, Ding LS. (2004). Advances in the studies on the chemical constituents and biologic activities for *Anemone* species. *Nat Prod Res Dev.* 16:581–584.
14. Zou ZJ, Liu HX, Yang JS. (2004). Phytochemical components and pharmacological activities of the genus *Anemone. Chin Pharm J.* 39:493–495.
15. Lipton RB, Göbel H, Einhäupl KM, Wilks K, Mauskop A. (2004). *Petasites hybridus* root (butterbur) is an effective preventive treatment for migraine. *Neurol.* 63(12):2240–2244.
16. Potter S. (1902). *A Compend of Materia Medica, Therapeutics, and Prescription Writing.*
17. Ballon L. (1904). Contribution à l'étude physiologique et thérapeutique des anémones. Thèse de Paris.

18. Pilcher JD, Burman DE, Delzell WR. (1916). The action of the so-called female remedies on the excised uterus of the guinea-pig. *Arch Intern Med.* 18(5):557–583.
19. Madaus G. (1938). *Lehrbuch der Biologischen Heilmittel.*
20. Saify ZS, Noor F, Mushtaq N, Dar A. (1998). Assessment of *Anemone pulsatilla* for some biological activities. *Pak J Pharma Sci.* 11(1):47–53.
21. Sun YX, Liu JC, Liu DY. (2011). Phytochemicals and bioactivities of *Anemone raddeana* Regel: A review. *Pharmazie.* 66:813–821.
22. Hao DC, Xiao PG, Ma H, Peng Y, He CN. (2015). Mining chemodiversity from biodiversity: Pharmacophylogeny of medicinal plants of the Ranunculaceae. *Chin J Nat Med.* 13:507–520.
23. Lee TH, Huang NK, Lai TC, Yang AT, Wang GJ. (2008). Anemonin, from *Clematis crassifolia*, potent and selective inducible nitric oxide synthase inhibitor. *J Ethnopharmacol.* 116:518–527.
24. Huang YH, Lee TH, Chan KJ, Hsu FL, Wu YC, Lee MH. (2008). Anemonin is a natural bioactive compound that can regulate tyrosinase-related proteins and mRNA in human melanocytes. *J Dermatol Sci.* 49(2):115–123.
25. Xiao K, Cao SR, Jiao le F, Lin FH, Wang L, Hu CH. (2016). Anemonin improves intestinal barrier restoration and influences TGF-β1 and EGFR signaling pathways in LPS-challenged piglets. *Innate Immun.* 22(5):344–352.
26. Duan H. (2006). Effect of anemonin on NO, ET-1 and ICAM-1 production in rat intestinal microvascular endothelial cells. *J Ethnopharmacol.* 104(3):362–366.
27. Jia D, Han B, Yang S, Zhao J. (2014). Anemonin alleviates nerve injury after cerebral ischemia and reperfusion (i/r) in rats by improving antioxidant activities and inhibiting apoptosis pathway. *J Mol Neurosci.* 53(2):271–279.
28. Martin ML, Ortíz de Urbina AV, Montero MJ, Carrón R, San Román L. (1988). Pharmacologic effects of lactones isolated from *Pulsatilla alpina* subsp. *Apiifolia*. *J Ethnopharmacol.* 24(2–3):185–191.
29. Tan C, Zhu W, Lu Y. (2002). Aloin, cinnamic acid and sophorcarpidine are potent inhibitors of tyrosinase. *Chin Med J* (Engl). 115(12):1859–1862.
30. Sun Y, Li M, Liu J. (2008). Haemolytic activities and adjuvant effect of *Anemone raddeana* saponins (ARS) on the immune responses to ovalbumin in mice. *Int Immunopharmacol.* 8:1095–1102.
31. Hao DC, Gu X, Xiao P. (2017). *Anemone* medicinal plants: Ethnopharmacology, phytochemistry and biology. *Acta Pharm Sin B.* 7(2):146–158.

32. Martin ML, Ortíz de Urbina AV, Montero MJ, Carrón R, San Román L. (1988). Pharmacologic effects of lactones isolated from *Pulsatilla alpina* subsp. *apiifolia*. *J Ethnopharmacol*. 24(2–3):185–191.
33. Martin ML, Ortíz de Urbina AV, Montero MJ, Carrón R, San Román L. (1988). Pharmacologic effects of lactones isolated from *Pulsatilla alpina* subsp. *apiifolia*. *J Ethnopharmacol*. 24(2–3):185–191.
34. Martin ML, Ortíz de Urbina AV, Montero MJ, Carrón R, San Román L. (1988). Pharmacologic effects of lactones isolated from *Pulsatilla alpina* subsp. *Apiifolia*. *J Ethnopharmacol*. 24(2–3):185–191.
35. Shi B, Liu W, Gao L, Chen C, Hu Z, Wu W. (2012). Chemical composition, antibacterial and antioxidant activity of the essential oil of *Anemone rivularis*. *J Med Plant Res*. 6:4221–4224.
36. Scudder JM. (1898). *The American Eclectic Materia Medica and Therapeutics*.
37. Mills S, Bone K. (2005). *The Essential Guide to Herbal Safety*. St Louis, MI: Elsevier-Churchill Livingstone.
38. Potter SOL. (1902). *A Compend of Materia Medica, Therapeutics, and Prescription*.
39. *The Pharmacopoeia of the United States of America*. (1890). 7th decennial rev. Philadelphia: National Convention for Revising the Phamacopoia [1893], p. 513.
40. Anonymous. (1996). *British Herbal Pharmacopoeia*. London: British Herbal Medicine Association.

Angelica sinensis

1. Hou TC. (2004). *Herbal Extracts*, vol. 1. Beijing: China Medical Scientific Technological Publishing Company, pp. 173–183.
2. Wu YC, Hsieh CL. (2011). Pharmacological effects of radix *Angelica sinensis* (*Danggui*) on cerebral infarction. *Chin Med*. 6:32.
3. Chen J, Chen T. (2004). Blood-tonifying herbs *Dang Gui* (*Radicis Angelicae sinensis*). *Chinese Med Herbol Pharmacol*. 17:3.
4. World Health Organization. (2001). *WHO Monographs on Selected Medicinal Plants*, vol 2. Geneva: WHO.
5. Suzuki A, Yamamoto M, Jokura H, Fujii A, Tokimitsu I, Hase T, Saito I. (2007). Ferulic acid restores endothelium-dependent vasodilation in aortas of spontaneously hypertensive rats. *Am J Hypertens*. 20:508–513.
6. Suzuki A, Yamamoto M, Jokura H, Fujii A, Tokimitsu I, Hase T, Saito I. (2007). Ferulic acid restores endothelium-dependent vasodilation in aortas of spontaneously hypertensive rats. *Am J Hypertens*. 20:508–513.

7. Yu Z, Ou-Yang JP, Liu YM, Zheng HQ, Yang JW, Tu SZ, Yang HL. (2000). The anti-atherogenetic effect of *Angelica* in rabbits aorta. *Zhongguo Dongmai Yinghua Zazhi*. 8(1):46–48.
8. Wang B, Ouyang J, Liu Y, Yang J, Wei L, Li K, Yang H. (2004). Sodium ferulate inhibits atherosclerogenesis in hyperlipidemia rabbits. *J Cardiovasc Pharmacol*. 43(4):549–554.
9. Lu GH, Chan K, Leung K, Chan CL, Zhao ZZ. et al. (2005). Assay of free ferulic acid and total ferulic acid for quality assessment of *Angelica sinensis*. *J Chromatogr A*. 1068(2):209–219.
10. Pen RX. (1981). Pharmacological effects of *danggui* (*Angelica sinensis*) on cardiovascular system. *Chin Trad Herb Drugs*. 12:321.
11. Cha L. (1981). Effects of *Angelica sinensis* on experimental arrhythmias. *Chin Pharmacol Bull*. 16:259.
12. Cha L, Chien CC, Lu FH. (1981). Antiarrhythmic effect of *Angelica sinensis* root, tetrandrine and *Sophora flavescens* root. *Chin Pharmacol Bull*. 16:53–54.
13. Wei ZM. (1985). A study on the electro-physiology in antiarrhythmia effect of *Angelica sinensis*. *J Beijing Coll Trad Chin Med*. 18:40–51.
14. Wang H, Peng RX. (1994). Sodium ferulate alleviated paracetamol-induced liver toxicity in mice. *Yao Hsueh Hsueh Pao*. 15:81–83.
15. Wu DF, Peng RX, Wang H. (1988). Sodium ferulate alleviates prednisolone-induced liver toxicity in mice. *Acta Pharmaceutica Sinica*. 30:801–805.
16. Wu DF, Peng RX. (1995). The effect of sodium ferulate on bromobenzene-induced liver injury in mice. *Zhongguo Yaoxue Zazhi*. 30:597–599.
17. Zuo AH, Wang L, Xiao HB. (2012). Research progress studies on pharmacology and pharmacokinetics of ligustilide. *Zhongguo Zhong Yao Za Zhi*. 37(22):3350–3353.
18. Haranaka K, Satomi N, Sakurai A, Haranaka R, Okada N, Kobayashi M. (1985). Antitumor activities and tumor necrosis factor producibility of traditional Chinese medicines and crude drugs. *Cancer Immunol Immunother*. 20(1):1–5.
19. Choy YM, Leung KN, Cho CS, Wong CK, Pang PK. (1994). Immunopharmacological studies of low molecular weight polysaccharide from *Angelica sinensis*. *Am J Chin Med*. 22(2):137–145.
20. Raman A, Lin ZX, Sviderskaya E, Kowalska D. (1996). Investigation of the effect of *Angelica sinensis* root extract on the proliferation of melanocytes in culture. *J Ethnopharmacol*. 54(2–3):165–170.
21. Kan WL, Cho CH, Rudd JA, Lin G. (2008). Study of the anti-proliferative effects and synergy of phthalides from *Angelica sinensis* on colon cancer cells. *J Ethnopharmacol*. 120(1):36–43.

22. Okuyama T, Takata M, Nishino H, Nishino A, Takayasu J, Iwashima A. (1990). Studies on the antitumor-promoting activity of naturally occurring substances. II. Inhibition of tumor-promoter-enhanced phospholipid metabolism by umbelliferous materials. *Chem Pharmacol Bull.* (Tokyo). 38(4):1084–1086.
23. Yin ZZ, Zhang LY, Xu LN. (1980). The effect of *Dang-Gui* (*Angelica sinensis*) and its ingredient ferulic acid on rat platelet aggregation and release of 5-HT. *Acta Pharmaceutica Sinica.* 15(6):321–326.
24. Lu GH, Chan K, Leung K, Chan CL, Zhao ZZ. et al. (2005). Assay of free ferulic acid and total ferulic acid for quality assessment of *Angelica sinensis*. *J Chromatogr A.* 1068(2):209–219.
25. Mei QB, Tao JY, Cui B. (1991). Advances in the pharmacological studies of radix *Angelica sinensis* (Oliv.) Diels (Chinese danggui). *Chinese Med J.* 104:776–781.
26. Ye YN, Liu ES, Shin VY, Koo MW, Li Y, Wei EQ, Matsui H, Cho CH. (2001). A mechanistic study of proliferation induced by *Angelica sinensis* in a normal gastric epithelial cell line. *Biochem Pharmacol.* 61(11):1439–1448.
27. Cho CH, Mei QB, Shang P, Lee SS, So HL, Guo X, Li Y. (2000). Study of the gastrointestinal protective effects of polysaccharides from *Angelica sinensis* in rats. *Planta Med.* 66(4):348–351.
28. Chou YP. (1979). The effect of *Angelica sinensis* on hemodynamics and myocardial oxygen consumption in dogs. *Acta Pharmaceutica Sinica.* 14:156–160.
29. Chen SG, Li CC, Zhuang XX. (1995). Protective effects of *Angelica sinensis* injection on myocardial ischemia/reperfusion injury in rabbits. *Zhongguo Zhong Xi Yi Jie He Za Zhi.* 15(8):486–488.
30. Yim TK, Wu WK, Pak WF, Mak DH, Liang SM, Ko KM. (2000). Myocardial protection against ischaemia-reperfusion injury by a *Polygonum multiflorum* extract supplemented 'Dang-Gui decoction for enriching blood', a compound formulation, ex vivo. *Phytother Res.* 14(3):195–199.
31. Kuang X, Yao Y, Du JR, Liu YX, Wang CY, Qian ZM. (2006). Neuroprotective role of Z-ligustilide against forebrain ischemic injury in ICR mice. *Brain Res.* 1102:145–153.
32. Hon PM, Lee CM, Choang TF, Chui KY, Wong HNC. (1990). A ligustilide dimer from *Angelica sinensis*. *Phytochem.* 29(4):1189–1191.
33. Hsu HY, Lin CC. (1996). A preliminary study on the radioprotection of mouse hematopoiesis by *dang-gui-shao-yao-san*. *J Ethnopharmacol.* 55(1):43–48.

34. Wang Y, Zhu B. (1996). The effect of *Angelica* polysaccharide on proliferation and differentiation of hematopoietic progenitor cells. *Chung Hua I Hsueh Tsa Chih*. 76:363–366.
35. Shi LF, Zheng XM, Cai Z, Wu BS. (1995). Comparison of influence of essential oil from *Ligusticum chuanxiong* Hort. on microcirculation in rabbit conjunctiva bulbar before and after decomposition of ligustilide. *Chin J Pharmcol Toxicol*. 9:157–158.
36. Lu GH, Chan K, Leung K, Chan CL, Zhao ZZ. et al. (2005). Assay of free ferulic acid and total ferulic acid for quality assessment of *Angelica sinensis*. *J Chromatogr A*. 1068(2):209–219.
37. Wang H, Li W, Li J, Rendon-Mitchell B, Ochani M. et al. (2006). The aqueous extract of a popular herbal nutrient supplement, *Angelica sinensis*, protects mice against lethal endotoxemia and sepsis. *J Nutr*. 136(2):360–365.
38. Liu SP, Dong WG, Wu DF, Luo HS, Yu JP. (2009). Protective effect of *Angelica sinensis* polysaccharide on experimental immunological colon injury in rat. *World J Gastroenterol*. 9(12):2786–2790.
39. Choy YM, Leung KN, Cho CS, Wong CK, Pang PK. (1994). Immunopharmacological studies of low molecular weight polysaccharide from *Angelica sinensis*. *Am J Chin Med*. 22(2):137–145.
40. Wilasrusmee C, Kittur S, Siddiqui J, Bruch D, Wilasrusmee S, Kittur DS. (2002). In vitro immunomodulatory effects of ten commonly used herbs on murine lymphocytes. *J Altern Complement Med*. 8(4):467–475.
41. Hirata JD, Swiersz LM, Zell B, Small R, Ettinger B. (1997). Does *dong quai* have estrogenic effects in postmenopausal women? A double-blind, placebo-controlled trial. *Fertil Steril*. 68(6):981–986.
42. Lau CB, Ho TC, Chan TW, Kim SC. (2005). Use of *dong quai* (*Angelica sinensis*) to treat peri- or postmenopausal symptoms in women with breast cancer: Is it appropriate? *Menopause*. 12(6):734–740.
43. Sun RY, Yan YZ, Zhang H, Li CC. (1989). Role of beta-receptor in the radix *Angelicae sinensis* attenuated hypoxic pulmonary hypertension in rats. *Chin Med J*. (Engl.). 102(1):1–6.
44. Ye TS, Zhang YW, Zhang XM. (2016). Protective effects of *Danggui Buxue Tang* on renal function, renal glomerular mesangium and heparanase expression in rats with streptozotocin-induced diabetes mellitus. *Exp Ther Med*. 11(6):2477–2483.
45. Shi M, Chang L, He G. (1995). Stimulating action of *Carthamus tinctorius* L., *Angelica sinensis* (Oliv.) Diels and *Leonurus sibiricus* L. on the uterus. *Chung Kuo Chung Yao Tsa Chih*. 20:173–175.

46. Pi XP. (1955). Effects of *Angelica sinensis* on uterus. *Nal Med J Chin.* 40:967.
47. Mei QB, Tao JY, Cui B. (1991). Advances in the pharmacological studies of radix *Angelica sinensis* (Oliv) Diels (Chinese dang gui). *Chin Med J.* 104:776–781.
48. Mei QB, Tao JY, Cui B. (1991). Advances in the pharmacological studies of radix *Angelica sinensis* (Oliv) Diels (Chinese dang gui). *Chin Med J.* 104:776–781.
49. Du J, Bai B, Kuang X, Yu Y, Wang C, Ke Y, Xu Y, Tzang AHC, Qian ZM. (2006). Ligustilide inhibits spontaneous and agonists- or K+ depolarization-induced contraction of rat uterus. *J Ethnopharmacol.* 108(1):54–58.
50. Chen JK, Chen TT, Crampton L. (2004). *Chinese Medical Herbology and Pharmacology.* City of Industry, CA: Art of Medicine Press.
51. Ko WC. (1980). A newly iolated antispasmodic—butylidenephthalide. *Jpn J Pharmcol.* 30(1):85–91.
52. Ozaki Y, Ma JP. (1990). Inhibitory effects of tetramethylpyrazine and ferulic acid on spontaneous movement of rat uterus in situ. *Chem Pharm Bull.* 38:1620–1623.
53. Du J, Bai B, Kuang X, Yu Y, Wang C, Ke Y, Xu Y, Tzang AHC, Qian ZM. (2006). Ligustilide inhibits spontaneous and agonists- or K+ depolarization-induced contraction of rat uterus. *J Ethnopharmacol.* 108(1):54–58.
54. Tao JY, Ruan YP, Mei QB, Liu S, Tian QL. et al. (1984). Studies on the antiasthmatic action of ligustilide of *dang-gui, Angelica sinensis* (Oliv.) Diels. *Yao Hsueh Hsueh Pao.* 19(8):561–565.
55. Wong AY, Chan KS, Lau WL, Tang LCH. (2007). Pregnancy outcome of a patient with atypical polypoid adenomyoma. *Fertil Steril.* 88(5):1438. e7–9.
56. World Health Organization. (2001). *WHO Monographs on Selected Medicinal Plants*, vol. 2. Geneva: WHO.
57. Mueller A. (1899). Versuche über die Wirkungsweise des Extrakts des chinesischen Emmenagogon *Tang-kui* (*Man-mu*) oder Eumenol-Merek. *Münchener Medizinische Wochenschrift.* 46:796–798.
58. Palm R. (1910). Erfahrungen mit Eumenol. *Münchener Medizinische Wochenschrift.* 1:23–25.
59. Buck P. (1899). Un nouveau remède spécifique contre la dysménorrhée: l'eumenol. *Belgique médicale.* 2:363–365.
60. Langes H. (1901). Beobachtungen bei der Verwendung einiger neuer Medikamente. Eumenol, Dionin und Stypticin. *Therapeutische Monatshefte.* 7:363.

61. Mueller A. (1899). Versuche über die Wirkungsweise des Extrakts des chinesischen Emmenagogon *Tang-kui* (*Man-mu*) oder Eumenol-Merek. *Münchener Medizinische Wochenschrift*. 46:796–798.
62. Gao YM, Zhang H, Duan ZX. (1988). Treatment of 112 cases of dysmenorrhea wuth *danggui jingyou* pill. *J Lanzhou Med Coll*. 1:36–38.
63. Gao YM, Zhang H, Duan ZX. (1988). Treatment of 112 cases of dysmenorrhea wuth *danggui jingyou* pill. *J Lanzhou Med Coll*. 1:36–38.
64. Chang HM, But PPH. (eds). (1986). *Pharmacology and Applications of Chinese Materia Medica*, vol. 1. Philadelphia: World Scientific Publishing.
65. Hirata JD, Swiersz LM, Zell B, Small R, Ettinger B. (1997). Does *dong quai* have estrogenic effects in postmenopausal women? A double-blind, placebo-controlled trial. *Fertil Steril*. 68(6):981–986.
66. Al-Bareeq RJ, Ray AA, Nott L, Pautler SE, Razvi H. (2010). *Dong Quai* (*Angelica sinensis*) in the treatment of hot flashes for men on androgen deprivation therapy: Results of a randomized double-blind placebo controlled trial. *Can Urol Assoc J*. 4(1):49–53.
67. Kupfersztain C, Rotem C, Fagot E, Kaplan B. (2003). The immediate effect of natural plant extract, *Angelica sinensis* and *Matricaria chamomilla* (Climex) for the treatment of hot flushes during menopause. A preliminary report. *Clin Exp Obst Gynec*. 30(4):203–206.
68. Burke BE, Olson RD, Cusack BJ. (2002). Randomized, controlled trial of phytoestrogen in the prophylactic treatment of menstrual migraine. *Biomed Pharmacother*. 56(6):283–288.
69. Fu YF, Xia Y, Shi YP, Sun NQ. (1988). Treatment of 34 cases of infertility due to tubal occlusion with compound *danggui* injection by irrigation. *Jiangsu J Trad Chin Med*. 9(1):15–16.
70. Terasawa K, Imadaya A, Tosa H, Mitsuma T, Toriizuke K. et al. (1985). Chemical and clinical evaluation of crude drugs derived from *Angelica acutiloba* and *A. sinensis*. *Fitoterapia*. 56(4):201–208.
71. Chen JK, Chen TT, Crampton L. (2004). *Chinese Medical Herbology and Pharmacology*. City of Industry, CA: Art of Medicine Press.
72. *Liao Ning Zhong Yi Za Zhi* (Liaoning Journal of Chinese Medicine) (1982). 6:40.
73. Bradley RR, Cunniff PJ, Pereira BJ, Jaber BL. (1999). Hematopoietic effect of radix *Angelicae sinensis* in a hemodialysis patient. *Am J Kidney Dis*. 134(2):349–354.
74. Liu YM, Zhang JJ, Jiang J. (2004). Observation on clinical effect of *Angelica* injection in treating acute cerebral infarction. *Zhongguo Zhongxiyi Jiehe Zazhi*. 24(3):205–208. In Chinese.

75. Xu J, Li G. (2000). Observation on short-term effects of *Angelica* injection on chronic obstructive pulmonary disease patients with pulmonary hypertension. *Zhongguo Zhong Xi Yi Jie He Za Zhi.* 20(3):187–189. In Chinese.
76. Zheng L. (1992). Short-term effect and the mechanism of radix *Angelicae* on pulmonary hypertension in chronic obstructive pulmonary disease. *Zhonghua Jie He He Hu Xi Za Zhi.* 15(2):95–97, 127. In Chinese.
77. Zhou QJ. (1985). Chinese medicinal herbs in the treatment of viral hepatitis. In: Chang HM, Yeung HW, Tso WW, Koo A. (eds). *Advances in Chinese Medicinal Materials Research.* Singapore: World Scientific Press, pp. 215–219.
78. Lo A, Chan K, Yeung JH, Woo KS. (1995). Danggui (*Angelica sinensis*) affects the pharmacodynamics but not the pharmacokinetics of warfarin in rabbits. *Eur J Drug Metab Pharmacokinet.* 20(1):55–60.
79. Fung FY, Wong WH, Ang SK, Koh HL, Kun MC, Lee LH, Li X, Ng HJ, Tan CW, Zhao Y, Linn YC. (2017). A randomized, double-blind, placebo-controlled study on the anti-haemostatic effects of *Curcuma longa*, *Angelica sinensis* and *Panax ginseng*. *Phytomed.* 32:88–96.
80. Zhu DP. (1987). Dong quai. *Am J Chin Med.* 15(3–4):117–125.
81. Pharmacopoeia Commission of the People's Republic of China. (1997). *Pharmacopoeia of the People's Republic of China*, English ed. Beijing: Chemical Industry Press.

Capsella bursa-pastoris

1. Grieve M. (1971). *A Modern Herbal.* New York: Dover Publications.
2. Bastien J.W. (1983). Pharmacopeia of Qollahuaya Andeans. *J Enthonopharmacol.* 8(1):97–111.
3. Kim H, Song MJ. (2013). Ethnomedicinal practices for treating liver disorders of local communities in the southern regions of Korea. *Evid Based Complement Alternat Med.* 869176.
4. Khare CP. (2007). *Indian Medicinal Plants: An Illustrated Dictionary.* New York: Springer Science & Business Media, p. 119.
5. Goodyer J. (trans.). (1959). *Dioscorides De materia Medica: The Greek Herbal of Dioscorides.* New York: Hafner Pub. Co.
6. Culpeper N, Ferrier WJ. (1932). *Culpeper's English Physician and Complete Herbal.* London: W. & G. Foyle.
7. Ellingwood F, Lloyd JU. (1983). *American Materia Medica, Therapeutics and Pharmacognosy*, 11th ed. [1898], repr. Portland: Eclectic Medical Publications.
8. Maisch JM. (1888). Notes on some old remedies. *Am J Pharm.* 16(7).

9. Fernie WT. (1897). *Herbal Simples Approved for Modern Uses of Cure.* Bristol: John Wright & Co.
10. Harste W. (1928). Die medizinische Wirkung der *Capsella Bursa pastoris* sowie der auf ihr lebenden Parasiten *Cystopus candidus* und *Peronospora parasitica* mit besonderer Berücksichtigung des Entwicklungsganges der beiden Pilze. *Arch Pharm.* 266(3):133–151.
11. Grieve M. (1971). *A Modern Herbal.* New York: Dover Publications.
12. Harste W. (1928). Die medizinische Wirkung der *Capsella Bursa pastoris* sowie der auf ihr lebenden Parasiten *Cystopus candidus* und *Peronospora parasitica* mit besonderer Berücksichtigung des Entwicklungsganges der beiden Pilze. *Arch Pharm.* 266(3):133–151.
13. Steinmetz EF. (1954). *Materia Medica Vegetabilis.* Amsterdam: Steinmetz, p. 81.
14. Weiss RF. (1988). *Herbal Medicine.* [Trans. by AR Meuss from the 6th German ed. of *Lehrbuch der Phytotherapie*]. Gothenburg: AB Arcanum.
15. Felter HW, Lloyd JU. (1898). *King's American Dispensatory.*
16. Chripkova M, Zigo F, Mojzis J. (2016). Antiproliferative efect of indole phytoalexins. *Molecules* (Basel). 21(12):1626.
17. Schuman E. (1939). Newer concepts of blood coagulation and control of haemorrhage. *Am J Obstet Gynecol.* 38:1002–1007.
18. Steinberg A. Segal HI, Parris HM. (1940). Role of oxalic acid and certain related dicarboxylic acids in the control of haemorrhage. *Ann Otol Rhinol Laryngol.* 49:1008–1021.
19. Vermathen M, Glasl H. (1993). Effect of the herb extract of *Capsella bursa-pastoris* on blood coagulation. *Planta Med.* 59(Supp.A):670.
20. Cha JM, Suh WS, Lee TH, Subedi L, Kim SY, Lee KR. (2017). Phenolic glycosides from *Capsella bursa-pastoris* (L.) Medik and their anti-inflammatory activity. *Molecules* (Basel). 22(6):1023.
21. Kuroda K, Kaku T. (1969). Pharmacological and chemical studies on the alcohol extract of *Capsella bursa-pastoris. Life Sci.* 8(3):151–155.
22. Al-Snafi AE. (2015). The chemical constituents and pharmacological effects of *Capsella bursa-pastoris*—A review. *Int J Pharmacol Toxicol.* 5:76–81.
23. Alizadeh H, Jafari B, Babae T. (2012). The study of antibacterial effect of *Capsella bursa-pastoris* on some of gram positive and gram negative bacteria. *J Basic Appl Sci Res.* 2(7):6940–6945.
24. Kuroda K, Akao M. (1981). Antitumor and anti-intoxication activities of fumaric acid in cultured cells. *Gann.* 72(5):777–782.
25. Kuroda K, Takagi K. (1968). Physiologically active substance in *Capsella bursa-pastoris. Nature.* 220(168):707–708.

26. Jurisson S. (1971). Determination of active substances of *Capsella bursa pastoris*. *Tartu Riiliku Ulikooli Toim*. 270:71–79.
27. Kuroda K, Takagi K. (1969). Studies on *Capsella bursa pastoris*. I. General pharmacology of ethanol extract of the herb. *Arch Int Pharmacodyn Ther*. 178(2):382–391.
28. Kuroda K, Kaku T. (1969). Pharmacological and chemical studies on the alcohol extract of *Capsella bursa-pastoris*. *Life Sci*. 8(3):151–155.
29. Alqasoumi SI, Al-Rehaily AJ, AlSheikh AM, Abdel-Kader MS. (2008). Evaluation of the hepatoprotective effect of *Ephedra foliate*, *Alhagi maurorum*, *Capsella bursa-pastoris* and *Hibiscus sabdariffa* against experimentally induced liver injury in rats. *Nat Prod Sci*. 14(2):95–99.
30. Alqasoumi SI. (2007). Isolation and chemical structure elucidation of hepatoprotective constituents from plants used in traditional medicine in Saudi Arabia. PhD thesis, College of Pharmacy, King Saud University.
31. European Medicines Agency. (2011). Assessment report on *Capsella bursa-pastoris* (L.) Medikus, herba.
32. Blumenthal M, Busse WR, Goldberg A, Gruenwald J, Hall T. et al. (eds). (1998). *The Complete German Commission E Monographs: Therapeutic Guide to Herbal Medicines*. Austin: American Botanical Council.
33. Jurisson S. (1971). Determination of active substances of *Capsella bursa pastoris*. *Tartu Riiliku Ulikooli Toim*. 270:71–79.
34. Jurisson S. (1971). Determination of active substances of *Capsella bursa pastoris*. *Tartu Riiliku Ulikooli Toim*. 270:71–79.
35. Grosso C, Vinholes J, Silva LR, de Pinho BG, Gonçalves RF, Valentão P, Jäger AK, Andrade PB. (2011). Chemical composition and biological screening of *Capsella bursa-pastoris*. *Braz J Pharmacog*. 21(4):635–644.
36. Shipochliev T. (1981). Uterotonic action of extracts from a group of medicinal plants. *Vet Med Nauki*. 18:94–98.
37. Kuroda K, Takagi K. (1968). Physiologically active substance in *Capsella bursa-pastoris*. *Nature*. 220(168):707–708.
38. Jurisson S. (1971). Determination of active substances of *Capsella bursa pastoris*. *Tartu Riiliku Ulikooli Toim*. 270:71–79.
39. Shipochliev T. (1981). Uterotonic action of extracts from a group of medicinal plants. *Vet Med Nauki*. 18:94–98.
40. Naafe M, Kariman N, Keshavarz Z, Khademi N, Mojab F, Mohammadbeigi A. (2018). Effect of hydroalcoholic extracts of *Capsella bursa-pastoris* on heavy menstrual bleeding: A randomized clinical trial. *J Altern Complement Med*. 24(7):694–700.

41. Ghalandari S, Kariman N, Sheikhan Z, Mojab F, Mirzaei M, Shahrahmani H. (2017). Effect of hydroalcoholic extract of *Capsella bursa pastoris* on early postpartum hemorrhage: A clinical trial study. *J Altern Complement Med.* 23(10):794–799.

Caulophyllum thalictriodes

1. Flannery M. (2012). Blue cohosh root *Caulophyllum thalictroides*: history. In A. Romm, R. Upton (eds). *American Herbal Pharmacopoeia and Therapeutic Compendium.* Scotts Valley, CA: American Herbal Pharmacopoeia.
2. Smith P. (1813). *The Indian Doctor's Dispensatory: being Father Smith's Advice Respecting Diseases and their Cure.* Cincinnati: Browne and Looker.
3. Erichsen-Brown C. (1979). *Medicinal and Other Uses of North American Plants.* New York: Dover Publications.
   Vogel VJ. (1970). *American Indian Medicine.* Norman, OK: University of Oklahoma Press.
4. Moerman D. (2000). *Native American Ethnobotany*, 3rd ed. Portland, OR: Timber Press.
5. Rafinesque C. (1828–1830). *Medical Flora: A Manual of the Medical Botany of the United States of North America*, 2 vols. Philadelphia: pub. unknown.
6. Bergner P. (2001). *Caulophyllum*: Cardiotoxic effects of blue cofosh on a fetus. *Med Herbalism.* 12(1):12–14.
7. Osol A, Farrar G. (1947). *The Dispensatory of the United States of America*, 24th ed. Philadelphia: J.B. Lippincott.
8. Lloyd J, Lloyd C. (1884–1887). *Drugs and Medicines of North America.* Bull. Lloyd Library of Botany, Pharmacy and Materia Medica. Reproduction Series No 9. Cincinnati, OH: Lloyd Library.
9. Scudder J. (1870). *Specific Medication and Specific Medicines.*
10. Felter H, Lloyd J. (1898). *King's American Dispensatory.*
11. King J. (1855). *American Eclectic Obstetrics.*
12. Lloyd J, Lloyd C. (1884–1887). *Drugs and Medicines of North America.* Bull. Lloyd Library of Botany, Pharmacy and Materia Medica. Reproduction Series No 9. Cincinnati, OH: Lloyd Library.
13. Ellingwood F. (1908). The true action of *Caulophyllum* (blue cohosh). *Ellingwood's Therapeutist.* 2(9):30.
14. Osol A, Farrar G. (1947). *The Dispensatory of the United States of America*, 24th ed. Philadelphia: J.B. Lippincott.
15. Allaire AD, Moos M-K, Wells SR. (2000). Complementary and alternative medicine in pregnancy: A survey of North Carolina certified nurse-midwives. *Obstet Gynecol.* 95(1):19–23.

16. Declercq ER, Sakala C, Corry MP, Applebaum S, Risher P. (2002). *Listening to Mothers: Report of the First National U.S. Survey of Women's Childbearing Experiences*. New York: Maternity Center Association.
17. Lothian JA. (2006). Saying "no" to induction. *J Perinatal Educ.* 15(2):43–45.
18. Bayles B. (2007). Herbal and other complementary medicine use by Texas midwives. *J Midwifery Women's Health.* 52(5):473–478.
19. McFarlin BL, Gibson MH, O'Rear J, Harman P. (1999). A national survey of herbal preparation use by nurse-midwives for labor stimulation. Review of the literature and recommendations for practice. *J Nurse-Midwifery.* 44(3):205–216.
20. Low Dog T. (2004). *Women's Health in Complementary and Integrative Medicine: A Clinical Guide*. St Louis, MO: Elsevier.
21. Rader JI, Pawar RS. (2013). Primary constituents of blue cohosh: Quantification in dietary supplements and potential for toxicity. *Analyt Bioanalyt Chem.* 405(13):4409–4417.
22. Schmeller T, Sauerwein M, Sporer F, Wink M, Müller, WE. (1994). Binding of quinolizidine alkaloids to nicotinic and muscarinic acetylcholine receptors. *J Nat Prod.* 57(9):1316–1319.
23. Flynn TJ, Kennelly EJ, Mazzola EP. et al. (1998). Screening of the dietary supplement blue cohosh for potentially teratogenic alkaloids using rat embryo culture [abstract]. *Teratology.* 57(4–5):219.
24. Scott CC, Chen KK. (1943). The pharmacological action of N-methylcytisine. *J Pharmacol Exp Ther.* 79:334.
25. Keeler R. (1976). Lupin alkaloids from teratogenic and nonteratogenic lupins. III. Identification of anagyrine as the probable teratogen by feeding trials. *J Toxicol Environ Health.* 1:887–898.
26. Eichelbaum M, Spannbrucker N, Steincke B. et al. (1979). Defective N-oxidation of sparteine in man: A new pharmacogenetic defect. *Eur J Clin Pharmacol.* 16:183–187.
27. Vinks A, Inaba T, Otton SV. et al. (1982). Sparteine metabolism in Canadian Caucasians. *Clin Pharmacol Ther.* 31(1):23–29.
28. El-Tahir K. (1991). Pharmacological actions of magnoflorine and aristolochic acid-1 isolated from the seeds of *Aristolochia bracteata*. *Int J Pharmacog.* 29:101.
29. Baillie N, Rasmussen P. (1997). Black and blue cohosh in labor. *NZ Med J.* 110:20–21.
30. Ferguson HC, Edwards LD. (1954). A pharmacological study of a crystalline glycoside of *Caulophyllum thalictroides*. *J Am Pharm Assoc.* 43:16–21.

31. Benoit PS, Fong HH, Svoboda GH, Farmsworth NR. (1976). Biological and phytochemical evaluation of plants XIV. Anti-inflammatory evaluation of 163 species of plants. *Lloydia*. 39(2–3):160–171.
32. Stanley B. (2007). *Caulophyllum thalictroides* induces mild bradycardia on frog hearts in situ. Thesis. St Paul, MN: Bethel University.
33. Chaudrasekhar K, Raa Vishwanath C. (1974). Studies on the effect of *Caulophyllum* on implantation in rats. *J Reprod Fertil*. 38:245–246.
34. Pilcher JD, Delzell WR, Burman GE. (1916). The action of the so-called female remedies on the excised uterus of the guinea-pig. *Arch Intern Med*. 18:557–583.
35. Ali Z, Khan IA. (2008). Alkaloids and saponins from blue cohosh. *Phytochem*. 69(4):1037–1042.
36. Berger J, DeGolier T. (2008). Pharmacological effects of the aqueous extract of *Caulophyllum thalictroides* (blue cohosh) on isolated Mus musculus uteri. *BIOS*. 79(3):103–114.
37. Chandler F. (ed.). (2000). *Herbs: Everyday Reference for Health Professionals*. Ottowa: Canadian Pharmacists Association, pp. 57–59.
38. Ferguson HC, Edwards LD. (1954). A pharmacological study of a crystalline glycoside of *Caulophyllum thalictroides*. *J Am Pharm Assoc*. 43(1):16–21.
39. Pilcher JD, Delzell WR, Burman GE. (1916). The action of various "female" remedies on the excised uterus of the guinea pig. *JAMA*. 67:490–492.
40. Pilcher J, Maurer R. (1918). The action of "female remedies" on intact uteri of animals. *Surg Gynecol Obstet*. 27:97–99.
41. Wu M, Hu Y, Ali Z, Khan IA, Verlangeiri AJ, Dasmahapatra AK. (2010). Teratogenic effects of blue cohosh (*Caulophyllum thalictroides*) in Japanese medaka (*Oryzias latipes*) are probably mediated through GATA2/EDN1 signaling pathway. *Chem Res Toxicol*. 23(8):1405–1416.
42. Hardin JW, Arena JM. (1974). *Human Poisoning from Native and Cultivated Plants*, 2nd ed. Durham, NC: Duke University Press, p. 60.
43. Rao RB, Hoffman RS. (2002). Nicotinic toxicity from tincture of blue cohosh (*Caulophyllum thalictroides*) used as an abortifacient. *Vet Hum Toxicol*. 44(4):221–222.
44. Jones TK, Lawson BM. (1998). Profound neonatal congestive heart failure caused by maternal consumption of blue cohosh herbal medication. *J Pediatr*. 132:550–552.
45. Finkel RS, Zarlengo KM. (2004). Blue cohosh and perinatal stroke. *N Engl J Med*. 351(3):302–303.

46. Finkel RS. (2004). More on blue cohosh and perinatal stroke/ The Author's Reply. *N Engl J Med.* 351(21):2239–2241.
47. Gunn TR, Wright IM. (1996). The use of black and blue cohosh in labour. *NZ Med J.* 109(1032):410–11.
48. Wright IMR. (1999). Neonatal effects of maternal consumption of blue cohosh. *J Pediatr.* 134(3):384–385.
49. Baillie N, Rasmussen P. (1997). Black and blue cohosh in labor. *NZ Med J.* 110(1036):20–21.
50. Satchithanandam S, Grundel E, Roach J, White KD, Mazzola E. et al. (2008). Alkaloids and saponins in dietary supplements of blue cohosh (*Caulophyllum thalictroides*). *J AOAC Int.* 91(1):21–32.
51. Smith P. (1813). *The Indian Doctor's Dispensatory: being Father Smith's Advice Respecting Diseases and their Cure.* Cincinnati: Browne and Looker.
52. Erichsen-Brown C. (1979). *Medicinal and Other Uses of North American Plants.* New York: Dover Publications.
53. Low Dog T. (2009). The use of botanicals during pregnancy and lactation. *Altern Ther Health Med.* 15(1):54–58.
Flannery M. (2012). Blue cohosh root *Caulophyllum thalictroides*: history. In A. Romm, R. Upton (eds). *American Herbal Pharmacopoeia and Therapeutic Compendium.* Scotts Valley, CA: American Herbal Pharmacopoeia.

Leonurus cardiaca

1. Dong Y, Liao J, Yao K, Jiang W, Wang J. (2017). Application of Traditional Chinese medicine in treatment of atrial fibrillation. *Evid Based Complement Alternat Med.* 1381732.
2. Shikov AN, Pozharitskaya ON, Makarov VG, Wagner H, Verpoorte R, Heinrich M. (2014). Medicinal plants of the Russian pharmacopoeia; their history and applications. *J Ethnopharmacol.* 154(3):481–536.
3. Fierascu RC, Fierascu I, Ortan A, Fierascu IC. et al. (2019). *Leonurus cardiaca* L. as a source of bioactive compounds: An update of the European Medicines Agency Assessment Report (2010). *BioMed Res Int.* 4303215.
4. Shikov AN, Tsitsilin AN, Pozharitskaya ON, Makarov VG, Heinrich M. (2017). Traditional and current food use of wild plants listed in the Russian *Pharmacopoeia*. *Front Pharmacol.* 8:841.
5. Gerard J. (1597). *The Herball or Generall History of Plants.*
6. Parkinson J. (1640). *Theatrum Botanicum.*

7. Culpeper N. (1652). *The English Physician*.
8. Moerman DE. (2009). *Native American Medicinal Plants: An Ethnobotanical Dictionary*. Portland, OR: Timber Press.
9. Cook W. (1869). *The Physio-medical Dispensatory*.
10. Felter HW, Lloyd JU. (1898). *King's American Dispensatory*.
11. Felter HW. (1922). *The Eclectic Materia Medica, Pharmacology and Therapeutics*.
12. Cheng K, Yip C, Yeung H, Kong Y. (1979). Leonurine, an improved synthesis. *Experientia*. 35(5):571–572.
13. Kong YC, Yeung HW, Cheung YM, Hwang JC, Chan YW. et al. (1976). Isolation of the uterotonic principle from *Leonurus artemesia*, the Chinese motherwort. *Am J Chin Med*. 4(4):373–382.
14. Wojtyniak K, Szymański M, Matławska I. (2013). *Leonurus cardiaca* L. (motherwort): A review of its phytochemistry and pharmacology. *Phytother Res*. 27(8):1115–1120.
15. Barnes J, Anderson LA, Phillipson JD. (2007). *Herbal Medicines*, 3rd ed. London: Pharmaceutical Press.
16. Rezaee-Asl M, Sabour M, Nikoui V, Ostadhadi S, Bakhtiarian A. (2014). The study of analgesic effects of *Leonurus cardiaca* L. in mice by formalin, tail flick and hot plate tests. *Int Schol Res Notices*. 687697.
17. Song X, Wang T, Zhang Z. et al. (2014). Leonurine exerts anti-inflammatory effect by regulating inflammatory signaling pathways and cytokines in LPS-induced mouse mastitis. *Inflammation*. 38(1):79–88.
18. Wu H, Dai A, Chen X. et al. (2018). Leonurine ameliorates the inflammatory responses in lipopolysaccharide-induced endometritis. *Internat Immunopharmacol*. 61:156–161.
19. Sadowska B, Micota B, Rozalski M, Redzynia M, Rozalski M. (2017). The immunomodulatory potential of *Leonurus cardiaca* extract in relation to endothelial cells and platelets. *J Innate Immunity*. 23(3):285–295.
20. Jafari S, Salaritabar A, Moradi A, Khanavi M, Samadi M. (2010). Antioxidant activity and total phenolic content of extracts and fractions of cultivated *Leonurus cardiaca* L. *Planta Med*. 76:376.
21. Matkowski A, Tasarz P, Szypuła E. (2008). Antioxidant activity of herb extracts from five medicinal plants from *Lamiaceae*, subfamily *Lamioideae*. *J Med Plants Res*. 2(11):321–330.
22. Rauwald HW, Savtschenko A, Merten A, Rusch C, Appel K, Kuchta K. (2015). GABAA receptor binding assays of standardized *Leonurus cardiaca* and *Leonurus japonicus* extracts as well as their isolated constituents. *Planta Med*. 81(12–13):1103–1110.

23. Ritter M, Melichar K, Strahler S. et al. (2010). Cardiac and electrophysiological effects of primary and refined extracts from *Leonurus cardiaca* L. (Ph. Eur.). *Planta Med*. 76(6):572–582.
24. Wojtyniak K, Szymański M, Matławska I. (2013). *Leonurus cardiaca* L. (motherwort): A review of its phytochemistry and pharmacology. *Phytother Res*. 27(8):1115–1120.
25. Arustamova FA. (1963). Hypotensive action of *Leonurus cardiaca* from Azerbaidzhan in experimental chronic hypertension of animals. *Izvest Akad Nauk Armyansk SSR Biol Nauki*. 16(7):47–52.
26. Seo DY, Lee SR, Heo JW, No MH, Rhee BD. et al. (2018). Ursolic acid in health and disease. *Kor J Physiol Pharmacol*. 22(3):235–248.
27. Xie X, Zhang Z, Wang X, Luo Z, Lai B. et al. (2018). Stachydrine protects eNOS uncoupling and ameliorates endothelial dysfunction induced by homocysteine. *Mol Med*. 24(1):10.
28. Kuang PG, Zhou XF, Zhang FY, Lang SY. (1988). Motherwort and cerebral ischemia. *J Tradit Chin Med*. 8(1):37–40.
29. Liu C, Yin H, Gao J, Xu X, Zhang T, Yang Z. (2016). Leonurine ameliorates cognitive dysfunction via antagonizing excitotoxic glutamate insults and inhibiting autophagy. *Phytomed*. 23(13):1638–1646.
30. Zou QZ, Bi RG, Li JM, Feng JB, Yu AM, Chan HP, Zhen MX. (1989). Effects of motherwort on blood hyperviscosity. *Am J Chin Med*. 17(1–2):65–70.
31. Xu D, Chen M, Ren X, Ren X, Wu Y. (2014). Leonurine ameliorates LPS-induced acute kidney injury via suppressing ROS-mediated NF-κB signaling pathway. *Fitoterapia*. 97:148–155.
32. Cheng H, Bo Y, Shen W. et al. (2015). Leonurine ameliorates kidney fibrosis via suppressing TGF-β and NF-κB signaling pathway in UUO mice. *Internat Immunopharmacol*. 25(2):406–415.
33. Yeung HW, Kong YC, Lay WP, Cheung KF. (1977). The structure and biological effect of leonurine—a uterotonic principle from the Chineses drug, *I-mu Ts'ao*. *Planta Med*. 31(1):51–56.
34. Kong YC, Yeung HW, Cheung YM, Hwang JC, Chan YW. et al. (1976). Isolation of the uterotonic principle from *Leonurus artemesia*, the Chinese motherwort. *Am J Chin Med*. 4(4):373–382.
35. Cheng F, Zhou Y, Wang M, Guo C, Cao Z, Zhang R, Peng C. (2020). A review of pharmacological and pharmacokinetic properties of stachydrine. *Pharmacol Res*. 155:104755.
36. Shikov AN, Pozharitskaya ON, Makarov VG, Demchenko DV, Shikh EV. (2011). Effect of *Leonurus cardiaca* oil extract in patients with arterial hypertension accompanied by anxiety and sleep disorders. *Phytother Res*. 25(4):540–543.

37. Liu W, Ma S, Pan W, Tan W. (2016). Combination of motherwort injection and oxytocin for the prevention of postpartum hemorrhage after cesarean section. *J Matern Fetal Neonatal Med.* 29(15):2490–2493.

Mitchella repens

1. United Plant Savers. (2012). Species At-Risk. Online. Available at http://www.unitedplantsavers.org/species-at-risk. [accessed 1 March 2015]
2. Scudder JM. (1870). *Specific Medication and Specific Medicines.*
3. Webster HT. (1996). Mitchella repens. *Eclectic Med J.* 2:23.
4. Niederkorn JS, Ellingwood F. (1908). *Ellingwood's Therapeutist,* vol. 2.
5. Niederkorn JS, Ellingwood F. (1908). *Ellingwood's Therapeutist,* vol. 2.
6. Felter HW, Lloyd JU. (1898). *King's American Dispensatory.*
7. Mills E, Duguoa JJ, Perri D, Koren G. (2006). *Herbal Medicines in Pregnancy and Lactation. An Evidence-Based Approach.* London: Taylor Francis.
8. Hooper S, Chandler R. (1984). Herbal remedies of the maritime Indians: Phytoesterols and triterpenes of 67 plants. *J Ethnopharmacol.* 10:181–194.
9. Felter HW. (1993). *The Eclectic Materia Medica, Pharmacology and Therapeutics* [1922]. Portland:OR: Eclectic Medical Publications.
10. Felter HW. (1993). *The Eclectic Materia Medica, Pharmacology and Therapeutics* [1922]. Portland:OR: Eclectic Medical Publications.
11. Ellingwood F. (1919). *The American Materia Medica, Therapeutics and Pharmacognosy.*
12. Horner S, DeGolier T. (2021). Mitchella repens (partridge berry) contracts uterine smooth muscle in isolated mouse tissues. *J Med Plant Sci.* 9(3):123–128.

Rubus ideaus

1. Gerard J. (1597). *The Herball or Generall History of Plants.*
2. Hamel PB, Chiltoskey MU. (1975). *Cherokee Plants and Their Uses.* Sylva NC: Herald Publishers.
Beckstrom-Sternberg SM, Moerman DE, Duke JA. (n.d.). The Medicinal Plants of Native America Database.
3. Thomson S. (1832). *New Guide to Health, or, Botanic Family Physician*, 8th ed. Columbus, OH: Pike, Platt & Co.
4. Coffin A I. (1866). *Treatise on Midwifery and the Diseases of Women and Children*, 13th ed. Repr. Windsor: Yesterday's Books, 1995.
5. Felter HW, Lloyd JU. (1898). *King's Amerian Dispensatory.*

6. Hool RL. (1918). *Health from British Wild Herbs*. Southport: WH Webb.
7. Fletcher-Hyde F. (1942). *Rubus idaeus*. *Herb Pract*. 3:4–5.
8. Pallivalappila AR, Stewart D, Shetty A, Pande B, McLay JS. (2013). Complementary and alternative medicines use during pregnancy: A systematic review of pregnant women and healthcare professional views and experiences. *Evid Based Complement Alternat Med*. 205639.
9. Byrne MJ, Semple S, Coulthard KP. (2002). Complementary medicine use during pregnancy. Interviews with 48 women in a hospital antenatal ward. *Aust Pharm*. 21:954–959.
10. Skouteris H, Wertheim EH, Rallis S, Paxton SJ, Kelly L, Milgrom J. (2008). Use of complementary and alternative medicines by a sample of Australian women during pregnancy. *Aust N Z J Obstet Gynaecol*. 48(4):384–390.
11. Frawley J, Adams J, Sibbritt D, Steel A, Broom A, Gallois C. (2013). Prevalence and determinants of complementary and alternative medicine use during pregnancy: Results from a nationally representative sample of Australian pregnant women. *Aust N Z J Obstet Gynaecol*. 53(4):347–352.
12. Forster DA, Denning A, Wills G, Bolger M, McCarthy E. (2006). Herbal medicine use during pregnancy in a group of Australian women. *BMC Pregnancy Child*. 6:21.
13. Mollart L, Skinner V, Adams J, Foureur M. (2018). Midwives' personal use of complementary and alternative medicine (CAM) influences their recommendations to women experiencing a post-date pregnancy. *Women Birth*. 31(1):44–51.
14. Whitehouse B. (1941). Fragarine: An inhibitor of uterine action. *BMJ*. 13:370–371.
15. Burn JH, Withell ER. (1941). A principle in raspberry leaves which relaxes uterine muscle. *Lancet*. 2:1–3.
16. Beckett AH, Belthle FW, Fell KR, Lockett MF. (1954). The active constituents of raspberry leaves. *J Pharm Pharmacol*. 6:785–794.
17. Bamford DS, Percival RC, Tothill AU. (1970). Raspberry leaf tea: A new aspect to an old problem. *Br J Pharmacol*. 40(1):161–162.
18. Rojas-Vera J, Patel AV, Dacke CG. (2002). Relaxant activity of raspberry (*Rubus idaeus*) leaf extract in guinea-pig ileum in vitro. *Phytother Res*. 16(7):665–658.
19. Olson A, Degolier T. (2016). Contractile activity of *Rubus idaeus* extract on isolated mouse uterine strips. *BIOS*. 87:39–47.

20. Zheng J, Pistilli MJ, Holloway AC, Crankshaw DJ. (2010). The effects of commercial preparations of red raspberry leaf on the contractility of the rat's uterus in vitro. *Reprod Sci.* 17(5):494–501.
21. Langhammer AJ, Nilsen OG. (2014). In vitro inhibition of human CYP1A2, CYP2D6, and CYP3A4 by six herbs commonly used in pregnancy. *Phytother Res.* 28(4):603–610.
22. Whitehouse B. (1941). Fragarine: An inhibitor of uterine action. *BMJ.* 13:370–371.
23. Simpson M, Parsons M, Greenwood J, Wade K. (2001). Raspberry leaf in pregnancy: Its safety and efficacy in labor. *J Midwif Women's Health.* 46(2):51–59.
24. Parsons M, Simpson M, Ponton T. (1999). Raspberry leaf and its effect on labour: Safety and efficacy. *Aust Coll Midwives Incorp J.* 12:20–25.
25. Nordeng H, Bayne K, Havnen GC, Paulsen BS. (2011). Use of herbal drugs during pregnancy among 600 Norwegian women in relation to concurrent use of conventional drugs and pregnancy outcome. *Complement Ther Clin Pract.* 17(3):147–151.
26. Cheang KI, Nguyen TT, Karjane NW, Salley KE. (2016). Raspberry leaf and hypoglycemia in gestational diabetes mellitus. *Obstet Gynecol.* 128(6):1421–1424.
27. Burn JH, Withell ER. (1941). A principle in raspberry leaves which RELAXES uterine muscle by. *Lancet.* 238(6149):1–3.
28. Beckett AH, Belthle FW, Fell KR. (1954). The active constituents of raspberry leaves; a preliminary investigation. *J Pharm Pharmacol.* 6(11):785–796.
29. Hastings-Tolsma M, Stoffel RT, Quintana AS, Kane RR, Turner J, Wang X. (2022). Effect of *Rubus idaeus* L. consumption during pregnancy on maternal mice and their offspring. *J Med Food.* 25(2):183–191.
30. Johnson J, Makaji E, Ho S. et al. (2009). Effect of maternal raspberry leaf consumption in rats on pregnancy outcome and the fertility of the female offspring. *Reprod Sci.* 16:605–609.
31. Makaji E, Ho SH, Holloway AC, Crankshaw DJ. (2011). Effects in rats of maternal exposure to raspberry leaf and its constituents on the activity of cytochrome p450 enzymes in the offspring. *Int J Toxicol.* 30(2):216–224.
32. Parsons M, Simpson M, Ponton T. (1999). Raspberry leaf and its effect on labour: Safety and efficacy. *Aust Coll Midwives Incorp J.* 12:20–25.
33. Bamford DS, Percival RC, Tothill AU. (1970). Raspberry leaf tea: A new aspect to an old problem. *Br J Pharmacol.* 40(1):161–162.

Thuja occidentalis

1. Parkinson J. (1640). *Theatrum Botanicum*.
2. Felter HW, Lloyd JU. (1898). *King's American Dispensatory*.
3. Remington JP, Wood HC. (1918). *The Dispensatory of the United States of America*.
4. Ellingwood F. (1919). *The American Materia Medica, Therapeutics and Pharmacognosy*.
5. Felter HW. (1922). *The Eclectic Materia Medica, Pharmacology and Therapeutics*.
6. Ellingwood F. (1908). *Ellingwood's Therapeutist*, vol. 2.
7. Wizenmann K. (1930). *Heilung und Heiligung*, vol. 4, p. 1386.
8. Madaus G. (1938). *Textbook of Biological Remedies*.
9. Alves LDS, Figueirêdo CBM, Silva CCAR, Marques GS, Ferreira PA. et al. (2014). *Thuja occidentalis* L. (Cupressaceae): Review of botanical, phytochemical, pharmacological and toxicological aspects. *Int J Pharm Sci Res*. 5:1163–1177.
10. Caruntu S, Ciceu A, Olah NK, Don I, Hermenean A, Cotoraci C. (2020). *Thuja occidentalis* L. (Cupressaceae): Ethnobotany, phytochemistry and biological activity. *Molecules* (Basel). 25(22):5416.
11. Gohla SH, Zeman RA, Bogel M, Jurkiewicz E, Schrum S. et al. (1992). Modification of the in vitro replication of the Human Immunodeficiency Virus HIV-1 by TPSg, a polysaccaride fraction isolated from the Cupressaceae *Thuja occidentalis* L. (Arborvitae). *Haematol Blood Transfus*. 35:140–149.
12. Gohla SH, Zeman RA, Gartner S, Popovic M, Jurkiewics E. et al. (1990). Inhibition of the replication of HIV-1 by TPSg, a polysaccharide-fraction isolated from the cupressaceae *Thuja occidentalis* L. *AIDS Res Hum Retrovir*. 6:131.
13. Frenkel M, Mishra BM, Sen S, Yang P, Pawlus A. et al. (2010). Cytotoxic effects of ultra-diluted remedies on breast cancer cells. *Int J Oncol*. 36:395–403.
14. Silva IS, Nicolau LAD, Sousa FBM, de Araújo S, Oliveira AP. et al. (2017). Evaluation of anti-inflammatory potential of aqueous extract and polysaccharide fraction of *Thuja occidentalis* Linn. in mice. *Int J Biol Macromol*. 105:1105–1116.
15. Stan MS, Voicu SN, Caruntu S, Nica IC, Olah NK. et al. (2019). Antioxidant and anti-inflammatory properties of a *Thuja occidentalis* mother tincture for the treatment of ulcerative colitis. *Antioxidants*. 8:416.

16. Bhargava SK, Singh TG, Mannan A, Singh S, Singh M, Gupta S. (2022). Pharmacological evaluation of *Thuja occidentalis* for the attenuation of neuropathy via AGEs and TNF-α inhibition in diabetic neuropathic rats. *Environ Sci Pollut Res Int.* 29(40):60542–60557.
17. Jahan N, Ahmad M, Mehjabeen, Zia-ul-haq M, Alam SM, Qureshi M. (2010). Antimicrobial screening of some medicinal plants of Pakistan. *Pak J Bot.* 42:4281–4284.
18. Jirovetz L, Buchbauer G, Denkova Z, Slavchev A, Stoyanova A, Schmidt E. (2006). Chemical composition, antimicrobial activities and odor descriptions of various *Salvia* sp. and *Thuja* sp. essential oils. *Ernährung Nutr.* 30:152–159.
19. Digrak M, Bagci E, Alma MH. (2002). Antibiotic action of seed lipids from five tree species grown in Turkey. *Pharm Biol.* 40:425–428.
    Gupta G, Srivastava AK. (2002). In-vitro activity of *Thuja occidentalis* Linn. against human pathogenic aspergilli. *Homoeopath Herit.* 27:5–12.
20. Tsiri D, Graikou K, Pobłocka-Olech L, Krauze-Baranowska M, Spyropoulos C, Chinou I. (2009). Chemosystematic value of the essential oil composition of *Thuja* species cultivated in Poland—antimicrobial activity. *Molecules* (Basel). 14:4707–4715.
21. Torres A, Vargas Y, Uribe D, Carrasco C, Torres C. et al. (2016). Proapoptotic and anti-angiogenic properties of the α/β-thujone fraction from *Thuja occidentalis* on glioblastoma cells. *J Neurooncol.* 128:9–19.
22. Siveen KS, Kuttan G. (2011). Augmentation of humoral and cell mediated immune responses by thujone. *Int Immunopharmacol.* 11:1967–1975.
23. Caruntu S, Ciceu A, Olah NK, Don I, Hermenean A, Cotoraci C. (2020). *Thuja occidentalis* L. (Cupressaceae): Ethnobotany, phytochemistry and biological activity. *Molecules* (Basel). 25(22):5416.
24. Dubey SK, Barta A. (2009). Antioxidant activities of *Thuja occidentalis* Linn. *Asian J Pharm Clin Res.* 2:73–76.
25. Aziz A, Khan IA, Ahmed MB, Munawar SH, Manzoor Z, Bashir S, Raza MA. (2014). Evaluation of antipyretic activity of *Thuja occidentalis* Linn. in PGE1 and TAB-vaccine induced pyrexia models in rabbits. *Int J Pharm Sci.* 4:481–484.
26. Dubey SK, Batra A. (2009). Role of phenolics in anti-atherosclerotic property of *Thuja occidentalis* Linn. *Ethnobot Leafl.* 13:791–800.
27. Won JN, Lee SY, Song DS, Poo H. (2013). Antiviral activity of the plant extracts from *Thuja orientalis*, *Aster spathulifolius*, and *Pinus thunbergii* against influenza virus A/PR/8/34. *J Microbiol Biotechnol.* 23(1):125–130.

28. Das S, Rani R. (2013). Antioxidant and gastroprotective properties of the fruits of *Thuja occidentalis*, Linn. *Asian J Biochem Pharm Res.* 3:80–87.
29. Ellingwood F. (1919). *The American Materia Medica, Therapeutics and Pharmacognosy.*
30. Dubey SK, Batra A. (2008). Hepatoprotective activity from ethanol fraction of *Thuja occidentalis* Linn. *Asian J Res Chem.* 1:32–35.
31. Saeed F, Jahan N, Mehjabeen S, Alam SM, Ahmad M. (2014). Effects of *Thuja occidentalis* extract on histo-pathological parameters in rabbits treated with and without carbon tetrachloride. *Br J Med Health Res.* 1:16–24.
32. Tyagi CK, Porwal P, Mishra N, Sharma A, Chandekar A. et al. (2019). Antidiabetic activity of the methanolic extracts of *Thuja occidentalis* twings in alloxan-induced rats. *Curr Trad Med.* 5(2):138–143.
33. Sunila ES, Hamsa TP, Kuttan G. (2011). Effect of *Thuja occidentalis* and its polysaccharide on cell-mediated immune responses and cytokine levels of metastatic tumor-bearing animals. *Pharm Biol.* 49(10):1065–1073.
34. Vömel T. (1985). Der Einfluss eines pflanzlichen Immunstimulans auf die Phagozytose von Erythrozyten durch das retikulohistozytäre System der isoliert perfundierten Rattenleber [Effect of a plant immunostimulant on phagocytosis of erythrocytes by the reticulohistiocytary system of isolated perfused rat liver]. *Arzneimittelforschung.* 35(9):1437–1439.
35. Sunila ES, Kuttan G. (2005). Protective effect of *Thuja occidentalis* against radiation-induced toxicity in mice. *Integr Cancer Ther.* 4(4):322–328.
36. Bodinet C, Freudenstein J. (1999). Effects of an orally applied aqueous-ethanolic extract of a mixture of *Thujae occidentalis* herba, *Baptisiae tinctoriae* radix, *Echinaceae purpureae* radix and *Echinaceae pallidae* radix on antibody response against sheep red blood cells in mice. *Planta Med.* 65:695–699.
37. Bodinet C, Lindequist U, Teuscher E, Freudenstein J. (2002). Effect of an orally applied herbal immunomodulator on cytokine induction and antibody response in normal and immunosuppressed mice. *Phytomed.* 9:606–613.
38. Bodinet C, Mentel R, Wegner U, Lindequist U, Teuscher E, Freudenstein J. (2002). Effect of oral application of an immunomodulating plant extract on influenza virus type A infection in mice. *Planta Med.* 68:896–900.

39. Joseph R, Pulimood SA, Abraham P, John GT. (2013). Successful treatment of *Verruca vulgaris* with *Thuja occidentalis* in a renal allograft recipient. *Indian J Nephrol.* 23(5):362–364.
40. Murali S, Saravanam PK, Dinakaran N. (2020). Role of *thuja* in the management of laryngeal papilloma. *BMJ Case Rep.* 13(12):e238846.
41. Reitz HD, Hergarten H. (1990). Immunmodulatoren mit pflanzlichen Wirkstoffen–2. Teil: eine wissenschaftliche Studie am Beispiel Esberitox® N. *Notabene Medici.* 20:304–306, 362–366.
42. Henneicke-von Zepelin HH, Hentschel C, Schnitker J, Kohnen R, Köhler G, Wüstenberg P. (1999). Efficacy and safety of a fixed combination phytomedicine in the treatment of the common cold (acute viral respiratory tract infection): Results of a randomised, double blind, placebo controlled, multicentre study. *Curr Med Res Opin.* 15:214–227.
43. Naser B, Lund B, Henneicke-von Zepelin HH, Köhler G, Lehmacher W, Scaglione F. (2005). A randomized, double-blind, placebo-controlled, clinical dose-response trial of an extract of *Baptisia*, *Echinacea* and *Thuja* for the treatment of patients with common cold. *Phytomed.* 12(10):715–722.
44. Stolze H, Forth H. (1983). Eine Antibiotikabehandlung kann durch zusätzliche Immunstimulierung optimiert werden. *Der Kassenarzt.* 23:43–48.
45. Hauke W, Köhler G, Henneicke-von Zepelin HH, Freudenstein J. (2002). Esberitox®N as supportive therapy when providing standard antibiotic treatment in subjects with a severe bacterial infection (acute exacerbation of chronic bronchitis). *Chemother.* 48:259–266.
46. Bendel R, Bendel V, Renner K, Carstens V, Stolze K. (1989). Zusatzbehandlung mit Esberitox N bei Patientinnen mit chemostrahlentherapeutischer Behandlung eines fortgeschrittenen Mammakarzinoms [Additional treatment with Esberitox N in patients with chemo-radiotherapy treatment of advanced breast cancer]. *Onkologie.* 12(Suppl. 3):32–38.
47. Bendel R, Bendel V, Renner K, Stolze K. (1988). Zusatzbehandlung mit Esberitox bei Patientinnen mit kurativer adjuvanter Bestrahlung nach Mammakarzinom [Supplementary treatment with Esberitox of female patients undergoing curative adjuvant irradiation following breast cancer]. *Strahlenther Onkol.* 164(5):278–283.
48. Cherepyuk O, Oktysyuk Y, Bazalytska A, Rozhko M. (2020). Correction of disordered oral immunity in children affected by dental caries with herbal immune modulator "Esberitox". *Pharmacia.* 67(4):347–450.

49. Saller R, Hellstern A, Hellenbrecht D. (1996). Chemische und toxikologische Eigenschaften von Thujon. *Internist Prax.* 36:553–556.
50. Hänsel R, Keller R, Rimpler H, Schneider G. (1994). *Hagers Handbuch der Pharmazeutischen Praxis: Drogen P–Z (Thuja)*, 5th ed. Berlin: Springer Verlag, pp. 955–966.
51. Felter HW, Lloyd JU. (1989). *King's American Dispensatory*.
52. Jungmichel G. (1932). Thuja-Vergiftung, todliche, durch Verwendung der Zweige als Abortivum. *Archives of Toxicology.* 3(1):89–90.
53. Bostelmann HC, Bödeker RH, Dames W, Henneicke-von Zepelin HH, Siegers CP, Stammwitz U. (2002). Immunmodulation durch pflanzliche Wirkstoffe. *Fortschr Med.* 120:119–123.
54. Henneicke-von Zepelin HH, Hentschel C, Schnitker J, Kohnen R, Köhler G, Wüstenberg P. (1999). Efficacy and safety of a fixed combination phytomedicine in the treatment of the common cold (acute viral respiratory tract infection): Results of a randomised, double blind, placebo controlled, multicentre study. *Curr Med Res Opin.* 15:214–227.
55. Naser B, Lund B, Henneicke-von Zepelin HH, Köhler G, Lehmacher W, Scaglione F. (2005). A randomized, double-blind, placebo-controlled, clinical dose-response trial of an extract of *Baptisia*, *Echinacea* and *Thuja* for the treatment of patients with common cold. *Phytomed.* 12(10):715–722.
56. Hauke W, Köhler G, Henneicke-von Zepelin HH, Freudenstein J. (2002). Esberitox®N as supportive therapy when providing standard antibiotic treatment in subjects with a severe bacterial infection (acute exacerbation of chronic bronchitis). *Chemother.* 48:259–266.
57. Reitz HD, Hergarten H. (1990). Immunmodulatoren mit pflanzlichen Wirkstoffen–2. Teil: eine wissenschaftliche Studie am Beispiel Esberitox® N. *Notabene Medici.* 20:304–306, 362–366.

Viburnum prunifolium

1. Scudder JM. (1870). *Specific Medication and Specific Medicines*.
2. Felter HW. (1922). *The Eclectic Materia Medica, Pharmacology and Therapeutics*.
3. Ellingwood F. (1908). *Ellingwood's Therapeutist*.
4. Cook W. (1869). *The Physio-medical Dispensatory*.
5. Shennan T. (1896). Experimental research into the action of *Viburnum Prunifolium* (Black Haw). *Trans Edinb Obstet Soc.* 21:34–48.
6. Felter HW, Lloyd JU. (1898). *King's American Dispensatory*.

7. The Pharmaceutical Society of Great Britain. (1911). *The British Pharmaceutical Codex: An Imperial Dispensatory for the Use of Medical Practitioners and Pharmacists.*
8. Cometa MF, Parisi L, Palmery M, Meneguz A, Tomassini L. (2009). In vitro relaxant and spasmolytic effects of constituents from *Viburnum prunifolium* and HPLC quantification of the bioactive isolated iridoids. *J Ethnopharmacol.* 123(2):201–207.
9. Hörhammer L, Wagner H, Reinhardt H. (1967). On new constituents from the bark of *Viburnum prunifolium* L. *J Am Pharm Assoc.* 34:205–207.
10. Jarboe CH, Zirvi KA, Nicholson JA, Schmidt CM. (1967). Scopoletin, an antispasmodic component of *Viburnum opulus* and *prunifolium. J Med Chem.* 10(3):488–489.
11. Cometa MF, Parisi L, Palmery M, Meneguz A, Tomassini L. (2009). In vitro relaxant and spasmolytic effects of constituents from *Viburnum prunifolium* and HPLC quantification of the bioactive isolated iridoids. *J Ethnopharmacol.* 123(2):201–207.
12. Munch JC, Pratt HJ. (1941). Studies on *Viburnum* XI: Bioassay methods. *Pharm Arch.* 12:88–91.
13. Grote IW, Woods M. (1947). Studies on *Viburnum* III: The uterine sedative action of various fractions. *J Am Pharm Assoc.* 36:191–192.
14. Evans WE, Harne WG, Krantz JC. (1942). A uterine principle from *Viburnum prunifolium. J Pharmacol.* 75:174–177.
15. Jarboe CH, Schmidt CM, Nicholson JA, Zirvi KA. (1966). Uterine relaxant properties of *Viburnum. Nature.* 212:837.
16. Cometa MF, Parisi L, Palmery M, Meneguz A, Tomassini L. (2009). In vitro relaxant and spasmolytic effects of constituents from *Viburnum prunifolium* and HPLC quantification of the bioactive isolated iridoids. *J Ethnopharmacol.* 123(2):201–207.
17. Balansard G, Chausse D, Boukef K. et al. (1983). Selection criteria for a Viburnum extract, *Viburnum prunifolium* L., as a function of its veinotonic and spasmolytic action. *Plantes Med Phytother.* 17(3):123–132.

Appendix: Vitamins and mineral, food sources

1. Fischer LM, da Costa KA, Kwock L, Galanko J, Zeisel SH. (2010). Dietary choline requirements of women: Effects of estrogen and genetic variation. *Am J Clin Nutr.* 92(5):1113–1119.

2. Lenton KJ, Sané AT, Therriault H, Cantin AM, Payette H, Wagner JR. (2003). Vitamin C augments lymphocyte glutathione in subjects with ascorbate deficiency. *Am J Clin Nutr.* 77(1):189–195.
3. Gambelunghe C, Rossi R, Micheletti A, Mariucci G, Rufini S. (2001). Physical exercise intensity can be related to plasma glutathione levels. *J Physiol Biochem.* 57(2):9–14.
4. Elokda AS, Nielsen DH. (2007). Effects of exercise training on the glutathione antioxidant system. *Eur J Cardiovasc Prev Rehabil.* 14(5):630–637.
5. Gulec M, Ozkol H, Selvi Y, Tuluce Y, Aydin A, Besiroglu L, Ozdemir PG. (2012). Oxidative stress in patients with primary insomnia. *Prog Neuropsychopharmacol Biol Psychiatry.* 37(2):247–251.
6. Jones DP, Coates RJ, Flagg EW, Eley JW, Block G, Greenberg RS, Gunter EW, Jackson B. (1992). Glutathione in foods listed in the National Cancer Institute's Health Habits and History Food Frequency Questionnaire. *Nutr Cancer.* 17(1):57–75.
7. Bianchini F, Vainio H. (2001). Allium vegetables and organosulfur compounds: Do they help prevent cancer? *Environ Health Perspect.* 109(9):893–902.
8. Bogaards JJ, Verhagen H, Willems MI, van Poppel G, van Bladeren PJ. (1994). Consumption of Brussels sprouts results in elevated alpha-class glutathione S-transferase levels in human blood plasma. *Carcinogenesis.* 15(5):1073–1075.
9. Soto C, Pérez J, García V, Uría E, Vadillo M, Raya L. (2010). Effect of silymarin on kidneys of rats suffering from alloxan-induced diabetes mellitus. *Phytomed.* 17(14):1090–1094.
10. Donatus IA, Sardjoko, Vermeulen NP. (1990). Cytotoxic and cytoprotective activities of curcumin. Effects on paracetamol-induced cytotoxicity, lipid peroxidation and glutathione depletion in rat hepatocytes. *Biochem Pharmacol.* 39(12):1869–1875.
11. Fischer LM, da Costa KA, Kwock L, Galanko J, Zeisel SH. (2010). Dietary choline requirements of women: Effects of estrogen and genetic variation. *Am J Clin Nutr.* 92(5):1113–1119.

INDEX

abnormal bleeding, 5, 8, 200
   Rubus ideaus, 290
   Vitex agnus-castus, 41
adenomyosis, 4, 5, 8, 31, 154
   Anemone pulsatilla, 263
   Herbs preclinical research, 173
AGC-US. *See* Atypical Glandular Cells of Undetermined Significance
atypical Glandular Cells of Undetermined Significance (AGC-US), 201
alkalinising herbs, 80
adaptogens, 34, 37, 56, 57, 81, 131, 132, 133, 186, 241, 204, 223, 234, 245
alopecia, 140
amenorrhoea, **46–65**, 12, 125
   Achillea millefolium, 18
   Actaea racemosa, 56, 57
   Alchemilla vulgaris, 58
   Anemone pulsatilla, 14
   Angelica sinensis, 22, 59
   anovulatory, 47, 48

   Artemisia vulgaris, 59
   causes of, 50–52
   control of menstrual cycle, 47
   dietary and lifestyle recommendations, 63–65
   Eclectics' recommendations, 61
   functional hypothalamic, 265
   herbal management of functional hypothalamic amenorrhoea, 55–57
   herbs research related to, 62–63
   information to gain, 48–49
   investigations, 49–50
   Leonurus cardiaca, 59, 60
   lifestyle, relaxation techniques and exercise, 65
   lignans and isoflavones intake, 63–64
   ovulatory, 47
   primary, 46
   red flags, 49
   Schisandra chinensis, 60
   secondary, 46–47

specific foods, 64
vitamins and minerals, 64
Zingiber officinale, 16
AMH. *See* anti-Müllerian hormone
anti-Müllerian hormone (AMH), 62, 69, 77, 84, 87, 129, 132, 135, 137, 149
anaerobic bacteria, vaginal, 94, 97, 105
analgesics, 5, 7, 22, 269
analgesics, herbal, 14, 161
   Achillea millefolium, 18, 252
   Actaea racemose, 166
   Andrographis paniculate, 173
   Anemone pulsatilla, 14, 261, 262, 263
   Calophyllum inophyllum, 236
   Foeniculum vulgare, 23
   Leonurus cardiaca, 283
   Myrtus communis, 113
   Rosa damascene fructus, 24
   Vitex agnus castus, 170
anti-androgenic herbs, 132, 137, 140
anti-inflammatory herbs, 12, 13, 38, 105, 123, 161, 162, 186, 204, 234
   Achillea millefolium, 18, 39, 251, 252
   Actaea racemosa, 18, 58, 166, 187
   Alchemilla vulgaris, 39, 58, 166, 256, 258
   Anemone pulsatilla, 167, 263, 264
   Angelica sinensis, 266, 267
   Arctostaphylos uva ursi, 105, **107**
   Calendula officinalis, 168
   Calophyllum inophyllum, 236
   Capsella bursa-pastoris, 40, 188, 273
   Caulophyllum thalictirodes, 278
   Cinnamomum zeylandicum, 41
   coconut oil, 237
   Curcuma longa, 174, 193, 206
   Filipendula ulmaria, 210
   Glycyrrhiza glabra, 189
   Humulus lupulus, 175
   Hydrocotyle asiatica, 170, 235
   lavender EO, 237
   Leonurus cardiaca, 284
   Matricaria chamomilla, 19, 237
   Myrtus communis, 210

Paeonia lactiflora, 175
Paeonia lactiflora and *Glycyrrhiza glabra*, 21
Phytolacca decandra, 223
resveratrol, 172
Ricinus communis, 192
Rosa damascene fructus, 21
Salix alba, 21
Thuja occidentalis, 297
Viburnum prunifolium, 15
Vitex agnus castus, 21, 170, 225
Zingiber officinale, 16, 42
anti-inflammatory foods/diet, 36, 38, 42. 149, 150, 177, 178, 196, 237
anti-oestrogenic, 221
   clomiphene, 77, 80, 81, 127
   letrozole, 77
   Depo-Provera, 68,
   Danazol, 68, 184, 221
   curcumin, 174
   Tamoxifen, 184
   smoking, 184
   Serenoa repens, 140
anti-haemorrhagic herbs, 36, 186
antispasmodic, 12, 13, 86, 161
antispasmodic, spasmolytic herbs
   Anemone pulsatilla, 261, 262
   Anethum graveolens, 22
   Dioscorea villosa, 19
   Leonurus cardiaca, 283
   Matricaria chamomilla, 19
   Paeonia lactiflora and *Glycyrrhiza glabra*, 20, 21
   Tanacetum parthenium, 176
   Valeriana officinalis, 15
   Viburnum prunifolium, 15, 170, 301, 302
   Zingiber officinalis, 16
antipruritics, 234
antimicrobial, herbs, 104, 105, 244
   Achillea millefolium, 252
   Arctostaphylos uva ursi, 107
   Calendula officinalis, 108
   Capsella bursa-pastoris, 273
   Hydrastis canadensis, 109, 110
   Melaleuca alternifolia, EO, 110

Pulsatilla chinensis and *Pulsatilla koreana*, 262
Thuja occidentalis, 295, 297
Thymus vulgaris, 111
anovulatory cycle, 30, 31, 34, 47, 48, 63, 87, 88, 89, 91, 125, 126, 243
aromatase, 47, 63, 128, 156, 157, 159, 182, 190
  increase, *Galega officinalis*, 147
  increase, *Paeonia lactiflora* & *Glycyrrhiza glabra*, 132, 163
  inhibit, berberine, 190
  inhibit, *Linum usitatissimum*, 152
  inhibit, resveratrol, 163, 172, 193
  inhibit, *Urtica dioica radix*, 148
ASC. *See* Atypical Squamous Cells
Atypical Squamous Cells, (ASC), 201
Asherman's syndrome, 47, 49
atypical polypoid adenomyoma, 59, 83, 268
autoimmune, 55, 159, 173, 175, 227, 232, 234, 236, 252
Avicenna, 43, 64

bacterial vaginosis (BV), 71, 79, 95, 96–98, 101, 103, 105 *See also* vaginal discharge
  Allium sativa, 106
  Calendula officinalis, 108
  clinical studies with specific food, 15–116
  clinical studies, vaginal applications, 113, 114
  conventional, treatment, 98
  herbal management, 104, 105
  Hydrastis canadensis, 110
  pathophysiology, 97–98
  probiotics, 112
  risk factors, 98
  Thymus vulgaris, 111
beer, 64, 194, 282
benign prostatic hyperplasia (BHP), 140
berberine, 87, 105, 110, 132, 142, 190, 210
17 beta-HSD. *See* 17 betahydroxysteroid dehydrogenase

17 betahydroxysteroid dehydrogenase (17 beta-HSD), 44, 138, 159, 184
betaine, 116, 303
BHP. *See* benign prostatic hyperplasia
bitters, 56, 204, 234, 244, 245
Blackwell, E., 256
Bombelon, 40, 272
brassica family vegetables, 311
breast disorders, benign, **215–230**
  Calendula officinalis, 223
  clinical trials, herbs, 225
  clinical trials, specific foods and nutrients, 229–230
  conventional treatment, 221
  cyclic mastalgia, 215–216
  dietary and lifestyle recommendations, 226–230
  differential diagnosis, 218–220
  fibrocystic breast changes, 215
  Ginkgo biloba, 223
  herbal management of, 222, 223
  herbs used in clinical practice, 223–225
  information obtained from case history, 216
  investigations, 217–221
  iodine and breast tissue, 226–227
  isoflavone phytoestrogen-rich foods, 228
  noncyclic mastalgia, 216
  non-proliferative lesions, 215
  pathophysiology of, 221–222
  physical examination, 216–217
  Phytolacca decandra, 223–224
  red flag, 217
  Vitex agnus-castus, 224–225
brenner tumours, 122. *See also* ovarian cysts
Bright's disease, 250
British Herbal Medicine Association (BHMA), x
British Herbal Pharmacopoeia (BHP), x
Burn, J. H., 291
BV. *See* bacterial vaginosis

Ca++ channel blocking activity, 12, 13, 18, 20, 22, 23
CA125. *See* cancer antigen, 125
calcium antagonists, 12. *See also* Ca++ channel blocking activity
cancer antigen, 125 (CA125), 120, 172, 175
cAMP. *See* 3′,5′-cyclic adenosine monophosphate
candidiasis, vaginitis, vulvovaginalis candidiasis, VVC, 94, 95, 98–99, 107, 110, 112. *See also* vaginal discharge
    achillea millefolium, 252
    Arctostaphylos uva ursi, 107
    clinical evidence, 113–114
    conventional treatment, 99
    dietary and lifestyle recommendation, 114–117
    Hydrastis canadensis, 110
    melaleuca alternifolia EO, 110
    probiotics, 112
    risk factors, 99
    symptoms, 98–99
    Thymus vulgaris, 111
castor oil, 192–193, 442
catechol-O-methyltransferase, 188, 195
CBT. *See* Cognitive Behavioral Therapy
cell adhesion, 159, 163, 171
cervical dysplasia, 100, **198–214**
    Astragalus membranaceus, 205
    Calendula officinalis, 209
    Camellia sinensis, 205–206
    categories of dysplasia, 199
    conventional treatment, 202–203
    Curcuma longa, 206
    dietary and lifestyle recommendations, 211–214
    Echinacea purpurea and *angustifolia*, 207
    Filipendula ulmaria, 210
    Ganoderma lucidum, 207–208
    herbal management of, 203–205
    herbs used in clinical practice, 205–211
    individual nutrients, 212–214
    internal treatment, 204
    investigations, 201–202
    Myrtus communis, 210
    Panax ginseng, 208
    pessary recipe, 211
    preclinical studies, 210–211
    prevention, 202
    risk factors for, 199–200
    symptoms, 200
    Thuja occidentalis, 208–209, 296, 299
    topical local treatment, 205
cervical intraepithelial neoplasia (CIN), 71, 201
cervical stenosis, 10, 47, 71
cervicitis, 10, 71, 102, 201
chancroids, 295
chlamydia, 5, 6, 95, 100, 102, 103, 106, 156, 182, 199, 295. *See also* vaginal discharge
chocolate cysts. *See* endometriomas
chocolate, 64, 228, 303, 306
choline, 241, 283, 303, 304, 311
CIN. *See* cervical intraepithelial neoplasia
cinnamic acid, 264
clomiphene, 58, 69, 77, 80, 81, 82, 88, 89, 92, 127, 136, 145, 148, 151
COCPs. *See* oral contraceptive pill
Coenzyme Q10, 92, 304–305
Coffin, A. I., 289
Cognitive Behavioral Therapy (CBT), 65
combined oral contraceptive pills (Cs). 33, 36, 99, 156. *See* oral contraceptive pill
conception, 58, 66, 74, 78, 82, 83, 89, 90, 91, 92, 146, 149, 160, 171, 256, 259, 293
Cook, W., 282
corpus luteum deficiency, luteal defect, luteal deficiency, luteal phase defect, 34, 37, 41, 54, 55, 61, 62, 63, 68, 74, 76, 78, 82, 83, 84, 85, 87, 136, 141, 160
corticotropin-releasing hormone (CRH), 53, 54, 60

costochondritis, 221
COX. *See* cyclooxygenase
Cox-2. *See* cyclooxygenase-2
CRH. *See* corticotropin-releasing hormone
CRP. *See* C-reactive protein
C-reactive protein, 143, 148, 149, 168, 196, 229
Culpeper, N., xi, 58, 59, 82, 250, 256, 260, 261, 282, 289
Curcuma longa, 105, 123, 162, 163, 164, 165, 166, 174, 185, 186, 204, 206, 234, 245, 305
curcumin, 113, 143, 164, 165, 171, 174, 193, 206, 213, 225, 238, 305
3′,5′-cyclic adenosine monophosphate (cAMP), 20, 222, 228, 230
cyclooxygenase (COX), 10, 11, 13, 16, 24, 26, 42, 156, 159, 166, 172, 174, 176, 193, 258
cyclooxygenase-2 (COX-2), 18, 20, 39, 156, 163, 165, 168, 169, 171, 172, 173, 252, 258, 284
cystadenocarcinoma, 122. *See also* ovarian cysts
cystadenomas, 122. *See also* ovarian cysts
cytokines, 29, 36, 38, 97, 150, 158, 159, 164, 168, 169, 171, 172, 176, 182, 183, 191, 284, 298

diary, 91, 149, 176, 177, 179, 194, 211, 227, 303, 304, 305, 306, 307, 308, 309, 310, 311
danazol, 68, 221
DASH diet, 149–150
dermatopontin (DPT), 186
dermoid cysts, 122. *See also* ovarian cysts
DES. *See* diethylstilbestrol
de Segovia, A. L., 39, 255
DHEA, 50, 51, 52, 84, 129, 141, 147
DHT. *See* dihydrotestosterone
diet,
    alkaline diet, 80
    anti inflammatory, 42, 178, 237
    dairy-rich diet, high fat diary, 91, 177, 194, 212

DASH diet, 149
diary free, 176, 179
gluten free, 176
high fat, 115
high fibre diet, 115, 149, 150, 151, 234, 244, 311
high-protein, 75, 150
isocaloric low glycaemic index, 404
ketogenic diet, 150
lignan-rich, 194
low carbohydrate/low-glycaemic index, 91, 116, 150
low fat, 222, 228
low FODMAP, 179
Mediterranean, 42, 90–91, 150, 177, 212
oils in, 226
phenolic/lignan phytoestrogen rich, 37, 63, 177, 194, 228
rich in fruits, vegetables, nuts and seeds, 26, 42, 63, 90, 105, 115, 177, 212, 226, 237, 242
diethylstilbestrol, (DES), 199
dihydrotestosterone, (DHT), 128, 232
Dioscorides, 15, 38, 59, 141, 186, 250, 261, 271
dioxin, 159–160
diuretic, 128, 222, 242, 251, 255, 273, 295, 296
docosahexaenoic acid, 150, 307
dopaminergic, 14, 18, 21, 37, 56, 57, 58, 61, 79, 131, 132, 166, 170–171, 185, 187, 190, 191, 204, 224, 241
DPT. *See* dermatopontin
DUB. *See* dysfunctional uterine bleeding
dysfunctional uterine bleeding (DUB), 30, 31, 33–45. *See also* menorrhagia
Achillea millefolium, 38–39
Alchemilla vulgaris, 39
Capsella bursa-pastoris, 40–41
causes of, 33–34
Cinnamomum zeylanicum, 41
contributing factors, 34–36

controlling bleeding using anti-haemorrhagics, 38
conventional treatment, 36
dietary and lifestyle recommendation, 42–45
endocrine dysregulation, 37
herbal approach, anovulatory/ovulatory cycle, 34
herbal management, 36–38
herbs, 38–42
Vitex agnus-castus, 41–42
with anovulatory cycles, 34
Zingiber officinale, 42
dysmenorrhoea, **3–27**, 31, 32, 35, 48, 68, 155, 157, 158, 161, 181, 186
Achillea millefolium, 18, 251, 254
Actaea racemosa, 18–19, 135
Anemone pulsatilla, 14, 264, 265
Angelica sinensis, 59, 83, 267, 269, 270
Atropa belladonna fol, 17
Cinnamomum zeylanicum, 41
clinical trials on nutrients, 26
conventional treatment, 11–12
dietary and lifestyle recommendations, 26–27
Dioscorea villosa, 19
empirically proven acute mixture, 17
flavonoids, 43
Glycyrrhiza glabra, 20–21
herbal management, 12–14
herbs used for, 14–25
information to gain in consultation, 3–6
Leonurus cardiaca, 283, 285
leukotriene levels, 10–11
Matricaria chamomilla, 19–20
Mitchella repens, 287
pathophysiology of primary dysmenorrhoea, 10–12
pelvic pain unrelated to menses, 6
primary dysmenorrhoea, 3, 4, 5, 6, 7
recommended investigations, 6
resveratrol, 172
risk factors, 11
Rubus ideaus, 293

secondary dysmenorrhoea, 3, 4, 5, 7, 8, 12, 32, 270, 302
secondary dysmenorrhoea differential diagnosis, 8–9
Thymus vulgaris, 111
Valeriana officinalis, 15
Viburnum prunifolium, 15, 170, 300, 301, 302
Vitex agnus-castus, 21
Zingiber officinale, 16, 171
dyspareunia, 5, 8, 9, 31, 32, 100, 102, 231

Eclectics, xi, 14, 17, 18, 19, 24, 25, 39, 41, 57, 59, 61, 81, 86, 107, 110, 111, 135, 170, 188, 189, 191, 208, 223, 250, 261, 265, 271, 277, 282, 283, 286, 288, 289, 295, 297, 300
ECM. *See* extracellular matrix
ectopic pregnancy, 3, 4, 6, 9, 73, 101, 102, 103, 104, 120, 121
EGCG. *See* epigallocatechin-3-gallate
EGF. *See* epidermal growth factor
Ellingwood, F., xi, 19, 40, 57, 61, 81, 86, 190, 191, 208, 271, 277, 287, 295, 297, 298, 300
emmenagogue(s), 12, 13, 14, 25, 35, 38, 40, 57, 59, 62, 80, 105, 111, 132, 186, 205, 251, 254, 261, 278, 283, 285, 296
eicosanoid, 12
emmolients, 234
emodin, 211
endocrine, 28, 33, 37, 53, 54, 74, 99, 125, 128, 147, 204, 241
endogenous opioids, 129–130
endometriomas, 6, 10, 122, 155. *See also* ovarian cysts
endometriosis, 3–6, 8, 31, 32, 34, 72, 73, 79, 91, 98, 103, 119, 120, 122, **154–179**, 184
Achillea millefolium, 254
Actaea racemosa, 166, 187
aetiologies, 157
Alchemilla vulgaris, 166–167, 256, 258, 259
Anemone pulsatilla, 167

Calendula officinalis, 168
Capsella bursa-pastoris, 275
clinical studies natural compounds, 172–173
conventional treatment, 156
dietary recommendations, 176–179
differential diagnosis, 156
Echinacea angustifolia/purpurea, 168–169
fertility, 160
Glycyrrhiza glabra, 169
herbal management of, 160–166
herbs, 166–171, 173–176
hormonal involvement, 159–160
Hydrastis canadensis, 189
Hydrocotyle asiatica, 170
immune system and inflammatory response, 158–159
investigations, 156
lifestyle, 179
mechanisms involved in, 162–166
nutrients and clinical effects, 178
pathophysiology of, 156–160
resveratrol, 193
retrograde menstruation, 157–158
surgical management, 156
symptoms, 155
Viburnum prunifolium, 170. 301
Vitex agnus-castus, 22, 170–171
Zingiber officinale, 171
environmental oestrogens, xeno-oestrogens, 159–160, 184, 242, 311
epidermal growth factor (EGF), 182, 183, 243
epigallocatechin-3-gallate (EGCG), 162, 165, 166, 174, 188, 189, 195, 197, 305
ER. *See* oestrogen receptors
oestradiol, 22, 44, 47, 53, 63, 64, 69, 71, 77, 81, 82, 87, 89, 121, 127, 131, 136, 138, 139, 140, 143, 144, 146, 147, 148, 152, 158, 159, 171, 174, 184, 193, 222, 257
extracellular matrix (ECM), 29, 163, 174, 182, 191, 196, 236

fertility, *See* infertility
FHA. *See* functional hypothalamic amenorrhoea; functional hypothalamic anovulation
fibre in foods, 115, 149, 150, 151, 234, 244, 311
fibrocystic breast changes, see breast disorders, benign
fibroids, uterine (leiomyomas) 3, 4, 5, 6, 9, 31, 33, 36, 43, 67, 73, 120, 179, **180–197**
   abnormal response to injury hypothesis, 182–183
   Achillea millefolium, 186–187, 254
   Actaea racemosa, 187
   Alchemilla vulgaris, 187–188, 256, 259
   Camellia sinensis, 188–189
   Capsella bursa-pastoris, 188, 275
   compounds in vegetables and fruit, 195–197
   conventional treatment, 181
   dietary and lifestyle recommendations, 194–197
   Glycyrrhiza glabra, 189, 190
   herb combinations and isolates, 193
   herbal management, 184–186
   herbs, 186–191
   Hydrastis canadensis, 189–190
   influence of sex hormones, 182
   investigations, 181
   Paeonia lactiflora & Glycyrrhiza glabra, 21
   Paeonia lactiflora, 190
   pathophysiology of, 182–184
   Punica granatum, pomegranate, 43
   Ricinus communis, 192–193
   risk factors, 183–184
   symptoms and complications, 180–181
   Thuja occidentalis, 191, 296
   Vitex agnus-castus, 191–192
fibromas, 122. *See also* ovarian cysts
Fitz-Hugh-Curtis syndrome, 103
flaxseed, 34, 79, 80, 83, 85, 132, 133, 134, 135, 147, 151, 177, 194, 212, 223, 225, 234, 241, 306

FODMAPs, see diet
follicle-stimulating hormone (FSH), 33, 34, 46, 47, 48, 50, 51, 52, 54, 58, 62, 64, 69, 74, 75, 76, 79, 82, 84, 86, 88, 89, 121, 123, 125, 126, 127, 128, 129, 135, 136, 139, 141, 142, 143, 145, 147, 148, 152, 166, 189, 244, 269
formononetin, 455
FSH. *See* follicle-stimulating hormone
functional cysts, 120, 121, 123, 124.
    See also ovarian cysts
functional hypothalamic amenorrhoea (FHA), 50, **52–65** *See also* amenorrhoea
    Actaea racemosa, 57–58
    Alchemilla vulgaris, 58
    Angelica sinensis, 59
    Artemesia vulgaris, 59
    conventional treatment, 55
    dietary and lifestyle reommendations, 63–65
    factors affecting GnRH, 54–55
    herbal management of, 55–57
    herbs in clinical practice, 57
    Leonurus cardiac, 59–60
    pathophysiology, 53–55
    Rhodiola rosea, 60
    Schisandra chinensis, 60
    symptoms, 52
    Vitex agnus-castus, 61
functional hypothalamic anovulation (FHA), 48, 49, 50

GABA. *See* γ-amino butyric acid
galactagogues, 131
gamma-aminobutyric acid. *See* γ-amino butyric acid
gamma-linolenic acid (GLA), 226, 229,
γ-amino butyric acid (GABA), 20, 58, 240, 284
Gardnerella vaginalis, 94, 97
genistein, 54, 57, 63, 176, 177, 195, 213, 337, 339, 342, 430, 445
Gerard, J., xi, 17, 59, 82, 261, 282, 289, 294

GH. *See* growth hormone
GI. *See* glycaemic index
GLA. *See* gamma-linolenic acid
glutathione (GSH), 136, 143, 151, 152, 214, 229, 253, 297, 305–306, 307
glycaemic index (GI). *See* diet
GnRH. *See* Gonadotropin-Releasing Hormone
GnRH-a. *See* Gonadotropin Releasing Hormone agonists
Gonadotropin-Releasing Hormone (GnRH), 47, 53, 54, 55, 57, 63, 129
    factors affecting secretion of, 54–55
Gonadotropin Releasing Hormone agonists (GnRH-a), 156
gonadotropins, 53, 77
gonorrhoea, 95, 100, 101, 102, 107, 110, 156, 261. *See also* vaginal discharge
granular ophthalmia, 295
Grieve, M., 40, 272
growth hormone (GH), 53, 126,
GSH. *See* glutathione
gymnemic acid, 85, 138, 139

haemoglobin A1C (HbA1C), 136, 139, 143, 144, 147, 152
HbA1C. *See* haemoglobin A1C
HDLs. *See* high density lipids
hepatics, 161, 185, 204
herbal vaginal applications, clinical studies, 113–114
HDL cholesterol, 136, 147, 148, 183, 297
HIF-1α. *See* hypoxia inducible factor
high density lipids see HDL
high-fibre foods. *See* diet.
high-grade Squamous Intraepithelial Lesions (HSIL), 202
high-protein diets. *See* diet.
Hill, J., 256
HIV. *See* human immunodeficiency virus
Hool, R. L., 290
hormonal herbs, x, 14, 243

hormonal modulators, 13, 123, 124
hormonal vaginitis, 95. *See also* vaginal discharge
hormone disrupting chemicals, 159–160, 184, 242, 311. *See also* environmental hormones
hormone dysregulation, 128–129
hormone producing cysts, 122. *See also* ovarian cysts
HPV. *See* human papillomavirus
HSIL. *See* high-grade Squamous Intraepithelial Lesions
human immunodeficiency virus (HIV), 100, 115, 200, 297
human papillomavirus (HPV), 198, 199, 200, 201, 202, 203, 205, 206, 207, 209, 210, 212, 213, 214
Hyde, F., 290
hyperandrogenism, 77, 125, 126, 128, 129, 130, 149
hyperinsulinaemia, 126, 128. *See also* insulin resistance
hyperprolactinemia, 41, 128–129, 140, 190
hyperthyroidism, hyperthyroid, 32, 34, 48, 49, 50, 51, 67, 68, 70, 79, 99, 227, 239,241, 232, 243
  herbs, 283, 285
hypertension, 149, 169, 183, 184, 189, 194, 250, 251, 285, 292
hypoglycaemic, 127, 131, 139, 292. *See also* insulin resistance, metabolic syndrome
hypothalamic-pituitary-ovarian axis, HPO axis, 56–57, 81, 129
hypothyroidism, hypothyroid, 32, 33, 48, 49, 50, 51, 53, 54, 55, 56, 67, 68, 69, 74, 99, 119, 129, 221, 227, 232, 239, 243, 244, 245
  herbs, 37, 57, 79, 81, 88, 131, 241
  iodine, 229
hypoxia, 29, 183, see also vasoconstriction
hypoxia inducible factor (HIF-1α), 36, 176

IBS. *See* irritable bowel syndrome
IFN. *See* interferon
IGF-1. *See* insulin-like growth factor
IL-1. *See* interleukin-1
immune-enhancing herbs, modulators, support, 106, 123, 161, 163,164, 165, 166–167, 173, 175, 191, 192, 204, 208, 213, 223, 227, 234, 266, 297, 298
immune system, 29, 70, 74, 95, 104, 116, 117, 157, 158–159, 160, 163, 164, 165, 178, 199, 200, 203, 204, 305
indole-3-carbinol, 188, 196, 211, 213, 273, 306
infertility, 5, 8, 31, 51, 52, 54, 59, 61, **66–93**, 98, 99, 100, 101, 102, 103, 118, 119, 122, 123, 125, 126, 127, 128, 132, 134, 136, 141, 145, 149, 154, 155, 160, 161, 180, 203, 303, 307
  Actaea racemosa, 81–82, 166
  Alchemilla vulgaris, 82, 255, 256
  Angelica sinensis, 82–83, 268
  Asparagus racemosus, 83
  Atropa belladonna, 86
  causes in women, 68–73
  clinical studies on nutrients, 92–93
  clinical studies, herbs, 84–85
  comprehensive approach to fertility optimization, 78–79, 86–89
  conception, 66
  conventional treatment, 77–78
  dietary and lifestyle recommendations, 89–93
  Dioscorea villosa, 83
  early evaluation criteria, 67
  Eclectic texts, 86
  factors affecting, 74–75
  factors affecting fertility, 74–75
  herbal management of, 78–81
  herbs used in clinical practice, 81
  information to gain, 67
  investigations, 76–77
  Linum sativum, 83

recurrent miscarriage, 74, 75, 93, 126, 287, 300, 301
Serenoa repens, 86
Viburnum prunifolium, 86
Vitex agnus-castus, 84
inflammatory markers, 143, 149, 158, 258, 297
insulin-like growth factor (IGF-1), 53, 150
insulin resistance/metabolic syndrome, 49, 51, 125, 126, 127, 128, 130–131, 133, 136, 137, 142, 143, 144, 149, 151, 152, 153, 239
interferon (IFN), 156, 168, 174, 176, 191, 208, 297
interleukin, 20, 163, 164, 172, 183
intrauterine contraceptive devices (IUD, IUCD), 4, 5, 9, 32, 36, 45, 98, 117, 158, 201
in vitro fertilisation (IVF), 68, 70, 74, 75, 76, 79, 88, 90, 92, 93, 142, 144
iodine and breast tissue, 226–227, 229
iodine, 131, 306
irritable bowel syndrome (IBS), 7, 179, 154
ischaemia
　cerebral, 263
　myocardial, 268
　myometrial, 10, 14
isoflavone, 44, 57, 63, 80, 133, 134, 152, 162, 166, 176, 177, 213, 225, 228, 269, 306
isoliquiritigenin, 189
IUCD. *See* intrauterine contraceptive devices
IVF. See *in vitro* fertilisation

KD. *See* ketogenic diet
ketogenic diet (KD), 150
King, J., xi, 277
King's American Dispensatory, 18, 59, 86, 283, 289
Kunzle, J., 256

Lactobacillus spp., species, 93, 94, 97, 104, 111, 112, 205, 212, 226
Large Loop Excision of the Transformation Zone (LLETZ), 203
LEEP. *See* Loop Electrosurgical Excision Procedure
leiomyomas see fibroids
leonurine, 59, 283, 284, 285
leptin, 53, 54, 55, 65, 128
　potential herb-effects on, 131, 135, 136, 141, 152
LETZ. *See* Loop Excision of the Transformation Zone
leukotriene, 10–11, 16, 20, 42, 171
LH. *See* luteinising hormone
lichen sclerosus (LS), **231–237**
　Calophyllum inophyllum, 236
　clinical studies with specific nutrients, 238
　clinical studies, herbs topically, 236–237
　conventional treatment, 233
　dietary and lifestyle recommendations, 237–238
　herbal management of, 233–234
　herbs in clinical practice, 234–237
　Hydrocotyle asiatica, 235–236
　investigation, 232
　oils for topical use, 237
　pathophysiology, 232
　specific nutrients, 238
　symptoms, 231–232
lignans, 34, 57, 63–64, 177, 194, 212, 238, 306
LLETZ. *See* Large Loop Excision of the Transformation Zone
Loop Electrosurgical Excision Procedure (LEEP), 203
Loop Excision of the Transformation Zone (LETZ), 203
low-carbohydrate diet. *See* diet, low-carbohydrate
low FODMAP diet, *See* diet, low FODMAP

low-glycaemic index *See* diet, low carbohydrate/low-glycaemic index
Low-grade Squamous Intraepithelial Lesions (LSIL), 202
LS. *See* lichen sclerosus
LSIL. *See* Low-grade Squamous Intraepithelial Lesions
luteal defect, *See* Corpus luteum deficiency
luteal deficiency, *See* Corpus luteum deficiency
luteal phase defect, *See* Corpus luteum deficiency
luteinising hormone (LH), 33, 34, 46, 47, 48, 50, 51, 54, 58, 63, 68, 71, 75, 76, 79, 82, 84, 85, 86, 87, 88, 89, 92, 121, 123, 125, 126, 127, 128, 131, 135, 136, 137, 139, 141, 142, 144, 145, 146, 147, 148, 166, 171, 244, 257, 269
lycopene, 195, 212, 213, 238, 304
lymphatic, 123, 157
    herbs, 106, 123, 161, 204, 222, 223, 295

mastalgia, 215, 216, 222, 226, 228, 242
    clinical trials, 225
    lifestyle, 230
    specific foods and nutrients, 229
    Trigonella foenumgraecum, 25
    Vitex agnus castus, 224, 225
mastalgia, noncyclic, 216. *See also* breast disorders, benign
matrix metalloproteinases (MMP), 29, 39, 156, 158, 159, 164, 169, 171, 172, 174, 175, 183, 189, 207, 252
Matthiolus, P. A., 256
Mediterranean diet, 42, 90–91, 150, 177, 212
mefenamic acid, 11, 15, 16, 22, 23, 24, 36, 41, 188, 274
melatonin, 21, 54, 93, 164, 170, 171, 191, 239, 242, 307

menopause, ix, 33, 36, 48, 51, 75, 76, 96, 121, 155, 183, 185, 216, 218, 219, **243–246**
    herbal management, 244–246, 269
    perimenopause, 31, 41, 48, 50, 239, 241, 243–244
    postmenopause, 244
    symptoms, 243
menorrhagia, 5, 8, 9, 11, 28–45, 155, 158, 161, 181, 185, 186, 200, see also dysfunctional uterine bleeding DUB
    achillea millefolium, 18, 38, 39, 250, 251, 254
    actaea racemose, 18, 81, 135
    Alchemilla vulgaris, 39, 58, 187, 256, 259
    angelica sinensis, caution, 270
    Arctostaphylos uva ursi, 107
    Capsella bursa-pastoris, 40, 188, 271, 273, 274, 275
    Caulophyllum thalictriodes, 277, 278
    causes, 32
    consideration, 30
    control of normal menstrual bleeding, 29–30
    conventional treatment, 33
    dietary and lifestyle recommendations, 42–43
    differential diagnosis, 31
    dysfunctional uterine bleeding, 33–42
    emergency, 30
    flavonoids, 43
    herb combinations and isolates, 193
    information to gain in consultation, 30
    investigations, 32–33
    nutrients, 44
    pomegranate, 43
    red flags, 32
    Rubus ideaus, 293
    specific nutrients, 43–45
    Vitex agnus castus, 41

518   INDEX

menstruation. *See also* amenorrhoea;
    menorrhagia, 4, 5, 7, 8, 10, 11,
    12, 16, 18, 20, 26, 27, 28, 33, 35,
    36, 38, 44, 46, 47, 48, 49, 52,
    55, 61, 62, 73, 83, 86, 97, 121,
    130, 132, 142, 154, 225, 244,
    250, 261, 267, 269, 282
  as injury, 183
  control of normal, 29–30
  retrograde, 157–159
metabolic/endocrine syndrome, 128,
    130–131
metabolic syndrome, 49, 51, 125, 126,
    127, 128, 130–131, 133, 136,
    137, 142, 143, 144, 149, 151,
    152, 153, 239
metformin, 84, 86, 87, 88, 89, 127, 130,
    137, 141, 142, 143, 144, 145, 147
microbiome, vaginal, endometrial, 36,
    78, 80, 93, 94–95, 98, 104,
    105, 205
microbiome, gut, 37, 105, 114, 115, 130,
    131, 132, 151, 179, 185, 204,
    222, 311
minerals, 26, 38, 63, 64, 90, 91, 92,
    212, 290
  boron, 26, 303
  calcium, 26, 92, 115, 194, 213,
    290, 303
  chromium, 151, 290, 304
  copper, 177
  food sources of, 303–310
  iodine, 131, 226–227, 229, 306
  iron, 32, 34, 36, 37, 38, 44, 64, 91, 92,
    115, 227, 290, 306
  magnesium, 26, 37, 64, 93, 290, 307
  selenium, 93, 151, 177, 214, 227, 229,
    290, 306, 308
  zinc, 16, 26, 64, 151, 177, 214,
    258, 311
miscarriage, 199, 293,
  herbs for threatened, 15, 83, 287, 300
  increased risk, 68, 69, 70, 72, 74, 75,
    76, 80, 91, 92, 93, 97, 160, 180
  recurrent, 74, 75, 93, 126, 287,
    300, 301

Mitchell, J., 286
MMP. *See* matrix metalloproteinases
mucous membrane restorative herbs,
    105, 204

N-acetylcysteine, 151, 307
naringenin, 162, 166, 174, 178
natural killer cells (NK), 158, 168, 173
neoplastic cysts, 122. *See also* ovarian
    cysts
nervine(s), 24, 34, 38, 56, 59, 81, 132,
    133, 161, 186, 194, 204, 223,
    234, 241, 245, 282, 283
neuropeptide Y (NPY), 53, 60
NF-kappaB. *See* nuclear factor-kappaB
NK. *See* natural killer
nonsteroidal anti-inflammatory drugs
    (NSAIDs), 10, 11, 12, 16, 156,
    171, 221, 252
NPY. *See* neuropeptide Y
NSAIDs. *See* nonsteroidal
    anti-inflammatory drugs
nuclear factor-kappaB (NF-κB), 158,
    165, 166, 169, 170, 173, 174,
    175, 176, 189
nutrients, specific, 26, 42, 43–45, 56,
    64, 74, 79, 90, 92, 115–116,
    150–151, 178, 204, 212–214,
    222, 229–230, 238, 241,
    303–310, 311

OCPs. *See* oral contraceptive pills
oestrogen, 12, 14, 29, 32, 34, 35, 37, 48,
    49, 50, 51, 52, 53, 54, 57, 58,
    63, 68, 74, 76, 77, 78, 79, 80,
    94, 105, 122, 123, 128, 129,
    159, 161, 166, 171, 190, 222,
    259, 268, 269
  agonist and antagonist, 14, 80, 172,
    174, 177
  amenorrhoea/oligomenorrhoea,
    46–47
  androgen to oestrogen conversion,
    33, 48, 51, 128, 129, 132, 159,
    163, 179, 182
  anti-oestrogenic, 221

benign breast disorders, 216
control normal bleeding and cycle, 29, 47
diet and lifestyle, influence, 74, 158, 178, 179, 184, 226, 228, 230, 242, 305, 307, 311
dysfunctional uterine bleeding, 33, 34
endometriosis, 154, 157, 159–160
environmental oestrogens, xeno-oestrogens, 159–160, 184, 242, 311
fibroid, 182, 183, 184
functional hypothalamic amenorrhoea, 52–54
lichen sclerosus, 232
melatonin influence, 171
menopause, 233, 243, 244, 245
oestrogen dominance/relative excess, 34, 37, 80, 99, 216, 129, 159, 184, 221
oestrogen-promoting herbs, 21, 57, 63, 80, 83, 141, 233, 234, 253
oestrogen, low, 46–47, 48, 49, 50, 51, 52, 96, 232, 244–245
PMS, 239, 240, 241, 242
stress, 50, 184
treatment relative oestrogen excess, 34, 35, 44, 80, 131, 148, 161, 185, 188, 194, 204, 222–223, 228, 241, 242, 305, 307, 311
unopposed oestrogen, 34, 41, 126, 184
weight, 35, 37, 50, 54, 128, 158, 184
oestrogen receptor(s)(ER), 14, 29, 79, 166, 172, 173, 223
oligomenorrhoea, **46–65**, 84, 87, 125, 141, 285, *See also* amenorrhoea
omega-3 fatty acids, 26, 36, 38, 63, 64, 90, 150, 178, 196, 213, 225, 229, 237, 307
oral contraceptive pills (OCPs), 12, 33, 36, 52, 84, 95, 96, 99, 105, 124, 156, 172, 184, 193, 200, 216, 221, 225
ovarian cancer, 120, 122, 170. *See also* ovarian cysts

ovarian cysts, 6, 10, **118–124**, 145, 148, 156
brenner tumours, 122
complications, 119
conventional treatment, 120
cystadenocarcinoma, 122
cystadenomas, 122
dermoid cysts, 122
endometriomas, 122
fibromas, 122
functional or physiologic cysts, 121
herbal management of, 123–124
hormone-producing cysts, 122
investigations, 120
neoplastic cysts, 122
ovarian cancer, 122
pathophysiology of, 121–122
polycystic ovary syndrome, 121–122
risk factors for, 119–120
symptoms, 119
theca lutein cysts, 122
ovarian function, 69, 78, 79

Papanicolaou test (Pap test), 201
papaya, 212, 304, 308
Pap test. *See* Papanicolaou test
Parkinson, J., 58, 82, 250, 256, 282, 294
Payne, R. L., 301
PCBs. *See* polychlorinated biphenyls
PCOS. *See* polycystic ovary syndrome
PDGF. *See* platelet-derived growth factor
pelvic circulation, 14, 37, 38, 56, 61, 80, 104, 105, 117, 123, 130, 132, 161, 186, 205, 233, 234, 254, 266, 270
pelvic inflammatory disease (PID), 4, 5, 6, 8, 31, 32, 33, 67, 73, 79, 98, 100, **101–104**, 120, 156, 182, 262, 264, *See also* vaginal discharge
Anemone pulsatilla, 262, 264
complications, 102–103
conventional treatment, 104
differential diagnosis, 103

investigations, 104
risk factors, 103
symptoms, 102
pelvic venous congestion, 3, 4, 9
pelvic venous varices, 3
pessary, 105, 111, 114, 211, 261
PGE2. *See* prostaglandin E2
physiologic cysts, 121. *See also* ovarian cysts
phytoestrogen, phenolic, 13, 14, 37, 57, 79, 131, 177, 185, 194, 204, 222, 226, 228, 234, 241, 244, 245, 311
PID. *See* pelvic inflammatory disease
platelet-derived growth factor (PDGF), 182
Pliny the elder, 38, 249, 250
PMDD, 240
PMS. *See* premenstrual syndrome
polychlorinated biphenyls (PCBs), 159. *See also* environmental oestrogens
polycystic ovarian syndrome (PCOS), 34, 51, 58, 62, 68, 76, 77, 79, 87, 121–122, **125–153**
  Actaea racemosa, 81, 135–136
  balancing stress response, 133
  Camellia sinensis, 153
  Cinnamomum zeylanicum, 136–137
  clinical studies, herbs, 84, 85, 87, 88, 89, 133–135, 142–146, 149–150
  conventional treatment, 127–128
  diagnosis, 126–127
  dietary and lifestyle recommendations, 91, 149–153
  differential diagnosis, 126–127
  digestive health and microbiome support, 132
  endogenous opioids, 129–130
  Glycine max, 152
  Glycyrrhiza spp., 137–138
  Gymnema sylvestre, 138–139
  herbal management of, 130–132
  hormone dysregulation, 128–129
  hormone modulation, 131
  investigations, 127
  Linum usitatissimum, 152
  long-term issues, 126
  menstruation regulation, 132
  Mentha spicata, 139–140
  metabolic syndrome, 128
  microbiome diversity, 130
  Paeonia lactiflora & *Glycyrrhiza glabra*, 140
  pathophysiology of, 128–130
  pelvic circulation, 132
  preclinical studies in PCOS models, 147–148
  reduce AMH concentrations, 132
  Serenoa repens/serrulata, 140–141
  stimulating ovulation, 131–132
  supplements in trials for PCOS, 150–151
  symptoms, 125–126
  treating insulin resistance, 130–131
  Vitex agnus-castus, 141
polycystic ovary syndrome, *See* polycystic ovarian syndrome (PCOS)
polyphenols, 38, 41, 43, 172, 213, 257,
pomegranate (*Punica granatum*), 26, 43, 305
prostanoid, 10, 12
premenstrual syndrome (PMS), ix, 5, 7, 11, 52, 64, 68, 223, 228, 229, **239–242**
  contributing factors, 239
  dietary recommendations, 242
  endogenous contributory factors, 239
  herbal management, 240–242
  Hypericum perforatum, 225
  predisposing factors, 239
  symptoms, 240
  Vitex agnus-castus, 21, 61, 130, 224
probiotics, 37, 93, 101, 104, 110, 112, 116, 212, 242, 307
progesterone, 35, 47, 62, 68, 76, 105, 121, 164, 182, 190, 433
  benign breast disorder, 221
  control menstrual bleeding, 29, 33, 34, 47

dysfunctional uterine bleeding, 34
dysmenorrhoea, 10, 12
endometriosis, 154, 160
fibroids, 182
herbs, 14, 21, 37, 61, 62, 63, 81, 84, 87, 88, 134, 136, 140, 141, 143, 144, 147, 148, 152, 171, 173, 185, 190, 204, 223, 241, 257, 258
hyperprolactinaemia, 54, 129
menopause, 243
nutrients, 223, 244
PMS, 239, 240
polycystic ovarian syndrome, 127, 129, 132
progesterone only pill, 36, 127
progesterone receptors, 159
progesterone-releasing IUCD, 9, 32, 158
receptors, 159, 36
relative progesterone deficiency, 37
selective progesterone receptor modulators, 181
stress, 55, 184
progesterone-releasing IUCD, 9, 32, 158
prostacyclin, 10, 11, 13, 26, 43
prostaglandin E2 (PGE2), 10, 11, 20, 23, 26, 29, 149, 157, 159, 165, 169, 175, 176, 178, 267
protoanemonin, 262, 264
puberty, delayed. *See* amenorrhoea
pulmonary hypertension, 268, 270

quercetin, 196, 211, 213, 238, 252, 257, 283, 290, 296

Rafinesque, C., 276, 277
resveratrol, 114, 162, 163, 164, 165, 166, 172, 185, 193, 238
retinoic acid, 196
retrograde menstruation, 157–158

salicin, 13, 15, 301
salpingitis, 102
scleroderma, 235, 236
scopoletin, 15, 301

sex hormone-binding globulin (SHBG), 37, 48, 51, 77, 127, 128, 131, 132, 139, 148, 149, 151, 152, 178, 179, 244
sexually transmitted disease/ infections, 73, 100, 101, 103, 106, 156, 295
SHBG. *See* sex hormone-binding globulin
Shennon, T., 301
Smith, P., 276, 277
SOD. *See* superoxide dismutase
spironolactone, 128, 138
stachydrine, 60, 283, 284, 285
Steinmetz, E. F., 272
steroidal saponins rich herbs, 14, 34, 56–57, 79, 80, 83, 85, 105, 124, 131, 146, 241
stress, 30, 33, 34, 37, 38, 47, 50, 51, 52, 53, 54, 55, 56, 60, 64, 65, 75, 76, 78, 81, 90, 91, 96, 116, 117, 129, 130, 133, 161, 169, 184, 185, 186, 194, 200, 204, 222, 223, 230, 232, 233, 234, 239, 274
stress, oxidative, 66, 143, 150, 151, 152, 158, 285, 297
sulforaphane, 196, 211, 214, 308

tamoxifen, 119, 184, 221
teratomas. *See* dermoid cysts. *See also* ovarian cysts
theca lutein cysts, 122. *See also* ovarian cysts
Thompson, S., 289
thyroid. *See* hypothyroid and hyperthyroid
tietze syndrome, 221
TNF-α. *See* tumour necrosis factor-α
tranexamic acid, 36, 43
trichomonas vaginalis, see trichomoniasis
trichomoniasis, 95, **99–101**. *See also* vaginal discharge
  Allium sativum, 106
  complications, 100
  conventional treatment, 100, 101

herbal treatment for, 114
herbal vaginal applications, 113
Hydrastis canadensis, 110
symptoms, 100
tryptophan-rich foods, 242
tumour necrosis factor-α (TNF-α), 20, 24, 130, 143, 150, 156, 165, 168, 169, 170, 171, 172, 175, 176, 182, 183, 189, 196, 208, 284
tyrosinase, 167, 259, 264,

ultrasound (US), 6, 33, 46, 50, 51, 76, 104, 118, 121, 126, 127, 145, 181, 217
uterine leiomyomas. *See* fibroids
uterine contractions, 12, 268, 289, 291
upper reproductive tract infections, 96–104. *See also* discharge
uterine tonic herbs, 205
uterine tonics, 12, 13, 14, 35, 37, 38, 56, 57, 80, 105, 123, 132, 186, 205, 251, 285, 286, 287, 293, 300, 301

vaginal discharge, 8, 94–117
  Allium sativum, 106–107
  Arctostaphylos uva ursi, 107
  bacterial vaginosis BV, 71, 79, 95–98, 101, 103, 105, 106, 108, 110, 111, 112, 113, 114, 115–116
  Baptisia tinctora, 108–109
  Calendula officinalis, 108
  candida vaginitis, 95, 98–99, 107, 110, 112, 252
  causes of changes in, 95–96
  clinical studies, 113–114, 115–116
  dietary and lifestyle recommendations, 114–117
  Echinacea angustifolia/purpurea, 108–109
  healthy vaginal microbiome, 94–95
  herbal vaginal applications, 112–114
  herbs used in clinical practice for vaginal infections, 106–114
  Hydrastis canadensis, 109–110
  lactobacillus-dominant vaginal flora, 104

  Melaleuca alternifolia EO, 110–111
  pelvic inflammatory disease, 101–104
  preclinical studies of interest, 114
  probiotics, 112
  risk factors, 96, 98, 99, 103, 116–117
  Thuja occidentalis, 108–109
  Thymus vulgaris, 111–112
  treatment principles of vaginal infections, 104–106
  trichomonas vaginalis, 99–101
  vaginal and upper reproductive tract infections, 96–104
vaginal lactobacilli, 93, 94, 97, 104, 111, 112, 114, 205, 212
vaginal microbiome. *See* microbiome, vaginal, endometrial
vaginal pessaries, 105, 106, 112, 205, 236
irritant vaginitis, 95. *See also* vaginal discharge
vascular endothelial growth factor (VEGF), 36, 166, 183, 267
vasoconstriction, 11, 29, 33, 38, 183
vasopressin, 10, 11, 12, 13, 16
vasostimulant, diffuse, 18, 39, 250, 251
VEGF. *See* vascular endothelial growth factor
vitamins, 42, 63, 90, 91, 177, 212, 213, 303, 311
  vitamin A, 44, 64, 93, 115, 177, 196, 213, 214, 227, 229, 238, 308. *See also* carotenoids
  vitamin B complex, 37, 44, 64, 309
  vitamin B9 (folate), 115, 177, 213, 214, 309
  vitamin B12, 64, 92, 116, 127, 214, 307, 309
  vitamin C, 44, 64, 115, 134, 136, 177, 213, 214, 229, 305, 306, 309
  vitamin D, 26, 64, 114, 151, 178, 189, 197, 213, 214, 238, 309–310
  vitamin K, 26, 45, 64, 310
  vitamin B2, 64
  vitamin B6, 26, 64, 189, 197, 230, 307, 308
  vitamin B1, 26, 308

vitamin E, 23, 26, 45, 64, 115, 177, 178, 213, 214, 226, 229, 230, 233, 234, 237, 238, 310
von Bingen, H., 255
vulvo vaginal candidiasis (VVC). *See* candidiasis, vaginal and vaginal discharge
VVC. *See* vulvo vaginal candidiasis

Weiss, R. F., 17, 40, 188, 262, 272

xeno-oestrogens, 159, 184, 242. *See also* environmental oestrogens, hormone disrupting chemicals.

zoladex, 36

HERB INDEX

Achillea millefolium, 249–254
  cervical dysplasia, 204, 210,
  dysmenorrhoea, 12, 13, 14, **18**
  endometriosis, 161
  fibroids, 186
  infertility, 80
  lichen sclerosus, 234
  menopause, 241, 245
  menorrhagia, 35, 38, **39**
  ovarian cysts, 123
  vaginal discharge, 105, 113
Actaea racemosa
  amenorrhoea/oligomenorrhea, 56, **57**
  benign breast disorders, 223, 225
  cervical dysplasia, 204, 205
  dysmenorrhoea, 13, 14, **18**
  endometriosis, 161, 162, 163, 164, 165, **166**, 171
  fibroids, 185, 186, **187**
  infertility, 79, 80, **81**, 84, 85
  lichen sclerosus, 234
  menopause, 245, 246
  menorrhagia, 34, 35, 37
  menstrual migraines, 269
  ovarian cysts, 123, 124
  PCOS, 130, 131, 132, 133, 134, **135**
  PMS, 241, 242
  use in labour, 281
  vaginal discharge, 105
Agnus castus see *Vitex agnus-castus*
Alchemilla vulgaris, 255–259
  amenorrhoea/oligomenorrhea, **58**
  cervical dysplasia, 205
  endometriosis, 161, 162, 163, **166**
  fibroids, 186, 187, **188**
  infertility, 80, **82**
  lichen sclerosus, 234
  menorrhagia, 35, 38, **39**
  ovarian cysts, 123
  vaginal discharge, 105
Allium sativum
  menopause, 245
  vaginal discharge, 105, **106**
Althea officinalis, 105

Aloe vera
    cervical dysplasia, 205
    infertility, 85
    PCOS, 133, 147
Andrographis paniculata
    endometriosis, 162, 163, 165, 166, 173
    vaginal discharge, 106
Anemone pulsatilla, 260–265
    dysmenorrhoea, 13, **14**, 17
    acute mix, 17
    endometriosis, 161, 162, 163, **167**
    fibroids, 186
    vaginal discharge, 109
Anethum graveolens
    dysmenorrhoea, 12, 13, 22
    infertility, 84, 85, 87
    vaginal discharge, 113
    PCOS, 134, 135, 142
Angelica sinensis, 266–270
    amenorrhoea, oligomenorrhoea, 56, **59**
    cervical dysplasia, 205
    dysmenorrhoea, 13, 14, 22
    endometriosis, 162, 163, 164, 165, 166
    infertility, 80, **82**
    menopause, 245
    menorrhagia, 35, 38
    ovarian cysts, 123
    PCOS, 133
Apium graveolens
    infertility, 80, 84, 85, 86
    PCOS, 134, 135, 142
Arctium lappa
    PCOS, 132
Arctostaphylos uva-ursi
    vaginal discharge, 105
Artemisia absinthium
    amenorrhoea, oligomenorrhoea, 56
    cervical dysplasia, 204, 205
    menopause, 245
    ovarian cysts, 123, 124
    PCOS, 132
    PMS, 241
    thujone, 297, 299
    vaginal discharge, 105

Artemisia vulgaris
    amenorrhoea, oligomenorrhoea, 56, **59**
    cervical dysplasia, 205
    infertility, 80
    ovarian cysts, 123
    PCOS, 132
    vaginal discharge, 105
Artichoke see *Cynara scolymus*
Ashwaganda see *Withania somnifera*
Astragalus membranaceus
    cervical dysplasia, 204, 205
    endometriosis, 161
    menopause, 245, 246
    ovarian cysts, 123
Asparagus racemosus
    infertility, 79, 80, **83**, 84, 85, 87
    lichen sclerosus, 234
    menopause, 245
    PCOS, 131, 132, 134, 135, 142
    vaginal discharge, 105
asparagus, 115, 305, 308, 309, 310
Atropa belladonna
    amenorrhoea, oligomenorrhoea, 61
    dysmenorrhoea, 14, 17
    infertility, 86
Avena sativa
    menopause, 145
    PMS, 241

Baptisia tinctoria
    cervical dysplasia, 204
    vaginal discharge, 106, 108, 109
    with thuja occidentalis, 296, 298, 299
Barberry see *Berberis vulgaris*
Bearberry see *Arctostaphylos uva-ursi*
belladonna see *Atropa belladonna*
Beth root see *Trillium erectum*
Berberis vulgaris
    benign breast disorders, 223
    cervical dysplasia, 204, 205
    menopause, 245
    ovarian cysts, 124
    PCOS, 142
    PMS, 241
    vaginal discharge, 105, 110

HERB INDEX 527

Baikal see *Scutellaria biacalensis*
Bilberry see *Vaccinium myrtillus*
Bladderwrack see *Fucus vesiculosus*
Black cohosh see *Actaea racemosa*
Black cumin see *Nigella sativa*
Black haw see *Viburnum prunifolium*
Blue cohosh see *Caulophyllum thalictroides*
Burdock, see *Arctium lappa*

Calendula officinalis
    benign breast disorders, 222, **223**
    cervical dysplasia, 204, 205, 209
    endometriosis, 161, 162, 163, 164, 165, **168**
    lichen sclerosus, 234
    ovarian cysts, 123
    vaginal discharge, 105, 106, **108**
    with achillea, 254
Calophyllum inophyllum
    lichen sclerosus, 234, **236**
Camellia sinensis
    cervical dysplasia, 204, 205, 213
    endometriosis, 162, 163, 166, 173, 174
    fibroids, 185, 186, **188**
    lichen sclerosus, 234
    menopause, 246
    menorrhagia, 42
    PCOS, 133, 134, 142, 153
    vaginal discharge, 114
Capsella bursa-pastoris, 271–275
    endometriosis, 162, 163
    fibroids, 186, **188**
    menorrhagia, 38, **40**
Capsicum spp
    composition essence, 290
    PMS, 241
    with raspberry leaf, 289
Carduus marianus see *Silybum marianum*
Cat's claw see *Uncaria tomentosa*
Caulophyllum thalictroides, 276–281
    amenorrhoea, oligomenorrhoea, 56, 61
    menorrhagia, 38
    PCOS, 132

Cayenne see *Capsicum spp*
celery see *Apium graveolens*
Centella asiatica see *Hydrocotyle asiatica*
Chamaelirium luteum
    amenorrhoea, oligomenorrhea, 56
    infertility, 80, 85
    menopause, 245
    menorrhagia, 38
    ovarian cysts, 124
    PCOS, 131
Chamomilla recutita see *Matricaria chamomilla*
Chasteberry see *Vitex agnus castus*
Chelidonium majus, 186
Chinese angelica see *Angelica sinensis*
Chilli see *Capsicum spp*
Cimicifuga racemosa see also Actaea racemosa
    compared to Anemone pulsatilla, 261
Cinnamon see *Cinnamomum zeylanicum/verum*
Cinnamomum cassia see also Cinnamomum zeylanicum/ verum
    amenorrhoea, oligomenorrhoea, 62, 63
    fibroids, 193
    infertility, 84, 85, 87
    PCOS, 144
Cinnamomum zeylanicum/verum
    amenorrhoea, oligomenorrhoea, 62
    composition essence, 290
    dysmenorrhoea, 13, 14, 22
    infertility, 85, 87, 89
    menorrhagia, 35, 38, **41**
    ovarian cysts, 123
    PCOS, 131, 133, 134, 135, **136**, 146
Commiphora molmol, 113, 211
Composition Essence, 290
Crampbark see *Viburnum opulus*
Crataegus spp.
    menopause, 245
    menorrhagia, 35, 38
Curcuma longa
    appendix, 305, 311
    cervical dysplasia, 204, **206**

528　HERB INDEX

endometriosis, 162, 163, 164, 165, 166, 174
fibroids, 185, 186
lichen sclerosus, 234
menopause, 245
menorrhagia, 42
ovarian cysts, 123
vaginal discharge, 105
Cynara scolymus
menopause, 245
PCOS, 132

Damiana see *Turnera diffusa*
Dill see *Anethum graveolens*
Dioscorea villosa
amenorrhoea, oligomenorrhea, 56
dysmenorrhoea, 13, 14, **19**
infertility, 79, 80, **83**, 85
menopause, 245
ovarian cysts, 124
PMS, 241

Echinacea angustifolia/purpurea
cervical dysplasia, 204, **207**
endometriosis, 161, 162, 163, 164, 165, **168**, 169
fibroids, 186
lichen sclerosus, 234
ovarian cysts, 123
vaginal discharge, 106, **108**, 109
with thuja, 191, 208, 209, 295, 296, 298, 299
Eleutherococcus senticosus
amenorrhoea, oligomenorrhea, 53
cervical dysplasia, 203, 204
menopause, 245, 246
PMS, 241
Equisetum arvense, 246

False Unicorn root see *Chamaelirium luteum*
Fennel see *Foeniculum vulgare*
Fenugreek see *Trigonella foenum-graceum*
Filipendula ulmaria
cervical dysplasia, 205, **210**
Flax see *Linum sativum*

Foeniculum vulgare
amenorrhoea, oligomenorrhoea, 62
dysmenorrhoea, 13, 14, 20, 23
infertility, 84, 85, 87
lichen sclerosus, 236
PCOS, 132, 134, 135, 143
vaginal discharge, 105, 114
Fucus vesiculosus, 131

Galega officinalis
PCOS, 131, 133, 147
Galium aperine, 222
Ganoderma lucidium
cervical dysplasia, 204, **207**
Garlic see also *Allium sativum*
appendix, 305, 307
benign breast disorders, 223, 229
PMS, 241
vaginal discharge, 105, 107, 111, 115
Gelsemium sempervirens, 261, 277, 281
Ginger see *Zingiber officinale*
Goat's rue see *Galega officinalis*
Gokhru see *Tribulus terrestris*
Gotu cola see *Hydrocotyle asiatica*
Ginkgo biloba
benign breast disorders, **222**
dysmenorrhoea, 13
menopause, 245
PMS, 242
Glycine max, 133, 152
Glycyrrhiza glabra
amenorrhoea, oligomenorrhoea, 56, 57, 63
benign breast disorders, 223
dysmenorrhoea, 14, 20, 21
endometriosis, 162, 163, 164, 165, **169**
fibroids, 185, 186, **189**
infertility, 80, 84, 85, 88, 89
lichen sclerosus, 234
menopause, 245
menorrhagia, 34, 37
PCOS, 132, 133, 134, 135, **137**, 140, 146
PMS, 241, 242
vaginal discharge, 105
Goldenseal see *Hydrastis canadensis*
Green tea see *Camellia sinensis*

Grifola frondosa
  infertility, 85, 88
  PCOS, 133, 134
Gymnema sylvestre
  PCOS, 131, 133, **138**, 139

Hamamelis virginiana
  composition essence, 290
Hawthorn berry/flowers see
  Crataegus spp.
Hen of the woods see *Grifola frondosa*
Hippophae rhamnoides
  endometriosis, 164, 165, 175
Hops see *Humulus lupulus*
Horsetail see *Equisetum arvense*
Humulus lupulus
  endometriosis, 175
  menopause, 245, 246
Hydrastis canadensis
  cervical dysplasia, 204, 205
  comparison to shepherd's purse, 272
  fibroids, 185, 186, 189
  PCOS, 142
  vaginal discharge, 105, **109**
  with thuja, 295
Hydrocotyle asiatica
  benign breast disorders, 223
  cervical dysplasia, 205
  endometriosis, 161, 162, 163, 164, 165
  fibroids, 186
  lichen sclerosus, 234, **235**
Hypericum perforatum
  benign breast disorders, 225
  endometriosis, 164, 166, 175
  menopause, 245
  PCOS, 146
  PMS, 241

Indigo, Wild see *Baptisia tinctoria*

Lady's mantle see *Alchemilla vulgaris*
Lavandula angustifolia
  dysmenorrhoea, 27
  lichen sclerosus, 236, 237
  PMS, 241
  vaginal discharge, 105
Lavender see *Lavandula angustifolia*

Lemonbalm see *Melissa officinalis*
Leonorus cardiaca, 282–265
  infertility, 81
Licorice see *Glycyrrhiza glabra*
Linum sativum/usitatissium
  amenorrhoea, oligomenorrhoea, 62
  benign breast disorders, 225, 228
  cervical dysplasia, 204
  infertility, **83**, 85
  menopause, 245
  PCOS, 131, 135, **152**
Liquorice see *Glycyrrhiza glabra*

Maitake see *Grifola frondosa*
Marjoram see *Origanum majorana*
Marigold see *Calendula officinalis*
Marshmallow see *Althea officinalis*
Matricaria chamomilla
  benign breast disorders, 225
  dysmenorrhoea, 12, 13, 18, **19**
  menorrhagia, 38
  PCOS, 133, 134, 135, 143
  PMS, 241
Matricaria recutita see matricaria
  chamomilla
Meadowsweet see *Filipendula ulmaria*
Melaleuca alternifolia
  vaginal discharge, 105, **110**
Melissa officinalis
  benign breast disorders, 223
  dysmenorrhoea, 14
  lichen sclerosus, 234
  menopause, 245
  menorrhagia, 38
  PMS, 241
Mentha piperata
  amenorrhoea, oligomenorrhoea, 62
  dysmenorrhoea, 13, 23
  PCOS, 139
Mentha spicata
  PCOS, 132, 134, 135, **139**, 147
Milk thistle see *Silybum marianum*
Mint see *Mentha piperata*
Mitchella repens, 286–288
  amenorrhoea, oligomenorrhoea, 56
  menorrhagia, 38
  PCOS, 132

Motherwort see *Leonorus cardiaca*
Mugwort see *Artemisia vulgaris*
Mullein see *Verbascum thapsus*
Myrtle see *Myrtus communis*
Myrtus communis
   cervical dysplasia, 205, **210**
   menorrhagia, 35, 38
   vaginal discharge, 113, 114

Nettle leaf see *Urtica spp folia*
Nettle root see *Urtica spp radix*
Nigella sativa
   amenorrhoea, oligomenorrhea, 57
   benign breast disorders, 225
   infertility, 79, 81, 85
   menorrhagia, 38
   PCOS, 131, 133, 134, 144
   PMS, 241
   vaginal discharge, 114

Oats see *Avena sativa*
Origanum majorana
   PCOS, 133, 134, 144

Paeonia lactiflora
   amenorrhoea, oligomenorrhea, 56, 57, 63
   benign breast disorders, 223
   dysmenorrhoea, 14, **20**
   endometriosis, 162, 163, 164, 165, 175
   fibroids, 185, 186, **190**, 193
   infertility, 79, 80, 84, 85, 87, 88, 89
   menopause, 245
   menorrhagia, 34, 37
   PCOS, 132, 134, 135, **140**, 144, 146
   PMS, 241, 242
   vaginal discharge, 105
Paeony see *Paeonia lactiflora*
Partridge berry see *Mitchella repens*
Peppermint see *Mentha piperata*
Panax ginseng
   cervical dysplasia, 204, **208**
   endometriosis, 162, 163, 164, 165, 166, 172
   infertility, 81, 88
   menopause, 245, 246

   PCOS, 131, 133, 148
   PMS, 241
Pasqueflower see *Anemone pulsatilla*
peach see *Prunus persicaria*
Phytolacca decandra/americana
   benign breast disorders, 222, **223**, 224
   cervical dysplasia, 204
   endometriosis, 161
   ovarian cysts, 123
   vaginal discharge, 106
Pimpinella anisum
   infertility, 84, 85, 86
   PCOS, 134, 135, 142
Plantago lanceolata, 204, 245
pomegranate see *Punica granatum*
Propolis, 114
Prunus persicaria, 193
Pulsatilla see *Anemone pulsatilla*
Punica granatum
   menorrhagia, 43
   vaginal discharge, 114

Red clover see *Trifolium pratense*
Rhodiola rosea
   amenorrhoea, oligomenorrhea, 53, 54, 56, **60**
   infertility, 81, 88
   PCOS, 131, 133
   PMS, 241
Rue see *Ruta graveolens*
Rosa damascena
   dysmenorrhoea, 13, 14, 24
Rosmarinus officinalis
   dysmenorrhoea, 13, 14, 24
   cervical dysplasia, 204, 210
Rubus idaeus, 289–293
   use in labour, 281
Rumex crispus, 241
Ruta graveolens
   amenorrhoea, oligomenorrhea, 56
   PCOS, 132

Sage see *Salvia officinalis*
Salix alba
   dysmenorrhoea, 13, 14, 24
Salvia officinalis
   menopause, 245, 246

ulcers, 254
vaginal discharge, 114
Salvia rosmarinus see *Rosmarinus officinalis*
Schisandra chinensis
   amenorrhoea, oligomenorrhea, 53, 54, **61**
   benign breast disorders, 223
   endometriosis, 161
   fibroids, 185
   menopause, 245
   PMS, 241
Scutellaria biacalensis
   endometriosis, 162, 165, 175
Scutellaria lateriflora, 241
Sea buckthorn see *Hippophae rhamnoides*
Serenoa serrulata/repens
   amenorrhoea, oligomenorrhea, 56, 61
   infertility, 86
   PCOS, 132, 134, **140**
Shatavari see *Asparagus racemosus*
Shepherd's purse see *Capsella bursa-pastoris*
Siberian ginseng see *Eleutherococcus senticosus*
Silybum marianum
   appendix, 305
   benign breast disorders, 223
   cervical dysplasia, 204, 211
   menopause, 245
   ovarian cysts, 124
   PCOS, 144
Slippery elm see *Ulmus fulva*
Soybean see *Glycine max*
Spearmint see *Mentha spicata*
St John's wort see *Hypericum perforatum*
Stachys betonica
   PMS, 241, 242
Stellaria media, 234
Symphytum officinale, 254

Tamanu see *Calophyllum inophyllum*
Tanacetum parthenium
   combined with achillea, 254
   endometriosis, 162, 163, 164, 165, 176
   PMS, 242

Taraxacum officinale radix
   benign breast disorders, 223
   cervical dysplasia, 204, 211
   fibroids, 185
   menorrhagia, 37
   menopause, 245
   PCOS, 132
   PMS, 241
Taraxacum officinale folia
   benign breast disorders, 222
   endometriosis, 169
   fibroids, 189
   PMS, 241, 242
Tea tree see *Melaleuca alternifolia*
Thuja occidentalis, 294–299
   benign breast disorders, 222
   cervical dysplasia, 204, 205, 207, **208**
   endometriosis, 161
   fibroids, 186, 191
   ovarian cysts, 123
   vaginal discharge, 106, **108**, 110
Thyme see *Thymus vulgaris*
Thymus vulgaris
   dysmenorrhoea, 13, 14, 25
   lichen sclerosus, 236
   vaginal discharge, 105, 107, **111**
Tribulus terrestris
   amenorrhoea, oligomenorrhea, 56, 57
   infertility, 79, 80, 85, 89
   PCOS, 131, 133, 134, 135, 145, 146
   vaginal discharge, 114
Trifolium pratense
   benign breast disorders, 225
   cervical dysplasia, 204
   infertility, 80, 85
   menopause, 245, 246
   PCOS, 131, 134, 135, 148
   PMS, 241
Trigonella foenum-graecum
   dysmenorrhoea, 14, 25
   infertility, 84, 85, 89
   menopause, 245
   PCOS, 131, 133, 134, 135, 144
Trillium erectum, 245
Turmeric see *Curcuma longa*
Turnera diffusa, 131, 241

Ulmus fulva
    PMS, 241
Uncaria tomentosa
    endometriosis, 162, 163, 164, 165, 176
Unicorn root, False see *Chamaelirium luteum*
Urtica spp folia
    infertility, 80
    menorrhagia, 38
Urtica spp radix
    PCOS, 131, 132, 148
Uva-ursi see *Arctostaphylos uva-ursi*

Vaccinium myrtillus
    dysmenorrhoea, 13
    lichen sclerosus, 234
    menorrhagia, 38
Valerian see *Valeriana officinalis*
Valeriana officinalis
    dysmenorrhoea, 12, 13, **15**
        acute mix, 17
    endometriosis, 161
    PMS, 241
Verbascum thapsus, 114
Verbena officinalis
    benign breast disorders, 223
    infertility, 81
    menopause, 245
    PCOS, 133
    PMS, 241
Vervain see *Verbena officinalis*
Viburnum opulus see also *Vib. prunifolium*
    endometriosis, 164, 165, 166, 170
    use in labour, 281
Viburnum prunifolium, 300–302
    amenorrhoea, oligomenorrhoea, 61
    dysmenorrhoea, 13, 14, **15**
        acute mix, 17
    endometriosis, 161, 163, 164, 165, 166, **170**
    fibroids, 186
    infertility, 86
Vitex agnus-castus
    amenorrhoea, oligomenorrhoea, 56, 57, **61**

benign breast disorders, **224**
cervical dysplasia, 204
dysmenorrhoea, 14, 18, 21
endometriosis, 161, 162, 163, 164, 166, **170**
fibroids, 185, 186, **191**
infertility, 79, 80, 81, **84**, 85
menopause, 245
menorrhagia, 34, 37, **41**
ovarian cysts, 124
PCOS, 130, 131, 132, 134, 135, 141
PMS, 241, 242
vaginal discharge, 105

Wild Indigo see *Baptisia tinctoria*
Wild Yam *Dioscorea villosa*
Witch hazel see *Hamamelis virginiana*
Withania somnifera
    amenorrhoea, oligomenorrhoea, 56, 57
    cervical dysplasia, 204
    endometriosis, 161
    infertility, 79, 81
    lichen sclerosus, 234
    menorrhagia, 38
    PCOS, 131, 133
    PMS, 241
Wormwood see *Artemisia absinthium*

Yam, Wild see *Dioscorea villosa*
Yarrow see *Achillea millefolium*

Zea mays, 245, 304
Zingiber officinale
    amenorrhoea, oligomenorrhea, 61
    cervical dysplasia, 204, 211
    dysmenorrhoea, 11, 13, 14, **16**
        acute mix, 17
    endometriosis, 161, 162, 163, 164, 165, 166, **171**
    menorrhagia, 35, 38, **42**
    ovarian cysts, 123
    PCOS, 133, 134, 148
    vaginal discharge, 114
    with achillea, 254

www.ingramcontent.com/pod-product-compliance
Ingram Content Group UK Ltd.
Pitfield, Milton Keynes, MK11 3LW, UK
UKHW020130260126
467176UK00005B/43

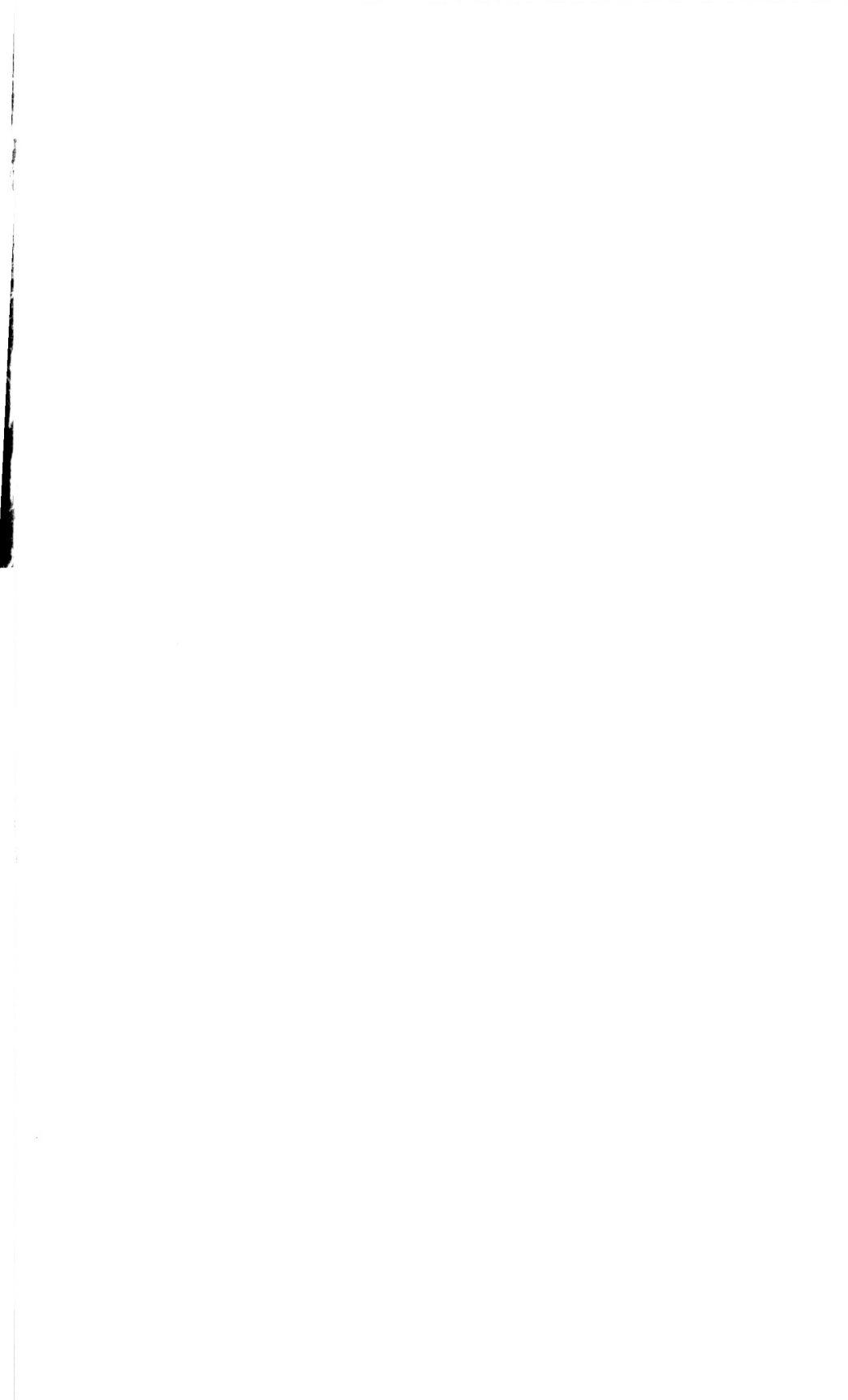